NATURAL THYROID TOOLKIT

Hashimoto's, Graves,' Iodine, Levothyroxine and Natural Desiccated Thyroid

JEFFREY DACH MD

Natural Thyroid Toolkit: Hashimoto's, Graves,' Iodine, Levothyroxine and Natural Desiccated Thyroid

Copyright 2023 Jeffrey Dach MD All Rights Reserved.
Published by Medical Muse Press

ISBN 978-1-732421-04-2 (Hardback)
ISBN 978-1-732421-02-8 (Paperback)
ISBN 978-1-732421-03-5 (Kindle EBook)

Author Contact information:
Jeffrey Dach, MD
7450 Griffin Road, Suite 180/190
Davie, Florida 33314
Office Telephone 954–792–4663
Website: www.jeffreydachmd.com

Disclaimer: The reader is advised to discuss the information found in these pages with his or her personal physicians and to act only upon the advice of his/her personal physician. This book is not intended as a substitute for the medical advice of a physician. The reader should regularly consult a physician in matters relating to his or her health, particularly in respect to any symptoms that may require diagnosis or medical attention. The authors and the publisher disclaim responsibility for any adverse effects resulting directly or indirectly from the information or advice contained in this book.

Cover Design: Yesna99 @ 99designs.com
Interior Design: Deborah Stocco

Dedication

This book is dedicated to my mom, Virginia Dale Dach, who died in 2020 at the age of 94. She underwent total thyroidectomy for a benign thyroid cyst at the age of 20 and took levothyroxine for 54 years. At the age of 74, I switched her thyroid medicine from levothyroxine to NDT, natural desiccated thyroid. One week later, my mom is feeling much better. She comes into my office, throws up her hands and says, "Why hasn't any other doctor done this for me before?"

Table of Contents

Note: Boldface has been added to portions of some quotations for emphasis.

Foreword by David Brownstein, MD

WESTERN PHYSICIANS HAVE BEEN DIAGNOS-ING and treating thyroid disorders for well over a century. In 1850, Dr. Thomas Curling, a surgeon at the London Hospital published a paper describing two severely hypothyroid (myxedematous) patients. The first patient's "growth was severely stunted...and had very little power of locomotion, with no power of speech." The second patient, a six months old infant "was plump...[and had] a large face with a small head and a very receding forehead. The tongue was large and protruding from the mouth."

Both patients succumbed to their underlying disease. At autopsy, no trace of the thyroid gland could be found on either patient. Dr. Curling stated, "I am not acquainted with any case on record in which a deficiency of the thyroid gland has been observed in the human body...." Before the discovery of treatment, severe hypothyroidism ran a fatal course. The 19th Century medical literature reported an average of 10 years from diagnosis to death.

It took Western physicians nearly 40 years to develop a treatment plan for hypothyroid patients. In 1891, George Murray, a pathologist in Newcastle, England successfully injected thyroid extract into a hypothyroid patient. The patient recovered and lived for almost 30 years. Shortly after George Murray's 1891 report, other physicians began using oral dosing of thyroid glands from animal sources. This is the same natural, desiccated thyroid that Dr. Dach describes in this book, "Natural Thyroid Toolkit." Natural thyroid hormone is one of the oldest medications in the Western world.

I have been practicing holistic medicine for over three decades. My first holistic patient was my father, Ellis, severely ill with coronary artery disease. Ellis suffered his first heart attack at age 40 and a second myocardial infarction at age 42. From that time on, he had progressive, worsening cardiac disease. Furthermore, he suffered from continual angina for over 25 years and had high cholesterol and diabetes. When I finished my residency and began treating patients, I was ready for the phone call that something terrible had happened to him.

Six months into practicing medicine, I ran across a book by Broda O. Barnes, "Hypothyroidism, the Unsuspected Illness." Dr. Barnes wrote about his career in treating hypothyroid patients. Dr. Barnes felt the primary cause of coronary artery disease was hypothyroidism. He described his experience with treating his cardiac patients with a small amount of natural desiccated thyroid hormone.

When I read Dr. Barnes' book, I was thinking of my dad. I drew blood tests and then put my father on a small amount of natural thyroid hormone. Within a week, Ellis' angina went away, never to return. Within a month his cholesterol level, which was consistently elevated above 300 mg/dL on cholesterol-lowering medications, fell below 200 mg/dL without changing his poor dietary habits. More importantly, he looked and acted much better. My father was suffering from heart disease for over 20 years due to an undiagnosed hypothyroid condition.

From that moment on, I began to test every patient for a hormonal imbalance. I have treated thousands of patients for thyroid disorders using similar protocols outlined by Dr. Jeffrey Dach in this book.

I have been involved in the Iodine Project with my mentor, Dr. Guy Abraham, for over 20 years. Over this time, my partners and I have successfully treated thousands of patients with iodine. My experience has led me to authoritatively state there is no better single nutrient therapy for my patients than correcting an iodine deficiency.

Iodine is one of the most misunderstood nutrients. Far too many holistic and conventional healthcare practitioners misunderstand how iodine works in the body. Here is a quote from my book, Iodine: Why You Need It, Why You Can't Live Without It... "Every cell in the body requires iodine to function optimally. Iodine is needed to make thyroid hormones and is needed to make all hormones produced in the body. Optimal iodine levels promote healthy immune and hormonal systems."

Many practitioners have the mistaken idea that iodine causes or worsens autoimmune thyroid disease. Rather it is iodine deficiency that causes or worsens autoimmune thyroid disease. Dr. Jeffrey Dach provides the scientific proof behind this concept. Only with a proper understanding of the importance of maintaining optimal iodine levels will we begin to reverse the epidemic of glandular diseases. This includes disorders of the thyroid, breast, ovary, uterus, prostate, and pancreas.

Dr. Jeffrey Dach has put tremendous effort into this book, and it shows. This book needs to be read by all physicians, and by all who are suffering from thyroid problems. I am a voracious reader. I have read hundreds of health books. Natural Thyroid Toolkit by Jeffrey Dach, MD is one of the best. It is a must-read.

David Brownstein, M.D.

Author of 17 books including Overcoming Thyroid Disorders, Iodine: Why You Need It, Why You Can't Live Without It, and The Miracle of Natural Hormones.

Center for Holistic Medicine
6089 W. Maple Road
West Bloomfield, MI 48322
Telephone 248-851-1600
www.drbrownstein.com

Introduction by Jeffrey Dach MD

DEPENDING ON WHICH SOURCE YOU read, between seven and thirty percent of the population has some kind of thyroid disorder. Many suffer needlessly with undiagnosed thyroid problems, a state of affairs expressed as a silent epidemic or an unsuspected illness. We have come a long way since 1891 when the first patient was treated with thyroid extract. The basic science of the humble thyroid gland has advanced a quantum leap since the primitive days of 1891. Although publicly available in the medical literature, current breakthroughs in thyroid science are largely ignored by mainstream medicine. The practice of thyroid endocrinology remains outdated, hampered by dogmatic reliance on older tests and treatments. Some might say financial interests are at stake, a result of "industry capture" by the pharmaceutical industry. For our purposes, let us remain oblivious to intimidating influences and bravely forge ahead with our task at hand, bringing the state of the art in thyroid diagnosis and treatment into the public realm with this book, Natural Thyroid Toolkit.

Medical Imaging of the Thyroid

The thyroid gland is superficial in the neck, lending itself to direct palpation by the examining doctor. Technological advances in medical imaging now allow more detailed examination using ultrasound and radionuclide scintigraphy. Thyroid medical imaging was my job for 25 years working in the hospital as a diagnostic and interventional radiologist doing thyroid ultrasound exams and ultrasound-guided biopsies of nodules. Of special interest to me was the field of nuclear medicine, thyroid imaging with radio-isotopes such as I-131, I-123, and technetium 99m. After 25 years of experience with medical imaging of the thyroid gland, I retired from radiology and opened an outpatient clinic treating thyroid patients. This book represents the culmination of about 20 years of experience prescribing natural desiccated thyroid (NDT) in the outpatient setting.

Apologies For Not Including Images

I must apologize for not including any of these above-mentioned medical images, except for the cover photomicrograph of the thyroid follicle architecture. You will find this on the front cover of this book. No worries, all these images are easy to find and view by typing into your favorite internet browser or search engine the type of imaging and the thyroid diagnosis. Click on the "Image" button to search for images. Hundreds of examples will pop up. First type in the word for the imaging technique such as ultrasound or nuclear medicine. Then type in the thyroid disorder, and voila, hundreds of representative images will pop up. This is especially useful in comparing the normal thyroid to Graves' disease, multinodular goiter, and Hashimoto's thyroiditis. For those with more curiosity and interest, try the YouTube animated videos on Thyroid. For example, for an animated explanation of the production of thyroid hormone discussed in Chapter 14, simply go to YouTube and type in the keywords: "production of thyroid hormone".

Laboratory Testing for the Thyroid

Laboratory testing is indispensable and provides a window into thyroid function. Serum TSH (thyroid stimulating hormone) is commonly mistaken as a thyroid hormone. TSH is not made by the thyroid and is not a thyroid hormone. TSH is made by the pituitary gland, the master endocrine controller at the base of the brain at the end of a long stalk resting in a bony indentation called the Sella Turcica. Serum tests for thyroid hormones are Free T3 and Free T4, and reverse T3, all produced by the thyroid gland, and controlled by the deiodinase system both within the thyroid gland and outside at the periphery. This deiodinase system is the paradigm shift in thyroid science and the ultimate controller of intracellular thyroid hormone levels. Unfortunately, we do not have a direct measurement of this deiodinase activity. We must use indirect measurements such as Free T3 to reverse T3 ratio to give us a window into the deiodinase system, useful for determining the efficacy of treatment. Two additional measurements useful in our armamentarium are serum selenium and spot urinary iodine. Selenium is a key nutrient for the proper functioning of both the anti-oxidant system, and the deiodinase system. Measurement of anti-TPO and anti-thyroglobulin antibodies warn us of an immune attack on the thyroid gland.

The Nuclear Reactor Accident Analogy

The thyroid gland is a small nuclear reactor in the neck. Most thyroid disorders, goiter, nodules, cancer, autoimmune thyroid disease, etc., can be understood by considering the analogy of a nuclear reactor accident. Let me explain. The nuclear reactor outside of town produces electricity for our homes and factories, functioning perfectly fine most of the time. However, if the graphite rod cooling system malfunctions, the nuclear reactor overheats with catastrophic meltdown and leakage of radiation into the environment. Past nuclear accidents in 1979 at Three Mile Island, 1986 at Chernobyl, and 2011 at Fukushima all resulted in reactor melt-down with the release of radiation into the environment.

Hydrogen Peroxide Production and Meltdown

Likewise, the cooling system for the thyroid is the selenoprotein anti-oxidant system, called glutathione peroxidase, and thioredoxin

reductase. Whereas radiation is the by-product of the nuclear reactor, hydrogen peroxide is the by-product of thyroid hormone production. Excessive hydrogen peroxide is highly volatile and destructive and may lead to the complete destruction of the thyroid gland in a process analogous to a nuclear reactor meltdown. Here, one is reminded of a syndrome called endemic myxedematous cretinism in Zaire, Africa, reported in 1990 by Dr. Jean Vanderpas. In this disease, the thyroid completely self-destructs resulting in profound hypothyroidism. (1-5)

Selenium-Based Anti-Oxidant System

Of course, the nuclear reactor has a graphite rod system to control the reaction and prevent a meltdown. The thyroid gland has a similar control system, the selenium-based anti-oxidant system that degrades excess hydrogen peroxide. If the capacity of the selenium anti-oxidant system is exceeded, then this results in thyroid inflammation and destruction, a scenario very similar to the nuclear meltdown. Indeed, excess hydrogen peroxide or lack of its degradation has been proposed in the etiology of various thyroid disorders. In 2007 Dr. Yue Song writes:

> H2O2 [hydrogen peroxide] …in thyroid cells, is a signal, a mitogen, a mutagen, a carcinogen, and a killer…various pathologies can be explained, at least in part, by overproduction and lack of degradation of H2O2 [hydrogen peroxide] (tumorigenesis, myxedematous cretinism, and thyroiditis) and by failure of the H2O2 generation or its positive control system (congenital hypothyroidism). (6)

TSH Elevation Generates Excess Hydrogen Peroxide

The next logical question is, what will cause the overproduction of hydrogen peroxide in the thyroid gland? The obvious answer is, an elevation of TSH (thyroid stimulating hormone) causes overproduction of hydrogen peroxide. As mentioned above, a good example of a "nuclear meltdown" in the thyroid is endemic myxedematous cretinism. In this syndrome, the thyroid gland is destroyed shortly after birth because of severe iodine and selenium deficiency leading to hypothyroidism and elevation of TSH. The high TSH then stimulates massive amounts of excess hydrogen peroxide. The combination of excess hydrogen peroxide generation and selenium deficiency leads to the complete destruction of the thyroid gland shortly after birth. An additional factor is dietary thiocyanate, a goitrogen that inhibits the uptake of iodide by the thyroid, worsening the underlying iodine deficiency. In 2007, Dr. Yue Song writes:

> Myxedematous endemic cretinism, caused by thyroid destruction after birth, has been linked to low iodine supply in early life, leading to intense stimulation [high TSH] and presumably H2O2 generation, to passage from low O2 to high O2 at birth, to selenium deficiency, and thus to decreases in GSH peroxidase and thioredoxin reductase activity and to dietary thiocyanate. The experimental reproduction of this scenario in newborn rats confirms the validity of these conclusions...**Interestingly, a similar scenario has been proposed for the physiopathology of [autoimmune] thyroiditis. Selenium dietary supplementation has therefore been proposed for the prevention and treatment of [autoimmune] thyroiditis and has indeed alleviated it.** (6) (1-10)

Benefits of TSH Suppression

If one considers the above mechanism correct, namely excess hydrogen peroxide generation secondary to TSH stimulation causes various thyroid disorders, then suppression of TSH is beneficial. Indeed, modern endocrinology uses TSH suppression to treat thyroid nodules and thyroid cancer.

Autoimmune Thyroid Disease

Extend this concept to autoimmune thyroid disease afflicting 5-7 percent of the global population as discussed above by Dr. Yue Song who proposes selenium supplementa-

tion to ensure a functioning selenium-based anti-oxidant system. One might also suggest TSH suppression for the autoimmune thyroid patient, as TSH suppression prevents excess hydrogen peroxide generation. Indeed, TSH suppression and selenium supplementation are critical elements of our treatment protocol for Hashimoto's thyroiditis, discussed in later Chapters. What about Graves' disease? How can we use TSH suppression to help the Graves' disease patient? The answer is the technique known as Block and Replace. This is the equivalent version of TSH suppression in the treatment of Graves' disease, as discussed in Chapters 15 and 16. (11-18)

Errors in Thyroid Endocrinology

This book discusses many of the errors in modern thyroid endocrinology. One might even think "Errors in Modern Thyroid Endocrinology" would make a good title for this book. After much deliberation, I decided this title was too negative, and changed it to Natural Thyroid Toolkit.

One of the errors of modern endocrinology is the dogmatic reliance on the TSH laboratory test. How do we know this is an error? Please do not take my word for it. Take the word of the past president of the American Thyroid Association, Dr. Antonio Bianco, in an interview with Endocrine News, saying:

> Do you know how many times I affirmed to my patients that their complaints of weight gain and poor memory associated with hypothyroidism were not thyroid related? And I explained that their serum TSH was normal, which meant that thyroid hormone economy had been normalized. Countless. Everybody did the same thing. And yet, even at that time, studies were showing that the basal metabolic rate was not fully restored with the normalization of serum TSH. We should have investigated this further. **Today, when I speak to those patients, I feel embarrassed.** (19-23)

A Second Error

A second error is the sole reliance on levothyroxine (T4-monotherapy) in the treatment of hypothyroidism. Again, Dr. Antonio Bianco admits to this error. Many patients benefit from a combination of T4 and T3. Dr. Bianco was surprised to learn 2 million Americans are using some form of combination of T3 and T4 treatment, such as NDT, natural desiccated thyroid, saying:

> Second, **many patients with residual symptoms do benefit from therapy containing a combination of LT4 [levothyroxine] and liothyronine (T3) [generic Cytomel].** This is supported by clinical trials. Physicians have been told not to use LT3 in the treatment of hypothyroidism because it is ineffective and because it could lead to cardiac arrhythmia and osteoporosis. Today there is good evidence that LT3 is effective for those patients that remain symptomatic on LT4, and when properly used at the indicated doses, it has been shown to be safe. I was surprised to learn that today there are almost 2 million patients in the USA using either LT3 or DTE [NDT, natural desiccated thyroid] for the treatment of hypothyroidism. (19-23)

These are only two of the many errors in modern thyroid endocrinology. A few more are discussed in the following Chapters of this book:

1. Sole reliance on TSH to monitor treatment.

2. TSH suppression may be needed for adequate treatment.

3. Reliance on T4 only-monotherapy (levothyroxine, generic Synthroid)

4. NDT– Natural desiccated thyroid is a better choice.

5. Shorter half-life makes NDT a safer choice.

6. Ignoring the beneficial effects of selenium, magnesium, vitamin D3, and a gluten-free diet for autoimmune thyroid disease.

7. Treating thyroid hormone levels while ignoring the autoimmune component of thyroid disease.

8. Failing to treat euthyroid Hashimoto's patients promptly with thyroid medication.

9. Failing to treat pregnant women with thyroid medication when anti-thyroid antibodies are elevated.

10. Failing to test for and treat with iodine because of "Medical Iodophobia," the irrational fear of using iodine. (24-26)

The Good News

There is good news! With a full understanding of thyroid hormone production, the deiodinase system, and the exact disease process affecting the thyroid gland, we can now offer improved treatments with better outcomes. This is the origin and motivation for this book, Natural Thyroid Toolkit. It has been a great learning experience for me to research and write Natural Thyroid Toolkit. I hope reading it will be for you as well. Join me and others at our online thyroid social community. Remember to sign up for a free monthly thyroid newsletter at www.jeffreydachmd.com.

♦ **References for Introduction**

1) Vanderpas, Jean B., et al. "Iodine and Selenium Deficiency Associated with Cretinism in Northern Zaire." The American Journal of Clinical Nutrition 52.6 (1990): 1087-1093."

2) Vanderpas, Jean-Baptiste, et al. "Iodine and Selenium Deficiency in Northern Zaire." The American Journal of Clinical Nutrition 56.5 (1992): 957-958."

3) Dumont, Jacques Emile, et al. "The Biochemistry of Endemic Cretinism: Roles of Iodine and Selenium Deficiency and Goitrogens." Molecular and Cellular Endocrinology 100.1-2 (1994): 163-166.

4) Contempre, Bernard, et al. "Selenium Deficiency Aggravates the Necrotizing Effects of a High Iodide Dose in Iodine-deficient Rats." Endocrinology 132.4 (1993): 1866-1868.

5) Contempré, Bernard, et al. "Thiocyanate Induces Cell Necrosis and Fibrosis in Selenium-and Iodine-deficient Rat Thyroids: A Potential Experimental Model for Myxedematous Endemic Cretinism in Central Africa." Endocrinology 145.2 (2004): 994-1002.

6) Song, Yue, et al. "Roles of Hydrogen Peroxide in Thyroid Physiology and Disease." The Journal of Clinical Endocrinology & Metabolism 92.10 (2007): 3764-3773

7) Kohrle, J., et al. "Selenium, the Thyroid, and the Endocrine System." Endocrine Reviews 26.7 (2005): 944-984.

8) Gärtner, Roland, et al. "Selenium Supplementation in Patients with Autoimmune Thyroiditis Decreases Thyroid Peroxidase Antibodies Concentrations." The Journal of Clinical Endocrinology & Metabolism 87.4 (2002): 1687-1691.

9) Duntas, Leonidas H., et al. "Effects of a Six-month Treatment with Selenomethionine in Patients with Autoimmune Thyroiditis." European Journal of Endocrinology 148.4 (2003): 389-393.

10) Willemin, Marie-Emilie, and Annie Lumen. "Thiocyanate: A Review and Evaluation of the Kinetics and the Modes of Action for Thyroid Hormone Perturbations." Critical Reviews in Toxicology 47.7 (2017): 543-569.

11) Ohye, Hidemi, and Masahiro Sugawara. "Dual Oxidase, Hydrogen Peroxide, and Thyroid Diseases." Experimental Biology and Medicine 235.4 (2010): 424-433.

12) Raad, Houssam, et al. "Thyroid Hydrogen Peroxide Production Is Enhanced by the Th2 Cytokines, IL-4 and IL-13, through Increased Expression of the Dual Oxidase 2 and Its Maturation Factor DUOXA2." Free Radical Biology and Medicine 56 (2013): 216-225.

13) Bednarek, Janusz, et al. "Oxidation Products and Anti-oxidant Markers in Plasma of Patients with Graves' Disease and Toxic Multinodular Goiter: Effect of Methimazole Treatment." Free Radical Research 38.6 (2004): 659-664."

14) Zuo, Ying, et al. "The Correlation between Selenium Levels and Autoimmune Thyroid Disease: A Systematic Review and Meta-analysis." Ann. Palliat. Med 10 (2021): 4398-4408.

15) Davcheva, Delyana M., et al. "Serum Selenium Concentration in Patients with Autoimmune Thyroid Disease." Folia Medica 64.3 (2022): 443-449.

16) Wood, Claire L., et al. "Randomized Trial of Block and Replace Vs Dose Titration Thionamide in Young People with Thyrotoxicosis." European Journal of Endocrinology 183.6 (2020): 637-645.

17) Vigone, M. C., et al. "Block-and-Replace" Treatment in Graves' Disease: Experience in a Cohort of Pediatric Patients." Journal of Endocrinological Investigation 43.5 (2020): 595-600.

18) Wiersinga, Wilmar M. "Graves' Disease: Can It Be Cured?" Endocrinology and Metabolism 34.1 (2019): 29-38.

19) Solving the Hypothyroidism Puzzle: Q&A: Antonio Bianco, MD, Ph.D. by Derek Bagley, Jan 2023, Endocrine News.

20) Idrees, Thaer, et al. "Liothyronine and Desiccated Thyroid Extract in the Treatment of Hypothyroidism." Thyroid 30.10 (2020): 1399-1413.

21) Ettleson, Matthew D., and Antonio C. Bianco. "Individualized Therapy for Hypothyroidism: Is T4 Enough for Everyone?" The Journal of Clinical Endocrinology & Metabolism 105.9 (2020): E3090-e3104.0 (2020): 1399-1413.

22) Jonklaas, Jacqueline, et al. "Evidence-based Use of Levothyroxine/Liothyronine Combinations in Treating Hypothyroidism: A Consensus Document." European Thyroid Journal 10.1 (2021): 10-38. (2020): 1399-1413.

23) Bianco, Antonio C. Rethinking Hypothyroidism: Why Treatment Must Change and What Patients Can Do. University of Chicago Press, 2022.

24) Abraham, Guy E. "The Wolff-Chaikoff Effect: Crying Wolf?" The Original Internist 12.3 (2005): 112-118. (2020): 1399-1413.

25) Abraham, Guy E. "The Safe and Effective Implementation of Orthoiodosupplementation in Medical Practice." The Original Internist 11.1 (2004): 17-36.

26) Atabek, M. E. "Medical Iodophobia Is Contagious." Journal of Pediatric Endocrinology & Metabolism 24 (2011): 861-862.

Chapter 1

Natural Thyroid as Anti-Aging

Anna Nicole Smith and Hashimoto's Hypothyroidism

IN 1993, ANNA NICOLE SMITH was Playboy's Playmate of the Year and later became a television and movie star. Unfortunately, fourteen years later at the age of 39, Anna Nicole Smith died at the Seminole Indian Hard Rock Hotel, a gambling casino in the shape of a giant guitar located not far from my office in Davie, Florida. Officially, her death was attributed to a drug overdose. However, the autopsy report described a low thyroid condition called Hashimoto's thyroiditis, an autoimmune thyroid disease. (1)

Natural Thyroid Instead of Growth Hormone?

Anna Nicole Smith was also taking human growth hormone (HGH). The obvious question is, why was Anna Nicole taking growth hormone when the autopsy report indicated she needed thyroid medication? Although the American Medical Association and the Institute of Medicine have opposed the use of HGH by aging baby boomers, the practice did have a brief period of popularity. I propose Anna Nicole Smith's real medical problem was thyroid deficiency rather than growth hormone deficiency. This may also apply to other baby boomers seeking anti-aging interventions. (2-7)

Human Growth Hormone at Cenegenics

In its day, the use of growth hormone as an anti-aging treatment was popularized by the Las Vegas Cenegenics Clinic run by Alan Mintz, M.D. Back in 2005, I was interested in learning about this field, so I spent a week doing a fellowship with Dr. Mintz at his clinic in Las Vegas. Dr. Mintz was famous for his 60 Minutes interview on CBS Television, highlighting his Cenegenics Clinic and human growth hormone treatment for aging baby boomers. Originally trained as a diagnostic radiologist, Dr. Mintz later entered the field of anti-aging medicine. Dr. Mintz was a visionary, and a pioneer who inspired many doctors, myself included. Sadly, Dr. Mintz passed away on June 3, 2007, less than a year after this 60-minute CBS television interview. (8-12)

Thyroid Hormone, The Missing Piece of the Puzzle

Over the years, various anti-aging protocols have included human growth hormone (HGH), dehydroepiandrosterone (DHEA), testosterone, estrogen, and progesterone. In addition, a basket of nutritional supplements is usually included. This type of hormone program is thought to have anti-aging properties. However, I would suggest thyroid hormone is the best and most effective anti-aging intervention. Treatment with thyroid hormone changes the body composition, skin, and hair quality and produces a more youthful appearance. In my experience, for patients with a low thyroid condition, these youthful changes with thyroid hormone treatment are much more profound than any other drug treatment. Yet, many doctors involved in so-called anti-aging medicine tend to be conservative when it comes to offering thyroid treatment. They usually decline to give thyroid medication if the TSH test is within the lab range, declaring the patient normal, without thyroid disease. If they prescribe thyroid hormone, it is typically synthetic levothyroxine instead of natural desiccated thyroid hormone (NDT). Natural thyroid is currently available as Armour thyroid from AbbVie/Allergan/Forrest

Labs or the NP Thyroid from Acella. Although available in the past, Nature-Throid from RLC Labs is not currently available as of the writing of this book. It is on back-order awaiting regulatory approval to resume production. AbbVie, the owner of Armour, also owns Synthroid.

Levothyroxine, also called generic Synthroid, contains only T4 (thyroxine). In contrast, the natural desiccated thyroid, NDT, contains both T3 and T4, accounting for the superior clinical results for natural desiccated thyroid. Mainstream medical practice relies on the TSH test to determine when to treat thyroid hormone so many people with low thyroid are missed and ignored by the medical system and are not given thyroid hormone medication. The Quest lab reference range for TSH is 0.40-4.50 mIU/L for adults. Endocrinologists at Walter Reed have found that patients prefer the NDT, natural desiccated thyroid, over levothyroxine (generic Synthroid). Of course, the benefits are greater when thyroid hormone is combined with a complete hormone replacement program, including estrogen, progesterone, and testosterone. (13-18)

Mark Starr and Type Two Hypothyroidism

A few months after the Cenegenics Clinic fellowship with Alan Mintz, M.D., I attended an ICIM (International College of Integrative Medicine) medical meeting in Grand Rapids, Michigan, where I met Mark Starr, M.D., a keynote speaker at the meeting. Dr. Starr presented his approach to diagnosing and treating the low thyroid condition, which he calls Type Two Hypothyroidism. Mark Starr's lecture and book on the same topic were an epiphany moment for me. I stood up and said, "Eureka". Dr. Starr's book claims that while 30% of the population are low thyroid, they are ignored and untreated by mainstream medicine. These unfortunate souls drag themselves from doctor to doctor with labels such as chronic fibromyalgia and chronic fatigue and suffer from hair loss, constipation, depression, and a host of other low thyroid symptoms. Dr. Starr explained why

thyroid blood tests such as the TSH (thyroid stimulating hormone) are unreliable. Dr. Starr instead relies on old-fashioned clinical judgment to decide if thyroid hormone is necessary and at what dosage. (19-23)

Clinical Signs and Symptoms of Hypothyroidism

The symptoms of hypothyroidism (listed below) are pathognomonic for a low thyroid condition. The astute clinician will find no difficulty making the diagnosis or at least harbor a high index of suspicion based on the patient exhibiting many of the typical symptoms listed below. Indeed, the low thyroid condition is associated with specific changes in facial features called myxedema, a characteristic puffy, swollen, coarse appearance of the face. Once the clinician recognizes this, it becomes easy to identify hypothyroid people in a crowd, such as when watching people go by at the train station or airport. They all share the same characteristic distinctive "puffiness" of the face. The astute physician may notice the following telltale signs and symptoms of hypothyroidism: dry skin, thinning of the outer eyebrows, slight fluid accumulation at the ankles, constipation, lack of sweating, weight gain, low body temperature (consistently below 97.9 F.), and high cholesterol.

Symptoms of Hypothyroidism

Weight Gain

Constipation

Puffy face, swelling of eyelids (myxedema)

Loss or thinning of eyebrows

Dry Hair and Skin

Hair Loss, Thinning Hair

Cold Intolerance

Low Libido

Chronic Fatigue

Fibromyalgia

Joint and/or Muscle Pain

Depression

Cold Hands or Feet

Low Body Temperature

Thickening of the Skin

Thinning, Splitting of Fingernails

The Long-term use of Acrylic Nails

Slow Heart Rate

Foggy Brain, Cognitive Impairment

Heavy or Irregular Menstrual Bleeding

The Delayed Tendon Reflex

Upon physical examination of the low thyroid patient, there may be noticeable changes in the skin, hair, and facial features related to myxedema, a peculiar skin infiltration with a gelatinous substance. There is also the delayed Achilles reflex time used in the "old days" for managing the thyroid patient before the invention of laboratory testing. The delay in relaxation is the delayed recovery time of the reflex. This is the finding indicating a low thyroid condition. Using a reflex hammer to check the Achilles reflex is still accepted by mainstream endocrinology as an indicator of low thyroid function. Other tendon reflexes, such as the brachioradialis in the forearm, are more convenient ways to elicit the reflex while the patient is comfortably seated. (24-30)

Physical Examination of the Thyroid

Palpation is useful in detecting the enlarged thyroid, also called goiter, and the presence of nodules or masses. Of course, thyroid ultrasound is much more accurate and sensitive. It can be used for confirmation of findings on physical examination. Portable laptop ultrasound machines are not expensive, and many endocrinologists include thyroid ultrasound as an office routine or complement to physical examination. A lucrative billing code for the procedure can be added to the patient encoun-

ter. The problem is that thyroid nodules are widespread in the population, and screening the population may lead to unnecessary biopsies. For this reason, in my office, we do not perform thyroid nodule screening with ultrasound. Instead, I reserve thyroid ultrasound based on clinical judgment, usually for confirmation or follow-up of thyroid nodules or masses on an individual basis. This is explained in Chapter 33 on The Thyroid Nodule Epidemic.

Thyroid Function Testing

Of course, no evaluation of the thyroid patient is complete without laboratory testing. A typical panel includes TSH, Free T3, Free T4, reverse T3, TPO, and thyroglobulin antibodies. If hyperthyroidism is suspected, the TSI and TRAb antibody tests are included. Remember, TSH is inverse to thyroid function. Hence, a high TSH, above the lab range, usually indicates a low thyroid condition. In most cases, the testing is straightforward and conclusive. However, in some cases, the labs may be difficult to interpret or "paradoxical." For example, the TSH may be "paradoxically" low even in some patients with a low thyroid condition, also called hypothalamic dysfunction. Jacob Teitelbaum MD reported hypothalamic dysfunction frequently in his chronic fatigue patients. In these cases, the patient actually has a low thyroid condition. Yet, TSH is usually below 3.0, which means no conventional endocrinologist would treat the patient with thyroid hormone. These are the unfortunate souls who remain untreated by the conventional medical system. (20-21) (31)

A Trial of Low-Dose Thyroid

Once it has been determined that thyroid hormone is likely beneficial, we may start a trial of low-dose thyroid NDT, natural desiccated thyroid. We begin with a half-grain tablet (30 mg) and gradually increase the dosage by half-grain increments every one to two weeks, assuming the patient tolerates the medication well. We educate the patient to observe for symptoms of thyroid excess, such as rapid heart rate, palpitations, feelings of warmth, anxiety, or insomnia. In addition, other supplements such as iodine, selenium, B12, iron, and magnesium are given based on laboratory testing. Suppose the patient experiences palpitations or any signs of thyroid excess. In that case, the patient is instructed to hold the thyroid medication and inform the prescribing physician. Typically for new patients, thyroid lab tests are repeated after 6 weeks, when dosage may be adjusted. The therapy goal is to relieve symptoms of the low thyroid condition. We typically see a resolution of low thyroid symptoms and improvement in the hair, skin, and facial features with adequate thyroid treatment.

Conclusion

Back in 2007, human growth hormone as an anti-aging treatment was a popular fad. I would argue the simple use of thyroid medicine would have been sufficient for many of these patients, simultaneously treating an undiagnosed low thyroid condition and serving as a robust anti-aging intervention.

♦ References for Chapter 1

1) Broward County Medical Examiner Autopsy on Vickie Lynn Marshall AKA Anna Nicole Smith DOB: 11/28/1967 Autopsy No: 07-0223 February 9, 2007 AGE: 39 Gertrude M. Juste, M.D. Associate Medical Examiner and Joshua A. Perper, M.D. Chief Medical Examiner

2) Aging Baby Boomers Turn to Hormone, Some Doctors Concerned about Growing 'Off-label' Use of Drug, by Sabin Russell, Chronicle Staff Writer, November 17, 2003, San Francisco Chronicle.

3) Human Growth Hormone Use Rises, but Is It Legal? May 9, 2007, By Caleb Hellerman, CNN.

4) Perls, Thomas T., et al. "Provision or Distribution of Growth Hormone for "Anti-Aging": Clinical and Legal Issues." JAMA 294.16 (2005): 2086-2090.

5) Liu, Hau, et al. "Systematic Review: The Safety and Efficacy of Growth Hormone in the Healthy Elderly." Annals of Internal Medicine 146.2 (2007): 104-115.

6) Anna Nicole Smith's Overdose -- a Prescription for Death by Dan Childs, ABC News Medical Unit

7) Anna Nicole Smith and Human Growth Hormone by Lynn Waddell 3/27/07 Newsweek

8) Cenegenics Las Vegas, 410 S. Rampart Blvd., Ste. 420 Las Vegas, NV 89145

9) Aging In The 21st Century 60-minutes by Daniel Schorn April 19, 2006, CBS News.

10) Obituary in Las Vegas Review: Alan P. Mintz, M.D., Co-Founder and CEO of Cenegenics Medical Institute, Passed Away June 3, 2007.

11) Conley, Kevin. "Warning: This Drug Reverses Aging." GQ Magazine, January 2006

12) Ginzburg, Enrique, et al. "Testosterone and Growth Hormone Normalization: A Retrospective Study of Health Outcomes." Journal of Multidisciplinary Healthcare 1 (2008): 79.

13) Acella Pharmaceuticals, 1880 McFarland Parkway Suite 110-B Alpharetta, GA 30005-1794

14) AbbVie-Allergan $63 Billion Deal Aided by Nestle, AstraZeneca Buys, Mon, January 27, 2020, Reuters News. Armour.

15) Hoang TD, et al. "Desiccated Thyroid Extract Compared with Levothyroxine in the Treatment of Hypothyroidism: A Randomized, Double-blind, Crossover Study. J Clin Endocrinol Metab. 2013 May;98(5):1982-90.

16) Shomon, Mary J. Living Well with Hypothyroidism: What Your Doctor Doesn't Tell You... That You Need to Know. Harper Collins, 2009.

17) Lowe, John C., and Gina Honeyman-Lowe. "Is Fibromyalgia a Thyroid-Related Condition?" Grenoble, France, May 6, 2000 (conference of the French Fibromyalgia Association of Région Rhône-Alpes) and in Toulon, France on May 11 (at the Centre Hospitalier Intercommunal).

18) Dach, Jeffrey. Bioidentical Hormones 101. iUniverse, 2011.

19) Mark, Starr. "Type 2 Hypothyroidism: The Epidemic." New Voice Publications, 2010.

20) Teitelbaum, Jacob. "Part 2--Protocols for Treating an Underactive Thyroid--Despite Normal Blood Tests." Townsend Letter for Doctors and Patients 241-242 (2003): 174-176.

21) Teitelbaum, Jacob. "Treat the Patient--not the Blood Tests!" Townsend Letter for Doctors and Patients 270 (2006): 117-120."

22) Mercola, Joseph M. "Experts Change Low Thyroid Diagnosis Criteria." Townsend Letter for Doctors and Patients 215 (2001): 28-28.

23) Wilson, Stephen A., et al. "Hypothyroidism: Diagnosis and Treatment." American Family Physician 103.10 (2021): 605-613.

24) Gillich, K. H., et al. "Validity of Achilles Tendon Reflex Measurement During Thyroid Gland Function Disorders." Medizinische Klinik 65.45 (1970): 1973-1982.

25) Kieffer, J., et al. "Diagnostic Value of the Achilles Tendon Reflex in Thyroid Diseases." Arquivos Brasileiros De Endocrinologia E Metabologia 15.1 (1966): 55-62.

26) Shafer, R. B., and F. Q. Nuttall. "Achilles Reflex in Thyroid Disorders: A 10-year Clinical Evaluation." The American Journal of the Medical Sciences 264.4 (1972): 313-317.

27) Goodman, E. "A Screening Test for Thyroid Function." Australian Family Physician 5.4 (1976): 550-561."

28) Franco, G., and T. Malamani. "Achilles Reflexogram and Hemodynamic Parameters in the Evaluation of Thyroid Function." Minerva Medica 67.51 (1976): 3325-3334.

29) Gaïdina, G. A., et al. "Changes in the Duration of the Achilles Reflex in Euthyroid Goiter in Children." Problemy Endokrinologii 33.3 (1987): 6-9."

30) Konrad Kail, N. D., and Robert F. Waters. "Managing Subclinical Hypothyroid Using Resting Metabolic Rate and Brachioradialis Reflexometry."

31) Teitelbaum, Jacob. "Highly Effective Treatment of Fibromyalgia and Chronic Fatigue Syndrome--Results of a Placebo-Controlled Study and How to Apply the Protocol." Townsend Letter for Doctors and Patients 231 (2002): 48-54.

Chapter 2

Why Natural Thyroid is Better than Synthetic Part One

In 2016, doctors prescribed 123 million prescriptions for Synthroid and its generic equivalent, levothyroxine, making it the most prescribed drug and the most prescribed thyroid drug in the U.S. Considering all this, how is it possible that a different thyroid drug called natural desiccated thyroid (NDT) is a better choice for many patients? Almost every day in my office, I find myself explaining to a patient why natural thyroid is superior to levothyroxine (generic Synthroid). (1)

What is Levothyroxine (Generic Synthroid)? And What is in it?

The thyroid gland secretes thyroid hormone into the bloodstream in response to TSH stimulation. The thyroid hormone consists of two subtypes called T4 (thyroxine) and T3, which refer to the number of iodine molecules attached to the tyrosine backbone. The thyroid gland secretes thyroid hormone into the bloodstream in a 14:1 ratio of T4:T3. However, serum levels are 4:1 due to peripheral conversion of T4 to T3 by the D1 deiodinase, as explained in later chapters. In 1949, the sodium salt of thyroxine was first introduced to the market. Thyroxine is the T4 component secreted by the thyroid consisting of a racemic mixture of isomers, levo, and dextro. Note: levo and dextro refer to the ability of the purified thyroxine molecule to rotate polarized light either to the left (levo) or the right (dextro). This is related to a slight difference in spatial configuration, such as the difference between the right and left hands. The L-isomer is more biologically active than the D-isomer. Levothyroxine, the generic form of Synthroid, is the L-isomer of thyroxine. The T3 component is available as liothyronine, (generic Cytomel). (1-2)

Difference Between T3 and T4

Thyroxine has one of the simplest chemical structures of all the hormones, consisting of two tyrosine molecules with either three or four iodine molecules added to the two-ring structure. T3 has three iodine atoms, and T4 has four iodine atoms. The numbers on T3 and T4 refer to the number of iodine atoms added to tyrosine. T4 is the prohormone that must be converted to T3 by the D1 and D2 deiodinase system, controlling the metabolic rate at the cellular level. This deiodinase enzyme contains selenium, explaining why selenium deficiency may result in the inability to convert T4 to T3.

Common brand names for levothyroxine in North America are Levoxyl, Synthroid, and Tiroscint. Outside of the U.S., common names are Thyrax, Euthyrox, Levaxin, and Eltroxin. Levothyroxine is a synthetic L-isomer of thyroxine, the more potent of the two isomers with similar biologic activity compared to the racemic mixture in natural thyroxine. (1-2)

What is Natural Desiccated Thyroid?

In 1891, George Murray published the first successful treatment of myxedema, hypothyroidism by injecting sheep thyroid extract into a hypothyroid patient. This thyroid extract derived from farm animal thyroid glands later became NDT, natural desiccated thyroid. It was the only thyroid medication available from 1891 to the 1970s when medicine shifted to T4-monotherapy with levothyroxine. Currently available NDT, natural desiccated thyroid, is made from desiccated porcine (pig) thyroid glands containing T4 and T3. On the other hand, Levothyroxine contains solely T4, with no T3. That is why levothyroxine is called T4-only monotherapy. (1-3)

From Medicine.Net: Answering a Viewer Question

Here is a question and answer quoted from a popular medical website called medicine.net.

Question: What is your feeling regarding natural vs. synthetic replacement therapy in hypothyroid situations? Armour, for example, vs. Synthroid? from L.H.

Doctor's Answer: While it is reasonable to assume that synthetic medications are less desirable than natural counterparts, in this case, natural thyroid hormone replacement is definitely not an ideal solution for the vast majority of people.

Here's why: Armour's thyroid is derived from a desiccated pig (porcine) thyroid gland. A number of years ago, these natural preparations were our only alternative. Replacement with desiccated thyroid creates dosing problems because there is no way to standardize the exact amount of the dose for each batch. As a matter of fact, these preparations do not report their dosage strength in milligrams but rather in grains of thyroid. This is because they don't really know the milligram equivalent in each dose. Dosing is also based on the assumption that each gland has equal amounts of hormones as the next gland and that the ratio of T4 and T3 (the more active hormone) are similar and constant in each gland from the pigs. There is no way to be certain of this, and patients on these preparations often have fluctuating hormone levels, which may or may not result in symptoms.

Regardless of symptoms, the goal of replacement therapy is to keep the hormone levels as stable as possible. This is much easier to achieve with synthetic preparations such as Levoxyl and Synthroid. These preparations come in a vast number of standardized doses, allowing for minute adjustments in hormone dosing. There is another comment that should be made. With all the issues surrounding "mad cow disease" and other ailments, I personally am reluctant to offer animal-based therapy to patients when a safe, effective well, studied synthetic preparation is widely available.

I hope this helps answer any questions you may have. Thank you for your question.

Medical Author: R.M., M.D. endquote medicine.net (4)

Contrary to the Medicine.net medical expert above, natural thyroid tablets are standardized and labeled in milligrams. The above statement is wrong about this. The label for the one-grain tablet says each tablet contains 60 mg of natural desiccated thyroid, 38 micrograms of T4, and 9 micrograms of T3.

The above medical expert claims levothyroxine (generic Synthroid) is standardized and stable, while NDT is not. Of course, this is nonsense based on taking points from drug company marketing. If the above statement is true, we expect to find that the FDA **has never** recalled Synthroid because of problems with stability or potency. We expect that the FDA **has** recalled NDT because the pills are unstable and vary in potency. So, let us ask the FDA about this. What do we find? The FDA has often said levothyroxine and Synthroid are unstable and vary in potency.

Is Synthroid (Levothyroxine) a Reliable and Stable Drug? No, Says the FDA.

Here is a 2001 quote from Pharmacy Today on Medscape:

Because Synthroid was marketed before 1962, it had never undergone FDA review. On August 14, 1997, FDA declared that no levothyroxine products had consistent potency and stability and called for companies that wished to continue marketing the drug to submit NDAs within 3 years.(5)

Synthroid was marketed in 1955 but was FDA-approved on July 24, 2002. The FDA sent a warning letter to Synthroid Manufacturer Knoll Pharmaceuticals on April 26, 2001, which informed them:

The history of potency failures...indicates that Synthroid has not been reliably potent and stable.

Levothyroxine is Unstable, and NOT of Consistent Potency from Lot to Lot

Here is an FDA document from August 14, 1997, Docket No. 97N-0314, which says Synthroid is unstable and varies in consistency from lot to lot:

The drug substance levothyroxine sodium (also called Synthroid**) is unstable in the presence of light, temperature, air, and humidity**. Unless the manufacturing process can be carefully and consistently controlled, orally administered levothyroxine sodium products **may not be fully potent through the labeled expiration date or be of consistent potency from lot to lot...** There is evidence from recalls, adverse drug experience reports, and inspection reports that even when a physician consistently prescribes the same brand of orally administered levothyroxine sodium, **patients may receive products of variable potency at a given dose**. Such variations in product potency present actual safety and effectiveness concerns...However, **no currently marketed orally administered levothyroxine sodium product has been shown to demonstrate consistent potency and stability**, and thus, no currently marketed orally administered levothyroxine sodium product is generally recognized as safe and effective. (6)

Natural Desiccated Thyroid Recalls

To be completely fair, there have also been many FDA recalls of various lots of natural desiccated thyroid NDT products for failing tests for potency and consistency. One was a recall of Forrest Lab's Armour thyroid in 2005. There have also been recalls of various lots of Nature-Throid from RLC labs and NP Thyroid from Acella.

Iodine is Highly Reactive

Iodine, bromine, chlorine, and fluorine are called halogens. These are highly oxidative and commonly used for water purification and household cleaning agents. This means any compound containing iodine, such as thyroid pills, is highly volatile and may readily decompose through oxidation. The reality is that both levothyroxine and NDT contain iodine which by nature is a volatile molecule easily oxidized, resulting in loss of potency. Any thyroid hormone product, regardless of type, will share this same instability problem with loss of potency over time. We depend on the manufacturer to compensate for this and provide a stable product. This explains why potency and consistency are a problem shared by all types of thyroid hormone products whether levothyroxine or natural desiccated thyroid. This is the volatile nature of iodine.

Conversion of T4 to T3 by Deiodinase Enzyme System

About 20% of patients do not feel well on levothyroxine. What is the explanation for this? The deiodinase system may be unable to efficiently convert T4 to T3. Levothyroxine contains T4, which must be converted to its active form T3 at the cell level. This conversion is done by the D1 and D2 deiodinase enzyme system, which, if not functioning optimally or malfunctioning, may cause poor conversion of T4 to T3. Laboratory studies may reveal a lower Free T3 and a higher Free T4 in patients on levothyroxine, suggesting an inability to convert. A higher reverse T3 in a patient on levothyroxine indicates the drug is being converted to an inactive metabolite and not working. Many of these patients feel better taking NDT, which contains T3 and T4. In my experience, most patients feel much better, with more energy and relief symptoms when switching from levothyroxine to NDT. This was confirmed by studies in 2013 by Hoang Thanh and in 2014 by Dr. Garry Pepper. In 2018, Dr. Gary Pepper studied patients who switched from levothyroxine to NDT, Armour thyroid. Dr. Pepper reported 78% of these patients preferred the NDT, Armour thyroid. (7-18)

Can I Get Mad Cow Disease from My Pig Thyroid Pill?

Millions of Americans have enjoyed ham sandwiches and pork products for decades without a single case of Mad Cow Disease ever reported. This invalidates the fear of Mad Cow Disease as an argument.

Free T3 and Free T4 Higher Diagnostic Performance

The Free T3 and Free T4 have replaced the older thyroid labs because of "higher diagnostic performance." If your doctor does not include Free T3 and Free T4 on your laboratory panel, you need a new doctor. In 2003, Dr. R. Sapin writes:

> Because of their higher diagnostic performance, free T4 (FT4) and free T3 (FT3) measurements have superseded total (free + bound) hormone determination. (19)

A Typical NDT Program: For diagnosis of low thyroid condition, we use a lengthy questionnaire that reviews over 70 symptoms of low thyroid, a complete thyroid blood panel including TSH, Free T3 and Free T4, reverse T3, thyroid antibodies, and a comprehensive physical examination. Laboratory studies include selenium, magnesium RBC, vitamin D3, Iron, and iodine levels. These supplements are given when found to be low. Once it has been determined that thyroid hormone is likely beneficial, the patient is started on a trial of low-dose NDT, Half Grain (30 mg) daily. The patient may report benefits of increased energy, clarity of mind, etc., or adverse effects such as palpitations, feeling of warmth, anxiety, or insomnia. The patient's symptoms are closely monitored. Dosage is increased weekly by half grain (30 mg.) increments. In the event of rapid heart rate or palpitations at rest, the patient is instructed to hold the daily dosage of thyroid medication and inform the physician. Labs are rechecked routinely at 6 weeks. This NDT program can be used to switch patients from levothyroxine to natural desiccated thyroid NDT. When switching, we simply stop the levothyroxine one day and start the NDT the next.

Instead of Natural Thyroid, Why Not Use Cytomel and Synthroid Together?

Liothyronine, generic Cytomel, is T3, and levothyroxine is T4, so why not prescribe the two in combination? The Cytomel provides the missing T3 to make a combination closer to the serum level for Free T3 and Free T4 from thyroid gland production and peripheral deiodinase activity. Some patients arrive at my office having been given this combination by the doctor. The advantage for the prescribing doctor is that levothyroxine and generic Cytomel are both available at the corner drugstore. Note: NDT is also widely available at all pharmacies.

Conclusion

One of the errors of modern endocrinology is reliance on T4 monotherapy with levothyroxine while ignoring the use of natural desiccated thyroid NDT. Another error is failing to use the Free T3 and Free T4 laboratory tests, which have superseded the older tests.

♦ References for Chapter 2

1) What is More Prescribed than Opioids? Weirdly, a Thyroid Drug. March 23, 2018, by Jacob Bell Senior Reporter, BioPharma Dive. https://www.biopharmadive.com/news/state-prescription-popularity-thyroid-opioid-drug/519870/

2) Mateo, Roselyn Cristelle I., and James V. Hennessey. "Thyroxine and Treatment of Hypothyroidism: Seven Decades of Experience." Endocrine 66.1 (2019): 10-17.

3) Murray, George R. "Note on the Treatment of Myxoedema by Hypodermic Injections of an Extract of the Thyroid Gland of a Sheep." British Medical Journal 2.1606 (1891): 796."

4) Natural vs. Synthetic Thyroid Medications for Thyroid Medical Editor: Medical Author: Ruchi Mathur, M.D. Medical Editor William C. Shiel Jr., MD, FACP, FACR Last Editorial Review: 1/11/2018 Medicine Net. https://www.medicinenet.com/natural_vs_synthetic_thyroid_medications/ask.htm

5) Unapproved Levothyroxine Products Hit in FDA Action, Pharmacy Today. 2001;7(8) American Pharmacists Association, Medscape August 1, 2001.

6) Federal Register: August 14, 1997 Volume 62, Number 157 [Notices][Page 43535-43538] Food and Drug Administration Notice Regarding Levothyroxine Sodium: William K. Hubbard, Associate Commissioner for Policy Coordination.

7) Idrees, Thaer, et al. "Liothyronine and Desiccated Thyroid Extract in the Treatment of Hypothyroidism." Thyroid 30.10 (2020): 1399-1413.

8) Bianco, Antonio C., et al. "Paradigms of Dynamic Control of Thyroid Hormone Signaling." Endocrine Reviews 40.4 (2019): 1000-1047.

9) Teitelbaum, Jacob. "Part 2--Protocols for Treating an Underactive Thyroid--Despite Normal Blood Tests." Townsend Letter for Doctors and Patients 241-242 (2003): 174-176.

10) Gomes-Lima, Cristiane, et al. "Can Reverse T3 Assay Be Employed to Guide T4 vs. T4/T3 Therapy in Hypothyroidism?" Frontiers in Endocrinology 10 (2019): 856.

11) Moskovich, Dotan, et. al. "Targeting the DIO3 Enzyme Using First-In-Class Inhibitors Effectively Suppresses Tumor Growth: A New Paradigm in Ovarian Cancer Treatment." Oncogene 40.44 (2021): 6248-6257.

12) Nappi, Annarita, et al. "Deiodinases and Cancer." Endocrinology 162.4 (2021).

13) Dentice, Monica, et. al. "Type 3 Deiodinase and Solid Tumors: An Intriguing Pair." Expert Opinion on Therapeutic Targets 17.11 (2013): 1369-1379.

14) Goemann, Luri Martin, et al. "Current Concepts and Challenges to Unravel the Role of Iodothyronine Deiodinases in Human Neoplasias." Endocrine-Related Cancer 25.12 (2018): R625-R645.

15) Willmington, Sunny, et al. "Treating Hypothyroidism Naturally." Townsend Letter for Doctors and Patients (2002): 80-81.

16) Pepper, Gary M., and Paul Y. Casanova-Romero. "Conversion to Armour Thyroid from Levothyroxine Improved Patient Satisfaction in the Treatment of Hypothyroidism." Journal of Endocrinology, Diabetes & Obesity 2 (2014): 1055-1060.

17) Hoang, Thanh D., et al. "Desiccated Thyroid Extract Compared with Levothyroxine in the Treatment of Hypothyroidism: A Randomized, Double-Blind, Crossover Study." The Journal of Clinical Endocrinology & Metabolism 98.5 (2013): 1982-1990.

18) Salvatore, Domenico, et al. "The Relevance of T3 in the Management of Hypothyroidism." The Lancet Diabetes & Endocrinology 10.5 (2022): 366-372.

19) Sapin, R., and J. L. Schlienger. "Thyroxine (T4) And Tri-Iodothyronine (T3) Determinations: Techniques and Value in the Assessment of Thyroid Function." Annales De Biologie Clinique. Vol. 61. No. 4. 2003.

Chapter 3

Why Natural Thyroid is Better than Synthetic Part Two

The Calcitonin and Parathyroid Connection

ALTHOUGH THE THYROID GLAND'S MAIN job is to produce thyroid hormone. Two other hormones are manufactured within the thyroid gland, calcitonin and parathyroid hormone, both involved in calcium metabolism. Parathyroid hormone (PTH) is produced by four small parathyroid glands, two embedded on each side. PTH hormone maintains the serum calcium within a very narrow range by mobilizing calcium from the bones into the blood stream. Any slight deviation from this narrow range for serum calcium is a serious medical problem, either hypercalcemia or hypocalcemia. Elevated parathyroid hormone levels, such as in parathyroid adenoma, causes increased urinary calcium excretion, hypercalcemia, and osteoporosis. Inadvertent removal of the parathyroid glands during thyroidectomy results in hypocalcemia, treated by giving the patient calcium tablets. (1-3)

Calcitonin is manufactured by the parafollicular cells (C cells) embedded deep within the thyroid gland. This hormone opposes the action of the parathyroid hormone, assists in maintaining good bone density, and prevents osteoporosis. One role of calcitonin is to protect the maternal skeleton during lactation. Measurement of serum calcitonin has been suggested for routine management of thyroid nodules since a high calcitonin level is an excellent marker for medullary thyroid cancer, which originates from parafollicular C-cells that produce calcitonin. In congenital hypothyroidism, there may be low or deficient calcitonin with associated loss of bone density. (4-16)

Thyroid Disorders Cause Destruction of Calcitonin Cells

Hashimoto's thyroiditis is a common cause of hypothyroidism and is associated with the destruction of the C-cells and loss of calcitonin production. The resulting calcitonin deficiency is a potential cause of bone resorption and osteoporosis. On the other hand, treatment with calcitonin nasal spray is an FDA-approved treatment for osteoporosis and has been shown to increase bone density. In 2000, Dr. Stamato studied the use of calcitonin nasal spray in 8 female hypothyroid patients treated with levothyroxine alone, and 8 treated with combined levothyroxine with calcitonin, finding the benefit of improved bone density in the group treated with the calcitonin. (17-21)

In 1998, Dr. Maria Borges writes:

We have found low basal and stimulated calcitonin values in patients with chronic autoimmune thyroiditis and thyroid enlargement, which represents an early phase of chronic autoimmune thyroiditis. Our data have also confirmed previous findings of deficient calcitonin secretion in advanced stages of chronic autoimmune thyroiditis in which thyroid atrophy is usually found. These findings may be associated with C-cell destruction following progressive, nonspecific follicular cell damage caused by lymphocytic infiltration and fibrosis of the gland. (18)

In 2002 in Thyroid, Dr. Angella Inzerillo writes:

Calcitonin was initially discovered as a hypocalcemic factor synthesized by thyroid parafollicular C cells. Early experiments demonstrated that calcitonin inhibited bone resorption and decreased calcium efflux from isolated cat tibiae, and subsequent histologic and culture studies confirmed the osteoclast as its major site of action. Its potent antiresorptive effect and analgesic action have led to its clinical use in the treatment of Paget's bone disease, osteoporosis, and hypercalcemia of malignancy. (10)

Hashimoto's, Radio-iodine, and Surgery

Total thyroidectomy may inadvertently result in hypoparathyroidism if the parathyroid glands are removed, rendering the patient hypo-calcemic in the postoperative period. The thyroid gland may be damaged by Hashimoto's thyroiditis or radioactive iodine. In this scenario, the parafollicular cells (C-cells) which make calcitonin may be damaged, inducing calcitonin deficiency and a greater risk for osteoporosis and fracture. Levothyroxine and T4-only medications do not provide the missing calcitonin. One might ask the obvious question, "Would giving calcitonin to these patients improve their quality of life and prevent osteoporosis?" (10-16)

Treating Hypothyroidism with Calcitonin

In 2019, Dr. Wedad Rahman from the University of Maryland in Baltimore asked this same question, "Can Calcitonin Replacement Improve the Quality of Life in Hypothyroid Patients?" Dr. Wedad Rahman noted that patients on levothyroxine after thyroidectomy do not feel well despite TSH in the normal range. He speculated this may be due to calcitonin deficiency. Underway at the University of Maryland is a small study of 11 hypothyroid patients treated with salmon calcitonin nasal spray. ClinicalTrials.gov Identifier: NCT03342001. We await the publication of those results. (16)

As you might guess, levothyroxine, Synthroid, and T4-only medications do not contain calcitonin. One could speculate that patients feel better on NDT because of the small amount of calcitonin present in NDT. However, this is mere speculation since we need more data to support this idea. I am unaware of any studies measuring the amount of calcitonin in NDT. I would guess the amount of calcitonin present in NDT is insignificant. Perhaps the real reason for the patient improvement when switching from levothyroxine to NDT is the added T3 in NDT, as we will discuss in the next chapter.

In 2021, Dr. Cvek did a retrospective study of basal calcitonin levels in 467 Hashimoto's thyroiditis patients from the Croatian Biobank, finding no significant difference in calcitonin levels in Hashimoto's compared to 184 healthy controls. (22-24)

After these negative studies, the endocrinology community seems to have lost interest in calcitonin nasal spray as a treatment for calcitonin deficiency for the maintenance of bone density in the autoimmune thyroid patient. However, the use of serum calcitonin testing remains a good screening test for medullary thyroid cancer in the workup of thyroid nodules. (25)

None of the Studies Used Natural Desiccated Thyroid

Unfortunately, all the medical studies that examine the bone-thyroid connection used T4-only medication, and none used NDT, desiccated natural thyroid, so we do not have a good comparison study to evaluate the long-term effect of NDT on bone density and osteoporosis. A good use of NIH research funding would be comparing the bone density and long-term fracture risk with natural desiccated thyroid compared to T4-only medications. However, for political reasons, we may never see NIH funding for this study using NDT.

The TSH Connection. TSH is Protective and Prevents Bone Resorption

Advances in our understanding of physiology and animal research have revealed that TSH hormone (thyroid stimulating hormone) directly affects bone cells, preventing bone resorption and, therefore, protecting bone density. This could explain the many studies correlating higher TSH with improved bone density. The problem with using TSH as a treatment for osteoporosis is that higher TSH is associated with an increased risk of coronary artery disease, as reported in 2008 by Dr. Bjørn O Åsvold's HUNT study. Higher TSH may also be associated with a host of low thyroid symptoms of fatigue, depression, loss of cognitive function, malaise, muscle aches, and pains. Patients feel better with a lower TSH and higher thyroid function, so cutting back on thyroid medication to let the TSH drift up may be good for bone density. However, it is not good for the patient. (26-29)

Will Thyroid Medication Give Me Osteoporosis?

In 2011, Dr. Marci Turner reported in the British Medical Journal that older women taking levothyroxine have increased fracture risk. (30)

In 2010 Dr. Murphy studied normal postmenopausal women correlating TSH levels with fracture risk. Dr. Murphy found a 35% increase in fracture risk in women with lower TSH values. In comparison, higher TSH values were protective against fracture. (1) Note: TSH=thyroid stimulating hormone. (31)

No Real Consensus on The Issue

To add confusion, a 2003 meta-analysis by Dr. Schneider reviewed 63 studies looking at the effect of thyroid medication (T4-only) on bone mineral density, finding no real consensus and concluding:

> Currently, debate still exists about the effects of thyroid hormone therapy on skeletal integrity, that is, the safety of levothyroxine use with respect to bone mineral density. (32)

More recent reviews by Dr. Alessandro Brancatella in 2020 and Dr. Prakar Poudel in 2022 found no deleterious effects on bone density in postmenopausal women taking TSH suppressive doses of levothyroxine. Dr. Bancatella writes:

> Fujiyama et al. evaluated 24 postmenopausal women treated with total thyroidectomy for DTC (thyroid cancer) and found no difference in the incidence of vertebral deformity nor in the rate of bone loss between patients and 179 age-matched controls. (33)

Dr. Prakar Poudel writes:

> Following an extensive evaluation, it was difficult to conclusively determine the association or effect of thyroxine or thyrotropin levels on bone mineral density in postmenopausal women. (34)

This topic is discussed in more detail in Chapter 7. TSH Suppression, Benefits, and Adverse Effects.

Good News About Bioidentical Hormones

The good news is that the TSH effect on bone density is relatively modest and is offset by the addition of estrogen, a bioidentical hormone, which increases bone density. Osteoporosis prevention employs a nutritional supplement program such as Calcium, Magnesium, Vitamin D3, Vitamin K2, and Vitamin C to protect and maintain bone density as reported in 1995 by Dr. Franklyn. (35)

Conclusion

One of the errors in modern thyroid endocrinology is ignoring the role of calcitonin produced by the thyroid gland's parafollicular cells (C-cells). The calcitonin-thyroid connection is largely ignored by conventional endocrinology. Will future medical treatment of the auto-immune thyroid patient include routine calcitonin testing and treatment with calcitonin nasal spray for the prevention of osteoporosis? Only time will tell. (36-53)

◆ References for Chapter 3

1) Tinawi, Mohammad. "Disorders of Calcium Metabolism: Hypocalcemia and Hypercalcemia." Cureus 13.1 (2021).

2) Schafer, Anne L., and Dolores M. Shoback. "Hypocalcemia: Diagnosis and Treatment." Endotext [Internet] (2016).

3) Carroll, Mary F., and David S. Schade. "A Practical Approach to Hypercalcemia." American Family Physician 67.9 (2003): 1959-1966.

4) Miller, Scott. "Calcitonin—Guardian of The Mammalian Skeleton, or Is It Just a Fish Story?" Endocrinology 147.9 (2006): 4007-4009.

5) Woodrow, Janine P., et al. "Calcitonin Plays a Critical Role in Regulating Skeletal Mineral Metabolism During Lactation." Endocrinology 147.9 (2006): 4010-4021.

6) Davey, Rachel A., et al. "Calcitonin Receptor Plays a Physiological Role to Protect Against Hypercalcemia in Mice." Journal of Bone and Mineral Research 23.8 (2008): 1182-1193.

7) Mirzaei, S., et al. "Possible Effect of Calcitonin Deficiency on Bone Mass After Subtotal Thyroidectomy." Acta Medica Austriaca 26.1 (1999): 29-31.

8) Cappelli, C., et al. "Bone Density and Mineral Metabolism in Calcitonin-Deficiency Patients." Minerva Endocrinologica 29.1 (2004): 1-10.

9) Barbot, N., et al. "Chronic Autoimmune Thyroiditis and C-Cell Hyperplasia. Study of Calcitonin Secretion in 24 Patients." Annales d'Endocrinologie. Vol. 52. No. 2. 1991.

10) Inzerillo, Angela M., et al. "Calcitonin: The Other Thyroid Hormone." Thyroid 12.9 (2002): 791-798.

11) Tobler, Paul H., et al. "Identity of Calcitonin Extracted from Normal Human Thyroid Glands with Synthetic Human Calcitonin-(1–32)." Biochimica et Biophysica Acta (BBA)-Protein Structure and Molecular Enzymology 707.1 (1982): 59-65.

12) Tashjian Jr, Armen H., et al. "Human Calcitonin: Immunologic Assay, Cytologic Localization and Studies on Medullary Thyroid Carcinoma." The American Journal of Medicine 56.6 (1974): 840-849.

13) Elisei, Rossella. "Routine Serum Calcitonin Measurement in the Evaluation of Thyroid Nodules." Best Practice & Research Clinical Endocrinology & Metabolism 22.6 (2008): 941-953.

14) Demeester Mirkine, Nelly, et al. "Calcitonin and Bone Mass Status in Congenital Hypothyroidism." Calcified Tissue International 46.4 (1990): 222-226.

15) Body, Jean-Jacques, et al. "Calcitonin Deficiency After Radioactive Iodine Treatment." Annals of Internal Medicine 109.7 (1988): 590-591.

16) Rahman, Wedad, et al. "Can Calcitonin Replacement Improve Quality of Life in Hypothyroid Patients?" Journal of the Endocrine Society 3. Supplement_1 (2019): MON-622.

17) Lima, Marcus A., et al. "Quantitative Analysis of C Cells in Hashimoto's Thyroiditis." Thyroid 8.6 (1998): 505-509.

18) Borges, Maria F., et al. "Calcitonin Deficiency in Early Stages of Chronic Autoimmune Thyroiditis." Clinical Endocrinology 49.1 (1998): 69-75.

19) Poppe, Kris, et al. "Calcitonin Reserve in Different Stages of Atrophic Autoimmune Thyroiditis." Thyroid 9.12 (1999): 1211-1214.

20) Trovas, G. P., et al. "A Randomized Trial of Nasal Spray Salmon Calcitonin in Men with Idiopathic Osteoporosis: Effects on Bone Mineral Density and Bone Markers." Journal of Bone and Mineral Research 17.3 (2002): 521-527.

21) Stamato, FJ da C., et al. "Effect of Combined Treatment with Calcitonin on Bone Densitometry of Patients with Treated Hypothyroidism." Revista da Associação Médica Brasileira 46 (2000): 177-181.

22) Cvek, M., et al. "Presence or Severity of Hashimoto's Thyroiditis Does Not Influence Basal Calcitonin Levels: Observations from CROHT Biobank." Journal of Endocrinological Investigation (2021): 1-9.

23) Maino, Fabio, et al. "Calcitonin Levels in Thyroid Disease Are Not Affected by Autoimmune Thyroiditis or Differentiated Thyroid Carcinoma." European Thyroid Journal 10.4 (2021): 295-305.

24) Grani, Giorgio, et al. "Interpretation of Serum Calcitonin in Patients with Chronic Autoimmune Thyroiditis." Endocrine Related Cancer 19.3 (2012): 345.

25) Broecker-Preuss, Martina, et al. "Update on Calcitonin Screening for Medullary Thyroid Carcinoma and the Results of a Retrospective Analysis of 12,984 Patients with Thyroid Nodules." Cancers 15.8 (2023): 2333.

26) Baqi, L. et al. "The Level of TSH Appeared Favorable in Maintaining Bone Mineral Density in Postmenopausal Women." Endocrine Regulations 44.1 (2010): 9-15.

27) Mazziotti, Gherardo, et al. "Recombinant Human TSH Modulates In Vivo C-Telopeptides of Type-1 Collagen and Bone Alkaline Phosphatase, But Not Osteoprotegerin Production in Postmenopausal Women Monitored for Differentiated Thyroid Carcinoma." Journal of Bone and Mineral Research 20.3 (2005): 480-486.

28) Karga, Helen, et al. "The Effects of Recombinant Human TSH on Bone Turnover in Patients After Thyroidectomy." Journal of Bone and Mineral Metabolism 28.1 (2010): 35-41.

29) Åsvold, Bjørn O., et al. "Thyrotropin Levels and Risk of Fatal Coronary Heart Disease: The HUNT Study." Archives of Internal Medicine 168.8 (2008): 855-860.

30) Turner, Marci R., et al. "Levothyroxine Dose and Risk of Fractures in Older Adults: Nested Case-Control Study." BMJ 342 (2011).

31) Murphy, Elaine, et al. "Thyroid Function Within the Upper Normal Range is Associated with Reduced Bone Mineral Density and an Increased Risk of Nonvertebral Fractures in Healthy Euthyroid Postmenopausal Women." The Journal of Clinical Endocrinology & Metabolism 95.7 (2010): 3173-3181.

32) Schneider, R., and C. Reiners. "The Effect of Levothyroxine Therapy on Bone Mineral Density: A Systematic Review of The Literature." Experimental and Clinical Endocrinology & Diabetes 111.08 (2003): 455-470.

33) Brancatella, Alessandro, and Claudio Marcocci. "TSH Suppressive Therapy and Bone." Endocrine Connections 9.7 (2020): R158-R172.

34) Poudel, Prakar, et al. "Effect of Thyroxine and Thyrotropin on Bone Mineral Density in Postmenopausal Women: A Systematic Review." Cureus 14.6 (2022).

35) Franklyn, J. A., et al. "Effect of Estrogen Replacement Therapy Upon Bone Mineral Density in Thyroxine-Treated Postmenopausal Women with a Past History of Thyrotoxicosis." Thyroid 5.5 (1995): 359-363.

36) Stall, Glenn M., et al. "Accelerated Bone Loss in Hypothyroid Patients Overtreated with L-Thyroxine." Annals Of Internal Medicine 113.4 (1990): 265-269

37) Meier, Christian, et al. "Restoration of Euthyroidism Accelerates Bone Turnover in Patients with Subclinical Hypothyroidism: A Randomized Controlled Trial." Osteoporosis International 15.3 (2004): 209-216.

38) Guo, Chun-Yuan, et al. "Longitudinal Changes of Bone Mineral Density and Bone Turnover in Postmenopausal Women on Thyroxine." Clinical Endocrinology 46.3 (1997): 301-307.

39) Baqi, L., et al. "Thyrotropin Versus Thyroid Hormone in Regulating Bone Density and Turnover in Premenopausal Women." Endocrine Regulations 44.2 (2010): 57-63.

40) Kumeda, Y., et al. "Persistent Increase in Bone Turnover in Graves' Patients with Subclinical Hyperthyroidism." Journal of Clinical Endocrinology and Metabolism 85 (2000): 4157-4161.

41) Chen, Cheng-Hsiung, et al. "Bone Mineral Density in Women Receiving Thyroxine Suppressive Therapy for Differentiated Thyroid Carcinoma." Journal of the Formosan Medical Association Taiwan Yi Zhi 103.6 (2004): 442-447.

42) Mazokopakis, Elias E., et al. "Changes of Bone Mineral Density in Pre-Menopausal Women with Differentiated Thyroid Cancer Receiving L-Thyroxine Suppressive Therapy." Current Medical Research and Opinion 22.7 (2006): 1369-1373.

43) Bauer, Douglas C., et al. "Risk for Fracture in Women with Low Serum Levels of Thyroid-Stimulating Hormone." Annals Of Internal Medicine 134.7 (2001): 561-568.

44) Mazziotti, Gherardo, et al. "Serum TSH Values and Risk of Vertebral Fractures in Euthyroid Postmenopausal Women with Low Bone Mineral Density." Bone 46.3 (2010): 747-751.

45) Wejda, B., et al. "Hip Fractures and The Thyroid: A Case-Control Study." Journal Of Internal Medicine 237.3 (1995): 241-247.

46) Hanna, F. W. F., et al. "Effect of Replacement Doses of Thyroxine on Bone Mineral Density." Clinical Endocrinology 48.2 (1998): 229-234.

47) Bauer, Michael, et al. "Bone Mineral Density During Maintenance Treatment with Supraphysiological Doses of Levothyroxine in Affective Disorders: A Longitudinal Study." Journal of Affective Disorders 83.2-3 (2004): 183-190.

48) Gyulai, Laszlo, et al. "Bone Mineral Density in Pre and Postmenopausal Women with Affective Disorder Treated with Long-Term L-Thyroxine Augmentation." Journal Of Affective Disorders 66.2-3 (2001): 185-191.

49) Larijani, B., et al. "Effects of Levothyroxine Suppressive Therapy on Bone Mineral Density in Premenopausal Women." Journal Of Clinical Pharmacy and Therapeutics 29.1 (2004): 1-5.

50) Muller, Carmen G., et al. "Possible Limited Bone Loss with Suppressive Thyroxine Therapy Is Unlikely to Have Clinical Relevance." Thyroid 5.2 (1995): 81-87.

51) Reverter, J. L., et al. "Lack of Deleterious Effect on Bone Mineral Density of Long-Term Thyroxine Suppressive Therapy for Differentiated Thyroid Carcinoma." Endocrine-related cancer 12.4 (2005): 973-981.

52) Sijanovic, S., and I. Karner. "Bone Loss in Premenopausal Women on Long-Term Suppressive Therapy with Thyroid Hormone." Medscape Women's Health 6.5 (2001): 3-3.

53) Adlin, E. Victor, et al. "Bone Mineral Density in Postmenopausal Women Treated With L-Thyroxine." The American Journal of Medicine 90.3 (1991): 360-366.

Chapter 4

Why Natural Thyroid is Better than Synthetic Part Three

IT HAS BEEN 132 YEARS since George Murray's 1891 paper on thyroid extract as a treatment for hypothyroidism, and since then, natural desiccated thyroid (NDT) has been prescribed with generally good results. In my opinion, NDT is the preferred thyroid medication, providing better results when compared to T4-only medications such as levothyroxine (generic Synthroid). Despite this, Endocrinology Societies such as the ATA (American Thyroid Association) have published guidelines advising doctors to avoid prescribing NDT for various reasons. The latest reason is that "there are no controlled trials" using NDT. Here is a quote from the 2012 ATA Guidelines:

> As of 2012, there are no controlled trials supporting the preferred use of desiccated thyroid hormone over synthetic L-thyroxine in the treatment of hypothyroidism or any other thyroid disease. (1-3)

A New Controlled Trial Comparing Natural Thyroid to Synthroid

This changed in 2013, as a controlled trial was published in the May 2013 Journal of Endocrinology by Dr. Thanh D. Hoang at the Walter Reed National Military Medical Center in Bethesda, Maryland. When a new patient on NDT comes to the Walter Reed Medical Center, their usual practice is to switch the patient over to levothyroxine (generic Synthroid). This is also generally true for most hospitals. However, occasionally, such a patient may not feel as well on levothyroxine, despite adequate dosing based on serum TSH levels. Dr. Thanh D Hoang writes:

> Patients on natural thyroid (desiccated thyroid extract, NDT), after being switched over to levothyroxine (L-T4), occasionally did not feel as well. (4)

This is precisely what I have found in actual clinical practice over the years. Patients who arrive in my office taking levothyroxine with lingering symptoms of hypothyroidism will typically feel much better when switched to NDT (natural desiccated thyroid).

Comparing Levothyroxine (generic Synthroid) to Natural Thyroid

Dr. Thanh D. Hoang's controlled study compared NDT with levothyroxine, finding roughly half the patients (48%) felt better on NDT, one-third had no preference, and one-fifth (18.6%) felt better on the levothyroxine (generic Synthroid). Clearly, the NDT wins the comparison test (48.6% vs. 18.6%). At the end of the study, 34 patients (48.6%) preferred NDT, 23 (32.9%) had no preference and 13 (18.6%) preferred levothyroxine (T4). Now that we have a controlled trial showing the natural thyroid is better, maybe the ATA should change its guideline. What is the explanation for the superiority of NDT for over half the patients? In my opinion, many of these patients are "poor converters," meaning they have poor conversion of T4 to T3 and need the small additional dose of T3 contained in NDT. Conversion of T4 to T3 depends upon peripheral deiodination, as shown below. (4)

Twenty Percent are Poor Converters

In 2011, Dr. Damiano Gullo in Catania, Italy, conducted a retrospective study of T4 to T3 conversion in 3,473 athyreotic patients in their thyroid clinic from 2000–2007 after undergoing total thyroidectomy for thyroid cancer. Note: athyreotic means having no thyroid gland.

Dr. Gullo writes the athyreotic patient is ideal for studying peripheral conversion (deiodination) of T4 to T3. Dr. Gullo found that about 20 percent of these patients had inadequate peripheral deiodination and could not maintain T3 or T4 in the reference range despite a normal TSH:

> Athyreotic patients do not secrete endogenous thyroid hormones, and all circulating T4 and T3 originate from replacement treatment with levothyroxine. These patients, therefore, are an ideal model to study peripheral tissues' capacity to produce the biologically active hormone T3 from the exogenous prohormone T4... More than 20% of these patients, despite normal TSH levels, do not maintain FT3 or FT4 values in the reference range, reflecting the inadequacy of peripheral deiodination to compensate for the absent T3 secretion. (5)

TSH Suppression Required

In agreement with Dr. Gullo is a 2012 study by Dr. Mitsuru Ito from Japan, who studied 135 patients after thyroidectomy treated with levothyroxine. To achieve the same Free T3 levels recorded before thyroidectomy, Dr. Mitsuru Ito found a suppressive levothyroxine dosage was needed. This dosage suppressed the TSH below the reference range. Dr. Ito writes:

> TSH-suppressive doses of levothyroxine are required to achieve preoperative native serum triiodothyronine levels in patients who have undergone total thyroidectomy. (6)

Two Types of D2 Deiodinase, Depending on Anatomic Location

What is the explanation for this? How can Dr. Gullo's and Dr. Ito's findings be explained? The explanation is as follows: There is a difference in the action of the D2 deiodinase depending on the anatomic location in the body. The D2 deiodinase located in the hypothalamic/pituitary region has a different action compared to the D2 deiodinase in the periphery. The key finding is the difference in hypothalamic vs. peripheral type 2 deiodinase (D2), demonstrated nicely by a 2015 study by Dr. Joao de Castro using mice in Dr. Antonio Bianco's laboratory at Rush Medical Center in Chicago. Dr. de Castro reported the D2 deiodinase enzyme in the hypothalamus controls TSH. However, the hypothalamic D2 is relatively **insensitive to inhibition by T4**, allowing D2 to rapidly convert T4 to T3, acting as a negative feedback mechanism that inhibits the production of TSH, leading to the suppression of TSH. However, the D2 **in the periphery is more sensitive to inhibition by T4.** This inhibits the peripheral conversion of T4 to T3, the active form of the hormone, causing peripheral hypothyroidism at the cellular level. This explains the lingering hypothyroid symptoms during treatment with levothyroxine despite TSH within the reference range. Combination therapy with both T3 and T4 is the solution. Dr. Joao de Castro writes:

> The current treatment for patients with hypothyroidism is levothyroxine (L-T4), along with normalization of serum thyroid-stimulating hormone (TSH). However, normalization of serum TSH with L-T4 monotherapy results in relatively low serum triiodothyronine (T3) and high serum T4/T3 ratio. .... Here, we determined that tissue-specific differences in D2 ubiquitination account for the high T4/T3 serum ratio in adult thyroidectomized (Tx) rats chronically implanted with subcutaneous L-T4 pellets. **While L-T4 administration decreased whole-body D2-dependent T4 conversion to T3, D2 activity in the hypothalamus was only minimally affected by L-T4....** in contrast to other D2-expressing tissues, **the hypothalamus is wired to have increased sensitivity to T4.** These studies reveal that tissue-specific differences in D2 ubiquitination are an inherent property of the TRH/TSH feedback mechanism and indicate that **only constant delivery of L-T4 and L-T3 fully normalizes T3-dependent metabolic markers** and gene expression profiles in Tx rats. (7)

I would mention here, that if Dr. De Castro had measured reverse T3 in his levothyroxine-treated laboratory mice, he would have found increased reverse T3, another indicator the deiodinase system is producing an undesirable result in the levothyroxine-treated patient. (8-11)

Free T4 and Reverse T3/Free T3 Ratio, A Useful Window into Status of Deiodinase System

In 1984, Dr. Shimada studied T3, T4, and reverse T3 in 61 hyperthyroid, 31 hypothyroid patients, 8 subacute thyroiditis, and 40 normal subjects. Dr. Shimada concluded "the relationship between serum T4 level and rT3/T3 ratio should be examined for adequate **information concerning the peripheral conversion of thyroid hormones** under various thyroid diseases." Examining the Free T4 and ratio of free T3 to reverse T3 is a useful window into the status of the deiodinase system. If the T4 in levothyroxine is being preferentially converted to reverse T3, this is useful information the levothyroxine is not working, and best to try a combination drug containing both T4 and T3 such as NDT. Dr. Shimada writes:

> In order to clarify the conversion of thyroxine (T4) to triiodothyronine (T3) or to reverse T3 (rT3), serum concentrations of T4, T3, rT3, thyrotropin (TSH), thyroxine-binding globulin (TBG) and values of T3 uptake (T3 U) were measured in 61 hyperthyroid and 31 hypothyroid patients, 8 patients with subacute thyroiditis, and 40 normal subjects. Then, free T4 index (FT4I), T3/T4, rT3/T4, and rT3/T3 ratio were calculated...The rT3/T3 ratio was high in the hyperthyroid patients and low in the hypothyroid patients compared with that in the normal subjects. ...Our results indicated that thyroid hormones themselves could regulate the conversion of T4 to T3 or rT3 by activating 5-monodeiodinase [D3 deiodinase] in hyperthyroidism and by activating 5'-monodeiodinase [D2 deiodinase] and suppressing 5-monodeiodinase [D3

deiodinase] in hypothyroidism. Serum rT3 level was a more sensitive parameter than serum T4 or T3 for evaluating thyroid dysfunction....we concluded that the relationship between serum T4 level and rT3/T3 ratio should be examined for adequate information concerning the peripheral conversion of thyroid hormones under various thyroid diseases. (10)

Genetic Mutation Explains Poor Peripheral Conversion of T4 to T3

In 2015, Elizabeth A. McAninch and Antonio Bianco at Rush Medical Center studied genetic variations, also called polymorphisms, in the D2 deiodinase enzyme system, explaining why levothyroxine, a T4-only medication, does not work in some patients. This is known as the Thr92Ala-D2 polymorphism present in up to 36 percent of the population, which impairs the peripheral conversion of T4 to T3. Dr. Elizabeth A. McAninch explains that people who harbor this mutation prefer combination therapy with both T3 and T4 rather than T4 alone. For example, NDT is a combination therapy since it contains both T3 and T4. Note: Levothyroxine is L-T4-only therapy. Dr. Elizabeth A. McAninch writes:

> A prevalent Thr92Ala-**D2 polymorphism** [between 12% and 36% of the population are homozygotes] ... Hypothyroid individuals carrying this polymorphism [in D2] were found to prefer a therapy that includes T3 vs monotherapy with L-T4 alone... (12)

Conclusion

Combination therapy with NDT is superior to T-4 monotherapy for two reasons as mentioned above. The first reason is Levothyroxine tends to suppress the TSH in spite of peripheral hypothyroidism. This is explained as a different mode of action for the D2 deiodinase system in the hypothalamus which is very sensitive to T4 inhibition vs. the periphery which is relatively insensitive to T4 inhibition. The second reason is the prevalence of genetic mutations in the

D2 enzyme system which explains why some people are poor converters and need the additional T3 in their thyroid medication. (13-14)

♦ **References for Chapter 4**

1) Murray GR. Myxoedema. In: Northumberland and Durham Med Soc Minute Book. University of Newcastle Archives; 1891; Feb 12:91–3

2) Slater, Stefan. "The Discovery of Thyroid Replacement Therapy. Part 3: A Complete Transformation." Journal of the Royal Society of Medicine 104.3 (2011): 100.

3) Garber, Jeffrey R., et al. "Clinical Practice Guidelines for Hypothyroidism in Adults: Cosponsored by the American Association of Clinical Endocrinologists and the American Thyroid Association." Endocrine Practice 18.6 (2012): 988-1028.

4) Hoang, Thanh D., et al. "Desiccated Thyroid Extract Compared with Levothyroxine in the Treatment of Hypothyroidism: A Randomized, Double-Blind, Crossover Study." The Journal of Clinical Endocrinology and Metabolism 98.5 (2013): 1982-1990.

5) Gullo, Damiano, et al. "Levothyroxine Monotherapy Cannot Guarantee Euthyroidism in All Athyreotic Patients." PLoS One 6.8 (2011): e22552.

6) Ito, Mitsuru, et al. "TSH-suppressive Doses of Levothyroxine Are Required to Achieve Preoperative Native Serum Triiodothyronine Levels in Patients Who Have Undergone Total Thyroidectomy." European Journal of Endocrinology 167.3 (2012): 373-378.

7) De Castro, Joao Pedro Werneck, et al. "Differences in Hypothalamic Type 2 Deiodinase Ubiquitination Explain Localized Sensitivity to Thyroxine." The Journal of Clinical Investigation 125.2 (2015): 769.

8) Wilson, Julian Bryant, and Theodore C. Friedman. "Reverse T3 in Patients with Hypothyroidism, Helpful or a Waste of Time?" Journal of the Endocrine Society 5. Supplement_1 (2021): A952-A952.

9) Gomes-Lima, Cristiane, et al. "Can Reverse T3 Assay Be Employed to Guide T4 vs. T4/T3 Therapy in Hypothyroidism?" Frontiers in Endocrinology 10 (2019): 856.

10) Shimada, T. "The Conversion of Thyroxine to Triiodothyronine (T3) or to Reverse T3 In Patients with Thyroid Dysfunction." Nihon Naibunpi Gakkai Zasshi 60.3 (1984): 195-206.

11) Exley, Sarah, Sonal Banzal, and Udaya Kabadi. "Low Reverse T3: A Reliable, Sensitive and Specific in Diagnosis of Central Hypothyroidism." Open Journal of Endocrine and Metabolic Diseases 11.7 (2021): 137-143.

12) McAninch, Elizabeth A., et al. "Prevalent Polymorphism in Thyroid Hormone-Activating Enzyme Leaves a Genetic Fingerprint That Underlies Associated Clinical Syndromes." The Journal of Clinical Endocrinology & Metabolism 100.3 (2015): 920-933.

13) Gorini, Francesca, et al. "Selenium: An Element of Life Essential for Thyroid Function." Molecules 26.23 (2021).

14 Drigo, Rafael Arrojo, and Antonio C. Bianco. "Type 2 Deiodinase at the Crossroads of Thyroid Hormone Action." The International Journal of Biochemistry & Cell Biology 43.10 (2011): 1432-1441.

Chapter 5

Errors in Modern Thyroid Endocrinology

POPULAR THYROID MESSAGE WEBSITES LIKE Janie Bowthorpe's, Stop the Thyroid Madness and Dana Trentini's Hypothyroid Mom has thousands of followers because they identify and alert readers to the "Errors in Modern Thyroid Endocrinology". Before we discuss these errors in detail, you might ask, "How is this possible that there could be errors in modern thyroid endocrinology?" We trust our doctors and medical institutions to practice medicine without errors. At least, we used to.

How Are Errors in Thyroid Medical Practice Possible?

The answer to this question becomes obvious, considering the money flowing from the drug industry to thyroid societies and doctors. Your doctor could be taking financial incentives from the drug industry, whether openly or secretly. For example, the American Thyroid Association, Endocrine Society, Endocrine Journals, Endocrine Research Grants, Endocrine Speakers Fees, and Endocrine Meetings are all heavily funded by the Major Drug Companies, including the ones that make Synthroid, levothyroxine, and T4-only thyroid medications. One might say the practice of endocrinology is "captured" by the drug industry. This is all public information. (75-85)

Creating Guidelines for the Benefit of the Benefactors

In 2012, the American Association of Clinical Endocrinologists (AACE) and the American Thyroid Association (ATA), published guidelines for prescribing thyroid pills, which says NDT, natural desiccated thyroid, should **NOT** be used:

There is no evidence to support using

desiccated thyroid hormone in preference to L-thyroxine monotherapy in the treatment of hypothyroidism, and therefore, desiccated thyroid hormone **should not be used** for the treatment of hypothyroidism. (1)

You might be surprised to know that these guidelines are wrong, which the ATA admitted when they came up with different guidelines in 2014. Nonetheless, the new guidelines still serve the drug industry's preference for their product, levothyroxine, over NDT. This preference serves a financial interest yet has no basis in medical science.

Follow the Money

Medical practice in the US is strongly influenced by guidelines promulgated by medical societies. So, when the ATA issues incorrect guidelines, you can understand how this leads to errors in the practice of thyroid endocrinology. By some strange coincidence. the ATA (American Thyroid Association) receives substantial financial support from AbbVie manufacturer of Synthroid, the same drug which is "Standard of Care" according to their "Guidelines." As of 2023, Acella, the current manufacturer of natural desiccated thyroid is listed alongside AbbVie as member of the Corporate Leadership Council for the ATA. Times are changing.

The Endocrine Society is proud to publicly disclose its funding which comes from (among others):

AbbVie Inc., Akrimax Pharmaceuticals, Alexion Pharmaceuticals, Inc., Amarin Pharma Inc., Bayer HealthCare, Boehringer Ingelheim Pharmaceuticals, Inc. & Lilly USA, LLC, Burroughs Wellcome Fund, Corcept Therapeutics Incorporated, Dexcom, Inc.,

Eisai Inc., Endo Pharmaceuticals Inc., Esaote North America, Inc., Ethicon Endo-Surgery, Inc., FNA Path Genentech, Inc., Janssen Pharmaceuticals, Inc., Lilly USA, LLC , Merck & Co., Inc., Mindray Thyroid Ultrasound by CSD, Novartis Pharmaceuticals Corporation, Noven Pharmaceuticals, Inc., Novo Nordisk Inc., NPS Pharmaceuticals, Inc., Pfizer, Inc., Salix Pharmaceuticals, Inc., Sanofi-Aventis U.S. Inc, Sanofi-Aventis U.S. Inc, Regeneron Pharmaceuticals Alliance, Takeda Pharmaceuticals U.S.A., Inc., Toshiba Head and Neck Ultrasound, Veracyte, Inc.

Of course, the fact their funding comes from the drug industry has nothing to do with any of the guidelines. Or does it? I think you are starting to get the idea. The above list of "2015 Leadership Donors" was proudly listed on the Endocrine Society website from 2015 to 2017. It may have been removed. No worries, a copy of this page from 2017 is still accessible using the Wayback Machine. Could this represent a conflict of interest? Of course not. How could you even think that? (75-86)

The Medical Board Has Some Questions

In 2012, prescribing NDT could trigger a medical board investigation and revocation of one's medical license. As of 2014, this all changed. It is perfectly OK for the humble country doctor to prescribe NDT as long as levothyroxine is "preferred." The updated ATA guidelines in 2014 said:

> We recommend that levothyroxine [T4 only] be considered as routine care for patients with primary hypothyroidism, in preference to use of thyroid extracts [NDT]. (2)

What happened between 2012 and 2014 to explain the change in ATA guidelines? Two publications in 2012 and 2013 by Antonio Bianco's group created a "Paradigm Shift" in endocrinology. This is the role of the deiodinase enzyme system and the need for combination therapy with both T3 and T4. Around this same time,

Dr. Bianco was on the board of directors of the ATA and, in 2015, served as president. (3-6)

The Paradigm Shift – The Deiodinase System

This "Paradigm Shift" in thyroid endocrinology is that the action of thyroid hormone on cellular metabolic rate is controlled by the intracellular deiodinase system. This was aptly described by Dr. Francesca Gorini, who writes in 2021:

> Virtually all tissues in the body receive the same signal by circulating T3; however, biological response and T4 to T3 conversion mainly depend on D2 and D3 [deiodinase] activities in the target tissues, in accord with the local metabolic request. (6)

Note: D1 and D2 convert T4 to T3, and D3 converts T4 to reverse T3, the inactive form. The deiodinase system and reverse T3 will be discussed in later chapters.

Why Won't My Endocrinologist Listen to Me?

Frequently, patients ask me a question: "Why won't my endocrinologist listen to me?" Many of these patients are escapees from the endocrinology office, having been ignored and mistreated by a succession of "cookie cutter" endocrinologists who give them minuscule amounts of T4-only medication (levothyroxine), which keeps the TSH in the "reference range". These poor miserable souls finally arrive in my office, where we switch them from levothyroxine to NDT, natural desiccated thyroid, in a dosage that gives them some relief from low thyroid symptoms. Two such NDT products currently available are NP Thyroid from Acella and Armour from Abbvie. A one-grain NDT tablet contains 38 mcg T4 and 9 mcg T3, a ratio of about 4:1 T4 to T3. Author's note: Before August 25, 2020, our office used Nature-Throid from RLC labs. However, this drug was voluntarily recalled on August 25, 2020, and has yet to be re-introduced. (7)

Patients Prefer NDT over Levothyroxine

Several cross-over studies published in the mainstream endocrinology literature reveal a subset of patients who don't feel well on T4-Only thyroid medication (Synthroid and levothyroxine). This subset reports they prefer and feel better taking NDT, natural desiccated thyroid. (8-9)

T3 Has Shorter Half-Life, This Makes Natural Thyroid a Safer Drug

The duration of activity of a drug is measured in half-life, the amount of time for drug blood levels to reduce by half, usually by metabolic breakdown in the liver or excretion by the kidneys. After one half-life, the peak blood level has been reduced in half. After two half-lives, only 25 percent of the drug remains in the bloodstream, etc. As it turns out, T3 has a 24-hour half-life, while T4 has a much longer one-week half-life. This difference in half-life explains why NDT is a safer choice than levothyroxine. (10-11)

The main adverse side effect of taking thyroid pills is thyroid excess, meaning the dosage is too high. Typical symptoms of thyroid excess are similar to thyrotoxicosis, namely, tachycardia, racing heart, anxiety, insomnia, tremor, and loose stools. The treatment is to stop taking thyroid pills. Thyroid excess symptoms resolve quickly for NDT within a few hours because of the short half-life of T3 in the NDT. However, for levothyroxine, it may take a week for symptoms to resolve because of the longer half-life of T4.

For this reason, NDT is safer than levothyroxine. In the event of thyroid excess, NDT is more forgiving and has more latitude than T4-only medications. Of course, this approach relies on a cooperative patient with good cognitive function who can participate in their care, recognize the rapid heart rate at rest, and then take a break from the thyroid pill. For example, a dementia patient or a young child could not be expected to cooperate and would not be a suitable candidate for NDT.

In the event the patient experiences any symptoms of thyroid excess, they will hold the NDT thyroid pill for a day. Because of the shorter half-life of the T3 in NDT, symptoms usually resolve after 6-12 hours. It is then safe to resume the NDT at a lower dosage the next day. We usually decrease in half-grain steps. We routinely check thyroid labs before starting thyroid medication and 6 weeks later. Initial labs include TSH, FT4, FT3, RT3, TPO and Thyroglobulin Antibodies, serum selenium, and spot urinary iodine.

Thyroid Hormone Ratios

The thyroid gland secretes T4 and T3 in a ratio of about 13:1. Peripheral conversion of T4 to T3 by D1 deiodinase maintains a serum level of about 4:1, (80 percent T4 and 20 percent T3). This serum ratio is closer to the ratio in NDT, natural desiccated thyroid. Each grain of NDT contains 38 micrograms of T4 and 9 micrograms of T3; this ratio is nearly 4:1. Authors note: actually, this ratio is 4.2:1. However, we average it out to 4:1. (12-14)

How is Thyroid Hormone Made? The Role of Selenium

Thyroid hormone is made by the organification of iodine, which involves adding iodine to tyrosine in the thyroglobulin protein. This occurs in the thyroid follicle at the apical membrane of the thyrocytes, forming a circular lining around the follicle. The organification process requires the oxidation of iodine by the TPO enzyme using hydrogen peroxide as a substrate. Hydrogen peroxide, as we all know, is highly oxidative and thus may damage adjacent cells. Hydrogen peroxide is available as a cleaning agent and topical antiseptic from the local drug store. The selenoprotein anti-oxidant system consisting of glutathione peroxidase, and thioredoxin reductase are necessary to degrade hydrogen peroxide. According to Dr. Song in 2007, various thyroid pathologies can be explained by over-expression or lack of degradation of this damaging hydrogen peroxide (H_2O_2). These thyroid pathologies include

Hashimoto's thyroiditis, autoimmune thyroiditis, thyroid nodules, thyroid cancer, etc. If the patient is selenium deficient, the seleno-protein anti-oxidant system may be dysfunctional, leading to oxidative injury or damage to the thyroid gland from excess hydrogen peroxide. (15-16)

The intracellular deiodinase enzyme system is also a seleno-protein. Dietary selenium deficiency will cause a dysfunctional deiodinase system, with intracellular hypothyroidism from the reduced conversion of T4 to T3 and higher serum T4/T3 ratio. Selenium deficiency is also associated with increased cancer risk and increased all-cause mortality. We routinely check the serum selenium level; those found low are given selenium supplements. As you will see below, ignoring the role of selenium is another error in modern endocrinology. (6) (17-19)

For more, see Chapter 14 the Production of Thyroid Hormone, and Chapters 20-22 on Selenium and the Thyroid.

The List of Errors in Thyroid Endocrinology

1. Sole Reliance on TSH to monitor treatment. (20)

2. TSH Suppression may be needed for adequate treatment. (21)

3. Reliance of T4 Only-Monotherapy (levothyroxine or Synthroid). (22)

4. NDT– Natural Desiccated Thyroid is a better choice. Shorter Half Life-makes NDT a safer choice. NDT Combines T3 and T4 – more robust for poor converters. (9)

5. Ignoring the Beneficial Effects of Selenium, Magnesium, Vitamin D3, and Gluten-Free Diet in Hashimoto's Autoimmune Thyroid Disease. (23-24)

6. Treating thyroid hormone levels while ignoring the autoimmune component of the thyroid disease. Importance of Gluten-Free Diet, Vitamin D3, and LDN. See Chapter 18.

7. Failing to promptly treat euthyroid Hashimoto's patients with thyroid medication. See Chapter 26.

8. Failing to treat pregnant women with anti-thyroid antibodies with thyroid medication. See Chapter 25.

9. Failing to test for iodine levels and supplement when low.

10. Ignoring iodine as a treatment for fibrocystic breast disease and breast cancer prevention. See Chapter 31 and 32.

The TSH Test Can Be Unreliable

The TSH can be unreliable in several medical conditions, such as Hypothalamic Dysfunction, Chronic Fatigue, and Fibromyalgia Patients (25-27)

More on this can be found in Chapter 10. The Unreliable TSH Lab Test.

Relying on TSH Within Reference Range

Despite normal TSH levels, many patients still have many nagging symptoms of hypothyroidism. In 2016, Antonio C. Bianco, MD, Ph.D., past president of the American Thyroid Association and past professor of medicine at Rush Medical School, published a study using 469 patients treated with levothyroxine (T4) compared to controls. The levothyroxine-treated patients were more likely to have higher T4:T3 ratios, higher BMI (Body Mass Index), and more likely to be taking Beta-Blockers drugs, statins, and SSRI anti-depressants. And they were more likely to suffer from cognitive impairment, also called "foggy brain." Dr. Bianco writes:

Patients complain of being depressed, slow, and having a foggy mind…They have difficulty losing weight. They complain of feeling sluggish and have less energy. Yet we doctors keep telling them, "I'm giving you the right amount of medication and your TSH is normal. You should feel fine"…Better medications [than levothyroxine] are needed to treat hypothyroidism….Patients who continue to have symptoms of levothyroxine monotherapy **might try a pill that contains both T3 and T4**. (20)

In the above quote, Dr. Bianco suggests trying a thyroid pill containing T3 and T4. I would add here we already have a pill that contains T3 and T4. This is called NDT, natural desiccated thyroid, available since 1891 and used by 20-30 percent of people on thyroid medication. Sadly, academic endocrinology has been transformed into a vending machine for the pharmaceutical industry. In order to be a good vending machine, we must give ourselves temporary amnesia, and when convenient forget about NDT, natural desiccated thyroid. To be fair, Dr. Bianco mentioned NDT in a different article in 2016. In 2018, Dr. Sarah Peterson reported the results of an online survey on thyroid medication usage (the ATA Hypothyroidism Treatment Survey). Of the 12,146 respondents, 62 percent were taking levothyroxine (T4 only), 9 percent a combination of levothyroxine and Cytomel (T3+T4), and 29 percent were taking natural desiccated thyroid, NDT (T3+T4). (28-30)

TSH Suppression May be Needed for Adequate Treatment

Dr. Mitsuru Ito is a thyroid expert at the Center for Excellence in Thyroid Care, Kuma Hospital, Kobe City, Japan. In 2012, Dr. Ito published his study treating athyreotic patients with levothyroxine after thyroidectomy. Note: athyreotic means having no thyroid gland. Dr. Ito found TSH suppressive doses of levothyroxine were needed in about 20 percent of patients to adjust the free thyroid hormone (Free T3) level back to the same historically normal level before the thyroidectomy. Dr. Ito explains this as "inadequacy of peripheral deiodination." In other words, the intra-cellular deiodinase system that converts T4 to T3 at the cellular level is not working well. Dr. Ito writes:

TSH-Suppressive doses of levothyroxine may be needed to achieve pre-operative

T3 levels after thyroidectomy. More than 20% of patients, despite normal TSH levels, do not maintain FT3 or FT4 values in the reference range, reflecting the inadequacy of peripheral deiodination to compensate for the absent T3 secretion. (21-22) (31)

Levothyroxine (L-T4) Alone Does not Resolve Symptoms of Hypothyroidism

In 2015, Dr. Elizabeth A. McAninch from Rush Medical School in Chicago writes:

Unfortunately, therapy with L-T4 [levothyroxine] alone does not resolve symptoms in all hypothyroid patients. Approximately 12% of the patients remain symptomatic despite normalizing serum TSH and TH [thyroid hormone] levels. Impaired cognition, fatigue, and difficulty losing weight are the main residual symptoms of these patients, **for which we lack understanding and have no mechanistic explanation.** (32)

Thanks to new research illuminating the deiodinase system, we now have a good understanding and a good mechanistic explanation of why levothyroxine alone does not resolve symptoms of hypothyroidism in many patients. This is related to how the deiodinase system works as discussed below.

Iodine Excess and Selenium Deficiency

As mentioned above, the seleno-protein anti-oxidant system protects the thyroid from oxidative damage. In 2018, Dr. Teng studied a mouse model of chronic iodine excess. In Dr. Teng's NOD autoimmune selenium-deficient mice, excessive iodine intake induced goiter, nodular enlargement of the thyroid gland, thyroiditis, lymphocytic infiltration, and oxidative damage to the thyroid follicular structure in a dose-dependent manner. However, the addition of selenium is protective in the NOD mouse model, alleviates iodine toxicity, and the anti-thyroid antibodies gradually decline. This mouse study highlights the importance of selenium supplementation. We routinely test selenium blood levels and give supplementations when found low. (34-45)

Iodine Suppresses Thyroid Function

Some patients read about high-dose iodine on the internet. And occasionally, we will see a patient in the office after taking high-dose iodine for a few months. These all report they feel fine. However, their thyroid labs are "out of whack," which disturbs their endocrinologist or primary care doctor. The TSH may be quite elevated (in the 40-70 mU/L range), caused by the suppressive effect of iodine on thyroid function. In 2006, Dr. Man studied the effect of iodine on thyroid function in a mouse model and writes:

> Moderate iodine excess continuously suppresses the thyroid iodine uptake and organification, which presents a mechanism for iodine-induced thyroid failure. (36-37)

Thankfully, this iodine-induced thyroid failure is temporary. Upon cessation of the high dose of iodine, the inhibitory effect promptly resolves, and thyroid labs return to normal. High-dose iodine reduces TPO activity, reduces iodine uptake, and reduces iodine organification by the thyroid gland. Autoimmune thyroid patients with Hashimoto's or Graves' disease are more sensitive to this suppressive effect of iodine. For example, for Graves' disease patients, iodine is commonly used in the hospital formulary as a pre-operative treatment in preparation for thyroidectomy. For the thyrotoxic Graves' disease patient, high-dose potassium iodide treatment suppresses thyroid function, allowing thyroidectomy to proceed. Historically, iodine was one of the first medicines used in 1863 when Armand Trousseau in Paris inadvertently used iodine to successfully treat a young woman suffering from thyrotoxicosis. (38-40)

Methimazole

Methimazole is currently the preferred mainstream thyroid-blocking drug used by endocrinologists to treat thyrotoxicosis in Graves' disease and toxic nodular goiter. Methimazole blocks the TPO enzyme, thus preventing the organification of iodine. For more on Graves' disease and ATDs (anti-thyroid drugs), see Chapters 15-17 on Treatment of Graves' Disease. (41-45)

Peripheral Conversion of T4 to T3

The intracellular deiodinase system is responsible for the peripheral conversion of T4 to its more biologically active form, T3. This is done by removing an iodine molecule from the tyrosine ring of thyroxine (T4), thus converting T4 to T3. However, in about 20% of patients, peripheral conversion of T4 to T3 is inadequate. In such patients taking levothyroxine, thyroid lab studies may show a higher T4 to T3 ratio than usually seen in the general population. The Free T3 will be at the lower end of the lab range, while the Free T4 will be higher than usually seen or at the high end of the normal range. These patients typically have a higher reverse T3. Why is T4 converted to reverse T3, the inactive form, instead of T3, the active form? The levothyroxine (T4) dose is interpreted at the cell level as excess T4, cellular hyperthyroidism. The cellular machinery attempts to protect the cell from excess T4 by converting T4 to reverse T3, the inactive form. Similarly, Graves's thyrotoxicosis has a high reverse T3 because of massive elevation of T4 with shunting of T4 to reverse T3 as a protective mechanism. In the hypothyroid patient on levothyroxine, the lab finding of shunting to reverse T3 predicts the patient will do well switching from levothyroxine to NDT (natural desiccated thyroid), which contains a combination of T3 and T4, the solution to T4 shunting to reverse T3. In these cases, the Free T4 may be higher than usually seen, and the Free T3 lower than usually seen. Unfortunately, the use of the reverse T3 test for this purpose has been ignored by conventional endocrinology which dogmatically clings to the idea that reverse T3 has no clinical utility in monitoring levothyroxine therapy. In 2019, Dr. Cristiane Gomes-Lima writes:

> Reverse T3 is physiologically relevant to thyroid economy. However, its clinical use as a biochemical parameter of thyroid function is very limited. Currently, no evidence supports the use of rT3 [reverse T3] to monitor levothyroxine therapy, either given alone or in combination with liothyronine. (46-47)

In my opinion, future studies will demonstrate the above conclusion to be in error, and the pattern of higher reverse T3, higher Free T4, and lower Free T3 (within the lab range) will be adopted as a valid strategy for predicting good outcomes when switching from T4 monotherapy to NDT or combination T4/T3 therapy.

Central Conversion of T4 to T3– Why TSH is Unreliable to Monitor Treatment with T4 Drugs

Here, it should be mentioned that the D2 deiodinase in the periphery is very sensitive to inhibition by Free T4. However, centrally, in the hypothalamus of the brain, which controls TSH, D2 deiodinase is relatively insensitive to inhibition by Free T4. This means that the hypothalamus of the brain promptly converts levothyroxine (T4) to T3. The brain will then recognize this intracellular T3 as thyroid excess and respond by lowering the TSH. Remember, TSH controls the production of thyroid hormone. A lower TSH suppresses the production of thyroid hormone by the thyroid gland.

To repeat the above discussion, T4 from the levothyroxine dose is sensed at the cellular level as "thyroid excess" and triggers a "protective effect" which downregulates the D2 deiodinase and upregulates the D3 deiodinase, shunting T4 to reverse T3. Yet because of the different sensitivity of central deiodinase, the TSH may be suppressed to quite low levels. This is the typical pattern of low TSH from levothy-

roxine treatment, yet persistent peripheral hypothyroidism causes low thyroid symptoms. The primary care physician or endocrinologist dogmatically looks solely at the TSH within the lab reference range and ignores the obvious fact the patient is still clinically hypothyroid. Typically, these patients are offered an SSRI anti-depressant with a pat on the back, or referral to a psychiatrist, obviously the wrong treatment. Under this scenario, these patients do much better switching from levothyroxine to natural desiccated thyroid, NDT, which allows for improved Free T3 levels at the cellular level and resolves the symptoms of a low thyroid condition. Another option is a combination of T3 and T4 by adding liothyronine, generic Cytomel, to the levothyroxine dose.

Note: TSH is a thyroid-stimulating hormone made by the pituitary under the control of TRH (thyroid-releasing hormone) made by the hypothalamus. When thyroid hormone blood levels are high, the hypothalamus instructs the pituitary to stop making TSH, which then plummets to low levels on lab testing. Without the stimulation of TSH, the thyroid stops making thyroid hormone. On the other hand, when thyroid hormone blood levels are low, the reverse occurs. The hypothalamus instructs the pituitary to make more TSH to stimulate the thyroid to make more thyroid hormone. In this case, the TSH blood test may show a very high TSH, which may reach 90-100 mU/L in severe cases of hypothyroidism. Note: Normal TSH lab reference range is 0.3 to 4.0 mU/L.

Reverse T3- The Inactive Form

Another deiodinase enzyme, called D3 or Type 3 deiodinase, converts T4 into reverse T3, the inactive form of T3. High reverse T3 can be found in thyrotoxicosis such as Graves' disease, toxic nodular goiter, and the autonomous thyroid nodule. The inactivation of T4 into reverse T3 is a built-in safety mechanism for protecting the body from thyrotoxicosis, the toxic effects of high thyroid hormone levels.

The low thyroid condition usually shows a high TSH and a low reverse T3 on lab testing.

In this scenario, the cells in the peripheral tissues upregulate the D2 deiodinase enzyme to increase the conversion of T4 to T3, its active form. At this same time, the D3 deiodinase enzyme is down-regulated to reduce the conversion of T4 to reverse T3, its inactive form. This allows more of the T4 to be converted to its active form, which is badly needed in the low thyroid patient. Remember, the deiodinase enzyme system is intracellular.

Euthyroid Sick Syndrome

High reverse T3 may also be found in a condition referred to as "euthyroid sick syndrome" in acute or chronic illness, starvation, and eating disorders. Although elevated reverse T3 in chronic illness can be observed, it is poorly understood. Treatment with T3 (liothyronine) is a matter of debate. Central hypothyroidism may resemble euthyroid sick syndrome, except that central hypothyroidism will have a low reverse T3. In contrast, euthyroid sick syndrome will have a high reverse T3, as an adaptation to protect the severely ill patient from excess thyroid hormone. (48-55)

After routinely measuring reverse T3 over the years, I have found this lab test usually confirms what we already know from the history, physical exam, and other routine labs. For example, high reverse T3 is a protective mechanism in the thyrotoxic patient. A different scenario is the reverse T3 in the normal range, yet higher than usually seen, a pattern found in patients who remain symptomatic while under treatment with levothyroxine, as discussed above. Alternatively, a low reverse T3 usually confirms hypothyroidism in the untreated patient or confirms central hypothyroidism with HPA dysfunction. Patients with central hypothyroidism typically show a low serum TSH even though they are clinically hypothyroid and have a low Free T3 and T4. These patients benefit from treatment with thyroid hormone.

Reverse T3 Elevated in Metastatic Cancer

Occasionally, it may be challenging to interpret a high reverse T3. For example, I recall an asymptomatic 85-year-old female patient in no acute distress. The thyroid labs were all normal except for an elevated reverse T3 of 28 ng/dL (normal range= 10 – 24 ng/dL). Since the patient seemed fine and the other thyroid labs were normal, I interpreted this as a lab error! A few weeks later, my office was informed the patient developed shoulder pain; subsequent x-rays, and bone scans by the orthopedic surgeon showed lytic bone lesions indicating extensive metastatic cancer. Sadly, the patient succumbed quickly to the extensive metastatic disease. In retrospect, the high reverse T3 was a marker for metastatic cancer. (56-63)

In 2021 Dr. Annarita Nappi found D3 deiodinase which converts T4 to inactive reverse T3, is barely detectable in adult tissues yet is upregulated in many cancer types and other chronic illnesses, thus explaining high reverse T3 levels in the cancer patient. Dr. Annarita Nappi writes:

> Although its expression is barely detectable in adult tissues, the D3 enzyme has been reactivated in several physiopathological conditions in which cell proliferation is enhanced, such as chronic inflammation, myocardial infarction, tissue repair, and critical illness... **Interestingly, in adult life, D3 is also re-expressed in cancer.** D3 was initially identified in various immortalized cell lines derived from adenocarcinoma, breast cancer, endometrium carcinoma, neuroblastoma basal cell carcinoma, ovarian cancer, and colon. Accordingly, D3 is upregulated in many murine and human tumors tissues, including the vascular tumors infantile hemangiomas and hepatic hemangioendothelioma as well as in various brain tumors, among which, gliosarcoma and glioblastoma multiforme. (60)

In 2013, Dr. Monica Dentice writes:

> Type 3 deiodinase (D3), the physiological inactivator of TH [thyroid hormone], is

an oncofetal protein whose re-activation in adult tissues has been correlated with **hyperproliferative states and with human solid tumors**. This suggests a link between deiodinase-mediated TH metabolism and carcinogenesis. (62-63)

Supraphysiologic Dosing T3?

According to Dr. Dayan in 2018, the human thyroid secretes T4 and T3 in a ratio is 14:1. The remainder of the peripheral T3 is produced by the deiodinase system. One grain tablet of natural desiccated thyroid (NDT) contains 38 mcg of T4 and 9 mcg of T3. This ratio is about 4:1.

Dr. Dayan's criticism of NDT, natural desiccated thyroid, is that the 4:1 T4/T3 ratio in the NDT provides excessive amounts of T3, producing "supra-physiologic dosing." In 2018 Thyroid Research, Dr. Dayan writes:

> The doses [for NDT] give a T4:T3 ratio of 4.2:1, significantly more T3 than the 14:1 secreted by the normal thyroid and the doses recommended above. This makes dosing difficult, as displayed by several studies which have shown supraphysiological T3 doses post-dose, fluctuating T3 levels during the day, and more hyperthyroid symptoms in subjects taking DTE [NDT] compared to LT4 monotherapy... Furthermore, it has also been shown that the majority of circulating T3 comes from peripheral conversion of T4 to T3 and not secretion of T3 from the thyroid, **hence a T4:T3 secretion ratio of approximately 14:1 appears average in humans**, suggesting only a small role for secreted T3. (64)

However, there is debate as to what the T4:T3 ratio should be. According to Dr Milner in 2007 Townsend Letter, the proper T4/T3 ratio for thyroid replacement is 4:1, not 14:1. This 4:1 ratio is closer to the Free T4 to Free T3 ratio reported in 2015 by Dr. Grmek in the Slovenian Medical Journal. Dr. Grmek studied the FT4 and FT3 blood levels in 225 patients with average age of 44 years. The mean Free T4 to Free T3 ratio was found to be 2.86 ± 0.52. This discrepancy in ratios can be explained by the peripheral conversion of T4 to T3. Of the circulating Free T3, about 20% comes from thyroid secretion, and the remaining 80% is from peripheral conversion of T4 to T3 via the D1 deiodinase enzyme, which is an intracellular system. D1 resides on cell membranes, while D2 resides inside the cell near the nucleus. Thus, D1 accounts for most of the peripheral circulating T3, while D2 accounts for the intracellular conversion of T4 to T3, acting on the nuclear compartment. (64-67)

The question remains, "Is there an issue with T3 supraphysiologic dosing with NDT"? Although studies show a transient rise in serum Free T3, 2-3 hours after ingestion of T3 (usually with liothyronine, generic Cytomel), patients rarely have a problem with this. If reported, then the dosage is decreased, and symptoms resolve. Likewise, we have patients taking 50 mcg of generic Cytomel a day (in 2 or three split doses), and most seem to do well with it. If there are symptoms of transient hyperthyroidism, then the dosage is decreased until symptoms resolve. In other words, we have not found "supraphysiologic dosing of T3" to represent a significant clinical problem with the short-acting T3 in liothyronine (generic Cytomel) or in NDT, natural desiccated thyroid. An occasional patient will report transient palpitations when first starting NDT, which can be avoided by gradually increasing dosage by small increments to allow acclimation. Patients are carefully instructed to hold the medication and then decrease dosage if excess thyroid symptoms are noted.

Compounded Slow Release T3

A strategy that avoids the peak in Serum T3 and avoids "supraphysiologic dosing" is the use of compounded slow-release T3. Some practitioners prefer to use a combination of T4 (levothyroxine) and compounded slow-release T3.

Dosing With NDT and Compounded Slow Release T3

In 2007, Dr. Martin Milner provides dosing schedules for NDT and compounded slow-release T3. (66-67)

Dosing with Combination Levothyroxine (T4) and Cytomel (T3)

In 2018 Dr. Colin Dayan provides a dosing schedule for the combination of levothyroxine and T3 (Liothyronine and generic Cytomel). (64-65)

Errors in Compounding T3 Capsules

When using compounded slow-release T3 preparations, one must be careful to select a high-quality pharmacy with experience making this product. If an error is made in the formulation with unusually high dosages of T4 or T3 in the capsule by mistake, this could lead to hospitalization for thyrotoxicosis. An FDA warning letter to a New Jersey Compounding pharmacy illustrates an error in compounded T3 formulation. The misbranded T3 capsules contained, by error, 2.5 mg T3 instead of the correct dosage of 2.5 micrograms T3, a dosage one thousand times higher than prescribed by the doctor. For this reason, I avoid prescribing compounded thyroid capsules with natural desiccated thyroid powder. I prefer manufactured thyroid tablets. This eliminates the possibility of human error in compounding thyroid capsules by hand. (68-70)

Note: a gram is a thousand milligrams, and a milligram is a thousand micrograms.

Various T4 and NDT Combinations

A number of practitioners and thyroid internet experts have written about adding a small dose of T4 (levothyroxine) to their NDT regimen. This idea is based on the difference in the T4:T3 ratio of NDT (4:1) and the ratio of secretion by the human thyroid (14:1). By adding a small dose of levothyroxine to the daily regimen, this ratio comes closer to the ideal 14:1, and more importantly, some patients report feeling better with it.

98:1 Ratio for T4:T3

In 2004, Dr. Kenneth Blanchard from Newton Lower Falls, Massachusetts, described the use of small doses of slow-release compounded T3 added to T4-only medication (levothyroxine). The dose he uses is less than 2.5 micrograms of compounded slow-release T3. Dr. Blanchard states that, in his opinion, higher doses of T3 (generic Cytomel), such as the 25 or 50 mcg tablets, are much too high, and explains the failure of mainstream endocrinology clinical trials using combinations of T4 and T3. The T3 dosage was too high! (71-72) (87)

Considerable Variation in T4:T3 Ratios

So, as we have seen above, expert practitioners claim success with T4:T3 ratios with a considerable range, from 4:1 all the way up to 98:1 (T4:T3) ratio. How do we reconcile these apparently contradicting treatment ratios? My best guess is that the D1/D2 deiodinase system for conversion of T4 to T3 is more robust than we had originally thought and can compensate for various T4:T3 ratios and keep things running smoothly. The one thing that causes problems is T4 monotherapy.

Many Do Well with T4 Monotherapy

Many of the millions of thyroid patients on T4 monotherapy with Synthroid or levothyroxine (generic Synthroid) are doing quite well with it. However, a subset of patients feels better when switched to NDT, natural desiccated thyroid containing T4:T3 in a 4:1 ratio. In my opinion, NDT is the preferred thyroid tablet. Two renowned physicians, Drs. Broda Barnes and William McK Jeffries found the 4:1 T4:T3 ratio in NDT quite satisfactory without the need to experiment with other ratios. (73-74)

Yet another smaller subset of patients feels better with the combination of NDT and levothyroxine providing a 14:1 ratio.

Yet another subset, according to Dr. Kenneth Blanchard, does well on T4 monotherapy with even smaller doses (1-2 mcg) of slow-release compounded T3. What is the correct ratio? My answer is: "The one that works for you!"

Medical Business Model Determines Thyroid Usage

We have two medical business models in the United States determining the type of thyroid medication prescribed. The first model is the Health Insurance Model used by mainstream medicine in which the medical office accepts the patient's health insurance. In this model, the doctor spends minimal time with the patient, 3-10 minutes per patient visit, and prescribes exclusively T4-only monotherapy with levothyroxine, generic Synthroid. Laboratory panels are limited to TSH and Free T4, and medication dosage is adjusted to maintain the TSH within the lab range (0.40-4.50 mIU/L Quest lab adult), being careful to avoid a "suppressed TSH" below the reference range. This is thyroid endocrinology made simple. So simple, one might say the doctor is overqualified to do this job. His many years of medical training are wasted. The doctor could be replaced by a high school student taught to do the same thing, adjust levothyroxine dosage based on TSH level.

The second model is the holistic/integrative medicine model, which does not accept health insurance. The patient pays cash for the office visit. In this model, NDT, natural desiccated thyroid, is used. The doctor spends more time with the patient, usually 30-60 minutes per office visit. The lab panel is more extensive, including TSH, FT3, FT4, RT3, TPO and thyroglobulin antibodies, serum selenium, magnesium, vitamin D3, and spot urine iodine. A suppressed TSH below the lab range is acceptable and may be required for adequate treatment. The doctor has more time to explain things, educate the patient about symptoms of thyroid excess and answer questions.

What is the Spot Urinary Iodine Test?

Quest, LabCorp and most other commercial labs will do a test called the spot urinary iodine. This is a single urine sample obtained at the same session as the blood draw. This is quick and easy way to get a measurement of the patient's iodine level. We do not use the lab reference range for this test. Instead, we use the WHO (World Health Organization) Guidelines. Under 100 mcg/L is iodine insufficiency. Under 50 mcg/L is iodine deficiency. Under 20 mcg/L is severe iodine deficiency. No need to do a 24-hour sample which requires the patient to carry around a collection bucket all day.

Conclusion

Errors in Modern Thyroid Endocrinology are understandable, considering the corrupting influence of industry funding of thyroid endocrine societies, meetings, research, and key opinion leaders. The first error is dogmatically insisting the TSH stays within the reference range when TSH suppression may be required for adequate therapy. The second error is dogmatically insisting on T4 monotherapy when naturally desiccated thyroid, containing both T3 and T4, is more effective and safer than T4 monotherapy. (75-85)

♦ **References for Chapter 5**

1) Garber, Jeffrey, R., et al. "ATA/AACE Guidelines for Hypothyroidism in Adults." Endocr Pract 18.6 (2012).

2) Jonklaas, Jacqueline, et al. "Guidelines for the Treatment of Hypothyroidism: Prepared by the American Thyroid Association Task Force on Thyroid Hormone Replacement." Thyroid 24.12 (2014): 1670-1751.

3) Bianco, Antonio C., et al. "Paradigms of Dynamic Control of Thyroid Hormone Signaling." Endocrine Reviews 40.4 (2019): 1000.

4) Bianco, Antonio C., and Sabina Casula. "Thyroid Hormone Replacement Therapy: Three 'Simple' Questions, Complex Answers." European Thyroid Journal 1.2 (2012): 88-98.

5) Drigo, Rafael Arrojo, et al. "Role of The Type 2 Iodothyronine Deiodinase (D2) in the Control of Thyroid Hormone Signaling." Biochimica Et Biophysica Acta (BBA)-General Subjects 1830.7 (2013): 3956-3964.

6) Gorini, Francesca, et al. "Selenium: An Element of Life Essential for Thyroid Function." Molecules 26.23 (2021).

7) FDA Announcement RLC Labs, Inc., Issues Voluntary Nationwide Recall of All Lots of Nature-Throid® and WP Thyroid® with Current Expiry Due to Sub Potency. September 3, 2020.

8) Pepper, Gary M., and Paul Y. Casanova-Romero. "Conversion to Armour Thyroid from Levothyroxine Improved Patient Satisfaction in the Treatment of Hypothyroidism." Journal of Endocrinology, Diabetes & Obesity 2 (2014): 1055-1060.

9) Hoang, Thanh D., et al. "Desiccated Thyroid Extract Compared with Levothyroxine in the Treatment of Hypothyroidism: A Randomized, Double-Blind, Cross-over Study." J Clin Endocrinol Metab 98.5 (2013): 1982-1990.

10) Jonklaas, Jacqueline, et al. "Single Dose T3 Administration: Kinetics and Effects on Biochemical and Physiologic Parameters." Therapeutic Drug Monitoring 37.1 (2015): 110.

11) Colucci, Philippe, et al. "A Review of the Pharmacokinetics of Levothyroxine for the Treatment of Hypothyroidism." European Endocrinology 9.1 (2013): 40.

12) Dayan, Colin, and Vijay Panicker. "Management of Hypothyroidism with Combination Thyroxine (T4) and Triiodothyronine (T3) Hormone Replacement in Clinical Practice: A Review of Suggested Guidance." Thyroid Research 11.1 (2018): 1-11.

13) Gomes-Lima, Cristiane, Leonard Wartofsky, and Kenneth Burman. "Can Reverse T3 Assay Be Employed to Guide T4 vs. T4/T3 Therapy in Hypothyroidism?" Frontiers in Endocrinology 10 (2019): 856.

14) Wiersinga, Wilmar M., et al. "2012 ETA Guidelines: The Use of L-T4+ L-T3 in the Treatment of Hypothyroidism." European Thyroid Journal 1.2 (2012): 55-71.

15) Song, Yue, et al. "Roles of Hydrogen Peroxide in Thyroid Physiology and Disease." The Journal of Clinical Endocrinology & Metabolism 92.10 (2007): 3764-3773

16) Ohye, Hidemi, and Masahiro Sugawara. "Dual Oxidase, Hydrogen Peroxide, and Thyroid Diseases." Experimental Biology and Medicine 235.4 (2010): 424-433.

17) Kobayashi, Ryohei, et al. "Thyroid Function in Patients with Selenium Deficiency Exhibits High Free T4 To T3 Ratio." Clinical Pediatric Endocrinology 30.1 (2021): 19.

18) Lang, Xueyan, et al. "FT3/FT4 Ratio Is Correlated with All-Cause Mortality, Cardiovascular Mortality, and Cardiovascular Disease Risk: NHANES 2007-2012." Frontiers in Endocrinology 13 (2022): 964822.

19) Dhas, Priya K., and G. Ramani. "Comparison of Selenium and Deiodinase Enzyme Among Healthy Controls and Hypothyroid Patients: A Pilot Study." International Journal of Health Sciences I: 6095-6103.

20) Peterson, Sarah J., Elizabeth A. McAninch, and Antonio C. Bianco. "Is a Normal TSH Synonymous With "Euthyroidism" in Levothyroxine Monotherapy?" The Journal of Clinical Endocrinology & Metabolism 101.12 (2016): 4964-4973.

21) Ito, Mitsuru, et al. "TSH-Suppressive Doses of Levothyroxine Are Required to Achieve Pre-Operative Native Serum Triiodothyronine Levels in Patients Who Have Undergone Total Thyroidectomy." European Journal of Endocrinology 167.3 (2012): 373-378.

22) Gullo, Damiano, et al. "Levothyroxine Monotherapy Cannot Guarantee Euthyroidism in All Athyreotic Patients." PLoS one 6.8 (2011): e22552.

23) Wang, W., et al. "Effects of Selenium Supplementation on Spontaneous Autoimmune Thyroiditis in NOD. H-2h4 Mice." Thyroid: Official Journal of the American Thyroid Association 25.10 (2015): 1137.

24) Liontiris, Michael I., and Elias E. Mazokopakis. "A Concise Review of Hashimoto Thyroiditis (HT) and the Importance of Iodine, Selenium, Vitamin D and Gluten on the Autoimmunity and Dietary Management of HT Patients. Points That Need More Investigation." Hell J Nucl Med 20.1 (2017): 51-56.

25) Teitelbaum, Jacob. "Effective Treatment of Chronic Fatigue Syndrome." Integrative Medicine 4.4 (2005): 23-29.

26) Holtorf, Kent. "Diagnosis and Treatment of Hypothalamic-Pituitary-Adrenal (HPA) Axis Dysfunction in Patients with Chronic Fatigue Syndrome (CFS) and Fibromyalgia (FM)." Journal of Chronic Fatigue Syndrome 14.3 (2007): 59-88.

27) Skinner GR, Thomas R, Taylor M, Sellarajah M, Bolt S, Krett S, et al. Thyroxine Should Be Tried in Clinically Hypothyroid but Biochemically Euthyroid Patients [Letter] BMJ. 1997; 314:1764.

28) McAninch, Elizabeth A., and Antonio C. Bianco. "The History and Future of Treatment of Hypothyroidism." Annals of Internal Medicine 164.1 (2016): 50-56.

29) Abraham, Guy E. "The History of Iodine in Medicine. Part II: The Search for and the Discovery of Thyroid Hormones." The Original Internist 13.2 (2006): 67-70.

30) Peterson, Sarah J., et al. "An Online Survey of Hypothyroid Patients Demonstrates Prominent Dissatisfaction." Thyroid 28.6 (2018): 707-721.

31) De Castro, Joao Pedro Werneck, et al. "Differences in Hypothalamic Type 2 Deiodinase Ubiquitination Explain Localized Sensitivity to Thyroxine." The Journal of clinical investigation 125.125 (2) (2015): 0-0.

32) McAninch, Elizabeth A., et al. "Prevalent Polymorphism in Thyroid Hormone-Activating Enzyme Leaves a Genetic Fingerprint That Underlies Associated Clinical Syndromes." The Journal of Clinical Endocrinology & Metabolism 100.3 (2015): 920-933.

33) Teng, X., et al. "Experimental Study on The Effects of Chronic Iodine Excess on Thyroid Function, Structure, and Autoimmunity in Autoimmune-Prone NOD. H-2h4 Mice." Clinical and Experimental Medicine 9.1 (2009): 51.

34) Xu, Jian, et al. "Supplemental Selenium Alleviates the Toxic Effects of Excessive Iodine on the Thyroid." Biological Trace Element Research 141.1-3 (2011): 110-118.

35) Wang, W., et al. "Effects of Selenium Supplementation on Spontaneous Autoimmune Thyroiditis in NOD. H-2h4 Mice." Thyroid: official journal of the American Thyroid Association 25.10 (2015): 1137.

36) Man, N., et al. "Long-Term Effects of High Iodine Intake: Inhibition of Thyroid Iodine Uptake and Organification in Wistar Rats." Zhonghua Yi Xue Za Zhi 86.48 (2006): 3420-3424.

37) Tajiri, Junichi, et al. "Studies of Hypothyroidism in Patients with High Iodine Intake." The Journal of Clinical Endocrinology & Metabolism 63.2 (1986): 412-417.

38) Trousseau, Armand. Clinical Medicine: Lectures Delivered at the Hôtel-Dieu, Paris. Vol. 2. P. Blakiston, Son, 1882.

39) Randle, Reese W., et al. "Impact of Potassium Iodide on Thyroidectomy for Graves' Disease: Implications for Safety and Operative Difficulty." Surgery 163.1 (2018): 68-72.

40) Reznick, David, et al. "Pre-Operative Optimization with Super Saturated Potassium Iodide Solution (SSKI) in Patients with Graves' Disease Undergoing Total Thyroidectomy." Ann Thyroid 4:7 (2019)

41) Azizi, Fereidoun, et al. "Control of Graves' Hyperthyroidism with Very Long-Term Methimazole Treatment: A Clinical Trial." BMC Endocrine Disorders 21 (2021): 1-7.

42) Barbesino, Giuseppe. "Long-Term, Low-Dose Methimazole Therapy Is Effective in Protecting Against Relapses in Graves' Disease." Clinical Thyroidology 35.2 (2023): 54-56.

43) Leech, Nicky J., and Colin M. Dayan. "Controversies in the Management of Graves' Disease." Clinical Endocrinology 49.3 (1998): 273-280.

44) Wiersinga, Wilmar M. "Graves' Disease: Can It Be Cured?" Endocrinology and Metabolism 34.1 (2019): 29-38.

45) Sjölin, Gabriel, et al. "The Long-Term Outcome of Treatment for Graves' Hyperthyroidism." Thyroid 29.11 (2019): 1545-1557.

46) Gomes-Lima, Cristiane, et al. "Can Reverse T3 Assay Be Employed to Guide T4 vs. T4/T3 Therapy in Hypothyroidism?" Frontiers in Endocrinology 10 (2019): 856.

47) Halsall, David J., and Susan Oddy. "Clinical and Laboratory Aspects of 3, 3', 5'-Triiodothyronine (Reverse T3)." Annals of Clinical Biochemistry 58.1 (2021): 29-37.

48) Ganesan, Kavitha, and Khurram Wadud. "Euthyroid Sick Syndrome." StatPearls Publishing, 2021.

49) Wartofsky, Leonard, and Kenneth D. Burman. "Alterations in Thyroid Function in Patients with Systemic Illness: The "Euthyroid Sick Syndrome." Endocrine Reviews 3.2 (1982): 164-217.

50) Exley, Sarah, et al. "Low Reverse T3: A Reliable, Sensitive and Specific in Diagnosis of Central Hypothyroidism." Open Journal of Endocrine and Metabolic Diseases 11.7 (2021): 137-143.

51) Lee, Sun, and Alan P. Farwell. "Euthyroid Sick Syndrome." Comprehensive Physiology 6.2 (2011): 1071-1080.

52) Liu, Huixin, et al. "Thyroid Hormone Replacement for Nephrotic Syndrome Patients with Euthyroid Sick Syndrome: A Meta-Analysis." Renal Failure 36.9 (2014): 1360-1365.

53) Wartofsky, Leonard, et al. "Trading One "Dangerous Dogma" For Another? Thyroid Hormone Treatment of the "Euthyroid Sick Syndrome." The Journal of Clinical Endocrinology & Metabolism 84.5 (1999): 1759-1762.

54) DeGroot, L. J. "Dangerous Dogmas in Medicine-Author's Response." Journal of Clinical Endocrinology & Metabolism 84.5 (1999): 1759-1760.

55) Shames, Richard, and Stuart Wenzel. "On the Fundamental Efficacy of Thyroid Hormone Therapy in Eating Disorders: Review of Mechanisms and Case Study." Journal of Restorative Medicine 12.1 (2022).

56) Ganesan, K., and K. Wadud. "Thyroid, Euthyroid Sick Syndrome." StatPearls [Internet]. Treasure Island (FL): StatPearls Publishing; 2018. Available from: https://www. ncbi. nlm. nih. gov/books/NBK482219/. Accessed: January 3 (2018).

57) Patki, Vinayak, et al. "Sick Euthyroid Syndrome: A Myth or Reality." Journal of Pediatric Critical Care 4.4 (2017): 44.

58) Peeters, Robin P., et al. "Serum 3, 3', 5'-Triiodothyronine (Rt3) And 3, 5, 3'-Triiodothyronine/Rt3 Are Prognostic Markers in Critically Ill Patients and Are Associated with Postmortem Tissue Deiodinase Activities." The Journal of Clinical Endocrinology & Metabolism 90.8 (2005): 4559-4565.

59) Moskovich, Dotan, et al. "Targeting the DIO3 Enzyme Using First-In-Class Inhibitors Effectively Suppresses Tumor Growth: A New Paradigm in Ovarian Cancer Treatment." Oncogene 40.44 (2021): 6248-6257.

60) Nappi, Annarita, et al. "Deiodinases and Cancer." Endocrinology 162.4 (2021): bqab016.

61) Goemann, Iuri Martin, et al. "Current Concepts and Challenges to Unravel the Role of Iodothyronine Deiodinases in Human Neoplasias." Endocrine-Related Cancer 25.12 (2018): R625-R645.

62) Dentice, Monica, et al. "Type 3 Deiodinase and Solid Tumors: An Intriguing Pair." Expert Opinion on Therapeutic Targets 17.11 (2013): 1369-1379.

63) Ciavardelli, Domenico, et al. "Type 3 Deiodinase: Role in Cancer Growth, Stemness, And Metabolism." Frontiers in Endocrinology 5 (2014): 215.

64) Dayan, Colin, and Vijay Panicker. "Management of Hypothyroidism with Combination Thyroxine (T4) and Triiodothyronine (T3) Hormone Replacement in Clinical Practice: A Review of Suggested Guidance." Thyroid Research 11.1 (2018): 1.

65) Grmek, Jernej, et al. "Usefulness of Free Thyroxine to Free Triiodothyronine Ratio for Diagnostics of Various Types of Hyperthyroidism." Slovenian Medical Journal 84.5 (2015).

66) Milner, Martin. "Hypothyroidism: Optimizing Medication with Slow-Release Compounded Thyroid Replacement." International Journal of Pharmaceutical Compounding 9.4 (2005): 268.

67) Milner, Martin. "Hypothyroidism: Optimizing Medication with Slow-Release Compounded Thyroid Replacement." Townsend Letter: The Examiner of Alternative Medicine 283 (2007): 80-86.

68) Khan, Wajid, et al. "Thyrotoxicosis Due To 1000-Fold Error in Compounded Liothyronine: A Case Elucidated by Mass Spectrometry." Clinical Mass Spectrometry 11 (2019): 8-11.

69) He, Zhiheng H., et al. "Thyrotoxicosis After Massive Triiodothyronine (LT3) Overdose: A Coast-To-Coast Case Series and Review." Drugs in Context 9 (2020).

70) FDA Warning Letter August 1, 2016, sent to Plainsboro Pharmacy, 9 Schalks Crossing Road Plainsboro, NJ 08536

71) Blanchard, Kenneth R. Functional Approach to Hypothyroidism: Bridging Traditional and Alternative Treatment Approaches for Total Patient Wellness by Hatherleigh Press. 2012.

72) Blanchard, Kenneth R. "Dosage Recommendations for Combination Regimen of Thyroxine And 3, 5, 3'-Triiodothyronine." The Journal of Clinical Endocrinology and Metabolism 89.3 (2004): 1486-7.

73) Barnes, Broda, Hypothyroidism: The Unsuspected Illness. Harper. First Edition (1976)

74) McK. Jefferies, William. Safe Uses of Cortisol. Charles C Thomas Pub Ltd; 3 edition 2004.

75) Irwig, Michael S., et al. "Financial Conflicts of Interest Among Authors of Endocrine Society Clinical Practice Guidelines." The Journal of Clinical Endocrinology & Metabolism 103.12 (2018): 4333-4338.

76) Murayama, Anju, et al. "Pharmaceutical Company Payments to Clinical Practice Guideline Authors." Integrity of Scientific Research: Fraud, Misconduct and Fake News in the Academic, Medical and Social Environment. Cham: Springer International Publishing, 2022. 451-468.

77) Khan, Rishad, et al. "Prevalence of Financial Conflicts of Interest Among Authors of Clinical Guidelines Related to High-Revenue Medications." JAMA Internal Medicine 178.12 (2018): 1712-1715.

78) Mooghali, Maryam, et al. "Financial Conflicts of Interest Among US Physician Authors of 2020 Clinical Practice Guidelines: A Cross-Sectional Study." BMJ open 13.1 (2023): e069115.

79) Grey, Andrew, et al. "Reporting of Conflicts of Interest in Oral Presentations at Medical Conferences: A Delegate-Based Prospective Observational Study." BMJ Open 7.9 (2017): E017019.

80) Nejstgaard, Camilla H., et al. "Association Between Conflicts of Interest and Favorable Recommendations in Clinical Guidelines, Advisory Committee Reports, Opinion Pieces, and Narrative Reviews: Systematic Review." BMJ 371 (2020).

81) Moynihan, Ray, et al. "Financial Ties Between Leaders of Influential US Professional Medical Associations and Industry: Cross Sectional Study." BMJ 369 (2020).

82) Neuman, Jennifer, et al. "Prevalence of Financial Conflicts of Interest Among Panel Members Producing Clinical Practice Guidelines in Canada and United States: Cross Sectional Study." BMJ 343 (2011).

83) Tabatabavakili, Sahar, et al. "Financial Conflicts of Interest in Clinical Practice Guidelines: A Systematic Review." Mayo Clinic Proceedings: Innovations, Quality & Outcomes 5.2 (2021): 466-475.

84) Endocrine Society List of Donors from 2017 available on the Wayback Machine at this URL: https://web.archive.org/web/20170724080955/http://www.endocrine.org/corporate-relations/corporate-liaison-board/leadership-donors

85) Endocrine Society Financial Disclosure URL: https://www.endocrine.org/ceu/ceu2019-miami/disclosures

86) American Thyroid Association List of Corporate Leadership Council Members URL: https://www.thyroid.org/professionals/partner-relations/

87) Blanchard, Ken, and Marietta Abrams Brill. What Your Doctor May Not Tell You About: Hypothyroidism: A Simple Plan for Extraordinary Results. Grand Central Publishing, 2004.

Chapter 6

TSH is Inadequate for Levothyroxine Dosing

Antonio Bianco MD Rattles a Few Cages in Mainstream Endocrinology

IN 2016, DR. ANTONIO BIANCO asked an important question, "Is a normal TSH synonymous with euthyroidism in levothyroxine monotherapy?" In other words, does a normal serum TSH indicate adequate treatment in patients given levothyroxine, T4-only monotherapy? Dr. Bianco is an endocrinologist and past president of the American Thyroid Association (ATA). (1-2)

Dr. Antonio Bianco studied 469 hypothyroid patients treated with T4 monotherapy, also called levothyroxine, generic Synthroid. The treated patients were compared to normal controls. Dr. Bianco found levothyroxine, T4-only, treated patients had difficulty converting T4 to T3, were more likely to be overweight, taking anti-depressants and statins, and had low thyroid symptoms despite the levothyroxine. Tragically, dogmatically clinging to the TSH reference range and levothyroxine as the only acceptable thyroid medicine are two errors of modern endocrinology. Dr. Bianco's report has freed endocrinology from the shackles of this false medical dogma. Many of my newsletters written over the years have stated that NDT, natural desiccated thyroid containing both T3 and T4, is a better choice when compared to levothyroxine (T4 monotherapy). In clinical practice using NDT, suppression of TSH below the reference range may be required to completely relieve hypothyroid symptoms. This is not unusual. For more on this, see Chapter 7. TSH Suppression Benefits and Adverse Effects.

Dr. Bianco's answer rattled a few cages in mainstream endocrinology, and we agree with his conclusions. Note: euthyroidism means having normal thyroid function. (1-2)

Dr. Antonio Bianco Found:

1) Levothyroxine (T4-only) treated patients "had higher serum free T4 and lower serum free T3 than healthy or matched controls."

My comment: T3 (tri-iodothyronine) is the active thyroid hormone, so a lower serum T3 means these patients have difficulty converting T4 into T3 and may suffer from low thyroid symptoms despite levothyroxine (T4).

2) Levothyroxine-treated patients were more likely to be overweight despite consuming fewer calories.

My comment: Weight gain is a common symptom of the low thyroid condition caused by a slow metabolic rate and failure to convert calories to energy. Instead of being used for energy, calories are stored up as weight gain.

3) Levothyroxine patients were "more likely to be taking anti-depressants and anti-cholesterol (statin) drugs compared to matched controls."

My comment: Lack of energy, fatigue, and depression are common symptoms of the low thyroid condition, all relieved by adequate thyroid dosage. Many publications, including the Hunt Study, show that elevated serum cholesterol is a symptom of a low thyroid condition. Providing a higher dosage of thyroid medicine is the correct treatment. This will suppress the TSH, reduce serum cholesterol, and prevent heart attacks. Instead of thyroid medicine, these patients may be treated with a statin anti-cholesterol drug which will reduce serum cholesterol without treating the low thyroid condition. This is the tragedy and error of mainstream medicine. (3-5)

Dr. Antonio Bianco Speaks Out

Dr. Antonio Bianco's study reports that levothyroxine dosage based on the TSH reference range does **NOT** necessarily provide symptom relief for many patients. That is because dosage based on TSH range may be inadequate, and a higher dosage with suppression of TSH may be needed for complete relief of low thyroid symptoms. (1-3)

Suppression of TSH May be Needed for Symptom Relief

We have found that suppression of TSH below the reference range is frequently needed for complete symptom relief in the low thyroid patient. Although endocrinology dogma opposes TSH suppression, the reality is endocrinologists commonly suppress the TSH long-term with thyroid medicine in two groups of patients, the post-thyroidectomy thyroid cancer patients and the thyroid nodule patients. Numerous published studies show no adverse effects of TSH suppression in both groups. For more, see Chapter 7 on TSH Suppression Benefits and Adverse Effects. (6-13)

The Low Thyroid Condition – Case Report

Mary is a 57-year-old female with chronic fatigue, dry, brittle hair, dry skin, muscle aches and pains, and depression, all obvious symptoms of a low thyroid condition. Mary has been to a number of endocrinologists, primary care doctors and even sought advice from her hairstylist. Her latest doctor prescribed a thyroid pill called levothyroxine (50 mcg) which has done little to relieve her symptoms. In addition, she has depression, and her psychiatrist prescribed an SSRI anti-depressant called Zoloft. She also takes Xanax for bouts of anxiety and insomnia. Mary came into the office frustrated with her conventional medical treatment, which was not helping her.

Routine Thyroid Panel

Our routine evaluation includes a full medical history, physical examination, and lab panel. Mary's lab panel showed a TSH of 5.2 uIU/mL, a Free T3 of 260 pg/mL and a Free T4 of 1.4 ng/dL. TPO antibodies, 1,100 IU/mL, were very elevated, indicating Hashimoto's Thyroiditis. Her spot urinary iodine level was 47 mg/dl indicating iodine deficiency, based on World Health Organization Guidelines.

Switching from Levothyroxine to Natural Thyroid

Mary was switched from levothyroxine to NDT, natural desiccated thyroid, and within a week reported improvement in clinical symptoms. Six weeks later, Mary's NDT dosage was gradually increased to Two and a Half Grains a day (one grain is 60 mg.) Mary reported improvement and could taper off her SSRI anti-depressants, as she no longer needs them.

Going to the OB/Gyne

Ten weeks later, Mary went to see her gynecologist for her annual exam, which included a TSH blood test with a low result of 0.1 uIU/mL, which is below the reference range. Her gynecologist looks at the TSH test result and then tells Mary she is taking too much thyroid medicine and needs to cut back. Mary then calls me at my office to relay this information. Two doctors are telling her different things, and Mary does not know whom to believe. This scenario plays out in my office with a different patient each week. The reality is that Mary is on the proper dosage of thyroid medication, and we expect to see a low or suppressed TSH result when this occurs.

In previous chapters, we discussed how NDT, natural desiccated thyroid is superior to levothyroxine (also called generic Synthroid, T4 monotherapy). That is why my office prefers NDT, Natural Desiccated Thyroid. The available NDT drugs are Armour Thyroid and NP Thyroid from Acella. Note: Nature-Throid has been recalled and is currently unavailable as of this date. NDT contains both T3 and T4 and is a more robust and safer thyroid medication when compared to T4-only medications such as levothyroxine and generic Synthroid. This is my assessment based on 15 years of clinical experience prescribing NDT. In addition, we have found that patients who have converted from levothyroxine to NDT are much happier with their treatment program. The mainstream medical literature is also in agreement.

Suppressed TSH may be Required

The TSH test is not reliable for monitoring treatment. When the patient reports complete relief of low thyroid symptoms, the patient may be taking a dosage that suppresses the TSH, meaning the TSH is below the lab reference range. This suppressed TSH may disturb the mainstream clinician who mistakenly believes the patient is taking too much thyroid medication. The issue can be settled simply by running a serum Free T3 and Free T4 lab test showing they are in the normal range, thus excluding any possibility of a "hyperthyroid state." Some physicians mistakenly believe that TSH is a thyroid hormone. It is not. The TSH is made by the pituitary gland, not the thyroid gland. This is a little piece of basic physiology from medical school long forgotten. Unfortunately, most conventional doctors do not order the Free T3 and Free T4 tests. They rely solely on the TSH to monitor medication dosage, another error in modern endocrinology. (2)

TSH Suppression – The TSH Test is Not a Reliable Monitor

Many patients do quite well on levothyroxine, generic Synthroid. However, about 20% (one-fifth) of patients on T4-only medications such as levothyroxine are not feeling well and have continued low thyroid symptoms. Why is that? A minuscule amount of T4 medication, such as 50 mcg of levothyroxine, may be sufficient to drive down the TSH. The endocrinologist will then consider the treatment dosage

adequate. Quite the contrary, it is not adequate, as explained by Dr. D.S. Oreilly and Dr. Henry Lindner, who claim that TSH suppression below the lab reference range may be needed for adequate treatment for the low thyroid condition. (14-25)

Japan in Agreement

In agreement is Dr. Mitsuru Ito from the Center for Excellence in Thyroid Care, Kuma Hospital, Japan, who writes:

> TSH-suppressive doses of levothyroxine are required to achieve pre-operative native serum triiodothyronine levels in patients who have undergone total thyroidectomy. (21)

Dr. Ito found that TSH suppression below the lab reference range is required for adequate treatment of the low thyroid condition. In this Kuma Hospital study, doctors found TSH-suppressive doses of Synthroid were needed in post-thyroidectomy patients to achieve the same normal serum T3 levels which were present on pre-operative laboratory tests.

NDT Natural Desiccated Thyroid

When NDT is prescribed for the first time, the dosage is gradually adjusted upwards, starting with a daily Half Grain tablet. Dosage is incremented weekly until reaching the dosage which provides complete relief of the patient's low thyroid symptoms. This represents the maintenance dosage. Thyroid labs are rechecked at six weeks or so. It is not unusual for the labs to show suppressed TSH, i.e., below the reference range (0.40-4.50 mIU/L), and free T3 at the upper end of the normal range (2.3-4.2 pg/mL, Quest Lab)

The low TSH is to be expected, is not disturbing, and assuming the Free T3 and Free T4 remain within the lab range, the suppressed TSH is not indicative of a hyperthyroid state. If the patient has any symptoms of thyroid excess, they are instructed to hold the thyroid pill for a day and resume the next day at a lower dosage. This protocol relies on a reliable patient with good cognitive function who can cooperate and assist in management. Otherwise, these patients are not candidates for this type of protocol and are instead referred to the endocrinologist for T4-only monotherapy.

Why Has Endocrinology Mismanaged the Low Thyroid Condition for Fifty Years?

If one follows the money trail, the answer is obvious. Levothyroxine, generic Synthroid, is America's fourth most prescribed drug, with 20 million patients. Massive drug industry profits are recycled back to fund Endocrinology Groups and Societies, medical meetings, and clinical research grants. They also fund the key opinion leaders to give lectures at conferences supporting levothyroxine (Synthroid) and the TSH test. This is all done despite the obvious clinical inferiority of T4-only medications such as levothyroxine and the unreliability of the TSH test to monitor the adequacy of treatment.

Conclusion

One of the errors of modern endocrinology is sole reliance on the TSH test to monitor levothyroxine therapy.

♦ References for Chapter 6

1) Peterson, Sarah J., Elizabeth A. McAninch, and Antonio C. Bianco. "Is a Normal TSH Synonymous with "Euthyroidism" in Levothyroxine Monotherapy?" The Journal of Clinical Endocrinology and Metabolism 101.12 (2016): 4964-4973.

2) Bianco, Antonio C. Rethinking Hypothyroidism: Why Treatment Must Change and What Patients Can Do. University of Chicago Press, 2022.

3) Rush University Medical Center. "Hypothyroidism Symptoms Linger Despite Medication Use, Normal Blood Tests." ScienceDaily. ScienceDaily, 12 October 2016. <www.sciencedaily.com/releases/2016/10/161012132038.htm>.

4) Åsvold, Bjørn O., et al. "Thyrotropin Levels and Risk of Fatal Coronary Heart Disease: The HUNT Study." Archives of Internal Medicine 168.8 (2008): 855-860.

5) Asvold, Bjørn O., et al. "The Association Between TSH Within the Reference Range and Serum Lipid Concentrations in a Population-Based Study. The HUNT Study." European Journal of Endocrinology 156.2 (2007): 181-186.

6) Reverter, J. L., et al. "Suppressive Therapy with Levothyroxine for Solitary Thyroid Nodules." Clinical Endocrinology 36.1 (1992): 25-28.

7) Gharib, Hossein, and Ernest L. Mazzaferri. "Thyroxine Suppressive Therapy in Patients with Nodular Thyroid Disease." Annals of Internal Medicine 128.5 (1998): 386-394.

8) Wémeau, Jean-Louis, et al. "Effects of Thyroid-Stimulating Hormone Suppression with Levothyroxine in Reducing the Volume of Solitary Thyroid Nodules and Improving Extraocular Nonpalpable Changes: A Randomized, Double-Blind, Placebo-Controlled Trial by the French Thyroid Research Group." The Journal of Clinical Endocrinology & Metabolism 87.11 (2002): 4928-4934.

9) Clark, Orlo H. "TSH Suppression in The Management of Thyroid Nodules and Thyroid Cancer." World Journal of Surgery 5.1 (1981): 39-46.

10) Grussendorf, M., et al. "Reduction of Thyroid Nodule Volume by Levothyroxine and Iodine Alone and in Combination: A Randomized, Placebo-Controlled Trial." J Clin Endocrinol Metab 96.9 (2011): 2786-2795.

11) Mainini, Edoardo, et al. "Levothyroxine Suppressive Therapy for Solitary Thyroid Nodule." Journal Of Endocrinological Investigation 18.10 (1995): 796-799.

12) Brabant, G. "Thyrotropin Suppressive Therapy in Thyroid Carcinoma: What Are the Targets?" The Journal of Clinical Endocrinology and Metabolism 93.4 (2008): 1167-1169.

13) Fitzgerald, Stephen P., and Henrik Falhammar. "Redefinition of Successful Treatment of Patients with Hypothyroidism. Is TSH the Best Biomarker of Euthyroidism?" Frontiers in Endocrinology 13 (2022).

14) Alevizaki, Maria, et al. "TSH May Not Be a Good Marker for Adequate Thyroid Hormone Replacement Therapy." Wiener Klinische Wochenschrift 117.18 (2005): 636-640.

15) Gullo, Damiano, et al. "Levothyroxine Monotherapy Cannot Guarantee Euthyroidism in All Athyreotic Patients." PLoS one 6.8 (2011): e22552.

16) O'Reilly, D. St J. "Thyroid Hormone Replacement: An Iatrogenic Problem." International Journal of Clinical Practice 64.7 (2010): 991-994.

17) Fraser, W. D., et al. "Are Biochemical Tests of Thyroid Function of Any Value in Monitoring Patients Receiving Thyroxine Replacement?" Br Med J (Clin Res Ed) 293.6550 (1986): 808-810.

18) Lindner, Henry H. "Against TSH-T4 Reference Range Thyroidology: The Case for Clinical Thyroidology." https://hormonerestoration.com/files/TSHHRsite.pdf

19) Tigas, Stelios, et al. "Is Excessive Weight Gain After Ablative Treatment of Hyperthyroidism Due to Inadequate Thyroid Hormone Therapy?" Thyroid 10.12 (2000): 1107-1111.

20) Meier, Christian, et al. "Serum Thyroid Stimulating Hormone in the Assessment of the Severity of Tissue Hypothyroidism in Patients with Overt Primary Thyroid Failure: Cross-Sectional Survey." BMJ 326.7384 (2003): 311-312.

21) Ito, Mitsuru, et al. "TSH-Suppressive Doses of Levothyroxine Are Required to Achieve Pre-Operative Native Serum Triiodothyronine Levels in Patients Who Have Undergone Total Thyroidectomy." European Journal of Endocrinology 167.3 (2012): 373-378.

22) Bianco, Antonio C., and Sabina Casula. "Thyroid Hormone Replacement Therapy: Three 'Simple Questions, Complex Answers." European Thyroid Journal 1.2 (2012): 88-98.

23) Biondi, Bernadette, and Leonard Wartofsky. "Combination Treatment with T4 And T3: Toward Personalized Replacement Therapy in Hypothyroidism?" The Journal of Clinical Endocrinology & Metabolism 97.7 (2012): 2256-2271.

24) Hoermann, Rudolf, et al. "Is Pituitary TSH an Adequate Measure of Thyroid Hormone-Controlled Homeostasis During Thyroxine Treatment." Eur J Endocrinol 168.2 (2013): 271-80.

25) Wiersinga, Wilmar M. "Paradigm Shifts in Thyroid Hormone Replacement Therapies for Hypothyroidism." Nature Reviews Endocrinology 10.3 (2014): 164-174.

Chapter 7

TSH Suppression Benefits and Adverse Effects

A FEW YEARS BACK, I attended a medical meeting that included a lecture on the diagnosis and treatment of thyroid disease. The speaker discussed the use of thyroid hormones to treat thyroid disorders, mentioning "the dangers of TSH suppression," advising the audience of doctors to avoid suppressing TSH with thyroid medication. In other words, always make sure the TSH stays within the laboratory reference range. Note: TSH suppression refers to a dosage of thyroid medication, levothyroxine or NDT, which causes the TSH to fall below the laboratory reference range (0.40-4.50 mIU/L for Quest Lab). The TSH is inverse with thyroid hormone dosage. As the dosage increases, the TSH goes down, and if the dosage is decreased, the TSH goes up.

Thyroid Excess and Thyrotoxicosis

The most disturbing adverse effect of taking thyroid hormone pills is thyroid excess. The patient is taking too many thyroid pills, causing iatrogenic thyrotoxicosis. This is to be avoided, as it may cause a clinical syndrome known as thyrotoxicosis, characterized by tachycardia, palpitations, insomnia, anxiety, panic attacks, etc. Tachycardia at rest is usually an early sign of thyroid excess, alerting the patient and physician to reduce thyroid dosage. If symptoms of thyroid excess are ignored and thyroid dosage is not reduced, then atrial fibrillation (A-fib) may ensue. A-fib is an atrial arrhythmia, one of the more severe complications of thyroid excess, best avoided. (1-5)

Take the Time to Go Over the Thyroid Excess List of Symptoms

We spend time with each patient in the office talking about thyroid excess signs and symptoms to look for. We give each patient a printout of this list to take home and post on their bulletin board to read every day. If the patient experiences any symptoms of thyroid excess, they are instructed to stop the thyroid pills for a day. Patient selection is also a factor here, as a patient with early dementia could not be expected to have the cognitive function to recognize thyroid excess and stop taking their thyroid pill. The patient must be able and willing to play a role in their health care. Otherwise, they are not a candidate for natural thyroid treatment. Instead, the patient is referred to your local friendly endocrinologist for levothyroxine to maintain TSH within the lab range.

Stop the Thyroid Pills

Thyroid excess is easily avoided by simply stopping the thyroid medication should signs of resting tachycardia occur. Resting tachycardia means a fast heart rate while at rest. Once the thyroid pill is stopped, symptoms resolve fairly quickly, usually within 6 hours. For T4 only levothyroxine, which has a longer half-life of one week, relief of thyroid excess symptoms may take a week to resolve. This explains why NDT is safer than T4-only medication. Symptoms of thyroid excess resolve faster with NDT, a combination of T3 and T4.

Is a Low TSH indicative of Thyroid Excess?

Mainstream endocrinology assumes that a suppressed TSH indicates thyroid excess and, by definition, thyrotoxicosis. This is true for the thyrotoxicosis of Graves' disease and Toxic Nodular Goiter. The TSH will be suppressed in these two thyroid disorders, and the Free T3 and Free T4 will be elevated. The reverse T3 will also be elevated. There may also be an elevation of serum calcium. In Graves' Disease with thyrotoxicosis, hypercalcemia from rapid bone turnover has been reported. The patient will have obvious symptoms of thyrotoxicosis with tachycardia, insomnia, anxiety tremor, etc. (6-8)

However, for the hypothyroid patients taking NDT, natural desiccated thyroid, a suppressed TSH merely indicates adequate treatment dosage with full clinical benefit and does not correspond with the clinical signs, symptoms, or laboratory findings of thyroid excess. The key difference is normal Free T3 and Free T4 levels, even though the TSH is suppressed. Note: TSH is a pituitary hormone and not a thyroid hormone. Many clinicians are unaware of this fact.

Iatrogenic Hyperthyroidism

Iatrogenic hyperthyroidism does exist when patients are taking excessive amounts of thyroid hormone. However, when the diagnosis is based solely on a TSH below the reference range, this is not iatrogenic hyperthyroidism, this is an error of modern endocrinology, the creation of a medical myth. The issue can be quickly resolved with additional lab testing showing normal Free T3, Free T4 levels, and reverse T3 levels. Examples of this abound in the medical literature. For example, in 2002 Dr. Cooper over-estimates the number of elderly patients diagnosed with iatrogenic hyperthyroidism, based solely on the TSH value, writing:

> From epidemiologic data it can be calculated that approximately 600,00 elderly individuals have iatrogenic hyperthyroidism from thyroid hormone overdose, putting them at risk for atrial fibrillation and osteoporosis. (2)

In order for these "estimated" 600,000 elderly individuals to actually have iatrogenic hyperthyroidism, the laboratory tests for Free T3 and Free T4 must be above the lab range. The problem is these two blood tests were not done. If they had been done, they would have been within the normal range, excluding any possibility of hyperthyroidism.

Monitoring the Other Labs and Clinical Status of the Patient

Of course, in addition to lab studies, the Free T3, Free T4, etc., the patient's clinical status is key to monitoring thyroid dosage. If the patient has no resting tachycardia nor any other symptoms of thyroid excess, then a suppressed TSH indicates adequate thyroid treatment, and by no stretch of the imagination could the patient possibly be in a state of thyroid excess or thyrotoxicosis. (9)

Adverse Health Effects of TSH Suppression

Another point mentioned at the medical meeting to persuade us clinicians not to suppress the TSH with thyroid medication was the idea that there are adverse health consequences when the TSH is suppressed. The major one is the loss of bone density, also called osteoporosis, which is a real consideration in long-standing Graves' Disease patients with thyrotoxicosis, however not so for the hypothyroid patient on NDT. (10-12)

Numerous studies have examined this idea in hypothyroid patients treated with NDT, natural desiccated thyroid hormone, and found this idea to be a medical myth. In our patient population, we see bone density improving, especially in women receiving bioidentical hormone replacement and bone supplements such as Vitamin D3, K2, magnesium, and calcium. (13-21)

TSH Suppression after Thyroidectomy for Thyroid Cancer

The idea that there must be some adverse health effects of a suppressed TSH has also been examined in two groups of patients on long-term TSH suppression with levothyroxine, and this idea has been found to be false. After total thyroidectomy for thyroid cancer, the patient will soon succumb to myxedema coma from thyroid failure unless given thyroid hormone replacement, usually with levothyroxine. How much levothyroxine dosage should be prescribed to these patients? Suppression of TSH with levothyroxine is thought useful to prevent cancer recurrence. In fact, TSH suppression after total thyroidectomy for thyroid cancer is a common practice in mainstream endocrinology. Several studies by Drs. Diane Schneider, Jordi Reverter, and Lara Vera, in this patient group, have found no adverse effects from long-term TSH suppression. (11) (21-24) (2) (16-18) (39)

DEXA Scan for Detection of Osteoporosis

DEXA scan is typically used to measure bone mineral density (BMD) for the detection of osteoporosis. In 2004, Dr. Cheng-Hsiung Chen studied bone mineral density in women treated with suppressive doses of levothyroxine post-thyroidectomy for thyroid cancer. He writes:

> Women with differentiated thyroid cancer who had long-term (7 +/- 3 years) T4 therapy and suppressed TSH levels had no evidence of lower Bone Mineral Density. (11)

Shrinking Thyroid Nodules with TSH Suppression

Mainstream endocrinologists commonly treat thyroid nodules with TSH suppression. In many cases, this treatment is successful when follow-up ultrasound shows the nodules remain stable or decrease in size. Again, studies have been done in this thyroid nodule group showing no adverse effects of TSH suppression on bone mineral density. (25-37)

In 2013, Dr. Flavio Zelmanovitz conducted a one-year prospective randomized trial using TSH suppression for thyroid nodules in 45 patients. Patients were treated with levothyroxine at 2.5–3.0 mg/kg per day to suppress TSH below 0.3 mIU/mL. After one year of TSH suppressive treatment, Dr. Flavio Zelmanovitz found no change in bone mineral density, writing:

> The data obtained in this study do not suggest any significant decrease in BMD [Bone Mineral Density] after 1 yr. of

treatment with suppressive doses of T4 [levothyroxine]… In conclusion, T4 treatment is associated with decreased nodule volume in 17% of patients and may inhibit growth in another 10%. (27)

No Adverse Effects from Low TSH Below Reference Range in Large Scale Study

In 2010, Drs. Graham Leese and Robert Flynn from the University of Dundee, UK, published their large-scale study showing no adverse effect of TSH suppression in the (.03-.40 mU/L) range. (13)

Suppressive Doses of Thyroid Hormone Needed for Adequate Therapy

In 2012, Dr. Mitsuru Ito from Japan studied patients before and after total thyroidectomy for thyroid cancer. Dr. Mitsuru Ito reported after thyroidectomy, TSH-suppressive doses of levothyroxine are required to achieve the same Free T3 levels before surgery. Dr. Ito writes that TSH is **not** an appropriate indicator of normal thyroid hormone levels (i.e., euthyroidism):

> serum TSH levels only reflect the feedback effect of thyroid hormones at the hypothalamic–pituitary level and, therefore, may not be an appropriate indicator of peripheral tissue euthyroidism. [Note: euthyroid means normal thyroid hormone levels.] (38)

In 2005, Dr. Alevizaki agrees with Dr. Ito (above), writing:

> TSH may not be a good marker for adequate thyroid hormone replacement therapy. (39)

In 2013, Dr. Rudolf Hoermann asks the question, is TSH an adequate measure of thyroid hormone homeostasis during thyroxine (levothyroxine) treatment? Dr. Rudolf Hoermann writes:

> (our) data reveal disjoints between FT4–TSH feedback and T3 production that persist even when sufficient T4 apparently restores euthyroidism. (40)

Thierry Hertoghe on Thyroid TSH Suppression

Dr. Thierry Hertoghe, possibly the most recognized thyroid expert on the planet, suppresses TSH in about 30% of his patients during treatment with thyroid hormone. (personal communication) In the May 2020 Townsend Letter, Dr. Hertoghe discusses his treatment protocol for Hashimoto's thyroiditis in women, writing levothyroxine treatment for Hashimoto's thyroiditis is most effective when enough dosage is given to suppress the TSH:

> Hormone treatments can decrease thyroid antibody levels by 20-70%. Thyroid treatment: Thyroid therapy is necessary not only to reduce thyroid antibodies but to relieve the patient's hypothyroid symptoms and the risks and severity of psychological and somatic disorders that often accompany autoimmune thyroiditis. Many studies have shown the efficacy of thyroxine treatment. **The best efficacy is reached when the dose is high enough to suppress the TSH level in the serum.** (41)

TSH suppression for Hashimoto's is discussed further below, and in Chapters 20-26.

Thyroid Hormone Receptor Mutation

Some patients harbor mutations in the thyroid hormone receptor, associated with peripheral resistance to thyroid hormone. This was hypothesized 30 years ago, and the exact genetic defect was identified in 2013. These patients may require TSH suppressive doses of thyroid medication to maintain the euthyroid state. (42)

Pregnancy May Have a Suppressed TSH

During pregnancy, HCG levels rise to very high levels. The high HCG inhibits the HPA (hypothalamic-pituitary axis), which results in a low or suppressed TSH. In pregnancy, suppression of TSH is normal and not indicative of a hyperthyroid state. In 2016, Dr. Offie Soldin writes:

> In up to 10–20% of normal pregnant women, serum TSH concentrations are transiently low or undetectable. (43-44)

There are many drugs that cause central hypothyroidism and suppress TSH, including metformin, glucocorticoids, dopamine agonists, somatostatin analogs, and rexinoids. (45-46)

Central Hypothyroidism

Both Drs. Kent Holtorf and Jacob Teitelbaum have devoted much of their careers to the study and treatment of chronic fatigue/fibromyalgia patients. One of the keys to understanding is the association between hypothalamic dysfunction and central hypothyroidism. In hypothalamic dysfunction, the TSH, may be paradoxically low, even though the patient is hypothyroid with chronic fatigue. According to Drs. Holtorf and Teitelbaum, the chronic fatigue patient may have central hypothyroidism with a suppressed TSH. Again, withholding thyroid hormone treatment from these patients because of a low or suppressed TSH would be a clinical error. (47-54)

Cancer treatment with cranial irradiation and chemotherapy may cause hypothalamic dysfunction and central hypothyroidism in cancer survivors. The TSH may be paradoxically low and unreliable in these cases. (55-60)

Hashimoto's Thyroiditis Autoimmune Thyroid Disease

It is common practice among endocrinologists to treat "euthyroid" Hashimoto's patients with levothyroxine. "Euthyroid" means the TSH is in the lab reference range. Studies show the benefits of thyroid hormone treatment in Hashimoto's patients even when the TSH is in the normal range, as mentioned above by Dr. Thierry Hertoghe in May 2020 Townsend Letter advocating TSH suppression for Hashimoto's patients. Such treatment with TSH suppression with thyroid hormone is thought beneficial in stabilizing the Hashimoto's autoimmune process and is recommended as soon as the diagnosis is established. (41) (61-66)

In 1999, Dr. Rink from Germany studied TSH suppression in Hashimotos' patients finding anti-thyroid antibody reduction was most significant in the TSH suppressed group. In addition, an iodine supplement dosage of 200 mcg/day is safe for Hashimotos' patients. Dr. Rink writes:

> The patients of the second collective [377 Hashimotos patients] revealed a significant decrease of the TgAb in the subgroups treated with up to 200 micrograms iodide/day, while **the reduction of the TPOAb depended on the thyrotropin level [TSH] and was most significant in the suppressed group** (p < 0.0001). ...A hormone therapy combined with a daily, low-dose iodine medication [200 mcg/day] is able to reduce the TgAb and the TPOAb levels even in patients with Hashimoto's thyroiditis. Note: Thyrotropin is TSH. (61)

Dr. Rink did not study the effect of higher iodine dietary intake in Hashimotos' patients on TSH suppressive doses of thyroid medication. In my opinion, based on my own clinical experience over the years, TSH suppression protects Hashimoto's patients from the toxic effects of excess iodine. For example, for women with fibrocystic breast disease in which higher doses of iodine (12.5 mg per day) are beneficial, TSH suppression allows the use of high-dose iodine without provoking increased anti-thyroid antibodies. This is my observation from clinical practice. Obviously, it would be nice to have supportive studies in the medical literature.

TSH Controls Hydrogen Peroxide Generation

The etiology of autoimmune thyroid disease is thought to be related to the overproduction or lack of degradation of hydrogen peroxide, the rate-limiting step in thyroid hormone production. Excess hydrogen peroxide causes antigenicity by damaging key proteins, TPO and thyroglobulin, as well as thyrocytes themselves. Since the generation of hydrogen peroxide is directly controlled by TSH, suppression of TSH turns off hydrogen peroxide generation. This is the crux of the benefit for Hashimoto's patients. Supplementing with selenium to improve anti-oxidant capacity to degrade hydrogen peroxide is beneficial as well. The peripheral deiodinase enzyme for the conversion of T4 to T3 is a selenium-based enzyme, so selenium deficiency will result in poor conversion of T4 to T3 with higher T4 levels and lower T3 levels. Selenium supplementation is beneficial for reversing all this. (67-68)

Estrogen for Prevention and Treatment of Post-Menopausal Bone Loss

In 1994, Drs. Diane Schneider and Elizabeth Barrett-Connor reported TSH suppression is safe in men and pre-menopausal women. However, the authors find that TSH suppression in post-menopausal women may be associated with loss of bone density, a finding also confirmed by Dr. Chen in 2004. Dr. Schneider found this loss of bone density is prevented by the concurrent use of estrogen, also called post-menopausal hormone replacement. This confirms the importance of estrogen hormone replacement in post-menopausal women to prevent the inevitable decline in bone density. More on post-menopausal hormone replacement can be found in my 2011 book, Bioidentical Hormones 101. (11) (16) (69-71)

In 1995, Dr. J. A. Franklyn used DEXA scans to study the effect of estrogen HRT (hormone replacement therapy) on bone mineral density in levothyroxine-treated post-menopausal women with a past history of thyrotoxicosis and levothyroxine use. Dr. Franklyn found that HRT, estrogen replacement, "abolished the reduction" in bone mineral density (BMD) seen in the control group without HRT. Franklyn writes estrogen replacement should be encouraged:

> Our results indicate that estrogen replacement therapy abolishes reduction in femoral and vertebral BMD [bone mineral density] in post-menopausal women with previous thyrotoxicosis and subsequent L-T4

[levothyroxine] therapy. This potentially beneficial influence of estrogen replacement upon both BMD and fracture risk in post-menopausal women with a history of thyroid disease suggests that estrogen administration should be encouraged in this group. (72)

In 1995, Dr. Fujiyama disputed Dr. Schneider's finding of bone loss in TSH-suppressed post-menopausal women. Dr. Fujiyama's point is that all post-menopausal women experience bone loss over time which is related to estrogen deficiency and is not accelerated by suppressive doses of thyroxine. He writes:

> Suppressive doses of thyroxine do not accelerate age-related bone loss in post-menopausal women. (19)

One is reminded that all post-menopausal women experience bone loss of 2-5 percent per year because of estrogen deficiency. In my opinion, the bone loss reported by Dr. Schneider is not due to TSH suppression from levothyroxine treatment. Rather, it is due to post-menopausal hormonal decline (i.e., estrogen deficiency). In my office, we offer HRT hormone replacement therapy to all post-menopausal women, including those on thyroid medication. We avoid the use of synthetic hormone preparations and instead use "bioidentical" hormones, which share the same molecular structure as our own hormones found in the human body. Any prudent physician would do the same. These patients also receive bone-building supplements containing Calcium, Vitamin D, Vitamin K, Magnesium, etc. As a result, we typically find bone density remaining stable or even increasing in our post-menopausal patients when studied with serial DEXA scans. (73-77)

In 2021, Dr. Anna Gosset advised estrogen replacement should be offered as first-line therapy for post-menopausal prevention of osteoporosis, writing the following:

> In conclusion, use of MHT [menopausal hormone therapy] should be reconsidered as a 1st therapeutic option to prevent osteoporosis in early postmenopausal women with a low- to moderate-risk of fracture where specific bone active medications are not warranted. It must be considered as a true primary preventive therapy to maintain bone mass and quality as well as decrease the risk of fracture at an age when this risk is not yet as high as later in life. (76-78)

Long Term TSH Suppression is Common

As mentioned above, the long-term suppression of TSH for the thyroid nodule patient and thyroid cancer patient is a common practice in mainstream endocrinology. Studies show no long-term adverse effects for men, pre-menopausal women, or post-menopausal women (on estrogen hormone replacement). The TSH test may not always reflect thyroid levels in the periphery or at the cellular level and may, in fact, be unreliable in a variety of medical conditions such as chronic fatigue, fibromyalgia, pregnancy, post-chemotherapy, autoimmune thyroid disease, hypothalamic dysfunction, central hypothyroidism, and various drugs. In 2014, Dr. Kent Holtorf writes:

> extreme caution should be used in relying on TSH or serum thyroid levels to rule out hypothyroidism in the presence of a wide range of conditions, including physiologic and emotional stress, depression, dieting, obesity, leptin insulin resistance, diabetes, chronic fatigue syndrome, fibromyalgia, inflammation, autoimmune disease, or systemic illness, as TSH levels will often be normal despite the presence of significant hypothyroidism. (53)

Conclusion

Dogmatically insisting on maintaining the TSH within the reference range and failing to recognize TSH suppression as beneficial in some patients is an error of modern endocrinology. (79-89)

♦ References Chapter 7

1) Abonowara, Abdulgani, et al. "Prevalence of Atrial Fibrillation in Patients Taking TSH Suppression Therapy for Management of Thyroid Cancer." Clinical and Investigative Medicine (2012): E152-E156.

2) Cooper, D. S., and E. C. Ridgway. "Thoughts on Prevention of Thyroid Disease in the United States." Thyroid 12 (2002): 925-929.

3) Bains, Ajay, et al. "Iatrogenic Thyrotoxicosis Secondary to Compounded Liothyronine." The Canadian Journal of Hospital Pharmacy 68.1 (2015): 57.

4) He, Zhiheng H., et al. "Thyrotoxicosis After Massive Triiodothyronine (LT3) Overdose: A Coast-To-Coast Case Series and Review." Drugs in Context 9 (2020).

5) Levine, Jeffrey M. "A Quality Improvement Study: Medication Error Leading to Thyrotoxicosis and Death." Journal of the American Medical Directors Association 5.6 (2004): 410-413.

6) Sharma, Anu, and Marius N. Stan. "Thyrotoxicosis: Diagnosis and Management." Mayo Clinic Proceedings. Vol. 94. No. 6. Elsevier, 2019.

7) Ozkaya, Hande Mefkure, et al. "Life-Threatening Hypercalcemia Due to Graves' Disease and Concomitant Adrenal Failure: A Case Report and Review of The Literature." Case Reports in Endocrinology 2015 (2015).

8) Clark, Lorna, et al. "Hyperthyroidism, An Overlooked Cause of Severe Hypercalcemia." Grand Rounds 10 (2010): 110-112.

9) Igoe, D., et al. "TSH as an Index of L-Thyroxine Replacement and Suppression Therapy." Irish Journal of Medical Science 161.12 (1992): 684-686.

10) Uzzan, B., et al. "Effects on Bone Mass of Long-Term Treatment with Thyroid Hormones: A Meta-Analysis." The Journal of Clinical Endocrinology & Metabolism 81.12 (1996): 4278-4289.

11) Chen, Cheng-Hsiung, et al. "Bone Mineral Density in Women Receiving Thyroxine Suppressive Therapy for Differentiated Thyroid Carcinoma." J Formos Med Assoc. 2004 Jun;103(6):442-7. PMID: 15278189.

12) Baqi, L., et al. "Thyrotropin Versus Thyroid Hormone in Regulating Bone Density and Turnover in Pre-Menopausal Women." Endocrine Regulations 44.2 (2010): 57-63.

13) Leese, Graham, and Robert Flynn. "Is It Safe for Patients Taking Thyroxine to Have a Low but Not Suppressed Serum TSH Concentration?" Endocrine Abstracts. Vol. 21. Bioscientifica, 2010.

14) Leese, G. P., et al. "Morbidity in Patients On L-Thyroxine: A Comparison of Those with a Normal TSH to Those with a Suppressed TSH." Clinical Endocrinology 37.6 (1992): 500-503.

15) Bauer, Douglas C., et al. "Low Thyrotropin Levels Are Not Associated with Bone Loss in Older Women: A Prospective Study." The Journal of Clinical Endocrinology & Metabolism 82.9 (1997): 2931-2936.

16) Schneider, Diane L., et al. "Thyroid Hormone Use and Bone Mineral Density in Elderly Women: Effects of Estrogen." JAMA 271.16 (1994): 1245-1249.

17) Marcocci, Claudio, et al. "Skeletal Integrity in Men Chronically Treated with Suppressive Doses of L-Thyroxine." Journal of Bone and Mineral Research 12.1 (1997): 72-77

18) Marcocci, Claudio, et al. "Carefully Monitored Levothyroxine Suppressive Therapy Is Not Associated with Bone Loss in Pre-Menopausal Women." The Journal of Clinical Endocrinology & Metabolism 78.4 (1994): 818-823.

19) Fujiyama, Kaoru, et al. "Suppressive Doses of Thyroxine Do Not Accelerate Age-Related Bone Loss in Late Post-Menopausal Women." Thyroid 5.1 (1995): 13-17.

20) Grant, David J., et al. "Suppressed TSH Levels Secondary to Thyroxine Replacement Therapy Are Not Associated with Osteoporosis." Clinical Endocrinology 39.5 (1993): 529-533.

21) Reverter, J. L., et al. "Lack of Deleterious Effect on Bone Mineral Density of Long-Term Thyroxine Suppressive Therapy for Differentiated Thyroid Carcinoma." Endocrine-Related Cancer 12.4 (2005): 973-981.

22) Reverter, Jordi L., and Eulàlia Colomé. "Potential Risks of the Adverse Effects of Thyrotropin Suppression in Differentiated Thyroid Carcinoma." Endocrinología y Nutrición 58.2 (2011): 75-83.

23) Reverter, Jordi L., et al. "Clinical Endocrinologists' Perception of the Deleterious Effects of TSH Suppressive Therapy in Patients with Differentiated Thyroid Carcinoma." Endocrinologia y Nutricion 57.8 (2010): 350-356.

24) Vera, Lara, et al. "Ten-Year Estimated Risk of Bone Fracture in Women with Differentiated Thyroid Cancer Under TSH-Suppressive Levothyroxine Therapy." Endokrynologia Polska 67.4 (2016): 350-358.

25) Gharib, Hossein, et al. "Suppressive Therapy with Levothyroxine for Solitary Thyroid Nodules." New England Journal of Medicine 317.2 (1987): 70-75.

26) Chen, Chiung-Ya, et al. "The Effect of Suppressive Thyroxine Therapy in Nodular Goiter in Post-Menopausal Women and 2 Year's Bone Mineral Density Change." Endocrine Journal 65.11 (2018): 1101-1109.

27) Zelmanovitz, Flávio, et al. "Suppressive Therapy with Levothyroxine for Solitary Thyroid Nodules: A Double-Blind Controlled Clinical Study and Cumulative Meta-Analyses." The Journal of Clinical Endocrinology & Metabolism 83.11 (1998): 3881-3885.

28) Clark, Orlo H. "TSH Suppression in the Management of Thyroid Nodules and Thyroid Cancer." World Journal of Surgery 5.1 (1981): 39-46.

29) Haymart, Megan Rist, et al. "Higher Serum TSH Level in Thyroid Nodule Patients is Associated with Greater Risks of Differentiated Thyroid Cancer and Advanced Tumor Stage." J Clin Endocrinol Metab 93.3 (2008): 809-14.

30) Welker, Mary Jo, and Diane Orlov. "Thyroid Nodules." American Family Physician 67.3 (2003): 559-566.

31) Wémeau, Jean-Louis, et al. "Effects of Thyroid-Stimulating Hormone Suppression with Levothyroxine in Reducing the Volume of Solitary Thyroid Nodules and Improving Extraocular Nonpalpable Changes: A Randomized, Double-Blind, Placebo-Controlled Trial by the French Thyroid Research Group." The Journal of Clinical Endocrinology & Metabolism 87.11 (2002): 4928-4934.

32) Castro, M. Regina, et al. "Effectiveness of Thyroid Hormone Suppressive Therapy in Benign Solitary Thyroid Nodules: A Meta-Analysis." The Journal of Clinical Endocrinology & Metabolism 87.9 (2002): 4154-4159.

33) Bennedbæk, Finn Noe, and Laszlo Hegedüs. "Management of the Solitary Thyroid Nodule: Results of a North American Survey." The Journal of Clinical Endocrinology & Metabolism 85.7 (2000): 2493-2498.

34) Filetti, Sebastiano, et al. "Nonsurgical Approaches to the Management of Thyroid Nodules." Nature Clinical Practice Endocrinology & Metabolism 2.7 (2006): 384-394.

35) Lima, Nicolau, et al. "Levothyroxine Suppressive Therapy is Partially Effective in Treating Patients with Benign, Solid Thyroid Nodules and Multinodular Goiters." Thyroid 7.5 (1997): 691-697.

36) Papini, E., et al. "A Prospective Randomized Trial of Levothyroxine Suppressive Therapy for Solitary Thyroid Nodules." Clinical Endocrinology 38.5 (1993): 507-513.

37) Cheung, Polly SY, et al. "Thyroxine Suppressive Therapy of Benign Solitary Thyroid Nodules: A Prospective Randomized Study." World Journal of Surgery 13 (1989): 818-821.

38) Ito, Mitsuru, et al. "TSH-Suppressive Doses of Levothyroxine Are Required to Achieve Pre-Operative Native Serum Triiodothyronine Levels in Patients Who Have Undergone Total Thyroidectomy." European Journal of Endocrinology 167.3 (2012): 373-378.

39) Alevizaki M, Mantzou E, et al. TSH May Not Be a Good Marker for Adequate Thyroid Hormone Replacement Therapy. Wiener Klinische Wochenschrift 2005 117 636–640.

40) Hoermann, Rudolf, et al. "Is Pituitary TSH an Adequate Measure of Thyroid Hormone-Controlled Homeostasis During Thyroxine Treatment?" European Journal of Endocrinology 168.2 (2013): 271-280.

41) Hertoghe, Thierry. Hashimoto's Thyroiditis, A Common Disorder in Women: How to Treat It, Part 2, Townsend Letter. #442 May 2020. https://www.townsendletter.com/article/hashimotos-thyroiditis-part-2/

42) Dumitrescu, Alexandra M., and Samuel Refetoff. "The Syndromes of Reduced Sensitivity to Thyroid Hormone." Biochimica et Biophysica Acta (BBA)-General Subjects 1830.7 (2013): 3987-4003.

43) Soldin, Offie P., et al "The Use of TSH In Determining Thyroid Disease: How Does It Impact the Practice of Medicine in Pregnancy?" Journal of Thyroid Research (2013): 148157.

44) Brotherton, Janet. "Suppression of Maternal Pituitary Thyroid-Stimulating Hormone During Pregnancy." Human Reproduction 5.4 (1990): 471-475.

45) Haugen, Bryan R. "Drugs that Suppress TSH or Cause Central Hypothyroidism." Best Practice & Research Clinical Endocrinology & Metabolism 23.6 (2009): 793-800.

46) Vigersky, Robert A., et al. "Thyrotropin Suppression by Metformin." The Journal of Clinical Endocrinology & Metabolism 91.1 (2006): 225-227.

47) Teitelbaum, Jacob. "Effective Treatment of Chronic Fatigue Syndrome." Integrative Medicine 10.6 (2011): 44.

48) Teitelbaum, Jacob. "Chronic Fatigue Syndrome, Fibromyalgia, and Myalgic Encephalomyelitis: A Clinical Perspective." Alternative Therapies in Health and Medicine 20.1 (2014): 45.

49) Teitelbaum, Jacob E., et al. "Effective Treatment of Chronic Fatigue Syndrome and Fibromyalgia—A Randomized, Double-Blind, Placebo-Controlled, Intent-To-Treat Study." Journal of Chronic Fatigue Syndrome 8.2 (2000): 3-15.

50) Teitelbaum, Jacob, et al. "Nutritional Intervention in Chronic Fatigue Syndrome and Fibromyalgia (CFS/FMS) A Unique Porcine Serum Polypeptide Nutritional Supplement." The Open Pain Journal 13.1 (2020).

51) Teitelbaum, Jacob. "Effective Treatment of Chronic Fatigue Syndrome." IMCJ 4.4 (2005): 24-29.

52) Holtorf, Kent. "Diagnosis and Treatment of Hypothalamic-Pituitary-Adrenal (HPA) Axis Dysfunction in Patients with Chronic Fatigue Syndrome (CFS) and Fibromyalgia (FM)." Journal of Chronic Fatigue Syndrome 14.3 (2007): 59-88.

53) Holtorf, Kent. "Peripheral Thyroid Hormone Conversion and Its Impact on TSH and Metabolic Activity." Journal of Restorative Medicine 3.1 (2014): 30-52.

54) Holtorf, Kent. "Thyroid Hormone Transport into Cellular Tissue." Journal of Restorative Medicine 3.1 (2014): 53-68.

55) Baronio, Federico, et al. "Central Hypothyroidism Following Chemotherapy for Acute Lymphoblastic Leukemia." (2011): 903-906.

56) Brabant, Georg, et al. "Hypothyroidism Following Childhood Cancer Therapy–An Under Diagnosed Complication." International Journal of Cancer 130.5 (2012): 1145-1150.

57) Wanaguru, Amy L., et al. "Central Hypothyroidism After Chemotherapy in Childhood Cancer Survivors: A Single Centre Series." Acta Oncologica (2022): 1-4.

58) Rose, Susan R., et al. "Diagnosis of Hidden Central Hypothyroidism in Survivors of Childhood Cancer." The Journal of Clinical Endocrinology & Metabolism 84.12 (1999): 4472-4479.

59) Rose, Susan R. "Cranial Irradiation and Central Hypothyroidism." Trends in Endocrinology and Metabolism 12.3 (2001): 97-104.

60) Beck-Peccoz, Paolo, et al. "Central Hypothyroidism—A Neglected Thyroid Disorder." Nature Reviews Endocrinology 13.10 (2017): 588-598.

61) Rink, T., et al. "Effect of Iodine and Thyroid Hormones in the Induction and Therapy of Hashimoto's Thyroiditis." Nuklearmedizin. Nuclear Medicine 38.5 (1999): 144-149.

62) Aksoy, Duygu Yazgan, et al. "Effects of Prophylactic Thyroid Hormone Replacement in Euthyroid Hashimoto's Thyroiditis." Endocrine Journal 52.3 (2005): 337-343.

63) Padberg, S., et al. "One-Year Prophylactic Treatment of Euthyroid Hashimoto's Thyroiditis Patients with Levothyroxine: Is There a Benefit?" Thyroid 11.3 (2001): 249-255.

64) Schmidt, Matthias, et al. "Long-Term Follow-Up of Anti-Thyroid Peroxidase Antibodies in Patients with Chronic Autoimmune Thyroiditis (Hashimoto's Thyroiditis) Treated with Levothyroxine." Thyroid 18.7 (2008): 755-760.

65) Hegedüs, Laszlo, et al. "Influence of Thyroxine Treatment on Thyroid Size and Anti-Thyroid Peroxidase Antibodies in Hashimoto's Thyroiditis." Clinical Endocrinology 35.3 (1991): 235-238.

66) Schumm-Draeger, P-M., et al. "Prophylactic Levothyroxine Therapy in Patients with Hashimoto's Thyroiditis." Experimental and Clinical Endocrinology and Diabetes 107.S 03 (1999): S84-S87.

67) Song, Yue, et al. "Roles of Hydrogen Peroxide in Thyroid Physiology and Disease." The Journal of Clinical Endocrinology and Metabolism 92.10 (2007): 3764-3773.

68) Kobayashi, Ryohei, et al. "Thyroid function in Patients with Selenium Deficiency Exhibits High Free T4 to T3 Ratio." Clinical Pediatric Endocrinology 30.1 (2021): 19-26.

69) Brancatella, Alessandro, and Claudio Marcocci. "TSH Suppressive Therapy and Bone." Endocrine Connections 9.7 (2020): R158-R172.

70) Ross DS, et al. Subclinical Hyperthyroidism and Reduced Bone Density as a Possible Result of Prolonged Suppression of the Pituitary-Thyroid Axis with L-Thyroxine. American Journal of Medicine 1987 82 1167–1170.

71) Dach, Jeffrey. Bioidentical Hormones 101. iUniverse, 2011.

72) Franklyn, J. A., et al. "Effect of Estrogen Replacement Therapy Upon Bone Mineral Density in Thyroxine-Treated Post-Menopausal Women with a Past History of Thyrotoxicosis." Thyroid 5.5 (1995): 359-363.

73) Tella, Sri Harsha, and J. Christopher Gallagher. "Prevention and Treatment of Post-Menopausal Osteoporosis." The Journal of Steroid Biochemistry and Molecular Biology 142 (2014): 155-170.

74) Nilas, L., and C. Christiansen. "The Pathophysiology of Peri- and Post-Menopausal Bone Loss." BJOG: An International Journal of Obstetrics & Gynaecology 96.5 (1989): 580-587.

75) Capozzi, Anna, et al. "Calcium, Vitamin D, Vitamin K2, and Magnesium Supplementation and Skeletal Health." Maturitas 140 (2020): 55-63.

76) Gosset, Anna, et al. "Menopausal Hormone Therapy for the Management of Osteoporosis." Best Practice & Research. Clinical Endocrinology & Metabolism 35.6 (2021): 101551.

77) Stuenkel, Cynthia A. "Menopausal Hormone Therapy and the Role of Estrogen." Clinical Obstetrics and Gynecology 64.4 (2021): 757-771.

78) Rozenberg, Serge, et al. "Is There a Role for Menopausal Hormone Therapy in the Management of Postmenopausal Osteoporosis?" Osteoporosis International 31 (2020): 2271-2286.

79) Bauer, Douglas C., et al. "Risk for Fracture in Women with Low Serum Levels of Thyroid-Stimulating Hormone." Annals of Internal Medicine 134.7 (2001): 561-568.

80) Cooper, David S. "TSH Suppressive Therapy: An Overview of Long-Term Clinical Consequences." Hormones (Athens) 9.1 (2010): 57-59.

81) Abo-Touk, Niveen A., and Dalia H. Zayed. "The Efficacy of Thyrotropin Suppression Therapy in Treatment of Differentiated Thyroid Cancer after Total Thyroidectomy." Forum of Clinical Oncology. Vol. 6. No. 2. 2015.

82) Pujol, Pascal, et al. "Degree of Thyrotropin Suppression as a Prognostic Determinant in Differentiated Thyroid Cancer." The Journal of Clinical Endocrinology & Metabolism 81.12 (1996): 4318-4323.

83) Biondi, Bernadette, and David S. Cooper. "Benefits of Thyrotropin Suppression Versus the Risks of Adverse Effects in Differentiated Thyroid Cancer." Thyroid 20.2 (2010): 135-146.

84) Samuels, M. H., et al. "Effects of Altering Levothyroxine (L-T4) Doses on Quality of Life, Mood, and Cognition In L-T4 Treated Subjects." The Journal of Clinical Endocrinology and Metabolism 103.5 (2018): 1997.

85) Poudel, Prakar, et al. "Effect of Thyroxine and Thyrotropin on Bone Mineral Density in Post-Menopausal Women: A Systematic Review." Cureus 14.6 (2022).

86) Zanella, André Borsatto, et al. "Effect of Suppressive Levothyroxine Therapy on Bone Mineral Density in Young Patients with Differentiated Thyroid Carcinoma." Metabolites 12.9 (2022): 842.

87) Wang, Shiwei, et al. "Effects of TSH Suppressive Therapy on Bone Mineral Density (BMD) and Bone Turnover Markers (Btms) in Patients with Differentiated Thyroid Cancer in Northeast China: A Prospective Controlled Cohort Study." Endocrine (2022): 1-12.

88) Sousa, B. É., et al. "Trabecular Bone Score in Women with Differentiated Thyroid Cancer on Long-Term TSH-Suppressive Therapy." Journal of Endocrinological Investigation 44.10 (2021): 2295-2305.

89) Muller, Carmen G., et al. "Possible Limited Bone Loss with Suppressive Thyroxine Therapy is Unlikely to Have Clinical Relevance." Thyroid 5.2 (1995): 81-87.

Chapter 8

Paradigm Shift from Levothyroxine to Combination T3/T4

As MENTIONED IN A PREVIOUS chapter, one of the errors in mainstream endocrinology is the dogmatic insistence on T4-monotherapy only. Only one single medicine, T4 only, may be prescribed to the hypothyroid patient. And what does this mean? T4 only means generic levothyroxine or brand name Synthroid, the most prescribed drug in America, with 123 million prescriptions in 2016. About 7% of the population is hypothyroid and needs treatment. In my opinion, NDT, natural desiccated thyroid, is preferable to T4-monotherapy. As we will see below, NDT is more robust, more effective, and safer than T4-monotherapy with levothyroxine.

A Subset of Patients Are Dissatisfied with T4-Monotherapy

The wheels of change are turning in medicine, as illustrated in 2018 by Angela M. Leung, MD writing on Medscape, the "Love-Hate Relationship with T4". This article caught my attention because it represents the beginning of a paradigm shift in mainstream endocrinology. With refreshing honesty, Angela M. Leung, MD, points out some patients are dissatisfied with T4-monotherapy and actively seek a combination of T3 and T4 treatment. Dr. Leung cites two reasons:

1) persistent hypothyroid symptoms even though the TSH is in the "normal range."

2) the possibility of a genetic mutation in the patient called a de-iodinase polymorphism which impairs the conversion of T4 to T3. (1)

Synthetic T3/T4 Combination

Dr. Angela Leung prescribes both T3 (liothyronine, generic Cytomel) and T4 (levothyroxine, generic Synthroid) in dosage that replicates the T3:T4 secretion ratio of the human thyroid. This will be named "Synthetic Combination." Dr. Leung writes:

> To best replicate the physiologic ratio of T3:T4 production, the separate prescriptions should be about 1:13-1:20 that of T3 to T4...A typical formula for a patient on 112 μg of synthetic T4 once daily, the new prescription is 5 μg of synthetic T3 twice daily and 100 μg of synthetic T4 daily. (1)

Some Patients Prefer (NDT) Natural Desiccated Thyroid

In another burst of refreshing honesty, Dr. Angela Leung admits that some patients prefer NDT, natural desiccated thyroid, whose first medical use dates to 1891, decades before the creation of the FDA (Food and Drug Administration). NDT was never actually FDA-approved as a new drug since it was "grandfathered in" in 1938 when Congress passed the Federal Food, Drug, and Cosmetic (FDC) Act. Thus, NDT natural desiccated thyroid is prescribed by physicians, dispensed by pharmacies and regulated by the FDA the same as any other drug. In 2020, Dr. Freddy Toloza writes:

> It is estimated that about 10–29% of patients with hypothyroidism use DTE [natural desiccated thyroid extract] as their primary thyroid hormone replacement medication in the US. (2-3)

Free T3 and Free T4 Are More Accurate and Preferred Laboratory Tests

In 2003, Dr. Sapin studied the T4:T3 ratio produced by the thyroid gland, finding this to be a 4:1 ratio. In addition, Dr. Sapin says the

Free T3 and Free T4 tests are more accurate and have replaced other thyroid hormone laboratory tests. Dr. Sapin writes:

> Hormonal production of the thyroid gland is constituted of thyroxine or T4 (80%) and triiodothyronine or T3 (20%). In the circulation, whole T4 originates from thyroid secretion but most of T3 (80%) is produced extra thyroidally from T4 deiodination... **Because of their higher diagnostic performance, free T4 (FT4) and free T3 (FT3) measurements have superseded total (free + bound) hormone determination.** (4)

Concerns About T4:T3 Ratio

In 2019, Dr. Peter Taylor studied T3 and T4 combination therapy stating that due to peripheral conversion of T4 to T3, the secretion ratio is around 14:1 T4 to T3, writing:

> Given the majority of circulating T3 comes from peripheral conversion of FT4 to FT3, a secretion ratio of FT4:FT3 in healthy individuals is ~14:1. (5-7)

Who is correct, Dr. Sapin or Dr. Taylor? How do we explain this contradiction?

Natural Desiccated Thyroid is 4:1, T4:T3

NDT, natural desiccated thyroid, contains T4 and T3 in a 4:1 ratio and can be regarded as another combination therapy. Although Dr. Leung reluctantly prescribes NDT, she will first try to dissuade the patient by disclosing drawbacks. Namely, Dr. Leung will argue NDT is suboptimal because the T4:T3 ratio in NDT is 4:1, while the thyroid secretion ratio ranges from 12:1 to 20:1. (5-7)

Opposing views in support of the 4:1 ratio can be found among prescribers of NDT. Although the thyroid gland T4:T3 secretion ratio is 12:1, only about 20% of serum T3 comes from thyroid secretion; the other 80% comes from peripheral conversion of T4 to T3. This means the final serum levels are closer to the 3:1 or 4:1 range found in NDT. Even though NDT does not replicate thyroid secretion ratio of 12:1, it does replicate the serum ratio of T4 to T3 (in the range of 3:1 to 4:1), which in my opinion, is the more relevant ratio. You can do this calculation on your own.

Do the Calculation from Your Own Lab Sheet

Average normal Free T4 is 1.0 ng/dl= 1000pcg/dl.

Average normal Free T3 is 300 pcg/dl.

FreeT4/Free T3 = 1000/300 = 3.3

The serum Free T4:T3 ratio in the average patient is 3.3:1, a value closer to the 4:1 found in NDT. Remember, after the thyroid pill is ingested and absorbed, it enters the circulating bloodstream as Free T3 and Free T4. Matching the serum T4:T3 ratio is the most logical dosing strategy.

127 Years of Use

In 20 years of clinical practice prescribing NDT to patients and family members, the 4:1 ratio in NDT has NEVER been a significant issue, so I would say this is an example of a medical myth, the creation of an "imaginary" objection. Another thing to think about is this: If there were any significant problems with natural desiccated thyroid requiring a black box warning or removal from the marketplace, it would have happened by now. Natural desiccated thyroid has been in use for over 127 years, representing the SOLE thyroid medication available from 1891 until 1955 (64 years), after which Synthroid entered the marketplace. One hundred twenty seven years of use for any drug is a very long track record attesting to safety and efficacy.

Reading the Comment Section

To give you an idea of the typical results we see every week prescribing NDT, read one of the comments by CM below Dr. Angela Leung's article on Medscape:

For over 15 years of treatment for hypothyroidism with various T4 medications, I complained about the continuation of hypothyroid symptoms, only to be told that my blood work was just fine. I finally found a doctor that was open to treating me with desiccated thyroid medication, and it completely changed my life. All of my symptoms have resolved. If patients speak, please listen and be opened minded enough to try a different medication instead of treating the lab values and not the patient. There are many people that have and would benefit from desiccated thyroid. Endquote Comment by CM in the comment section for (1)

Note: in the above comment, there is no mention of a problem with the NDT T4:T3 ratio, which is 4:1.

My Mom, First Thyroid Patient

My first thyroid patient, about 20 years ago, was a 70-year-old female on Synthroid for 50 years since her total thyroidectomy for a "benign cyst" at age 20. An operation, which in retrospect, was probably unnecessary. Three weeks after switching her to NDT, natural desiccated thyroid, she came back into the office, threw up her hands, and exclaimed:

> I feel so much better! Why hasn't any other doctor done this for me before?

This was my mom. My very first thyroid patient was my mother. Over the years, these results are routine when switching from T4 monotherapy to NDT, natural desiccated thyroid.

Natural Desiccated Thyroid – 6 Problems

Although NDT has stood the test of time as a good combination of T4/T3 therapy, we must remember that nothing is perfect. To be fair, let us review six problems with NDT, courtesy of Weston Childs in his article, "Six problems with NDT. " Dr. Weston Childs writes:

1) Changing formula. The formula may change from time to time, mostly involving the fillers. However, this may affect the absorption and potency of the final product.

2) Backlogs. Manufacturers may encounter problems with production which may cause backlogs making the product difficult to obtain. Local pharmacies may not carry the product when this happens. This may be related to the scarcity of raw materials for the factory or interruption of manufacturing during the transition to a newer, larger manufacturing facility.

3) Ratio of T3 to T4 in NDT is fixed at 1:4. Rarely, a patient may require a different ratio of T3 to T4.

4) Sensitive to T3 component. Some patients are hypersensitive to T3 and react with transient symptoms of thyroid excess after each dose. (These are rapid heart rate, tachycardia, anxiety, panic attack, loose stools, etc.)

5) Allergies. Rarely a patient will find they are allergic to a component in natural desiccated thyroid.

6) Under-Dosing. Most doctors do not routinely prescribe natural desiccated thyroid. If you are able to convince your doctor to prescribe it for you, they may commonly make the error of under-dosing. (8)

Conclusion

There is no question the winds of medicine are changing in endocrinology regarding dogmatic insistence on T4 monotherapy. However, in medicine, the wheels of change turn slowly, so I would not hold my breath waiting for the local friendly endocrinologist to change their prescribing practices anytime soon. Thank goodness for that, since otherwise, I would have nothing to do! (9-26)

♦ **References for Chapter 8**

1) Leung, Angela M. The Love-Hate Relationship with Levothyroxine. Medscape. October 25, 2018 https://www.medscape.com/viewarticle/903788

2) Slater, Stefan. "The Discovery of Thyroid Replacement Therapy. Part 3: A Complete Transformation." Journal of the Royal Society of Medicine 104.3 (2011): 100-106.

3) Toloza, Freddy JK, et al. "Patient Experiences and Perceptions Associated with the Use of Desiccated Thyroid Extract." Medicina 56.4 (2020): 161.

4) Sapin, R., and J. L. Schlienger. "Thyroxine (T4) and Tri-Iodothyronine (T3) Determinations: Techniques and Value in the Assessment of Thyroid Function." Annales De Biologie Clinique. Vol. 61. No. 4. 2003.

5) Taylor, Peter N., et al. "Combination Thyroid Hormone Replacement; Knowns and Unknowns." Frontiers in Endocrinology (2019): 706.

6) Dayan, Colin, and Vijay Panicker. "Management of Hypothyroidism with Combination Thyroxine (T4) and Triiodothyronine (T3) Hormone Replacement in Clinical Practice: A Review of Suggested Guidance." Thyroid Research 11.1 (2018): 1-11.

7) Wiersinga, Wilmar M., et al. "2012 ETA Guidelines: The Use Of L-T4+ L-T3 in the Treatment of Hypothyroidism." European Thyroid Journal 1.2 (2012): 55-71

8) Six Problems with Natural Desiccated Thyroid Hormone by Westin Childs, DO. https://www.restartmed.com/6-problems-with-natural-desiccated-thyroid-hormone/

9) Jonklaas, Jacqueline, et al. "Guidelines for The Treatment of Hypothyroidism: Prepared by the American Thyroid Association Task Force on Thyroid Hormone Replacement." Thyroid 24.12 (2014): 1670-1751.

10) Gereben, Balázs, et al. "Scope and Limitations of Iodothyronine Deiodinases in Hypothyroidism." Nature Reviews Endocrinology 11.11 (2015): 642-652.

11) Lum, S. M., et al. "Peripheral Tissue Mechanism for Maintenance of Serum Triiodothyronine Values in a Thyroxine-Deficient State in Man." The Journal of Clinical Investigation 73.2 (1984): 570-575.

12) Wouters, Hanneke JCM, et al. "No Effect of the Thr92Ala Polymorphism of Deiodinase-2 on Thyroid Hormone Parameters, Health-Related Quality of Life, and Cognitive Functioning in a Large Population-Based Cohort Study." Thyroid 27.2 (2017): 147-155.

13) Butler, Peter W., et al. "The Thr92Ala 5' Type 2 Deiodinase Gene Polymorphism is Associated with a Delayed Triiodothyronine Secretion in Response to the Thyrotropin-Releasing Hormone–Stimulation Test: A Pharmacogenomic Study." Thyroid 20.12 (2010): 1407-1412.

14) Bianco, Antonio C., and Brian S. Kim. "Pathophysiological Relevance of Deiodinase Polymorphism." Current Opinion in Endocrinology, Diabetes, and Obesity 25.5 (2018): 341.

15) Garber, Jeffrey R., et al. "Clinical Practice Guidelines for Hypothyroidism in Adults: Cosponsored by the American Association of Clinical Endocrinologists and the American Thyroid Association." Thyroid 22.12 (2012): 1200-1235.

16) Medicines Use and Spending in the U.S. A Review Of 2016 and Outlook to 2021. IQVIA Institute for Human Data Science. May 4, 2017. Source Accessed October 15, 2018.

17) Hennessey, James V. "Historical and Current Perspective in the Use of Thyroid Extracts for the Treatment of Hypothyroidism." Endocrine Practice 21.10 (2015): 1161-1170.

18) Samuels, Mary H., et al. "Effects of Altering Levothyroxine (L-T4) Doses on Quality of Life, Mood, and Cognition in L-T4 Treated Subjects." The Journal of Clinical Endocrinology and Metabolism 103.5 (2018): 1997-2008.

19) Leung, Angela M. "Levothyroxine Dose Adjustment Resulting in Mild Variations of Serum TSH Levels Within or Near the Normal Range Has No Effect on Quality of Life, Mood, and Cognition in Hypothyroid Individuals." Clinical Thyroidology 30.6 (2018): 263-265.

20) Peterson, Sarah J., et al. "An Online Survey of Hypothyroid Patients Demonstrates Prominent Dissatisfaction." Thyroid 28.6 (2018): 707-721.

21) Stevens EW, Leung AM. "A Patient Survey of Hypothyroid Individuals Demonstrates Dissatisfaction with Treatment and with Managing Physicians." Clin Thyroidol. 2018; 30:175-178.

22) Hoang TD, et al. "Desiccated Thyroid Extract Compared with Levothyroxine in the Treatment of Hypothyroidism: A Randomized, Double-Blind, Crossover Study." J Clin Endocrinol Metab. 2013; 98:1982-1990. Abstract

23) Alexander, Erik K., et al. "2017 Guidelines of the American Thyroid Association for the Diagnosis and Management of Thyroid Disease During Pregnancy and the Postpartum." Thyroid 27.3 (2017): 315-389.

24) Wiersinga WM, et al. "2012 ETA Guidelines: The Use Of L-T4 + L-T3 In the Treatment of Hypothyroidism." Eur Thyroid J. 2012; 1:55-71.

25) McAninch, Elizabeth A., and Antonio C. Bianco. "The Swinging Pendulum in Treatment for Hypothyroidism: From (And Toward?) Combination Therapy." Frontiers in Endocrinology (2019): 446.

26) Hennessey, James V. "Historical and Current Perspective in the Use of Thyroid Extracts for the Treatment of Hypothyroidism." Endocrine Practice 21.10 (2015): 1161-1170.

Chapter 9

Which Thyroid is Best, Natural, Synthetic, or Combination?

SUSAN IS A 42-YEAR-OLD PROFESSOR of Literature at the local liberal arts college. Susan was crying in my office as she told her story of frustration. About four years ago, she was treated with radioactive iodine, a form of thyroid ablation for Graves' Disease. Susan now requires lifelong thyroid replacement. After seeing four different endocrinologists who prescribed four different doses of thyroid medication, Susan is still unhappy with her treatment. The last endocrinologist prescribed 175 mcg of levothyroxine, and Susan's TSH is suppressed down to a very low 0.01 mIU/L. However, Susan continues to suffer chronic fatigue, depression, weight gain, foggy thinking, and constipation, all typical symptoms of a low thyroid condition.

T4 Only Medication Cannot Guarantee Euthyroid State.

T4 medication, levothyroxine, is a prohormone and must be converted to its active form, T3. This is done by the D1 and D2 deiodinase enzyme system inside our cells which converts T4 to T3. The endocrinologist assumes levothyroxine (T4-only) is converted to T3 by the peripheral tissues at the proper rate to produce normal thyroid levels. This assumption is incorrect, as shown by studies in Dr. Antonio Bianco's laboratory at Rush Medical Center. The paradigm shift in thyroid endocrinology is understanding the deiodinase enzyme system controls the conversion of T4 to T3 at the cellular level. The deiodinase control of T3 has been ignored by mainstream endocrinology, leading to several errors, one of which is the dogmatic perpetuation of T4-monotherapy. (1-7)

Defective T4 to T3 Conversion

In 2011, Dr. Damiano Gullo from Italy reported T4 to T3 conversion is defective in about 20% of patients treated with levothyroxine (T4 monotherapy) after thyroid ablation (athyreotic patients). Dr. Gullo writes:

> Athyreotic patients have a highly heterogeneous T3 production capacity from orally administered levothyroxine. More than 20% of these patients, despite normal TSH levels, do not maintain FT3 or FT4 values in the reference range, reflecting the inadequacy of peripheral deiodination to compensate for the absent T3 secretion. A more physiological treatment than levothyroxine monotherapy may be required in some hypothyroid patients. (8-9)

Indeed, Susan's labs showed a high normal Free T4 of 1.6 ng/dL and a low normal Free T3 of 240 ng/dL, indicating poor conversion of T4 to T3, "reflecting the inadequacy of peripheral deiodination to compensate for the absent T3 secretion". Several animal studies have been done to answer why peripheral conversion of T4 to T3 is reduced. (8)

T4 – Monotherapy Explained

The key to understanding the failings of T4-monotherapy lies with the D2 deiodinase enzyme system, which resides in our cells and plucks an iodine molecule off T4, converting it to T3, the active form of the hormone. In a 2013 report, Dr. Antonio Bianco writes this intracellular D2 deiodinase enzyme system is the master controller for thyroid levels. Knowledge of the deiodinase system creates a new paradigm in our understanding of thyroid function:

Thyroid hormone–responsive metabolic

processes are turned on and off by thyroid hormone via deiodination pathways that are taking place inside the target cells, seemingly invisible from the plasma viewpoint... deiodination supports a new paradigm in which hormones are activated or inactivated in a controlled fashion in specific thyroid hormone-target tissues. (3)

D2 in the Pituitary (Centrally) Acts Differently from D2 in Periphery

According to a 2015 animal study by Dr. De Castro, the D2 deiodinase enzyme system in the pituitary acts differently from the D2 in the peripheral tissues. In the peripheral tissues, D2 is inactivated by T4. High T4 levels inactivate D2 deiodinase as a safety mechanism to protect the cells from local hyperthyroidism. Elevated T4 levels inactivate the D2 enzyme in the peripheral tissues, thereby preventing the conversion of T4 to its active form, T3.

However, the D2 in the hypothalamus and pituitary is **a different type that is not inactivated by T4**. In the hypothalamus and pituitary, the abundant T4 in circulation is promptly converted to intracellular T3, which then suppresses the TSH to low levels. This results in the pattern we see with Susan's labs, relatively higher serum T4 and relatively lower serum T3. In the periphery, cells are starved of T3 because of the inactivation of the D2 enzyme by T4, thus inhibiting the conversion of T4 to T3 in the peripheral tissues. In his mouse study, Dr. De Castro found that only constant infusion of both T4 and T3 normalized thyroid levels. Dr. De Castro writes:

> in contrast to other D2-expressing tissues, the hypothalamus is wired to have increased sensitivity to T4... only constant delivery of L-T4 and L-T3 fully normalizes T3 -dependent metabolic markers and gene expression profiles in thyroidectomized rats. (4)

Levothyroxine Suppresses TSH, While Leaving Periphery in Hypothyroid State

In most tissues, exposure to T4 inactivates the D2 deiodinase, which decreases the conversion of T4 to T3 and decreases the peripheral production of T3. Similarly, this also occurs in the brain, where the elevated serum T4/T3 ratio results in hypothyroid brain cells. However, the exception to this rule is the hypothalamus, where the D2 deiodinase is less susceptible to T4-induced inactivation. This means levothyroxine T4 monotherapy suppresses TSH. However, in the periphery, T4 conversion to T3 via D2 is inhibited by T4, creating a hypothyroid state. This explains the findings in thyroidectomized mice in which T4 treatment normalizes TSH, yet there is reduced peripheral T3. **This also explains the failings of Susan's T4-only monotherapy with levothyroxine which suppresses her TSH while leaving the peripheral tissues in a hypothyroid state.** (1-9)

Combination Treatment with T3 andT4

If T4 monotherapy leads to cellular hypothyroidism in the periphery, while the TSH is suppressed centrally, what is the solution? Combined therapy with both T3 and T4 may resolve this problem. The past dogmatic insistence on T4 monotherapy seems to be changing as more and more endocrinologists are embracing a combination of T3 and T4 therapy. In 2014, Dr. Wilmar Wiersinga writes:

> Levothyroxine plus liothyronine [generic Cytomel, T3] combination therapy is gaining in popularity....in some of the 14 published trials; this combination was definitely preferred by patients and associated with improved metabolic profiles. (1)

In 1995 and 1996, Dr. Escobar studied thyroidectomized mice and found that T3 and T4 levels could not be normalized with T4 monotherapy alone. Rather, a steady infusion of both drugs, T3 and T4, was needed to maintain a euthyroid state. In addition, a number of human studies show that patients prefer combination therapy. (9-10)

Adverse Effects of Thyroid Pills

Adverse effects of thyroid excess are similar for all three types of thyroid medication, levothyroxine, NDT, and combination therapy with T3 and T4. Rapid heart rate at rest (tachycardia) is the symptom we are most concerned about. The patient is instructed to watch for this symptom and hold the thyroid pill if this is noted. Other symptoms of thyroid excess to watch out for include anxiety, insomnia, and loose stools. Although these side effects are identical for NDT and levothyroxine, their half-lives are quite different. For the T3 component of NDT, the half-life is 24 hours. For T4, the half-life is one week. This means a more rapid resolution of symptoms within 6 hours when holding the NDT dose when compared to levothyroxine which may take a week for symptoms to abate. (11-12)

Which type of thyroid pill do you prefer?

1. Synthetic T4 and T3. Mainstream endocrinology uses levothyroxine (T4) combined with Cytomel (T3) in a ratio of (12:1).

2. T4 plus a slow-release compounded T3 to avoid supraphysiologic dosing of T3, which peaks 2 hours after ingestion.

3. NDT, Natural Desiccated Thyroid, which contains T4:T3 in the ratio of 4:1.

4. NDT plus T4 levothyroxine. Some patients prefer a 12:1 ratio of T4 to T3, so adding an appropriate dose of T4 to NDT will do the trick.

Here is a sample dosing schedule:
One Grain tablet of NDT provides 9 mcg of T3 and 38 mcg of T4. Add another 75 mcg of levothyroxine (T4) to obtain the desired T4:T3 ratio of (113: 9) = (12.5:1). We have found a few patients after thyroid ablation may prefer adding T4 to obtain this combination.

Option 1) Combined T3 and T4 (Levothyroxine and Cytomel)

Dr. Colin Dayan discusses this option in 2018 Thyroid Research. Dr. Dayan prefers a T4:T3 ratio of (14:1) because this matches the secretion rate of the thyroid gland. In 2018, Dr. Dayan writes:

> The doses [for NDT] give a T4:T3 ratio of 4.2:1, significantly more T3 than the 14:1 secreted by the normal thyroid and the doses recommended above. This makes dosing difficult, as displayed by several studies which have shown supraphysiological T3 doses post-dose, fluctuating T3 levels during the day, and more hyperthyroid symptoms in subjects taking DTE compared to LT4 monotherapy... Furthermore, it has also been shown that the majority of circulating T3 comes from peripheral conversion of T4 to T3 and not secretion of T3 from the thyroid, hence a T4:T3 secretion ratio of approximately 14:1 appears average in humans, suggesting only a small role for secreted T3...Practicing clinicians will be able to identify a group of patients not satisfied on LT4 monotherapy which makes up a small subset of all their patients on LT4.... Both ATA and ETA suggest that in an appropriate clinical setting (see below), combination therapy may be trialed to determine if it is beneficial for the individual patient.... despite recommendations and guidelines from various specialist bodies, the use of combination T4/T3 therapy appears significant in most developed countries. (13)

Dr. Colin Dayan's routine is to give T3 (liothyronine, generic Cytomel) to a patient already on "adequate LT4 monotherapy" (usually 75-150 mcg levothyroxine) yet still having symptoms of hypothyroidism. Dr. Dayan will then remove some of the T4 dose (usually 50-75 mcg of T4) and replace it with (5 – 20) mcg of T3. Usually, generic Cytomel (Liothyronine) in a split dose is given twice a day to avoid or reduce "supraphysiologic dosing."

Option 2 Slow Release T3

Dr. Martin Milner describes his routine using compounded slow-release T3 in his article in the 2005 Townsend Letter. In order to avoid supraphysiologic dosing with T3, Dr. Milner suggests using slow-release compounded T3. (14-15)

Option 3: Synthetic T3 and T4 Combination

Which T4:T3 Ratio do You Prefer, 14:1 or 4:1? As mentioned above, a major objection to NDT, (natural desiccated thyroid) is the T4:T3 ratio, which is 4:1, providing a much larger T3 bolus compared to the 14: 1 ratio (T4:T3) ratio discussed by Dr. Colin Dayan in his 2018 article. (13)

Others, such as Dr. Martin Milner, disagree and prefer to use the 4:1 (T4:T3) ratio commonly found in NDT. Perhaps Dr. Milner is right since this 4:1 (T4:T3) ratio is closer to the serum (T4:T3) ratio for the average patient, which is 3.3:1. Dr. Jernej Grmek, in the 2015 Slovenian Medical Journal, studied the free thyroxine to free triiodothyronine ratios (FT4:FT3) in 225 patients, reporting this mean ratio was 2.86 ± 0.52.(41) This discrepancy between serum T4:T3 (3.3:1) ratio and secreted T4:T3 (14:1) ratio can be explained by the fact that 80% (most) of our T3 comes from peripheral conversion of T4 to T3 via the intra-cellular D1 deiodinase enzyme. Of the circulating Free T3, only 20 % comes from thyroid secretion, the remaining 80% from peripheral conversion of T4 to T3 via the D1 de-iodinase enzyme. (13-16)

5:1 Ratio Combination T4:T3 Wins the Contest

in 2005, Dr. Bente Appelhof studied two different T4:T3 synthetic combination ratios, 5:1 and 10:1 ratio, and compared them to T4 monotherapy in a randomized, double-blind study of 141 patients with Hashimoto's hypothyroidism. About 47 patients were randomized to each treatment group, T4 monotherapy, 5:1 combination, and lastly, 10:1 combination

therapy. **The patients most preferred the 5:1 ratio.** Please note this T4:T3 (5:1) ratio synthetic combination most closely approximates the 4:1 ratio found in NDT Natural Desiccated Thyroid. (17)

Which Thyroid Pill is Best, Synthetic Combination or NDT?

In 2018 Dr. Anam Tariq from Johns Hopkins examined this question. Dr. Tariq performed a retrospective observational study of 100 patients from an endocrinology clinic in Pennsylvania over six years, comparing T4 monotherapy to synthetic T3, T4 combination therapy, and NDT, natural desiccated thyroid. Patients on T4 monotherapy for a year who continued to complain of hypothyroid symptoms were candidates for combination therapy. The starting dose for T3 was:

> 5 micrograms [T3 per day] in conjunction with an appropriate decrease of 12.5 micrograms in LT4 to achieve the standard physiological circulating FT4:FT3 ratio of nearly 14:1. (18)

The maximum dose of T3 was 12.5 mcg. For NDT, the starting dose was 15 mg (quarter grain), and then titrated up. The T4:T3 ratio was, of course, 4:1 for NDT. The authors also checked and optimized all patients' B12 and Vitamin D levels.

The average dose of DTE (NDT) was 30 mg. The average LT4/LT3 dose was 75 µg/5 µg to obtain physiologic thyroid levels. Fifty-two percent had Hashimoto's disease, 22% had surgical hypothyroidism, 10% had ablation for either Graves' disease or thyroid cancer, and 16% had miscellaneous etiologies.

I found it remarkable that the mean TSH for all treated patients was in the 1.8 to 1.9 mIU/L range, regardless of what combination of thyroid medication was used. Likewise, the Free T3 and Free T4 levels were remarkably similar across all treatment modalities. The adverse effects of synthetic combination therapy were:

6.7% of the 100 patients complained of palpitations and anxiety and had confirmed TSH <0.35 µIU/mL without atrial arrhythmias. (18)

Many patients reported feeling better on combination therapy (NDT or Synthetic T3, T4) compared to levothyroxine monotherapy. Both combination therapies seemed equally safe and effective. The authors conclude:

> Combination therapy of LT4 and LT3 has remained an experimental treatment that can be used at the physician's discretion. Our observational study concludes that for a subset of patients who feels suboptimal on LT4 monotherapy, synthetic therapy [LT4 and LT3] is beneficial and safe in controlling hypothyroid symptoms and improving quality of life. (18)

Genetic Mutations in the D2 Deiodinase

As mentioned above, the D2 deiodinase enzyme is the control mechanism for the tissue-level conversion of T4 to T3. What if the patient harbors a polymorphism, a mutation, in the D2 deiodinase gene? Will this affect the T4 to T3 peripheral conversion ability? And, if so, would these patients prefer combination therapy? Dr. Allan Carle says yes, of course. In 2017, Dr. Carle studied 45 autoimmune hypothyroid patients on levothyroxine using genetic analysis of the D2 gene. 60 percent of patients harboring D2 gene polymorphisms preferred combination therapy with both T3 and T4. If two SNPs (single nucleotide polymorphisms) were present, all of these (100%) patients preferred combination therapy. (6-7) (19-22)

Major Objection to NDT – High Peak T3 levels

Mainstream endocrinology's major objection and reason for rejecting NDT is the high T3 peak for a few hours after ingesting the thyroid pill. However, this argument also applies to combination therapy with levothyroxine and generic Cytomel (liothyronine), which has recently become acceptable for mainstream endocrinologists. In 2012, Dr. Wiersinga writes about the combination of T4 and T3 therapy:

> It is suggested to start combination therapy in an L-T4/L-T3 dose ratio between 13:1 and 20:1 by weight (L-T4 once daily and the daily L-T3 dose in two doses). Currently, available combined preparations all have an L-T4/L-T3 dose ratio of less than 13:1 and are not recommended. (23)

This argument seems rather vacuous since many patients do well with NDT, which contains a T4:T3 ratio of 4:1. In addition, many patients do well on synthetic combination T4 and T3 with the 5:1 ratio as described above by Dr. Bente Appelhof in 2005. This is very similar and essentially the same ratio found in NDT, natural desiccated thyroid, which is 4:1. If one objects to the T3 in NDT, then one must object equally to T3 in synthetic combinations used by conventional endocrinologists. The reality is that many patients do well on both. (17)

Back to the Patient

Susan was switched to NDT, natural desiccated thyroid, starting with half a grain daily and gradually increasing the dosage by half a grain weekly increment until reaching a maintenance dose of 3 grains a day. Susan's thyroid labs at 3 grains showed a suppressed TSH of 0.25 mIU/L, and both the serum T3 and T4 were in the normal range. Serum T3 was 320 ng/dL, and serum T4 was 1.1 ng/dL. More importantly, Susan was now feeling back to her normal self with the resolution of hypothyroid symptoms and no adverse effects of thyroid excess. Note: Blood testing is done while fasting early in the AM, near the opening time for the blood draw station. The patient is instructed to hold the AM thyroid medication until after the blood draw.

Conclusion

Of the 7% of the population suffering from hypothyroidism, most will do well on T4-only thyroid medication such as levothyroxine with the local endocrinologist. However, a subset

(20%) of these patients will continue to suffer from low thyroid symptoms despite being on levothyroxine. These will feel better on a combination of T3 and T4, synthetic T3 and T4 at their local endocrinologist or NDT, natural desiccated thyroid used by integrative medical practitioners. The 5:1 or 4:1 ratio of T4 to T3 is preferred. However, a smaller subset of patients will prefer the 12:1 ratio, which can be obtained by adding T4 to NDT or a synthetic combination of T4 and T3 in the proper ratio. (24-47)

♦ **References for Chapter 9**

1) Wiersinga, Wilmar M. "Paradigm Shifts in Thyroid Hormone Replacement Therapies for Hypothyroidism." Nature Reviews Endocrinology 10.3 (2014): 164.

2) Abdalla, Sherine M., and Antonio C. Bianco. "Defending Plasma T3 is a Biological Priority." Clinical Endocrinology 81.5 (2014): 633-641.

3) Bianco, Antonio C. "Cracking the Code for Thyroid Hormone Signaling." Transactions of the American Clinical and Climatological Association 124 (2013): 26.

4) De Castro, Joao Pedro Werneck, et al. "Differences in Hypothalamic Type 2 Deiodinase Ubiquitination Explain Localized Sensitivity to Thyroxine." The Journal of Clinical Investigation 125.2 (2015): 769.

5) Bianco, Antonio C., and Brian W. Kim. "Deiodinases: Implications of the Local Control of Thyroid Hormone Action." Journal of Clinical Investigation 116.10 (2006): 2571.

6) Jo, Sungro, et al. "Type 2 Deiodinase Polymorphism Causes ER Stress and Hypothyroidism in the Brain." The Journal of Clinical Investigation 129.1 (2019): 230-245.

7) Wang, Xichang, et al. "The Type 2 Deiodinase Thr92Ala Polymorphism is Associated with Higher Body Mass Index and Fasting Glucose Levels: A Systematic Review and Meta-Analysis." BioMed Research International 2021 (2021).

8) Gullo, Damiano, et al. "Levothyroxine Monotherapy Cannot Guarantee Euthyroidism in All Athyreotic Patients." PLoS One 6.8 (2011): e22552.

9) Escobar-Morreale, Hector F., et al. "Replacement Therapy for Hypothyroidism with Thyroxine Alone Does Not Ensure Euthyroidism in All Tissues, as Studied in Thyroidectomized Rats." The Journal of Clinical Investigation 96.6 (1995): 2828-2838.

10) Escobar-Morreale, Héctor F., et al. "Only the Combined Treatment with Thyroxine and Triiodothyronine Ensures Euthyroidism in all Tissues of the Thyroidectomized Rat." Endocrinology 137.6 (1996): 2490-2502.

11) Colucci, Philippe, et al. "A Review of the Pharmacokinetics of Levothyroxine for the Treatment of Hypothyroidism." European Endocrinology 9.1 (2013): 40.

12) Jonklaas, Jacqueline, et al. "Single Dose T3 Administration: Kinetics and Effects on Biochemical and Physiologic Parameters." Therapeutic Drug Monitoring 37.1 (2015): 110.

13) Dayan, Colin, and Vijay Panicker. "Management of Hypothyroidism with Combination Thyroxine (T4) and Triiodothyronine (T3) Hormone Replacement in Clinical Practice: A Review of Suggested Guidance." Thyroid Research 11.1 (2018): 1.

14) Milner, Martin. "Hypothyroidism: Optimizing Medication with Slow-Release Compounded Thyroid Replacement." International Journal of Pharmaceutical Compounding 9.4 (2005): 268.

15) Milner, Martin. "Hypothyroidism: Optimizing Medication with Slow-Release Compounded Thyroid Replacement." Townsend Letter: The Exam

16) Grmek, Jernej, et al. "Usefulness of Free Thyroxine to Free Triiodothyronine Ratio for Diagnostics of Various Types of Hyperthyroidism." Slovenian Medical Journal 84.5 (2015).

17) Appelhof, Bente C., et al. "Combined Therapy with Levothyroxine and Liothyronine in Two Ratios, Compared with Levothyroxine Monotherapy in Primary Hypothyroidism: A Double-Blind, Randomized, Controlled Clinical Trial." The Journal of Clinical Endocrinology & Metabolism 90.5 (2005): 2666-2674.

18) Tariq, Anam, et al. "Effects of Long-Term Combination LT4 and LT3 Therapy for Improving Hypothyroidism and Overall Quality of Life." Southern Medical Journal 111.6 (2018): 363.

19) Carlé, Allan, et al. "Hypothyroid Patients Encoding Combined MCT10 And DIO2 Gene Polymorphisms May Prefer L-T3+ L-T4 Combination Treatment–Data Using a Blind, Randomized, Clinical Study." European Thyroid Journal 6.3 (2017): 143-151.

20) Ahmed, Ziyan, et al. "Improvement of Treatment-Resistant Depression in a Patient with Primary Hypothyroidism and Thr92Ala5'Type 2 Deiodinase Gene Polymorphism with Multiple Daily Doses of Triiodothyronine." Journal of the Endocrine Society 5. Supplement_1 (2021): A937-A937.

21) Panicker, Vijay, et al. "Common Variation in The DIO2 Gene Predicts Baseline Psychological Well-Being and Response to Combination Thyroxine Plus Triiodothyronine Therapy in Hypothyroid Patients." The Journal of Clinical Endocrinology & Metabolism 94.5 (2009): 1623-1629.

22) Ahmed, Ziyan S., et al. "Improvement of Depression in a Patient with Hypothyroidism and Deiodinase Polymorphism with LT3 Therapy." Clinical Case Reports 10.4 (2022): e05651.

23) Wiersinga, Wilmar M., et al. "2012 ETA Guidelines: The Use Of L-T4+ L-T3 in the Treatment of Hypothyroidism." European Thyroid Journal 1.2 (2012): 55-71.

24) Surks, Martin I., et al. "A New Radioimmunoassay for Plasma L-Triiodothyronine: Measurements In Thyroid Disease and in Patients Maintained On Hormonal Replacement." The Journal of Clinical Investigation 51.12 (1972): 3104-3113.

25) Hoang, Thanh D., et al. "Desiccated Thyroid Extract Compared with Levothyroxine in the Treatment of Hypothyroidism: A Randomized, Double-Blind, Crossover Study." The Journal of Clinical Endocrinology & Metabolism 98.5 (2013): 1982-1990.

26) Biondi, Bernadette, and Leonard Wartofsky. "Combination Treatment with T4 and T3: Toward Personalized Replacement Therapy in Hypothyroidism?" The Journal of Clinical Endocrinology & Metabolism 97.7 (2012): 2256-2271.

27) Snyder, Scott. "Bioidentical Thyroid Replacement Therapy in Practice: Delivering a Physiologic T4:T3 Ratio for Improved Patient Outcomes with the Listecki-Snyder Protocol." Int J Pharm Compd 16 (2012): 376-380.

28) Kotwal, Anupam, and Donald SA McLeod. "Role of Levothyroxine/Liothyronine Combinations in Treating Hypothyroidism." Endocrinology and Metabolism Clinics of North America 51.2 (2022): 243-263.

29) Schmidt, Ulla, et al. "Peripheral Markers of Thyroid Function: The Effect of T4 Monotherapy Versus T4/T3 Combination Therapy in Hypothyroid Subjects in a Randomized Cross-Over Study." Endocrine connections (2013): EC-12.

30) Benvenga, Salvatore. "When Thyroid Hormone Replacement Is Ineffective?" Current Opinion in Endocrinology, Diabetes, and Obesity 20.5 (2013): 467-477.

31) Samuels, Mary H., et al. "The Effects of Levothyroxine Replacement or Suppressive Therapy on Health Status, Mood, And Cognition." The Journal of Clinical Endocrinology and Metabolism 99.3 (2014): 843.

32) Hennemann, G., et al. "Thyroxine Plus Low-Dose, Slow-Release Triiodothyronine Replacement in Hypothyroidism: Proof of Principle." Thyroid 14.4 (2004): 271-275.

33) Escobar-Morreale, Hector F., et al. "Treatment of Hypothyroidism with Combinations of Levothyroxine Plus Liothyronine." The Journal of Clinical Endocrinology & Metabolism 90.8 (2005): 4946-4954.

34) Escobar-Morreale, Héctor F., et al. "Thyroid Hormone Replacement Therapy in Primary Hypothyroidism: A Randomized Trial Comparing L-Thyroxine Plus Liothyronine with L-Thyroxine Alone." Annals of Internal Medicine 142.6 (2005): 412-424.

35) Ling, C., et al. "Does TSH Reliably Detect Hypothyroid Patients?" Annals of Thyroid Research 4.1 (2018): 122.

36) Saravanan, Ponnusamy, et al. "Partial Substitution of Thyroxine (T4) with Tri-Iodothyronine in Patients on T4 Replacement Therapy: Results of a Large Community-Based Randomized Controlled Trial." The Journal of Clinical Endocrinology & Metabolism 90.2 (2005): 805-812.

37) Braverman, Lewis E., et al. "Effects of Replacement Doses of Sodium-L-Thyroxine on the Peripheral Metabolism of Thyroxine and Triiodothyronine in Man." The Journal of Clinical Investigation 52.5 (1973): 1010-1017.

38) Desouza, Lynette A., et al. "Thyroid Hormone Regulates Hippocampal Neurogenesis in The Adult Rat Brain." Molecular and Cellular Neuroscience 29.3 (2005): 414-426.

39) Montero-Pedrazuela, Ana, et al. "Modulation of Adult Hippocampal Neurogenesis by Thyroid Hormones: Implications in Depressive-Like Behavior." Molecular Psychiatry 11.4 (2006): 361.

40) Burmeister, Lynn A., et. al. "Thyroid Hormones Inhibit Type 2 Iodothyronine Deiodinase in the Rat Cerebral Cortex by Both Pre- and Posttranslational Mechanisms." Endocrinology 138.12 (1997): 5231-5237.

41) Beard, John L., et al. "Plasma Thyroid Hormone Kinetics Are Altered in Iron-Deficient Rats." The Journal of Nutrition 128.8 (1998): 1401-1408.

42) Martínez-Iglesias, Olaia, et al. "Hypothyroidism Enhances Tumor Invasiveness and Metastasis Development." PLoS one 4.7 (2009): e6428.2017

43) Jonklaas, Jacqueline. "Persistent Hypothyroid Symptoms in a Patient with a Normal Thyroid Stimulating Hormone Level." Current Opinion in Endocrinology, diabetes, and obesity 24.5 (2017): 356.

44) Hennessey, James V., and Ramon Espaillat. "Current Evidence for the Treatment of Hypothyroidism with Levothyroxine/Levotriiodothyronine Combination Therapy Versus Levothyroxine Monotherapy." International Journal of Clinical Practice 72.2 (2018): e13062.

45) Peterson, S. J., et al. "An Online Survey of Hypothyroid Patients Demonstrates Prominent Dissatisfaction." Thyroid: Official Journal of the American Thyroid Association (2018).

46) Wiersinga, W. M. "Therapy of Endocrine Disease: T4 + T3 Combination Therapy: Is There a True Effect?" European Journal of Endocrinology 177.6 (2017): R287.

47) Hannoush, Zeina C., and Roy E. Weiss. "Thyroid Hormone Replacement in Patients Following Thyroidectomy for Thyroid Cancer." Rambam Maimonides Medical Journal 7.1 (2016).

Chapter 10

The Unreliable TSH Lab Test

A Woman with a Low Thyroid Condition

SUZY IS A 59-YEAR-OLD POST-MENOPAUSAL woman with low thyroid function. About three months ago, she started her bio-identical hormone program and NDT, natural desiccated thyroid. After starting the program, she was doing well with more energy, better sleep, improved appearance of skin and hair, and resolution of her menopausal symptoms of hot flashes and sweats. However, about 12 weeks into her program, Suzy visited her primary care doctor, who did a follow-up thyroid panel. Her primary care doctor informed Suzy that her TSH test result was below the normal lab range; therefore, her thyroid dose was too high and should be reduced. (Note: TSH is Thyroid Stimulating Hormone made by the pituitary gland, not the thyroid gland).

Too Many Cooks Spoil the Soup

Suzy called me at the office, distraught and confused. Two doctors were telling her two different things, and she did not know whom to believe. Her primary care doctor was telling her one thing, and I was telling her another. I explained to Suzy that her primary care doctor was incorrect in relying slavishly on the TSH test. Even though her TSH test was 0.15 mU/L which is below the lab reference range of 0.3 mU/L, this was perfectly acceptable and indicated her thyroid medicine was suppressing the TSH to a low level which was perfectly fine. This test interpretation means she is taking thyroid pills, and the pills are working. It does not mean she is "hyperthyroid" by any stretch of the imagination.

No Clinical Evidence of Thyrotoxicosis

I also informed Suzy that her primary care doctor is mistakenly relying on the TSH test to determine her thyroid dosage. The TSH test is an indirect measure of thyroid function and can be unreliable in monitoring thyroid dosage. A more accurate indicator of thyroid function is the Free T3, which in her case was 375 pg/mL, well within the normal range of 240 to 420 pg/mL. The Free T4 was 1.2 ng/dl, also normal. The Free T3 and Free T4 lab tests, together with the absence of any signs or symptoms of thyroid excess, indicate the patient is taking the proper dosage. What are the symptoms of thyroid excess we are looking for? These are the symptoms of resting tachycardia, rapid heartbeat, or palpitations, and Suzy reported no such symptoms. In fact, Suzy said she felt fine, and now that she understands it, she did not want to go back to feeling tired or sluggish before she started the thyroid pills. Suzy was relieved that the low TSH result was perfectly acceptable, and there was nothing to worry about. This kind of TSH discussion is a recurring event at my office.

Conventional Docs Slavishly Rely on the TSH Test

The thyroid laboratory panel used by conventional primary care doctors is limited to the TSH and Free T4. They usually do not do the Free T3, the most informative thyroid lab test. Instead, mainstream endocrinology relies on the TSH test, which is not a direct measure of thyroid function and can, in fact, be unreliable. The TSH is not made by the thyroid gland; it is made by the pituitary, a small gland at the end of a stalk at the base of the brain sitting within a bony landmark called the sella turcica.

Most conventional doctors are unfamiliar with the use of NDT, natural desiccated thyroid, which contains both T3 and T4, and instead use levothyroxine, generic Synthroid, which contains only T4. This is called T4 monotherapy.

The Health Insurance Model

In the Health Insurance Business Model, the primary care doctor's office fee is billed to the patient's health insurance. This could be private health insurance or Medicare, the U.S. government health insurance for citizens over 65. Regardless, the insurance company has its own guidelines and fee schedules for reimbursement, usually a ridiculously small amount, squeezing the doctor financially. To compensate, the doctor must see more patients daily, with less time per patient. The office visit is brief, usually 3-5 minutes. In this short time, primary care doctors can provide only the most basic care, which is a quick glance at the TSH lab report. If the TSH is below the lab reference range, the doctor gives a new prescription for less levothyroxine dosage. If the TSH is above the reference range, the levothyroxine dosage is increased. It is that easy. This is the over-simplification of thyroid endocrinology, a consequence of accepting health insurance.

Talking with a Neighboring Endocrinologist

One day, I found myself talking on the phone with an endocrinologist at a large medical clinic in south Florida, explaining why the TSH blood test can be unreliable. He informed me I was wrong and that he used the TSH test as the gold standard. We agreed to disagree and parted company as friends. I have found that, in general, endocrinologists and mainstream doctors rely heavily on TSH to diagnose the low thyroid condition.

Recommending a Few Thyroid Books

I recommend a book by Dr. Barry Durrant Peatfield, "Your Thyroid and How to Keep It Healthy." After serving as a general practi-

tioner in the British National Health Service, Dr. Peatfield traveled to the United States to train at the Broda Barnes Institute. Dr. Peatfield later returned to England to start his own thyroid clinic. His book was written at the end of a long career and contains the wisdom of 25 years of diagnosing and treating thyroid conditions. One section of the book is devoted to the unreliable TSH. Here is a quote from Dr. Peatfield:

> 1) Anxiety in the medical establishment about rules and dogma has led to a slavish reliance on blood tests, such as the TSH, which are often unreliable and can actually produce a false picture.
>
> 2) Very few doctors can accept the fact that a normal or low TSH may still occur with low thyroid function.
>
> 3) As a result of this test [TSH], thousands are denied treatment for low thyroid condition. (1)

Dr. Peatfield's Reward After a Lifetime of Service

After a lifetime of work serving his community, you might imagine the honors and accolades for such a knowledgeable thyroid physician as Dr. Peatfield, yet quite the opposite happened. Dr. Peatfield's license was suspended in 2001 at the age of 68 by the General Medical Council of England (GMC). The GMC ruling was based on "unfavorable testimony" from competing endocrinologists who "slavishly rely on the TSH test" to measure thyroid function, diagnose the low thyroid condition, and monitor treatment with levothyroxine. Sadly, this sort of "Witch Hunt" has kept medical science in the "Dark Ages" regarding treating the low thyroid condition. (2)

Broda Barnes and the Low Thyroid Condition

Another helpful book recommended to you was written by Broda Barnes, M.D., on the low thyroid condition. Broda Barnes, M.D. reported 40 years ago on the same problem of his medical colleagues relying too heavily on thyroid blood tests. His 1976 book, "Hypothyroidism: The Unsuspected Illness," is a medical classic and should be required reading for every medical student and doctor. I have read the book many times. The book contains the condensed wisdom of a lifetime of research and clinical experience with the thyroid. It rings true today as it did in 1976. (3)

Hypothyroidism the Unsuspected Illness, by Broda Barnes MD

In 2013, Dr. Bjørn Åsvold from Norway published the HUNT study estimating 9 percent of females and 3 percent of males suffer from a low thyroid condition. Dr. Broda Barnes estimated a larger number; 40 percent of the population suffers from a low thyroid condition and would benefit from thyroid medication. Of course, Barnes' opinion differed from that of mainstream medicine of his time, which relied dogmatically on thyroid blood tests to make the diagnosis of low thyroid. Barnes felt the blood tests were unreliable and instead used the basal body temperature, history, and physical examination. This medical debate regarding the unreliability of thyroid blood testing continues today. (4-8)

Being an astute clinician, Dr. Barnes makes several observations about the low thyroid condition. Firstly, low thyroid is associated with reduced immunity to infectious diseases such as T.B. (tuberculosis). In the 1940s, before the advent of modern antibiotics, most low-thyroid children succumbed to infectious diseases before reaching adulthood. Secondly, low thyroid is associated with a peculiar form of skin thickening called myxedema which causes a characteristic appearance of the face, puffiness around the eyes, fullness under the chin, loss of outer eyebrows, and hair thinning or hair loss. (9-11)

A third observation by Dr. Barnes is that low thyroid is associated with menstrual irregularities, miscarriages, and infertility. Dr. Barnes treated thousands of young women with thyroid pills which restored menstrual cycle reg-ularity and fertility. In his day, the medical system resorted to the drastic measure of hysterectomy for uncontrolled menstrual bleeding. Although today's use of birth control pills to regulate the menstrual cycles is admittedly a far better alternative, Dr. Barnes found that the simple administration of NDT, natural desiccated thyroid served quite well. Again, Barnes noted that blood testing was usually normal in these cases which respond to thyroid medication. (12-14)

A lengthy chapter is devoted to heart attacks and the low thyroid condition. Based on autopsy data from Graz, Austria, Barnes concluded that low thyroid patients who previously would have succumbed to infectious diseases in childhood go on years later to develop heart disease. Barnes also found that thyroid treatment was protective in preventing heart attacks, based on his own clinical experience. Likewise, for diabetes, Dr. Barnes found that adding thyroid medication was beneficial in preventing the onset of vascular disease in diabetics. Again, blood tests are usually normal. (15)

Important Point: A low thyroid condition is a serious risk factor for heart disease. This is discussed in Chapter 13, Thyroid Hormone Prevents Heart Attacks.

Dr. Barnes devotes separate chapters in the book to the discussion of chronic fatigue, migraine headaches, and emotional/behavioral disorders, all of which respond to treatment with thyroid medication.

The final chapter describes Dr. Barnes's work on obesity when he presided over a hospital ward of volunteer obese patients and monitored everything they ate. He found that obese patients invariably ate a high carbohydrate diet and avoided fat. Barnes added fat back into the menu and reduced the refined carbohydrates, and found that his obese patients lost 10 pounds a month with no hunger pangs.

Missing from the Dr. Barnes classic book expanded by later authors, Hypothyroidism Type Two by Mark Starr, and Your Thyroid and How to Keep it Healthy by Barry Durrant

Peatfield. Discussions of Iodine supplementation are covered in books by David Derry and David Brownstein. Adrenal Fatigue and Cortisol are covered by The Safe Uses of Cortisol by William McK. Jefferies and Wilson's book on Adrenal Fatigue. (1-3) (16-21)

More on the Unreliability of the TSH Lab Test

In 2013, Dr. A.D. Toft, a physician at the Endocrine Department Royal Infirmary of Edinburgh, writes in the British Medical Journal about the need for TSH suppression in some patients:

> We have long taken the view that most hypothyroid patients are content with a dose of thyroxine that restores serum concentrations of thyroid stimulating hormone (TSH) to the low normal range. However, some achieve a sense of well-being **only when serum thyroid stimulating hormone is suppressed** when we take care to ensure that serum tri-iodothyronine (Free T3) is unequivocally normal...Until valid evidence shows that such a policy is detrimental, we will continue to treat patients holistically rather than insist on adherence to a biochemical definition of adequacy of thyroxine replacement. The issue of whether a little too much thyroxine is dangerous is likely to evaporate when appropriate preparations become available to allow treatment of hypothyroidism with both tri-iodothyronine and thyroxine (T3 and T4 combinations). (4)

Classic Example of Misapplication of a Laboratory Test

Thanks to Jonathan Wright, MD, for bringing to my attention an article in the June 2010 International Journal of Clinical Practice by Dr. O'Reilly, which summarizes the medical literature on this question of the reliability of the TSH test. In 2010, Dr. O'Reilly reviewed the medical literature and the history of thyroid medicine, providing the medical studies showing that Dr. Barnes and Dr. Peatfield were right all along. Dr. O'Reilly writes:

Thyroid hormone replacement is one of the very few medical treatments devised in the 19th century that still survive. It is safe, very effective, and hailed as a major success by patients and clinicians. Currently, it is arguably the most contentious issue in clinical endocrinology. The current controversy and patient disquiet began in the early 1970s when on theoretical grounds and without proper assessment, the serum thyrotropin (TSH) concentration was adopted as the means of assessing the adequacy of thyroxine replacement. The published literature shows that the serum TSH concentration is a poor indicator of clinical status in patients on thyroxine. The adequacy of thyroxine replacement should be assessed clinically, with the serum T3 being measured when required to detect over-replacement....The use of the TSH measurement to assess thyroid status in patients on thyroxine [levothyroxine, generic Synthroid] replacement could be considered a classic example of the misapplication of a laboratory test...The adequacy of thyroxine replacement should be assessed clinically, with the serum T3 being measured when required to detect over-replacement. (5)

In 1994, Dr. J.A. Franklyn writes in the Journal of Clinical Endocrinology & Metabolism:

> Undetectable TSH results, even in a third-generation assay, are not diagnostic of overt hyperthyroidism but are also found in subjects with treated thyroid disease and NTI [Non-Thyroidal Illness = euthyroid sick syndrome]. (22-25)

Health Freedom Law in Florida

Despite the obvious need for a better approach to the low thyroid condition, there has been very little movement to rehabilitate mainstream endocrinology, which dogmatically clings to the TSH test and synthetic T4-only medications such as levothyroxine. Here in the state of Florida, we are fortunate in 2001 the state legislature passed a Health Freedom Law which protects doctors and patients from unwarranted abuse or harassment for utilizing "outside of mainstream medical practices," such as correct diagnosis and treatment of the low thyroid condition based on the wisdom of Drs. Broda Barnes, Barry Peatfield, DS O'Reilly, Jonathan Wright, David Brownstein, and many others. (16-21) (26)

Conclusion

Dogmatically clinging to and slavishly relying on the TSH test to diagnose hypothyroidism and monitor levothyroxine therapy is an error of modern thyroid endocrinology. (27-30)

♦ References for Chapter 10

1) Durrant-Peatfield, Barry. Your Thyroid and How to Keep it Healthy: The Great Thyroid Scandal and How to Avoid It. Hammersmith Books Limited, 2012.

2) Investigation into Thyroid Doctor. BBC News, May 17, 2001. Dr. Barry Durrant-Peatfield.

3) Barnes, Broda Otto, and Lawrence Galton. Hypothyroidism: The Unsuspected Illness. New York: Harper & Row, 1976.

4) Toft, A. D., and G. J. Beckett. "Thyroid Function Tests and Hypothyroidism: Authors' Reply." BMJ 326.7398 (2003): 1087.

5) O'Reilly, D. St J. "Thyroid Hormone Replacement: An Iatrogenic Problem." International Journal of Clinical Practice 64.7 (2010): 991-994.

6) Åsvold, Bjørn Olav, et al. "Changes in the Prevalence of Hypothyroidism: the HUNT Study in Norway." European Journal of Endocrinology 169.5 (2013): 613-620.

7) Unnikrishnan, Ambika Gopalakrishnan, et al. "Prevalence of Hypothyroidism in Adults: An Epidemiological Study in Eight Cities of India." Indian Journal of Endocrinology and Metabolism 17.4 (2013): 647.

8) Sichieri, Rosely, et al. "Low Prevalence of Hypothyroidism Among Black and Mulatto People in a Population-Based Study of Brazilian Women." Clinical Endocrinology 66.6 (2007): 803-807.

9) Wall, Cristen Rhodes. "Myxedema Coma: Diagnosis and Treatment." American Family Physician 62.11 (2000): 2485-2490.

10) Montesinos, María del Mar, and Claudia Gabriela Pellizas. "Thyroid Hormone Action on Innate Immunity." Frontiers in Endocrinology 10 (2019): 350.

11) De Vito, Paolo, et al. "Thyroid Hormones as Modulators of Immune Activities at the Cellular Level." Thyroid 21.8 (2011): 879-890.

12) Foster, Ruth C., and Thornton, Madeline J. "Thyroid in the Treatment of Menstrual Irregularities." Endocrinology 24.3 (1939): 383-388.

13) Rosenberg, Isadore N. "Menstrual Instability in Thyroid Disease." Clinical Obstetrics and Gynecology 12.3 (1969): 755-770.

14) Verma, Indu, et al. "Prevalence of Hypothyroidism in Infertile Women and Evaluation of Response of Treatment for Hypothyroidism on Infertility." International Journal of Applied and Basic Medical Research 2.1 (2012): 17.

15) Barnes, Broda Otto, and Charlotte W. Barnes. Solved the Riddle of Heart Attacks. Robinson Press, 1976.

16) Starr, Mark. M.D., Hypothyroidism Type 2: The Epidemic. New Voice Publications, 2010.

17) Jefferies, William McK. Safe Uses of Cortisol. Charles C Thomas Publisher, 2004.

18) Wilson, James L., and Jonathan V. Wright. Adrenal Fatigue: The 21st-Century Stress Syndrome. Smart Publications, 2001.

19) Derry, David Michael. Breast Cancer and Iodine. Bloomington, IN: Trafford, 2001.

20) Brownstein, David. Iodine: Why You Need It, Why You Can't Live Without It. Medical Alternatives Press, 2008.

21) Brownstein, David. Overcoming Thyroid Disorders. Medical Alternatives Press, 2008.

22) Franklyn, J. A., et al. "Comparison of Second and Third Generation Methods for Measurement of Serum Thyrotropin in Patients with Overt Hyperthyroidism, Patients Receiving Thyroxine Therapy, and Those with Nonthyroidal Illness." The Journal of Clinical Endocrinology & Metabolism 78.6 (1994): 1368-1371.

23) McDermott, Michael T. "Non-Thyroidal Illness Syndrome (Euthyroid Sick Syndrome)." Management of Patients with Pseudo-Endocrine Disorders: A Case-Based Pocket Guide (2019): 331-339.

24) Ganesan, Kavitha, and Khurram Wadud. "Euthyroid Sick Syndrome." StatPearls [Internet]. StatPearls Publishing, 2021.

25) Krysiak, Robert, et al. "Euthyroid Sick Syndrome: An Important Clinical Problem." Wiadomosci Lekarskie (Warsaw, Poland: 1960) 70.2 pt 2 (2017): 376-385.

26) State of Florida Health Freedom Law: CHAPTER 2001-116 Senate Bill No. 1324 An act relating to health care; creating s. 456.41, F.S.; amending s. 381.026, F.S.; Ch. 2001-116 (S.B. 1324) Effective May 31, 2001.

27) Fraser, W. D., et al. "Are Biochemical Tests of Thyroid Function of Any Value in Monitoring Patients Receiving Thyroxine Replacement?" Br Med J (Clin Res Ed) 293.6550 (1986): 808-810.

28) Wheatley, T., et al. "Thyroid Stimulating Hormone Measurement by an Ultrasensitive Assay During Thyroxine Replacement: Comparison with Other Tests of Thyroid Function." Annals of Clinical Biochemistry 24 (1987): 614-619.

29) O'Reilly, Denis St J. "Thyroid Function Tests—Time for a Reassessment." BMJ 320.7245 (2000): 1332-1334.

30) O Reilly, D. St J. "Thyroid Function Tests-Time for a Reassessment." Hong Kong Practitioner 23.5 (2001): 212-216.

Chapter 11

Hypothyroidism and Reversible Cardiomyopathy

JIM IS A 47-YEAR-OLD ACCOUNTANT under the care of his cardiologist for cardiomyopathy, a dilated baggy heart with poor contractility. Jim's echocardiogram revealed a dilated left ventricle with an ejection fraction of 20 percent (Normal = 50-60 percent). Jim's nuclear stress test was normal, indicating no flow-limiting lesions in the coronary arteries. However, Jim is short of breath with minimal exertion and sometimes wakes up at night with shortness of breath. Examination shows mild edema of the lower extremities and normal breath sounds on auscultation. Laboratory evaluation shows low serum selenium of 105, high TSH of 10.2 µIU/ml, low Free T3 of 240, and low Free T4 of 0.6 ng/dl. Jim was treated with selenium 200 mcg/day and NDT one grain (60mg) per day. Three months later, his lab tests have improved, and Jim reports his symptoms have resolved, and his follow-up echocardiogram showed his ejection fraction had improved from 20 percent to 38 percent.

Reversible cardiomyopathy may be caused by hypothyroidism, and the TSH can be quite high in these cases. In 2018, Dr. Rastogi reported a young female with a TSH of 313 µIU/ml (normal 0.4-4.0) and Free T4 of only 0.22 ng/dl (normal 0.8-1.6). The cardiomyopathy showed significant improvement after 5 months of thyroid hormone therapy. (1)

Reversible Cardiomyopathy Due to Hypothyroidism

In 2016, Dr. Samuel Roberto reported a case of reversible heart failure due to hypothyroidism in a 65-year-old male with symptoms of heart failure, shortness of breath, worse with exertion, and fatigue. The patient had a history of Graves' Disease treated with I-131 radioactive iodine. After the thyroid ablation, the patient became hypothyroid and was prescribed levothyroxine but ran out and stopped taking his medication. Initial labs showed creatinine phosphokinase (CPK) of 1158 IU/L. Echocardiogram revealed a left ventricular ejection fraction of only 15% (normal 55%) and severe global hypokinesis. Nuclear stress testing was negative for myocardial ischemia. Thyroid stimulating hormone was markedly elevated at 150.20 µIU/mL, and Free T4 was very low at 0.3 ng/dL. Oral levothyroxine was restarted at 50 micrograms daily and later increased to 112 µg/day. The patient felt better within 48 hours. Follow-up labs at six weeks showed improvement in TSH 17.28 µIU/mL and FT4 1.0 ng/dL, and the levothyroxine dose was increased to 150 µg/day. Final thyroid labs at 12 weeks showed TSH 1.00 µIU/mL, FT4 1.2. Repeat echocardiography at six months showed an improved ejection fraction of 45%. Dr. Samuel Roberto writes:

> Heart failure precipitated by dilated cardiomyopathy due to hypothyroidism is unique for its potential reversibility following thyroid hormone supplementation. Administration of thyroid hormone can restore contractile function. (2)

How Does Hypothyroidism Cause Reversible Cardiomyopathy?

In 2019, Dr. Sahin, in Bucharest, did an animal study of drug-induced hypothyroidism, finding oxidative and inflammatory changes in the cardiac tissue. Dr. Sahin writes:

> Hypothyroidism increases oxidative stress and causes inflammatory alterations in cardiac tissue. In addition, our study also suggested that thyroid hormone

deficiency would increase the amounts of cardiac NLRP3 and caspase-1 protein, which indicates that hypothyroidism exerts its destructive effects through sterile inflammation. Elucidation of sterile inflammation-associated pathways may produce promising results in the treatment of hypothyroidism-induced cardiac damage. (3)

In 2016, Dr. Nasra Ayuoba studied an animal model of hypothyroid-induced cardiomyopathy. The anti-inflammatory botanical, thymoquinone, protected against hypothyroid-induced cardiac inflammatory histopathology. (4)

The Heart is Dependent on Circulating T3

The membrane-bound D1 deiodinase system converts T4 to T3 in the periphery and is responsible for most of the circulating T3. Heart muscle is dependent on serum T3 to maintain activity. Unlike other organ systems that take up T4 from the circulation and convert it to T3 with intracellular D2 deiodinases, myocytes have no significant deiodinase activity. Instead, myocytes take up T3, not T4, to maintain intracellular T3 levels. Thus, myocytes depend on a good peripheral T3 level in circulation to maintain their function. The heart is a special case and will develop reversible dilated cardiomyopathy in response to low Free T3 levels. In 2007, Dr. Irwin Klein writes:

> The heart relies mainly on serum T3 because no significant myocyte intracellular deiodinase activity takes place, and it appears that T3, and not T4, is transported into the myocyte... T3 exerts its cellular actions through binding to thyroid hormone nuclear receptors (T.R.s). (5-6)

Combined Low Free T3 and Selenium Deficiency

In 2019, Dr. Magdalena Fraczek-Jucha found low free T3 levels (low T3 syndrome) and selenium deficiency were highly prevalent in heart failure patients, writing:

Low fT3 levels [free T3 levels] and fT3/fT4 ratio are associated with more advanced H.F. [heart failure], reflected by echocardiographic variables. Another finding was a high incidence of selenium deficiency in our H.F. patients (74.6%) ... Low T3 syndrome is frequently found in patients with HFrEF [heart failure with reduced ejection fraction] and is associated with a poor outcome. Selenium deficiency is highly prevalent in severe H.F. patients. (7-8)

Selenium deficiency is linked to cardiomyopathy in two ways. Firstly, selenium is a component of the D1 deiodinase enzyme, which converts T4 to T3 to maintain peripheral T3 levels. Selenium is also a component of glutathione peroxidase, the major intracellular anti-oxidant. Selenium deficiency has been found to be a reversible cause of cardiomyopathy, and selenium supplements will frequently reverse the condition. (9-15)

Coenzyme Q-10 Deficiency

Coenzyme Q-10 deficiency is common in cardiomyopathy patients and has been implicated in the etiology of congestive heart failure. Treatment involves eliminating statin drug culprit that depletes coenzyme Q10. Secondly, the patient is given coenzyme Q10 supplements (300 mg per day) to restore the depleted coenzyme Q10 serum levels. Further benefits can be obtained with a cocktail of mitochondrial nutrients such as selenium, D-ribose, L-carnitine, alpha lipoic acid, thiamine (benfotiamine), and magnesium (glycinate). This nutritional protocol is beneficial for improving cardiac function and reversing cardiomyopathy. The occurrence of statin induced cardiomyopathy is much greater than reported. In my opinion, cardiologists are in a state of denial and in many cases will fail to recognize statin-induced cardiomyopathy in their patient population, even when pointed out. I personally have seen a patient with complete reversal from an ejection fraction of 20 percent on statins to complete recovery with an ejection fraction of 55 percent within 12 weeks after statin withdrawal and coenzyme Q10 replacement, based on the 2019 report by Dr. Peter Langsjoen. (16-23)

Atrial Fibrillation Frequently Associated with Dilated Cardiomyopathy

In 2021, Dr. Karolina Zawadzka reviewed the role of thyroid hormones in dilated cardiomyopathy, in which there is a compensatory increase in D2 deiodinase activity which converts T4 to T3, leading to a local hyperthyroid state within the myocardium. This local hyperthyroidism in the myocardium can explain the association of atrial fibrillation with dilated cardiomyopathy. In an animal model, treatment with PTU (propyl thiouracil), which inhibits D2 deiodinase conversion of T4 to T3, improves cardiac function. Other drugs which inhibit T4 to T3 conversion are amiodarone, propranolol, and corticosteroids. Indeed, the benefits of amiodarone for atrial fibrillation may lie in its inhibition of deiodinase, thus reducing T3 levels in the myocardium. Dr. Karolina Zawadzka writes:

> In contrast, Wang et al. showed **increased D2 activity, leading to a local hyperthyroid state within the myocardium despite unchanged serum T3 levels...** Admittedly, D2 mRNA is physiologically expressed in the human myocardium but not in the heart of a healthy rodent. Nevertheless, Wang et al., by means of real-time quantitative reverse transcriptase-polymerase chain reaction analyses, showed that D2 was overexpressed in the heart of DCM [Dilated Cardiomopathy] mice... **Additionally, treatment with the anti-thyroid drug propylthiouracil improved cardiac function in DCM mice, reduced the expression of the abovementioned hypertrophic markers, and prevented cardiac enlargement. Likewise, the use of propylthiouracil was accompanied by an improvement in ejection fraction and extended lifespan of the DCM animals.** (24-31) (49)

Amiodarone for Atrial Fibrillation

In 1986, Dr. Wiegand studied the effect of amiodarone on the ventricular myocardium of the rat, finding the drug induces a hypothyroid state, inducing redistribution of iso myosins similar to hypothyroidism while simultaneously inducing a low T3 syndrome. Note: Myosin is the main contractile protein in heart muscle. Amiodarone changes the various forms of myosin (iso myosins) produced by the heart muscle cells to a pattern that resembles that seen with hypothyroidism. Dr. Wiegand writes:

> Due to the similar electrophysiological effects of amiodarone and hypothyroidism in the myocardium, **the induction of a local hypothyroid state has been proposed as the mechanism of action of amiodarone**... We conclude that **amiodarone induces a hypothyroid-like state** in the ventricular myocardium of rats by inhibiting the action of T3--an effect which cannot be attributed to an antagonism at the T3 nuclear receptor level. (32-40)

In 1999, Dr. Shiva Shahrara writes:

> Amiodarone, a powerful antiarrhythmic drug, **may exert its effect by antagonism of the thyroid hormone**, probably at the receptor level... In conclusion, this study shows that amiodarone subtype selectively downregulates the T.R. mRNA [thyroid hormone receptor messenger RNA] levels in mouse myocardium in a dose-dependent manner. These results support a thyroid hormone-dependent action of amiodarone. (33-40)

Based on the above studies, one might speculate atrial fibrillation in the cardiomyopathy patient is a result of the upregulation of D2 deiodinase conversion of T4 to T3 with local hyperthyroidism in the myocardium. Amiodarone, structurally similar to thyroid hormone, addresses this local hyperthyroidism within the myocyte by antagonizing thyroid hormone locally within the myocyte.

Cardiologists commonly use amiodarone for arrhythmias, including patients with dilated cardiomyopathy and low ejection fraction who go into atrial fibrillation. Given the above, once the patient's ejection fraction has returned to normal and the atrial fibrillation resolved, the amiodarone should be carefully tapered and then discontinued, since there is no further need to induce a local hypothyroid state in the myocardium. Indeed, as discussed above, hypothyroidism itself is a major cause of reversible cardiomyopathy. In addition. adverse effects of amiodarone such as corneal deposits may limit use. (41-44)

Conclusion

Dilated cardiomyopathy caused by hypothyroidism is remarkable in that it can be completely reversed by the administration of thyroid hormone. A more robust program includes selenium, coenzyme Q10, L-carnitine, D-ribose, and magnesium. Statin-induced cardiomyopathy is a common problem and is mostly denied and ignored by the cardiology community, easily reversible by stopping the statin drug and giving the patient the missing coenzyme Q10. Selenium deficiency is another cause of cardiomyopathy frequently missed by the medical system completely reversible with selenium supplements. (45-63)

♦ References for Chapter 11

1) Rastogi, P., et al. "Hypothyroidism-Induced Reversible Dilated Cardiomyopathy." Journal of Postgraduate Medicine 64.3 (2018): 177.

2) Roberto, E. Samuel, et al. "Differential Reversibility in Heart Failure Due to Hypothyroidism: A Series of Contrasting Cases with Review of Literature." International Journal of Case Reports and Images (IJCRI) 7.1 (2016): 1-6.

3) Sahin, E., et al. "Hypothyroidism Increases Expression of Sterile Inflammation Proteins in Rat Heart Tissue." Acta Endocrinologica (Bucharest) 15.1 (2019): 39.

4) Ayuoba, Nasra N., et al. "Thymoquinone Protects Against Hypothyroidism-Induced Cardiac Histopathological Changes in Rats Through a Nitric Oxide/Antioxidant Mechanism." Biomedical Research 27.1 (2016): 93-102.

5) Klein, Irwin, and Sara Danzi. "Thyroid Disease and the Heart." Circulation 116.15 (2007): 1725-1735.

6) Sabatino, Laura, et al. "Deiodinases and the Three Types of Thyroid Hormone Deiodination Reactions." Endocrinology and Metabolism 36.5 (2021): 952-964.

7) Fraczek-Jucha, Magdalena, et al. "Low Triiodothyronine Syndrome and Selenium Deficiency-Undervalued Players in Advanced Heart Failure? A Single-Center Pilot Study." BMC Cardiovascular Disorders 19.1 (2019): 1-9.

8) Lisco, Giuseppe, et al. "Congestive Heart Failure and Thyroid Dysfunction: The Role of the Low T3 Syndrome and Therapeutic Aspects." Endocrine, Metabolic & Immune Disorders-Drug Targets 20.5 (2020): 646-653.

9) Burke, Michael Philip, and Kenneth Opeskin. "Fulminant Heart Failure Due to Selenium Deficiency Cardiomyopathy (Keshan Disease)." Medicine, Science and the Law 42.1 (2002): 10-13.

10) Li, Guangsheng, et al. "Keshan Disease: An Endemic Cardiomyopathy in China." Human Pathology 16.6 (1985): 602-609.

11) Marinescu, Victor, and Peter A. McCullough. "Nutritional and Micronutrient Determinants of Idiopathic Dilated Cardiomyopathy: Diagnostic and Therapeutic Implications." Expert Review of Cardiovascular Therapy 9.9 (2011): 1161-1170.

12) Fleming, C. Richard, et al. "Selenium Deficiency and Fatal Cardiomyopathy in a Patient on Home Parenteral Nutrition." Gastroenterology 83.3 (1982): 689-693.

13) Burke, Michael Philip, and Kenneth Opeskin. "Fulminant Heart Failure Due to Selenium Deficiency Cardiomyopathy (Keshan Disease)." Medicine, Science and the Law 42.1 (2002): 10-13.

14) Johnson, Robert Arnold, et al. "An Occidental Case of Cardiomyopathy and Selenium Deficiency." New England Journal of Medicine 304.20 (1981): 1210-1212.

15) Saliba, W., et al. "Heart Failure Secondary to Selenium Deficiency, Reversible After Supplementation." International Journal of Cardiology 141.2 (2010): e26-e27.

16) Filipiak, Krzysztof J., et al. "Heart Failure—Do We Need New Drugs or Have Them Already? A Case of Coenzyme Q10." Journal of Cardiovascular Development and Disease 9.5 (2022): 161.

17) Jankowski, Jerzy, et al. "Coenzyme Q10–A New Player in the Treatment of Heart Failure?" Pharmacological Reports 68.5 (2016): 1015-1019.

18) Sharma, Abhinav, et al. "Coenzyme Q10 and Heart Failure: A State-Of-The-Art Review." Circulation: Heart Failure 9.4 (2016): e002639.

19) Sinatra, Stephen T. "Metabolic Cardiology: Management of Congestive Heart Failure." Nutritional and Integrative Strategies in Cardiovascular Medicine. CRC Press, 2022. 189-216.

20) Okuyama, Harumi, et al. "Statins Stimulate Atherosclerosis and Heart Failure: Pharmacological Mechanisms." Expert Review of Clinical Pharmacology 8.2 (2015): 189-199.

21) Bolog, Mihaela Ioana. "Coenzyme Q10 and Selenium in Heart Failure–A New Perspective." Internal Medicine 16.5 (2019): 41-51.

22) Mortensen, Svend A., et al. "The Effect of Coenzyme Q10 on Morbidity and Mortality in Chronic Heart Failure: Results From Q-SYMBIO: A Randomized Double-Blind Trial." JACC: Heart Failure 2.6 (2014): 641-649.

23) Langsjoen, Peter H., et al. "Statin-Associated Cardiomyopathy Responds to Statin Withdrawal and Administration of Coenzyme Q10." The Permanente Journal 23 (2019).

24) Zawadzka, Karolina, et al. "Thyroid hormones—An Underestimated Player in Dilated Cardiomyopathy?" Journal of Clinical Medicine 10.16 (2021): 3618.

25) Wang, Yuan-Yuan, et al. "Up-Regulation of Type 2 Iodothyronine Deiodinase in Dilated Cardiomyopathy." Cardiovascular Research 87.4 (2010): 636-646.

26) Lindenmeyer, M., et al. "Does Amiodarone Affect Heart Rate by Inhibiting the Intracellular Generation of Triiodothyronine from Thyroxine?" British Journal of Pharmacology 82 (1984): 275-280.

27) Forfar, J. C., et al. "Occult Thyrotoxicosis: A Correctable Cause of Idiopathic Atrial Fibrillation." The American Journal of Cardiology 44.1 (1979): 9-12.

28) Pachucki, Janusz, et al. "Type 2 Iodothyronine Deiodinase Transgene Expression in the Mouse Heart Causes Cardiac-Specific Thyrotoxicosis." Endocrinology 142.1 (2001): 13-20.

29) Rosene, Matthew L., et al. "Inhibition of the Type 2 Iodothyronine Deiodinase Underlies the Elevated Plasma TSH Associated with Amiodarone Treatment." Endocrinology 151.12 (2010): 5961-5970.

30) Kerin, Nicholas Z., et al. "Relation of Serum Reverse T3 to Amiodarone Antiarrhythmic Efficacy and Toxicity." The American Journal of Cardiology 57.1 (1986): 128-130.

31) Kozdag, Guliz, et al. "Relation Between Free Triiodothyronine/Free Thyroxine Ratio, Echocardiographic Parameters and Mortality in Dilated Cardiomyopathy." European Journal of Heart Failure 7.1 (2005): 113-118.

32) Wiegand, V., G. Wagner, and H. Kreuzer. "Hypothyroid-like Effect of Amiodarone in the Ventricular Myocardium of the Rat." Basic Research in Cardiology 81 (1986): 482-488.

33) Shahrara, Shiva, and Viktor Drvota. "Thyroid Hormone A1 and B1 Receptor mRNA Are Downregulated by Amiodarone in Mouse Myocardium." Journal of Cardiovascular Pharmacology 34.2 (1999): 261-267.

34) Perret, Gérard, et al. "Amiodarone Decreases Cardiac B-Adrenoceptors Through an Antagonistic Effect On 3, 5, 3'triiodothyronine." J Cardiovasc Pharmacol 19 (1992): 473-478.

35) Hartong, R., W. M. Wiersinga, and T. A. Plomp. "Amiodarone Reduces the Effect of T3 On Beta-Adrenergic Receptor Density in Rat Heart." Hormone and metabolic research 22.02 (1990): 85-89.

36) Paradis, Pierre, et al. "Amiodarone Antagonizes the Effects of T3 at the Receptor Level: An Additional Mechanism for Its In Vivo Hypothyroid-Like Effects." Canadian Journal of Physiology and Pharmacology 69.6 (1991): 865-870.

37) Gotzsche, Liv Bjorn-Hansen, and Hans Ørskov. "Cardiac Triiodothyronine Nuclear Receptor Binding Capacities in Amiodarone-Treated, Hypo- And Hyperthyroid Rats." European Journal of Endocrinology 130.3 (1994): 281-290.

38) Drvota, Viktor, et al. "Amiodarone is a Dose-Dependent Noncompetitive and Competitive Inhibitor of T3 Binding to Thyroid Hormone Receptor Subtype Beta 1, Whereas Disopyramide, Lignocaine, Propafenone, Metoprolol, Dl-Sotalol, and Verapamil Have No Inhibitory Effect." Journal of Cardiovascular Pharmacology 26.2 (1995): 222-226.

40) Mohr-Kahaly, S., et al. "Cardiovascular Effects of Thyroid Hormones." Zeitschrift fur Kardiologie 85 (1996): 219-231.

41) Qin, Dingxin, et al. "Mortality Risk of Long-Term Amiodarone Therapy for Atrial Fibrillation Patients Without Structural Heart Disease." Cardiology Journal 22.6 (2015): 622-629.

42) Glover, Benedict M., and Adrian Baranchuk. "Amiodarone for Atrial Fibrillation: Friend or Foe?" Cardiology Journal 22.6 (2015): 603-604.

43) Torp-Pedersen, Christian, et al. "The Safety of Amiodarone in Patients with Heart Failure." Journal of cardiac failure 13.5 (2007): 340-345.

44) Adelstein, Evan C., et al. "Amiodarone is Associated with Adverse Outcomes in Patients with Sustained Ventricular Arrhythmias Upgraded to Cardiac Resynchronization Therapy—Defibrillators." Journal of Cardiovascular Electrophysiology 30.3 (2019): 348-356.

41) Khalife, Wissam I., et al. "Treatment of Subclinical Hypothyroidism Reverses Ischemia and Prevents Myocyte Loss and Progressive LV Dysfunction in Hamsters with Dilated Cardiomyopathy." American Journal of Physiology-Heart and Circulatory Physiology 289.6 (2005): H2409-H2415.

42) Zawadzka, Karolina, et al. "Thyroid Hormones—An Underestimated Player in Dilated Cardiomyopathy?" Journal of Clinical Medicine 10.16 (2021): 3618.

43) Chen, Xiaoai, et al. "Effectiveness and Safety of Thyroid Hormone Therapy in Patients with Dilated Cardiomyopathy: A Systematic Review and Meta-analysis of RCTs." American Journal of Cardiovascular Drugs (2022): 1-10.

44) Khochtali, I., et al. "Reversible Dilated Cardiomyopathy Caused by Hypothyroidism." International Archives of Medicine 4.1 (2011): 20.

45) Seol, Myung Do, et al. "Dilated Cardiomyopathy Secondary to Hypothyroidism: A Case Report with a Review of The Literature." Journal Of Cardiovascular Ultrasound 22.1 (2014): 32-35.

46) Santos, Alvani D., et al. "Echocardiographic Characterization of the Reversible Cardiomyopathy of Hypothyroidism." The American Journal of Medicine 68.5 (1980): 675-682.

47) Gerdes, A. Martin. "Restoration of Thyroid Hormone Balance: A Game Changer in the Treatment of Heart Failure?" American Journal of Physiology-Heart and Circulatory Physiology 308.1 (2015): H1-H10.

48) Santi, Adriana, et al. "Overt Hypothyroidism Is Associated with Blood Inflammatory Biomarkers Dependent of Lipid Profile." Journal of Applied Biomedicine 14.2 (2016): 119-124.

49) Lubrano, V., et al. "Relationship Between Triiodothyronine and Proinflammatory Cytokines in Chronic Heart Failure." Biomedicine & pharmacotherapy 64.3 (2010): 165-169.

50) Madan, Nidhi, et al. "Hypothyroid Heart: Myxoedema as a Cause of Reversible Dilated Cardiomyopathy." Case Reports 2015 (2015): bcr2015212045.

51) Minhas, Simran, et al. "Big Heart Problems: A Case of Reversible Nonischemic Cardiomyopathy Due to Severe Hypothyroidism." Circulation 146.Suppl_1 (2022): A15510-A15510.

52) Sunkara, Anusha, et al. "A Curious Case of the Dilated Heart: A Case of Reversible Dilated Cardiomyopathy Due to Severe Hypothyroidism Caused by Hashimoto's Thyroiditis." Journal of the American College of Cardiology 73.9S1 (2019): 2703-2703.

53) Do Seol, Myung, et al. "Dilated Cardiomyopathy Secondary to Hypothyroidism: Case Report with a Review of Literature." Journal of Cardiovascular Ultrasound 22.1 (2014): 32-35.

54) Shah, Nisarg, and Stasia Miaskiewicz. "Hypothyroidism: A Reversible Cause of Heart Failure." Endocrine Abstracts. Vol. 41. Bioscientifica, 2016.

55) Yang, F. Y., et al. "Keshan Disease—An Endemic Mitochondrial Cardiomyopathy in China." Journal of Trace Elements and Electrolytes in Health and Disease 2.3 (1988): 157-163.

56) Boldery, Rachel, et al. "Nutritional Deficiency of Selenium Secondary to Weight Loss (Bariatric) Surgery Associated with Life-Threatening Cardiomyopathy." Heart, Lung, and Circulation 16.2 (2007): 123-126.

57) Reeves, William C., et al. "Reversible Cardiomyopathy Due to Selenium Deficiency." Journal of Parenteral and Enteral Nutrition 13.6 (1989): 663-665.

58) Massoure, P. L., et al. "Bilateral Leg Edema After Bariatric Surgery: A Selenium-Deficient Cardiomyopathy." Obesity Research & Clinical Practice 11.5 (2017): 622.

59) Quercia, Robert A., et al. "Selenium Deficiency and Fatal Cardiomyopathy in a Patient Receiving Long-Term Home Parenteral Nutrition." Clinical Pharmacy 3.5 (1984): 531-535.

60) Loscalzo, Joseph. "Keshan Disease, Selenium Deficiency, and the Selenoproteome." New England Journal of Medicine 370.18 (2014): 1756-1760.

61) Chen, Jun-Shi. "An Original Discovery: Selenium Deficiency and Keshan Disease (An Endemic Heart Disease)." Asia Pacific Journal of Clinical Nutrition 21.3 (2012): 320-326.

62) Oropeza-Moe, Marianne, et al. "Selenium Deficiency Associated Porcine and Human Cardiomyopathies." Journal of Trace Elements in Medicine and Biology 31 (2015): 148-156.

63) Benstoem, Carina, et al. "Selenium and Its Supplementation in Cardiovascular Disease—What Do We Know?" Nutrients 7.5 (2015): 3094-3118.

Chapter 12

Hypothyroidism and the Immune System

Low Thyroid Condition Reduces Immunity to Infectious Diseases

BRODA BARNES, M.D. (1906-1988) WAS perhaps the most outstanding American thyroid scientist and physician of his time. Dr. Barnes obtained his PhD on thyroid gland at the University of Chicago, and MD degree from Rush Medical College. Dr. Barnes was professor of medicine at the University of Illinois, and his papers and memorabilia are preserved in the University of Chicago Library. In 1942, Dr. Barnes published in JAMA his "Barnes Basal Temperature Test" which I find useful on a daily basis. Low basal body temperature is a marker for the low thyroid condition. An astute clinician, Dr. Barnes observed the low thyroid condition associated with reduced immunity to infectious diseases, as well as greater risk of mortality from infection, findings reported in his 1976 book, "Hypothyroidism, the Unsuspected Illness." Unfortunately, the mainstream endocrinologists of his time rejected Dr. Barnes's teachings, including this one about hypothyroidism associated with reduced immunity to infection. (1) (20)

The Hypothyroid Mouse and Infectious Disease

In 2014, Dr. Cristiana Perrotta from Milan, Italy, used hypothyroid mice to show Dr. Barnes was right all along. Dr. Cristiana Perrotta studied the ability of hypothyroid mice to battle and withstand an infectious insult. The hypothyroid mice were challenged with intra-peritoneal injection of gram-negative endotoxin. This induced fatal endotoxemia, with 90% mortality after 96 hours. However, when the hypothyroid mice were injected with T3 (thyroid hormone) for five days before the challenge

with gram-negative endotoxemia, they fared better with only 30% mortality. This was an impressive demonstration of the importance of thyroid hormone for boosting the immune system and protecting from infectious diseases. (2)

Thyroid Hormone and Cancer Immunity

Stress-Induced Model of Lymphoma

If thyroid hormone enhances our immune system and protects us from infectious disease, one might predict thyroid hormone confers similar protection from cancer, called immune surveillance. (3)

In 2009, Dr. Luciana Frick studied a stress-induced mouse lymphoma model. Mice were injected with lymphoma cells and then subjected to chronic stress by restraining them in a narrow confinement tube. These restrained diseased mice were compared to control mice. The restrained mice exhibited impaired T-cell mediated immunity and accelerated progression of lymphoma. However, thyroid hormone treatment of the mice with levothyroxine enhanced their immune systems, improved the impaired T cell immunity, and suppressed lymphoma cell proliferation. Dr. Luciana Frick agrees with the teachings of Dr. Broda Barnes, stating:

> These results show that thyroid hormones are regulators of tumor evolution, acting through the modulation of T-cell mediated immunity affected by chronic stress...These findings also indicate a potential therapeutic action of thyroxin in the adjuvant treatment of stress-related disorders such as immunosuppression and cancer...Results presented herein are consistent with prior evidence that demonstrates that **experimental hypothyroidism leads to a general depression of the immune system.** (4-5)

In 2009, Dr. Clare Hodkinson studied the relationship between thyroid hormone levels and immunity in healthy men and women, writing:

> Overall, the current study provides preliminary evidence to suggest that higher concentrations of T3 and T4, within normal physiological ranges, enhance innate and adaptive immunity through maintenance of specific cell populations and greater responsiveness to immune stimuli. (6)

In 2011, Dr. Julia Rubingh found activation of the immune system depends on thyroid status, writing:

> In general, a hyperthyroid state leads to a more activated immune system, whereas hypothyroidism leads to a less activated immune system. (7)

In 2021, Dr. Roberto De Luca studied thyroid hormone with the immune response, finding that hyperthyroidism increased the immune response, while hypothyroidism had the opposite effect, writing:

> Newly synthesized T.H.s [thyroid hormones] induce leukocyte [immune cell] proliferation, migration, release of cytokines, and antibody production, triggering an immune response against either sterile or microbial insults...The existence of a bidirectional crosstalk between the endocrine and the immune system, in which THs and cytokines represent the key players, is well documented. A central role of T.H.s in the modulation of the immune system is confirmed by the influence of T3 and T4 in cytokine maturation and release... Abnormal T.H.s secretion, hyperthyroidism, autoimmune thyroiditis, and hypothyroidism can affect immunological functions. Hyperthyroidism correlates with increased humoral and immune cell responses. Opposite effects were found in hypothyroidism. (8)

Immune Cells Make TSH

In 2021, Dr. Roberto De Luca made the striking observation that specific immune cells (T and B lymphocytes) are capable of synthesizing and releasing TSH (thyroid stimulating hormone), which then stimulates the thyroid gland and plays a decisive role in the immune response, writing:

> T and B lymphocytes [immune cells] are capable of synthesizing and releasing TSH, which might affect healthy and abnormal thyroid cells expressing the TSH receptor. This novel and unexpected non-pituitary source of TSH could also be decisive in affecting immune response during infections and chronic inflammation. Initial reports of TSH and immune cells appeared more than 20 years ago. Bacterial toxins or in vitro TRH [Thyrotropin Releasing Hormone] administration enhance TSH production and release from leukocytes. The work of Blalock et al. (1984) showed that TSH induced a strong cellular and humoral response, thus enhancing the lymphocyte proliferation by inducing the production of endogenous inflammatory factors: IL-6 and monocyte chemoattractant protein-1 (MCP-1). Moreover, in vitro and in vivo studies showed that TSH treatments significantly increased T3 levels in thymocytes and other immune cells. Experiments performed in mice lacking the pituitary gland (unable to produce central TSH) showed increased TSH levels during inflammation. (8)

Hypothyroidism and Increased Susceptibility to Infectious Disease

In 2022, Dr. Christina Wenzek reported on the interplay of thyroid hormones with the immune system, admitting Dr. Broda Barnes had been right all along, hypothyroidism is associated with increased susceptibility to infectious disease, writing:

> hypothyroidism has been associated with increased susceptibility to infectious diseases... hypothyroidism was identified as a risk factor for periprosthetic joint infections

based on a meta-analysis of institutional databases on patients with arthroplasty. In line with this, increased mortality of hypothyroid rats was observed in a caecal ligation and puncture model of sepsis... In recent years, there is growing evidence for a direct influence of T.H.s [thyroid hormones] on the immune system. Cells of both the innate and adaptive immune systems express a variety of components involved in local T.H. action and are sensitive to T.H.s affecting immune cell function. (9)

In 1995, Dr. Philip Schoenfeld reported a case of a 71-year-old man with hypothyroidism and suppressed cell-mediated immunity and bacteremia (bacteria growing in the blood stream). Serial lymphocyte studies showed gradual improvement in lymphocyte function as the patient's thyroid status improved. Dr. Philip Schoenfeld writes:

> A 71-year-old man had severe hypothyroidism, chronic autoimmune thyroiditis, and bacteremia due to Edwardsiella tarda. A review of the literature identified the hypothesis that E tarda infections may occur more frequently in immunocompromised patients. Previous animal studies have shown decreases in lymphocyte function during hypothyroidism, with the return of normal lymphocyte function during euthyroid states. Therefore, lymphocyte transformation studies were obtained, demonstrating severe decreases in our patient's lymphocyte function. Except for chronic autoimmune thyroiditis, other immune system abnormalities were excluded. Serial lymphocyte transformation studies showed gradual improvement in lymphocyte function during a gradual return to euthyroid state. (10)

Conclusion

Recent Studies in the medical literature show that Dr. Broda Barnes was correct. The low thyroid condition is associated with impaired immunity to infection. Ignoring the link between the immune system and thyroid function is another error of conventional endocrinology. (11-19)

◆ **References for Chapter 12**

1) Barnes, Broda Otto, and Lawrence Galton. Hypothyroidism: The Unsuspected Illness. New York: Harper & Row, 1976.

2) Perrotta, Cristiana, et al. "The Thyroid Hormone Triiodothyronine Controls Macrophage Maturation and Functions: Protective Role During Inflammation." The American Journal of Pathology 184.1 (2014): 230-247.

3) Swann, Jeremy B., and Mark J. Smyth. "Immune Surveillance of Tumors." The Journal of clinical investigation 117.5 (2007): 1137-1146.

4) Frick, Luciana Romina, et al. "Involvement of Thyroid Hormones in the Alterations of T-Cell Immunity and Tumor Progression Induced by Chronic Stress." Biological Psychiatry 65.11 (2009): 935-942.

5) Frick, L. R., et al. "Chronic Restraint Stress Impairs T-Cell Immunity and Promotes Tumor Progression in Mice." Stress 12.2 (2009): 134-143.

6) Hodkinson, Clare F., et al. "Preliminary Evidence of Immune Function Modulation by Thyroid Hormones in Healthy Men and Women Aged 55–70 years." Journal of Endocrinology 202.1 (2009): 55-63.

7) Rubingh, Julia, et al. "The Role of Thyroid Hormone in the Innate and Adaptive Immune Response During Infection." Comprehensive Physiology 10.4 (2011): 1277-1287.

8) De Luca, Roberto, et al. "Thyroid Hormones Interaction with Immune Response, Inflammation and Non-Thyroidal Illness Syndrome." Frontiers in Cell and Developmental Biology 8 (2021): 614030.

9) Wenzek, Christina, et al. "The Interplay of Thyroid Hormones and the Immune System—Where We Stand and Why We Need to Know About It." European Journal of Endocrinology 186.5 (2022): R65-R77.

10) Schoenfeld, Philip S., et al. "Suppression of Cell-Mediated Immunity in Hypothyroidism." Southern medical journal 88.3 (1995): 347-349.

11) De Vito, Paolo, et al. "Thyroid Hormones as Modulators of Immune Activities at The Cellular Level." Thyroid 21.8 (2011): 879-890.

12) Alamino, V. A., et al. "The Thyroid Hormone Triiodothyronine Reinvigorates Dendritic Cells and Potentiates Anti-Tumor Immunity." OncoImmunology 5.1 (2016): e1064579.

13) G Ahmed, R., et al. "Nongenomic Actions of Thyroid Hormones: From Basic Research to Clinical Applications. an Update." Immunology, Endocrine & Metabolic Agents in Medicinal Chemistry 13.1 (2013): 46-59.

14) Kim, Won Gu, and Sheue-yann Cheng. "Thyroid Hormone Receptors and Cancer." Biochimica et Biophysica Acta (BBA)-General Subjects 1830.7 (2013): 3928-3936.

15) Klecha, Alicia J., et al. "Integrative Study of Hypothalamus–Pituitary–Thyroid–Immune System Interaction: Thyroid Hormone-Mediated Modulation of Lymphocyte Activity Through the Protein Kinase C Signaling Pathway." Journal of Endocrinology 189.1 (2006): 45-55.

16) Montesinos, María del Mar, and Claudia Gabriela Pellizas. "Thyroid Hormone Action on Innate Immunity." Frontiers in Endocrinology 10 (2019): 350.

17) Jara, Evelyn L., et al. "Modulating the Function of the Immune System by Thyroid Hormones and Thyrotropin." Immunology Letters 184 (2017): 76-83.

18) Van der Spek, et al. "Thyroid Hormone and Deiodination in Innate Immune Cells." Endocrinology 162.1 (2021): bqaa200.

19) Van Der Spek, Anne H., et al. "Regulation of Intracellular Triiodothyronine is Essential for Optimal Macrophage Function." Endocrinology 159.5 (2018): 2241-2252.

20) Barnes, Broda. "Basal Temperature Versus Basal Metabolism." Journal of the American Medical Association 119.14 (1942): 1072-1074.

Chapter 13

Thyroid Hormone Prevents Heart Attacks

The Low Thyroid Condition and Heart Disease

IN 1976, DR. BRODA BARNES observed heart disease and heart attacks associated with a low thyroid condition and wrote his classic book, Solved the Riddle of Heart Attacks. Dr. Barnes discovered this connection during summer vacations in Graz, Austria. Dr. Barnes knew the area around Graz had a high prevalence of thyroid disorders, and for the past 100 years, authorities mandated autopsies on every citizen of Graz, yielding a wealth of autopsy data for study by Dr. Barnes. While studying the autopsy files every summer, Dr. Barnes discovered low thyroid patients survived the usual childhood infectious diseases thanks to the invention of antibiotics. However, many of these same low thyroid patients died of heart disease years later. Barnes also found that thyroid hormone was protective in preventing heart attacks. Likewise, for diabetes, Dr. Barnes found thyroid hormone beneficial for preventing vascular disease in diabetics. (1)

The Hunt Study – Thyroid Function and Heart Disease

The 2008 Hunt Study from Norway by Dr. Bjørn Åsvold creates a paradigm shift in thyroid treatment and confirms that Dr. Broda Barnes was right all along. The 2008 Hunt Study published in the Archives of Internal Medicine examined TSH's correlation with mortality from coronary heart disease (CHD). Dr. Bjørn Åsvold concludes:

> The results indicate that relatively low but clinically normal thyroid function may increase the risk of fatal CHD [coronary heart disease]. (2-4)

The Hunt Study measured TSH levels in 17,000 women and 8,000 men with no known underlying thyroid disease or heart disease. All patients had "normal TSH" levels meaning the TSH values were in the lab reference range of 0.5 to 3.5 mU/L. The women were stratified into three groups, lower TSH, intermediate, and upper TSH levels, and mortality from heart disease was recorded over an 8-year observation period.

70% Increase in Heart Disease Mortality for TSH in Upper Normal Range

The Hunt study found that the group with the higher TSH had a 70% increased mortality from heart disease compared to the lower TSH group. Remember, all these TSH values were in the normal lab range.

	TSH	Death from Heart Disease
Group 1	0.50-1.4	Baseline Risk
Group 2	1.5-2.	40% higher than Baseline
Group 3	2.5-3.5	70% higher than Baseline

This mortality benefit is mind-boggling and far exceeds any drug intervention available. One may then ask the next most logical question. Can the use of thyroid hormone to reduce TSH to the low end of "normal" (0.5 mU/L) similarly reduce mortality from cardiovascular disease? We will try to answer this question below.

Thyroid Hormone also improves LDL Lipo-Proteins

Another report from the Hunt Study published in 2007 showed that LDL cholesterol was linearly associated with TSH levels. The best way to normalize the lipoprotein profile and reduce mortality from heart disease is to reduce TSH to the lower end of the normal range. A TSH in the upper end of the normal range is associated with increased cardiovascular mortality and elevations in LDL lipoprotein measurements. A TSH at the lower end of the normal range is associated with protection from heart disease. (2-4)

Statin Drugs or Thyroid to Prevent Heart Disease in Women?

Decades of published statin drug studies show that statin drugs simply do not work for women. Yes, statin drugs reduce cholesterol levels. However, there is no health benefit for women to reduce cholesterol levels with statin drugs, with no reduction in all-cause nor cardiovascular mortality. On the other hand, the HUNT study shows that TSH levels in the lower normal range provide a 70% reduction in heart disease mortality for women. Could this same reduction in mortality be accomplished with thyroid medication for women with elevated TSH? If so, then this is good news for women with elevated TSH concerned about preventing heart disease. Thyroid hormone replacement is an alternative to statin drugs that is far more effective. Rather than levothyroxine, generic Synthroid, we prefer to use natural desiccated thyroid, NDT, because clinical results are better. (5-6)

Natural Thyroid Adverse Effects of Palpitations

Although natural thyroid is safe, there is always the possibility of adverse effects from thyroid excess, defined as too much thyroid medication. The earliest sign of thyroid excess is usually a rapid heart rate at rest or perhaps palpitations at rest. Thyroid hormone intensifies the Beta-adrenergic effect on the heart, increasing the heart rate (sinus tachycardia). This effect can be reversed by the judicious use of a Beta Blocker drug such as propranolol, commonly prescribed for Graves' disease patients in thyrotoxicosis. (7-9)

Instructions for the Patient

We spend about five minutes at the office reviewing this adverse effect before starting patients on thyroid medication. Usually, patients will notice the resting heart rate going up as the first sign. Once recognized, the patient is instructed to stop the thyroid medication. Symptoms usually resolve within 6 hours for natural desiccated thyroid, NDT. However, this is not true for levothyroxine (T4 only), which has a longer half-life and may take a week for symptoms to resolve. It is perfectly safe to stop the NDT thyroid medication at any time, as there will be no acute changes, merely a gradual reversion to the original state that existed before starting the thyroid pills.

Some patients are very sensitive to thyroid medication and will have excess thyroid symptoms such as rapid heart rate and palpitations from small amounts of thyroid medication. These are usually the elderly with underlying heart disease and/or magnesium deficiency, and we usually avoid giving thyroid medication to these patients. We also liberally supplement everyone with magnesium if their RBC magnesium levels are low. Another group of patients, those with low cortisol or impaired adrenal function, may have difficulty tolerating small doses of thyroid hormone. This is discussed in Chapter 34 Adrenal Insufficiency, HPA Dysfunction, and Fatigue.

About 5 percent of our patients initially started on thyroid medication will notice symptoms of thyroid excess with a rapid heart rate. They will stop the medication for a day or two and restart at a lower dosage with no problem. This is more common in Hashimoto's patients whose own production of thyroid hormones may fluctuate from month to month. This problem of fluctuating thyroid hormone levels resolves when the Hashimoto's patient is on a suitable dose of thyroid medication that suppresses the TSH. Patients with magnesium deficiency or HPA dysfunction (with low AM cortisol output on salivary testing), will also tend to be more sensitive to small amounts of thyroid medication, so caution is also advised in these groups.

Adrenal Insufficiency and Adrenal Crisis

Autoimmune adrenal insufficiency is commonly associated with autoimmune thyroid disease. It is important to recognize adrenal insufficiency prior to prescribing thyroid hormone medication since thyroid hormone may precipitate adrenal crisis in these cases. Treatment with glucocorticoids may reverse hypothyroidism in these cases, and thyroid hormone may not be needed. Low AM cortisol, high ACTH, and inability to tolerate small doses of thyroid hormone are possible tip-offs that underlying adrenal insufficiency may be present. (10-19)

In 2005, Dr. Roberto Salvatori writes:

> In patients [with adrenal insufficiency] who are also hypothyroid, thyroid hormones should never be replaced before administering glucocorticoids; euthyroidism may trigger an adrenal crisis by accelerating the metabolism of cortisol. (17)

This is discussed more completely in Chapter 34 on Adrenal Insufficiency, HPA Dysfunction, and Chronic Fatigue.

Thyroid Excess Can Rarely Cause Atrial Fibrillation

So far, our office patients have been fortunate to avoid atrial fibrillation from excess thyroid medication. Avoiding atrial fibrillation is important, and that is why we spend a great deal of time with each patient discussing the symptoms of thyroid excess and the importance of stopping the thyroid medication if these symptoms are noted. The main symptom we are looking for is rapid heart rate at rest. If the patient notices this, they are instructed to hold the thyroid pill for a day, and once symptoms resolve resume at a lower dosage.

Mainstream Doctors Do Not Have Time to Discuss Adverse Effects

Perhaps one of the reasons the mainstream conventional doctors will give only a minuscule amount of levothyroxine, generic Synthroid, to the low thyroid patient is that they simply do not have the time to discuss thyroid excess and cannot afford an adverse event which is more likely if the patient does not have a clue about what to watch out for. In addition, mainstream medical doctors may not recognize the patient with HPA dysfunction and low cortisol output or magnesium deficiency, so they can run into problems with thyroid excess without understanding why. This also makes them cautious, tending to undertreat. (20)

Atrial Fibrillation

In patients with underlying heart disease prone to cardiac arrhythmias, thyroid excess can cause atrial fibrillation with characteristic irregular heart rate and EKG findings. Atrial fibrillation can be a problem because if it becomes chronic and does not resolve on its own, the cardiologist will try a maneuver called cardioversion, the application of an electrical shock to restart a normal cardiac rhythm. Catheter ablation is another form of treatment for chronic atrial fibrillation. A commonly prescribed cardiology drug for atrial fibrillation is amiodarone discussed in Chapter 19. Iodine-Induced Hyperthyroidism. Amiodarone contains iodine and one of the adverse effects is hyperthyroidism. Because atrial fibrillation causes stagnant blood and clot formation in the left atrium, blood thinners are prescribed to prevent a stroke from cerebral embolization (CVA cerebrovascular accident). Blood thinners carry the risk of bleeding. One may avoid atrial fibrillation by simply stopping the thyroid pills whenever symptoms of rapid heart rate or palpitations are noted at rest. Exercise-induced tachycardia, rapid heart rate, does not count since that is a normal cardiovascular response to exercise. (21-22)

HUNT Study Repeated in the United States

Dr. Kosuke Inoue Suggests Re-evaluation of TSH reference Range

In 2016, Dr. Kosuke Inoue repeated the HUNT study in the United States by following a prospective cohort of 12,584 U.S. adults over 20 years of age with normal TSH levels. After 19 years of follow-up and 3,395 deaths, Dr. Kosuke Inoue found high normal TSH associated with increased all-cause and cardiovascular mortality, as demonstrated in the HUNT study. Dr. Kosuke Inoue writes:

> A significantly higher risk of all-cause mortality (adjusted hazard ratio HR 1.27), and cardiovascular mortality (HR 1.30), and cancer mortality (HR 1.43) was observed in the high normal TSH group than in the medium normal TSH group... Conclusions: High normal TSH levels compared with medium normal TSH levels were associated with **increased risk of all-cause, cardiovascular, and cancer mortalities over a long-term follow-up period among U.S. adults**. This study indicates that the reference range for TSH levels may require re-evaluation. (6)

Subclinical Hypothyroidism

Subclinical hypothyroidism (SCH) is defined as elevated TSH with normal thyroid hormone levels. In 2012, Dr. Salman Razvi studied patients with subclinical hypothyroidism, finding treatment with levothyroxine was associated with fewer cardiac ischemic events in younger people (40-70 yrs.) with SCH. (23)

A Review of the Medical Literature

In 2020, Dr. Negar Omidi reviewed the medical literature on thyroid hormone replacement in cardiovascular disorders, agreeing with Dr. Broda Barnes that hypothyroidism is associated with an increased risk for cardiovascular disease. For the hypothyroid patient suffering from chest pain (angina) from atherosclerotic coronary artery disease, Dr. Negar Omidi feels treatment with levothyroxine will resolve angina and halt the progression of coronary artery disease. Caution with levothyroxine is advised in the elderly. Even subclinical hypothyroidism (SCH) is a risk factor for cardiovascular disease. However, Dr. Omodi is not convinced patients with subclinical hypothyroidism (SCH) require treatment with thyroid medication. Dr. Negar Omidi writes:

> Studies on patients with overt hypothyroidism and those with myxedema coma demonstrated an increased rate of atherosclerosis among these patients compared with controls... Subclinical hypothyroidism is a clinically asymptomatic state of the disease with abnormal laboratory findings, i.e., a TSH level above the normal cutoff range with normal thyroid hormone levels. The condition has a considerable prevalence of 4.3% to 9.5% in the United States... a meta-analysis of 11 prospective cohort studies has revealed an association between subclinical hypothyroidism and increased risk of cardiovascular complications such as coronary heart disease and mortality. In addition, another meta-analysis by Singh et al. demonstrated that subclinical hypothyroidism was significantly related to coronary artery disease and cardiovascular mortality. **As a result, even subclinical hypothyroidism can be considered as a risk factor for cardiovascular disorders, although further evidence on this matter seems necessary**...Treating **overt hypothyroidism** with levothyroxine improves a large portion of the cardiovascular dysfunction caused by the disease, including a lipid profile, diastolic dysfunction, cardiomyopathy, hypertension, heart rate, and its variability during exercise. **Levothyroxine is also effective for interrupting the progression of atherosclerosis in these patients...A large study on hypothyroid subjects suggested that angina may improve or at least stop recurring in these patients after treatment with levothyroxine**...With regard to subclinical hypothyroidism, the evidence is present but not enough to conclude treatment with thyroid hormones...(24-25)

Low Free T3 Associated with Increased Coronary Artery Calcification

Coronary artery calcification can be measured with a CAT scan which yields the coronary calcium score, the most sensitive and accurate predictor of heart attack risk. The cholesterol panel has largely been replaced by the calcium score, as discussed in 2018, Heart Book, by Jeffrey Dach MD (one of my previous books). (26-30)

In 2014, Dr. Zhu from China showed a low Free T3 (FT3) level is associated with increased coronary artery calcification and increased major cardiac events (MACE). Dr. Zhu writes:

> FT3 levels are associated with coronary artery calcification scores and the incidence rate of MACE in patients with suspected coronary artery disease. A low FT3 level is considered an important risk factor for high calcification scores and MACE. (31)

Many other studies using calcium score or coronary angiography confirm the association of low Free T3 levels with the severity and progression of coronary artery disease, while higher free T3 levels are protective. (32-35)

In 2019, Dr. Madalena von Hafe reviewed the impact of hypothyroidism on ischemic heart disease stating that low thyroid hormone levels are a risk factor for atherosclerotic coronary artery disease, and thyroid hormone replacement may reverse atherosclerosis, and improve blood flow to the heart. Thyroid hormone replacement is a promising treatment for patients with ischemic heart disease. Dr. Madalena von Hafe writes:

> in ischemic heart disease, abnormalities in thyroid hormone levels are common and are an important factor to be considered. In fact, low thyroid hormone levels should be interpreted as a cardiovascular risk factor.... **TH replacement therapy may reverse atherosclerosis**, lower peripheral vascular resistance and improve myocardial perfusion in patients with hypothyroidism... **TH replacement treatment exhibits anti-**

ischemic and cardioprotective effects, acting as a promising target for ischemic heart disease. (37-38)

Conclusion

Back in the 1960s, Dr. Broda Barnes recognized the link between hypothyroidism and coronary artery disease, recommending thyroid hormone replacement as prevention and treatment for ischemic heart disease. Decades later, many independent studies have finally confirmed that Dr. Barnes was right all along. Ignoring the link between coronary atherosclerosis and thyroid function is another error of conventional endocrinology. (38-63)

♦ **References for Chapter 13**

1) Barnes, Broda Otto, and Charlotte W. Barnes. Solved the Riddle of Heart Attacks. Robinson Press, 1976.

2) Åsvold, Bjørn O., et al. "Thyrotropin Levels and Risk of Fatal Coronary Heart Disease: The HUNT Study." Archives Of Internal Medicine 168.8 (2008): 855-860.

3) Asvold, Bjørn O., et al. "The Association Between TSH Within the Reference Range and Serum Lipid Concentrations in a Population-Based Study. The HUNT Study." European Journal of Endocrinology 156.2 (2007): 181-186.

4) Åsvold, Bjørn O., et al. "Thyroid Function and the Risk of Coronary Heart Disease: 12-Year Follow-Up of the HUNT Study in Norway." Clinical Endocrinology 77.6 (2012): 911-917.

5) Walsh, Judith ME, and Michael Pignone. "Drug Treatment of Hyperlipidemia in Women." Jama 291.18 (2004): 2243-2252.

6) Inoue, Kosuke, et al. "Association Between Serum Thyrotropin Levels and Mortality Among Euthyroid Adults in The United States." Thyroid 26.10 (2016): 1457-1465.

7) Marrakchi, S., et al. "Arrhythmia and Thyroid Dysfunction." Herz 40. Suppl 2 (2015): 101-9.

8) Hoit, Brian D., et al. "Effects of Thyroid Hormone on Cardiac B-Adrenergic Responsiveness in Conscious Baboons." Circulation 96.2 (1997): 592-598.

9) Williams, Lewis T., et al. "Thyroid Hormone Regulation of Beta-Adrenergic Receptor Number." Journal of Biological Chemistry 252.8 (1977): 2787-2789.

10) Kasperlik-Załuska, Anna A., et al. "Autoimmunity as the Most Frequent Cause of Idiopathic Secondary Adrenal Insufficiency: Report of 111 Cases." Autoimmunity 36.3 (2003): 155-159.

11) Papierska, Lucyna, and Michał Rabijewski. "Delay in Diagnosis of Adrenal Insufficiency Is a Frequent Cause of Adrenal Crisis." International Journal of Endocrinology 2013 (2013).

12) Choudhary, Nidhi, et al. "Thyroxine Replacement Precipitating Adrenal Crisis." Endocrine Abstracts. Vol. 19. Bioscientifica, 2009.

13) Fonseca, V., et al. "Acute Adrenal Crisis Precipitated by Thyroxine." British Medical Journal (Clinical Research ed.) 292.6529 (1986): 1185.

14) Davis, Julian, and Michael Sheppard. "Acute Adrenal Crisis Precipitated by Thyroxine." British Medical Journal (Clinical research ed.) 292.6535 (1986): 1595.

15) Osman, I. A., and Peter Leslie. "Addison's Disease. Adrenal Insufficiency Should Be Excluded Before Thyroxine Replacement Is Started." BMJ: British Medical Journal 313.7054 (1996): 427.

16) Murray, Jonathan Stephen, et al. "Deterioration of Symptoms After Start of Thyroid Hormone Replacement." BMJ 323.7308 (2001): 332-333.

17) Salvatori, Roberto. "Adrenal Insufficiency." JAMA 294.19 (2005): 2481-2488.

18) Abdullatif, Hussein D., and Ambika P. Ashraf. "Reversible Subclinical Hypothyroidism in the Presence of Adrenal Insufficiency." Endocrine Practice 12.5 (2006): 572-575.

19) Kasperlik-Załuska, A. A., et al. "Secondary Adrenal Insufficiency Associated with Autoimmune Disorders: A Report of Twenty-Five Cases." Clinical Endocrinology 49.6 (1998): 779-783.

20) Ho, Timothy, et al. "Post-Visit Patient Understanding About Newly Prescribed Medications." Journal of General Internal Medicine (2021): 1-4.

21) Abonowara, Abdulgani, et al. "Prevalence of Atrial Fibrillation in Patients Taking TSH Suppression Therapy for Management of Thyroid Cancer." Clinical and Investigative Medicine (2012): E152-E156.

22) Papaleontiou, Maria, et al. "Thyroid Hormone Therapy and Incident Stroke." The Journal of Clinical Endocrinology & Metabolism 106.10 (2021): e3890-e3900.

23) Razvi, Salman, et al. "Levothyroxine Treatment of Subclinical Hypothyroidism, Fatal and Nonfatal Cardiovascular Events, and Mortality." Archives of Internal Medicine 172.10 (2012): 811-817.

24) Omidi, Negar, et al. "The Role of Thyroid Diseases and their Medications in Cardiovascular Disorders: A Review of the Literature." Current Cardiology Reviews 16.2 (2020): 103-116.

25) Palmieri, Emiliano A., et al. "Subclinical Hypothyroidism and Cardiovascular Risk: A Reason to Treat?" Treatments in Endocrinology 3 (2004): 233-244.

26) Hecht, Harvey S., et al. "Relation of Coronary Artery Calcium Identified by Electron Beam Tomography to Serum Lipoprotein Levels and Implications for Treatment." The American Journal of Cardiology 87.4 (2001): 406-412.

27) Hecht, Harvey S. "Coronary Artery Calcium Scanning: Past, Present, and Future." JACC: Cardiovascular Imaging 8.5 (2015): 579-596.

28) Nicoll, Rachel, et al. "The Coronary Calcium Score is a More Accurate Predictor of Significant Coronary Stenosis than Conventional Risk Factors in Symptomatic Patients: Euro-CCAD Study." International Journal of Cardiology 207 (2016): 13-19.

29) Greenland, Philip, et al. "Coronary Calcium Score and Cardiovascular Risk." Journal of the American College of Cardiology 72.4 (2018): 434-447.

30) Dach, Jeffrey. Heart Book. How to Keep Your Heart Healthy, Medical Muse Press, 2018.

31) Zhu, Lijie, et al. "Relationship of Serum-Free T3 With the Coronary Artery Calcification and Major Adverse Cardiac Events in Patients with Suspected Coronary Artery Disease." Zhonghua Xin Xue Guan Bing Za Zhi 42.12 (2014): 1017-1021.

32) Yu, Na, et al. "The Association of Thyroid Hormones with Coronary Atherosclerotic Severity in Euthyroid Patients." Hormone and Metabolic Research 54.01 (2022): 12-19.

33) Abdu, Fuad A., et al. "Low Free Triiodothyronine as a Predictor of Poor Prognosis in Patients with Myocardial Infarction with Non-Obstructive Coronary Arteries." Frontiers in Endocrinology 12 (2021).

34) Zhou, Bing-Yang, et al. "Free Triiodothyronine in Relation to Coronary Severity at Different Ages: Gensini Score Assessment in 4206 Euthyroid Patients." Journal of Geriatric Cardiology: JGC 13.12 (2016): 978.

35) Gholampourdehaki, Mehrzad. "Relationship Between Thyroid Hormones Levels and Coronary Artery Disease in Euthyroid Individuals." EBNESINA 23.2 (2021): 92-99.

36) Zhang, Baowei, et al. "A Low FT3 Level as a Prognostic Marker in Patients with Acute Myocardial Infarctions." Internal Medicine 51.21 (2012): 3009-3015.

37) Von Hafe, Madalena, et al. "The Impact of Thyroid Hormone Dysfunction on Ischemic Heart Disease." Endocrine Connections 8.5 (2019): R76.

38) Lev-Ran, Arye. "Thyroid Hormones and Prevention of Atherosclerotic Heart Disease: An Old-New Hypothesis." Perspectives in Biology and Medicine 37.4 (1994): 486-494.

39) Lang, Xueyan, et al. "FT3/FT4 Ratio Is Correlated with All-Cause Mortality, Cardiovascular Mortality, and Cardiovascular Disease Risk: NHANES 2007-2012." Frontiers in Endocrinology 13 (2022): 964822.

40) Yuan, Deshan, et al. "Predictive Value of Free Triiodothyronine (FT3) to Free Thyroxine (FT4) Ratio in Long-Term Outcomes of Euthyroid Patients with Three-Vessel Coronary Artery Disease." Nutrition, Metabolism and Cardiovascular Diseases 31.2 (2021): 579-586.

41) Coceani, Michele, et al. "Thyroid Hormone and Coronary Artery Disease: From Clinical Correlations to Prognostic Implications." Clinical Cardiology: An International Indexed and Peer-Reviewed Journal for Advances in the Treatment of Cardiovascular Disease 32.7 (2009): 380-385.

42) Ertaş, Faruk, et al. "Low Serum Free Triiodothyronine Levels Are Associated with the Presence and Severity of Coronary Artery Disease in the Euthyroid Patients: An Observational Study." Anatolian Journal of Cardiology/Anadolu Kardiyoloji Dergisi 12.7 (2012).

43) Daswani, Ravi, et al. "Association of Thyroid Function with Severity of Coronary Artery Disease in Euthyroid Patients." Journal Of Clinical and Diagnostic Research: JCDR 9.6 (2015): OC10.

44) Zhang, Yiyi, et al. "Thyroid Hormones and Coronary Artery Calcification in Euthyroid Men and Women." Arteriosclerosis, Thrombosis, and Vascular Biology 34.9 (2014): 2128-2134.

45) Park, Hye-Jeong, et al. "Association of Low Baseline Free Thyroxin Levels with Progression of Coronary Artery Calcification Over 4 Years in Euthyroid Subjects: The Kangbuk Samsung Health Study." Clinical Endocrinology 84.6 (2016): 889-895.

46) Imaizumi, Misa, et al. "Risk for Ischemic Heart Disease and All-Cause Mortality in Subclinical Hypothyroidism. Journal of Clinical Endocrinology & Metabolism 89.7 (2004): 3365-3370.

47) Kim, Eun Sook, et al. "Association Between Low Serum Free Thyroxine Concentrations and Coronary Artery Calcification in Healthy Euthyroid Subjects." Thyroid 22.9 (2012): 870-876.

48) Rajagopalan, Viswanathan, et al. "Safe Oral Triiodo-L-Thyronine Therapy Protects from Post-Infarct Cardiac Dysfunction and Arrhythmias Without Cardiovascular Adverse Effects." PLoS one 11.3 (2016): e0151413.

49) Suh, Sunghwan, and Duk Kyu Kim. "Subclinical Hypothyroidism and Cardiovascular Disease." Endocrinology and Metabolism 30.3 (2015): 246.

50) Kvetny, J. et al. "Subclinical Hypothyroidism Is Associated with a Low-Grade Inflammation, Increased Triglyceride Levels and Predicts Cardiovascular Disease in Males Below 50 Years." Clinical endocrinology 61.2 (2004): 232.

51) Hak, A. Elisabeth, et al. "Subclinical Hypothyroidism Is an Independent Risk Factor for Atherosclerosis and Myocardial Infarction in Elderly Women: The Rotterdam Study." Ann Intern Med 132 (2000): 270-278.

52) Tseng, Fen-Yu, et al. "Subclinical Hypothyroidism Is Associated with Increased Risk for All-Cause and Cardiovascular Mortality in Adults." Journal of the American College of Cardiology 60.8 (2012): 730-737.

53) Rhee, Connie M., et al. "Hypothyroidism and Mortality Among Dialysis Patients." Clinical Journal of the American Society of Nephrology (2012): CJN-06920712.

54) Razvi, Salman, et al. "The Incidence of Ischemic Heart Disease and Mortality in People with Subclinical Hypothyroidism: Reanalysis of the Whickham Survey Cohort." The Journal of Clinical Endocrinology and Metabolism 95.4 (2010): 1734-1740.

55) Rodondi, Nicolas, et al. "Subclinical Hypothyroidism and the Risk of Coronary Heart Disease and Mortality." JAMA: the Journal of the American Medical Association 304.12 (2010): 1365.

56) Langen, Ville L., et al. "Thyroid-Stimulating Hormone and Risk of Sudden Cardiac Death, Total Mortality and Cardiovascular Morbidity." Clinical Endocrinology 88.1 (2018): 105-113.

57) Ortolani Jr, Pedro D., et al. "Association of Serum Thyrotropin Levels with Coronary Artery Disease Documented by Quantitative Coronary Angiography: A Transversal Study." Archives of Endocrinology and Metabolism 62 (2018): 410-415.

58) Seo, Suk Min, et al. "Thyroid Stimulating Hormone Elevation as a Predictor of Long-Term Mortality in Patients with Acute Myocardial Infarction." Clinical Cardiology 41.10 (2018): 1367-1373.

59) Sue, Laura Y., and Angela M. Leung. "Levothyroxine for the Treatment of Subclinical Hypothyroidism and Cardiovascular Disease." Frontiers In Endocrinology 11 (2020): 591588.

60) Udovcic, Maja, et al. "Hypothyroidism and the Heart." Methodist DeBakey Cardiovascular Journal 13.2 (2017): 55.

61) Corona, G., et al. "Thyroid and Heart, a Clinically Relevant Relationship." Journal of Endocrinological Investigation 44.12 (2021): 2535-2544.

62) Shi, Hongshuo, et al. "Efficacy and Safety of Thyroxine Therapy on Patients with Heart Failure and Subclinical Hypothyroidism: A Protocol for Systematic Review and Meta-Analysis." Medicine 100.3 (2021).

63) Biondi, Bernadette. "Is There Any Reason to Treat Subclinical Hypo and Hyperthyroidism?" Annales d'Endocrinologie. Vol. 82. No. 3-4. Elsevier Masson, 2021.

Chapter 14

The Production of Thyroid Hormone

SUCCESSFUL TREATMENT OF THYROID DISORDERS requires a solid understanding of the production of thyroid hormone and how this relates to thyroid disorders and their treatments. In this chapter, we take a deep dive into the molecular biology and pathophysiology of the thyroid gland production of thyroid hormone at the cellular and biochemical levels. In addition, we will explore how drug treatment for thyroid disease affects thyroid hormone production.

What is Thyroid Hormone?

The main job of the thyroid gland is to produce thyroid hormone and release it into the bloodstream. The serum ration of T4 to T3 is about 4:1. Once secreted into the bloodstream by the thyroid cells called thyrocytes, T4 thyroid hormone is transported to a trillion cells in our body, called the periphery. Once the T4 thyroid hormone reaches the peripheral cell, it must be taken up and converted to T3, its active form. This conversion from T4 to T3 is done by the D1 and D2 deiodinase enzymes. T4 is a pro-hormone with four iodine atoms attached to two tyrosine rings. The D2 deiodinase enzyme is intracellular and removes one iodine from T4, thus converting T4 into T3. This intracellular T3 is the active form of thyroid hormone which increases intracellular energy and serves as a "major endocrine controller of metabolic rate," as discussed below. The membrane-bound D1 deiodinase also converts T4 to T3 and is responsible for most of the circulating T3. Lastly, the D3 deiodinase converts T4 to an inactive form, reverse T3. This is a protective mechanism to prevent hyperthyroidism at the cellular level.

The Major Controller of Metabolic Rate

The thyroid has far-reaching effects on health from fetal development to adulthood, which cannot be overstated. In 2014, Dr. Carla Portulano discussed the significance of thyroid function for overall human health, writing:

> The significance of the thyroid gland for human health is difficult to overstate, given the wide-ranging effects of the thyroid hormones on prenatal and early development as well as on intermediary metabolism at all stages of life. (1)

Increases Size and Number of Mitochondria

Thyroid hormones have been described as "the major endocrine controllers of metabolic rate." Higher thyroid hormone levels increase the metabolic rate, primarily from effects on mitochondria, stimulating increased numbers and size of mitochondria, called mitochondriogenesis, as well as respiratory chain components within the mitochondria. In 2008, Dr. Mary Ellen Harper discussed the effect of thyroid hormone on mitochondria, writing:

> thyroid hormones stimulate mitochondriogenesis and thereby augment cellular oxidative capacity. Thyroid hormones induce substantial modifications in mitochondrial inner membrane protein and lipid compositions. Results are consistent with the idea that thyroid hormones activate the uncoupling of oxidative phosphorylation through various mechanisms involving inner membrane proteins and lipids. Increased uncoupling appears to be responsible for some of the hypermetabolic effects of thyroid hormones. (2)

In 2022, Dr. Federica Cioffi discussed how thyroid hormones increase specific components of the mitochondrial respiratory chain, writing:

almost all components of the respiratory chain [within mitochondria] are directly or indirectly affected by iodothyronines [thyroid hormones]. In some cases, the actions result in an activation of specific biochemical pathways, while in others, the effects would result in an increase in mRNA or protein levels of specific components of the respiratory chain. (3)

The Thyrocyte and Follicular Lumen:

Thyrocytes are worker bees of the thyroid gland, arranged circumferentially around the follicles, the round "storage tanks" filled with pink staining colloid, also called thyroglobulin, a precursor converted to thyroid hormone by adding iodine molecules. This process is called organification. The cover of this book shows a photomicrograph of the thyroid gland demonstrating the architectural pattern of hundreds of follicles lined by thyrocytes.

The NIS Sodium Iodide Symporter

The thyrocytes are roughly triangular-shaped and have a specific orientation. The apex is nearest the lumen of the follicle and contains the villous apical membrane involved in organification. The basal membrane of the thyrocyte contains the NIS, the sodium iodide symporter, the active transport mechanism which takes up iodide from the bloodstream and concentrates iodide 20-50 times that of plasma in normal people, and 100 times in Graves' disease. (4)

Five Steps of Thyroid Hormone Synthesis

In 2022, Dr. Muhammad Shahid discussed the five steps of thyroid synthesis. (5)

Step One: Synthesis of Thyroglobulin:
Thyrocytes lining the thyroid follicles produce a protein called thyroglobulin (TG), the precursor to thyroid hormone. TG is secreted by exocytosis into the follicles where it is stored for later use. Initially, thyroglobulin has no iodine molecules attached. However, over time, the thyrocyte attaches iodine to the thyroglobulin in a process called organification. This is done at the apical villous membrane, the work area.

Step Two: Uptake of Iodide, the Sodium Iodide Symporter:
TSH stimulation causes increased activity of the Sodium Iodide Symporter (NIS), the active transport of iodide into the thyrocyte. The NIS is a protein embedded within the basolateral membrane of the thyrocyte, actively pumping iodide into the cell, maintaining a concentration 20 to 50 times higher than in the bloodstream. In Graves' hyperthyroidism, this ratio is increased to greater than 100 times higher due to massive TSH receptor stimulation by TSI and TRAb antibodies. In Graves' disease, this increased concentration of iodide within the thyrocyte is rapidly converted to thyroid hormone by a process called organification, the addition of iodine to thyroglobulin, discussed below. Extremely high thyroid hormone levels cause thyrotoxicosis and TSH suppression to near-zero blood levels. Normal thyroids will stop producing thyroid hormone if the TSH is near zero. However, in Graves' disease, TSH receptor antibodies continue to uncontrollably stimulate thyroid hormone production. (6-16)

Concentrating Lithium and Bromine

The NIS in the thyrocyte basal membrane will also concentrate other ions, such as lithium and bromine. Lithium is discussed in its own Chapter 17. Bromine is toxic, and if concentrated in the thyroid gland, this may interfere with iodine uptake and concentration, leading to iodine deficiency and hypothyroidism. Bromine is present in certain soft drinks which contain BVO (brominated vegetable oil), and is present in the environment as flame retardants and food fumigants. This is discussed in Chapter 29. Bromine Detoxification with Unrefined Sea Salt. (17)

The iodide is pumped into the thyrocyte by the NIS at the basolateral membrane and diffuses through the thyrocyte towards the apical membrane, where it is pumped by the Pendrin transporter into the follicular lumen. Note: the role of Pendrin is still a question for debate. (18-28)

Step Three: Iodination of Thyroglobulin:

Thyroglobulin provides the polypeptide backbone for the synthesis and storage of thyroid hormone within the follicle. The thyrocyte manufactures thyroglobulin within the endoplasmic reticulum and uses exocytosis to secrete the thyroglobulin into the follicular lumen. Once in the follicular lumen, thyroglobulin is called colloid. Thyroglobulin is converted to thyroid hormone by the addition of iodine in a process called organification, carried out by the thyroperoxidase (TPO) enzyme, a heme-containing molecule with a porphyrin ring structure similar to hemoglobin. Simply stated, organification is the addition of iodine to thyroglobulin to make thyroid hormones.

TPO is secreted into the follicular lumen at the thyrocyte apex villous membrane and has three functions:

1) oxidation of iodide(I-) to iodine (I2).

2) organification of iodine, the attachment of iodine(I2) to thyroglobulin.

3) coupling together of two tyrosine residues to make T4, thyroxine.

Once iodide (I-) is oxidized by TPO to molecular iodine (I2), the molecular iodine then combines with ring-like Tyrosine residues on the thyroglobulin to form MIT and DIT (mono-io-do-tyrosine and di-iodothyronine).

Oxidation of Iodide to Iodine: TPO uses hydrogen peroxide to oxidize iodide (I-) to iodine (I2). The hydrogen peroxide is generated by NADPH oxidases, dual oxidases 1 and 2 (DUOX1 and DUOX2) located in the villous apex of the thyrocyte. Iodide, a negative ion, is oxidized to molecular iodine (I2) by the TPO thyroperoxidase enzyme using hydrogen peroxide as a substrate. This all takes place inside the follicles at the micro-villous surface of the apical membrane of the thyrocytes, the working area where the DUOX enzyme system generates hydrogen peroxide.

Organification: Iodine (I2) spontaneously attaches to tyrosine residues of thyroglobulin protein, generating monoiodotyrosine (MIT, one iodine) and di-iodotyrosine (DIT, two iodines)

Coupling reaction: Iodinated tyrosine residues are coupled by TPO making triiodothyronine (T3) and tetraiodothyronine (T4) also called thyroxine. T4 is made from 2 DITs coupled together. T3 is made from MIT and DIT coupled together.

Step Four: Storage: Thyroid hormones (T3 and T4) are stored in the follicular lumen bound to thyroglobulin as colloid, a combination of free and iodinated thyroglobulin.

Step 5: Release of thyroid hormone into circulation: Iodinated thyroglobulin is taken up at the apex of the thyrocytes within vesicles via endocytosis and travels back towards the basal membrane. While in transit, these vesicles are fused with lysosomes containing acid and proteolytic enzymes, which digest the thyroglobulin, freeing the T3 and T4, subsequently released at the basolateral membrane into the capillary bloodstream. Any extra iodine is salvaged and returned to the intracellular iodine pool. (18-28)

Hashimoto's Thyroiditis, Seropositive and Seronegative

In Hashimoto's thyroiditis, blood tests show elevated antibodies to the TPO (thyroperoxidase) enzyme and to thyroglobulin. All three proteins, TPO enzyme, thyroglobulin, and DUOX H2O2 generation are all located near the apical villous membrane inside the follicle, so they can all interact together. One hypothesis is that damage caused by excess hydrogen peroxide to TPO and thyroglobulin creates antigenicity and autoimmunity. Microscopic examination of the thyroid gland in Hashimoto's patients shows lymphocytic infiltration with both B-cells and T-cells, indicating an autoimmune process. In a small percentage of cases of Hashimoto's thyroiditis, the TPO and thyroglobulin tests will be negative. This is called seronegative Hashimoto's, found in about 5% of cases in population studies. In 1987, Dr. Betterly found 2.8% of the 144 seronegative controls showed subclinical hypothyroidism, which could be cases of seronegative Hashimoto's. In 2018, Dr. Emre Sedar Saygili from Turkey evaluated 670 thyroidectomy surgical specimens. In 89 cases the pathology findings were compatible with Hashimoto's thyroiditis (CTL). Of these 89 cases, 25 percent were seronegative Hashimoto's thyroiditis. Dr. Emre Sedar Saygili writes:

> In our study, although all our cases were histopathologically diagnosed with CLT [chronic lymphocytic thyroiditis, Hashimoto's disease], in approximately **one of four patients, both anti-Tg [anti-thyroglobulin] and anti-TPO [anti-thyroperoxidase] negativities were detected**. Histologically detection rate of Hashimoto thyroiditis is much higher than that of CLT diagnosed on the basis of serologic tests. Despite the availability of highly sensitive measurement methods, **in some patients with hypothyroidism, these antibodies cannot be detected**. Since hypoechoic thyroid pattern is observed in most of these patients during ultrasonographic examination, they have been considered to have seronegative autoimmune thyroiditis (SN-AIT). In population-based studies, the prevalence of SN-AIT has been estimated to be 5%. (29-32)

Immune Complexes Deposited Along Basement Membrane

In both Graves' and Hashimoto's disease, electron microscopy may show electron-dense deposits along the basement membrane of the follicular cells. These are immune complexes when visualized with immunofluorescent staining. These deposits could represent antibodies to the NIS, which is discussed in 2020 by Dr. Anna-Marie Eleftheriadou. When present, this may cause dysfunction of the NIS in these disease entities. (33-36)

Immunofluorescent staining in Hashimoto's with high titers of TPO antibodies shows intense staining of the cytoplasm of thyrocytes without staining of colloid in follicles. This is the location where TPO is manufactured. In cases with high thyroglobulin antibody titers, there is diffuse staining of colloid within the follicles. This is where the thyroglobulin is stored. (37-38)

Organification Defect in Hashimoto's – Perchlorate Discharge

Hashimoto's disease results in organification defect, a decreased ability to organify iodine. This is called "inability to organify iodine" and explains the low iodine content of the thyroid gland in Hashimoto's patients and the rapid washout of iodine with the perchlorate discharge test. Perchlorate is a competitive inhibitor of the NIS, sodium iodide symporter, and blocks iodide uptake, so any non-organified iodine remaining in the thyroid gland will "wash out." The test is useful for identifying an organification defect. (39-46)

Perchlorate Washout Test

In patients with lymphocytic thyroiditis, also called Hashimoto's thyroiditis, their perchlorate discharge test will show a positive test, meaning a large amount of iodine will wash out and not be retained by the thyroid. This indicates an organification defect. However, in normal patients, the iodide is oxidized to iodine by TPO and H202 and then organified, i.e., bound to Tyrosine residues on thyroglobulin. This organified iodine stays within the follicles and cannot "wash out." However, if the iodine is not organified, then it will wash out, as demonstrated by a perchlorate discharge test. A more sensitive version of this test is the "iodide-perchlorate" discharge test. (39-46)

Hypothyroidism From High Iodide Intake

High dietary iodine intake from seaweed consumption is commonplace in the Japanese diet. Most are able to compensate with no adverse effects. However, an occasional Japanese individual is unable to compensate and develops a high TSH from the suppressive effects of iodine on thyroid function. These patients harbor subclinical Hashimoto's thyroiditis. In 1986, Dr. Junichi Tajiri studied hypothyroidism (high TSH) induced by high iodine intake in 22 Japanese patients. Hypothyroidism was reversible for about half the patients using an iodine-restricted diet. In the other half, in which the hypothyroidism was irreversible, 9 out of 10 patients had a positive perchlorate discharge test, indicating an underlying organification defect. Thyroid biopsies showed the reversible patients had milder lymphocytic thyroiditis (autoimmune thyroiditis). On the other hand, those with irreversible hypothyroidism had more severe thyroid destruction. An organification defect is playing a major role in patients with lymphocytic thyroiditis (i.e., Hashimoto's thyroiditis). Dr. Junichi Tajiri found patients who are unable to compensate for a high-iodine Japanese diet usually have subclinical autoimmune thyroiditis with an organification defect. The authors write:

> **The patients with reversible hypothyroidism had focal lymphocytic thyroiditis changes in the thyroid biopsy specimen, whereas those with irreversible hypothyroidism had more severe destruction of the thyroid gland.** These results indicate the existence of a reversible type of hypothyroidism sensitive to iodine restriction and characterized by relatively minor changes in lymphocytic thyroiditis histologically. Attention should be directed to this type of hypothyroidism because thyroid function may revert to normal with iodine restriction alone. (46)

Methimazole Thyroid Blocking Drug

Methimazole (MMI), the first-line thyroid-blocking drug, works by irreversibly binding to and blocking the function of the TPO enzyme, thus inhibiting the organification of iodine. This inability to organify induced by methimazole bears a similarity to Hashimoto's thyroiditis which also has an organification defect. In addition, methimazole inhibits the DUOX enzyme, thus inhibiting hydrogen peroxide formation, a beneficial feature that prevents excess hydrogen peroxide damage to the thyrocytes.

When starting MMI for Graves' disease, it takes about six weeks (plus or minus two weeks) for thyroid hormone levels to normalize. It takes this amount of time for all the preformed thyroid hormones stored in follicles to be secreted and metabolized. Adverse side effects include rash and agranulocytosis, and these are dose-related. Agranulocytosis is serious and can induce fatal immunosuppression. MMI is about 10 times more potent than PTU (Propylthiouracil) in blocking thyroid function. Although MMI partially inhibits the DUOX enzyme, which generates hydrogen peroxide, it does not block the D1 deiodinase enzyme, which converts T4 to T3 in the periphery, as does PTU, corticosteroids, and the Beta Blocker, propranolol. Most of the circulating T3 is a result of the D1 deiodinase conversion of T4 to T3. In Graves' disease, the D1 deiodinase is upregulated, so blocking D1 with one of these drugs is beneficial for treating thyrotoxicosis. MMI has a long duration of action, allowing for once-a-day dosing. (47-51)

Methimazole Immunomodulatory Effects

There has been considerable study and interest in the immunomodulatory effects of methimazole which could explain long-term remission in a subset of Graves' disease patients, with normalization of TRAb antibodies and thyroid function. In my opinion, the inhibition of H2O2 generation by MMI may explain the immunomodulatory effects with gradual reduction of anti-thyroid antibody levels on long-term MMI treatment leading to remission. However, the exact mechanism MMI induces complete curative remission in Graves' disease is still a matter of debate. (52-59)

Methimazole Differences with KI or Lithium Carbonate

A major difference in the thyroid-blocking function of methimazole vs. potassium iodide (KI) or lithium carbonate is this: methimazole (MMI) does not block the release of thyroid hormone from the thyroid gland. However, **both KI and lithium block the release of thyroid hormone from the thyroid gland.** This feature is useful in some patients resistant to MMI, as it provides a different mechanism of action that may remain effective despite resistance to MMI. In Painless Thyroiditis (PT), MMI is ineffective. Other agents PTU, Corticosteroids, and Beta Blockers are more useful, as these inhibit D1 deiodinease and block conversion of T4 to T3. This is discussed in more detail in later Chapters on iodine and lithium for the treatment of Graves' Disease, Chapters 15-17.

Loss of Auto-Regulation in Hashimoto's

As mentioned above, the thyroid gland in Hashimoto's patients has lost the autoregulation needed to escape from the suppressive effects of KI dietary excess, rendering these patients more sensitive to "Iodine Blockade" described by Wolff and Chaikoff as the suppressive effect of iodide on thyroid function. In normal thyroid glands, downregulation of the NIS symporter RNA by iodide and direct inhibition of NIS within the basal membrane leads to eventual escape from the suppressive effects of KI within days. When autoregulatory activity is functioning normally, the thyroid compensates for the excess iodide by reducing iodide uptake and concentration at the NIS at the basolateral membrane. Although the normal healthy thyroid gland may escape from the inhibitory effects of excess iodide, there is no similar escape from thyroid blockade with methimazole or lithium. (60-63)

As mentioned above, after TPO antibody, the second antibody in Hashimoto's disease is the anti-thyroglobulin antibody. Additional antibodies against the NIS (sodium iodide symporter) and against Pendrin have also been discovered. However, lab tests for NIS and Pendrin are not yet available for clinicians. (6)(22)

Graves' Disease, TSI, and TRAb Antibodies

In Graves' disease, the TSI and TRAb antibodies stimulate the TSH receptor causing the signs and symptoms of Graves' hyperthyroidism. About 70-85 percent of Graves' disease patients also have thyroperoxidase (TPO) and thyroglobulin antibodies. These are Hashimoto's antibodies. Indeed, some authors believe Graves' and Hashimoto's' are two extremes of the same disease process with different manifestations. In 2023, Dr. Masahito Katahira found the presence of thyroglobulin antibodies was associated with milder disease and shorter time to remission, while presence of TPO antibodies in Graves' disease was associated with more severe disease with higher TRAb levels and longer time to remission writing:

> Patients positive for TgAbs [thyroglobulin antibodies] develop GD [Graves' disease] with lower TRAb titers and undergo earlier remission than those negative for TgAbs. Patients positive for TPOAbs [thyroperoxidase antibody] develop GD with high TRAb titers and need a long time to achieve remission. (64) (149-150)

Methimazole-Antithyroid Medication

Methimazole (MMI) works by irreversibly inactivating the thyroid peroxidase enzyme (TPO), thus preventing organification, a necessary step for thyroid hormone synthesis. In 2019, Dr. Yoshihara found MMI and PTU both inhibit the intrathyroidal D1 deiodinase in cultured rat thyrocytes. However, in 1975, Dr. Saberi found in humans, only PTU but not MMI inhibits peripheral D1 activity, reducing serum Free T3 levels in T4-treated patients (using levothyroxine). In 1999, working in vitro, Dr.

Sugawara found MMI increases TPO mRNA, resulting in greater amounts of TPO enzyme in the thyroid gland. Thus, upon stopping or decreasing the MMI or PTU drug, there may be a rebound phenomenon with worsening hyperthyroidism. This is discussed further in Chapter 16. Iodine Treatment of Graves' Disease Part Two. (25) (51) (151-152)

Genetic Mutation in Thyroperoxidase

Failure to organify iodine can be found in those harboring genetic mutations in the thyroperoxidase enzyme. In these cases, iodide in the thyroid gland cannot be oxidized and/or bound to the thyroglobulin protein, as reported by Dr. Wu in 2002. (24)

Selenium, Selenoproteins, and Hydrogen Peroxide

The normal thyroid gland has a high selenium content due to the high concentration of selenoproteins, glutathione peroxidases, thioredoxin reductases, and deiodinases. The selenium-based anti-oxidants protect the thyrocytes from oxidative damage associated with hydrogen peroxide production, which is needed for thyroid hormone biosynthesis.

Iodination of thyroglobulin, or organification, is the critical step of thyroid hormone biosynthesis. It is catalyzed by thyroid peroxidase (TPO) and occurs within the follicular space at the apical plasma membrane. Hydrogen peroxide-generating enzymes, called DUOX (Dual Oxidase), are also found at this same location, at the villous apical membrane of the thyrocyte just within the follicular lumen. Both enzyme systems (TPO and DUOX) are needed for the organification of iodine to tyrosine residues in the thyroglobulin. Various thyroid pathologies, including Hashimoto's thyroiditis, can be explained by overproduction and lack of degradation of hydrogen peroxide (H2O2), causing damage to the thyrocyte structures. (20) (26-28)

Wolff-Chaikoff Effect – Excess Iodine Intake Inhibits Organification

Seventy-four years after first described, the Wolff-Chaikoff effect is still not well understood. The best way to describe the Wolff-Chaikoff effect is the inhibition by iodide of its own organification. This effect describes the inhibition of hydrogen peroxide (H2O2) generation caused by iodide itself. The intake of excess iodide limits the oxidation and binding of I2 (iodine) to thyroglobulin because of the reduced availability of hydrogen peroxide at the apical membrane. As mentioned previously, in Hashimoto's thyroiditis, autoregulatory functions are lost. These patients are more sensitive to the inhibitory effect of iodine excess on thyroid function. Give them potassium iodide, and the TSH will go up. The inhibitory effect of iodide on thyroid function can be seen in Graves' disease. However, normal healthy people have no trouble escaping from the inhibitory effects of iodide. After a few days, TSH returns to normal. This is called the "Escape from the Wolff-Chaikoff Effect." The mechanism for escape is thought to be the generation of iodolactones and reduction in NIS activity and NIS mRNA.

Iodine Supplements at the Health Food Store

Occasionally, an apparently normal healthy person will visit my office because they have a very high TSH after consuming an iodide/iodine supplement from the health food store. These people have subclinical (euthyroid) autoimmune thyroid disease and are unable to escape from the inhibitory effects of the iodide (the Wolff-Chaikoff Effect). In 2002, Dr. K. Markou discussed this same exact point, writing:

> However, in a few apparently normal individuals, in newborns and fetuses, in some patients with chronic systemic diseases, euthyroid patients with autoimmune thyroiditis, and Graves' disease patients previously treated with

radioimmunoassay (RAI), surgery or anti-thyroid drugs, **the escape from the inhibitory effect of large doses of iodides is not achieved and clinical or subclinical hypothyroidism ensues**. (73)

TSH Stimulates Hydrogen Peroxide Generation

In 1988, Dr. Bernard Corvilain studied the Wolff-Chaikoff effect in dog thyroid slices in vitro, finding elevated TSH stimulates hydrogen peroxide generation and organification. Excess iodide had the opposite effect, greatly inhibiting hydrogen peroxide generation as well as organification via reduction of intracellular signaling from TSH (The Wolff-Chaikoff Effect), writing:

> In dog thyroid slices, **thyrotropin [TSH] and** carbamylcholine **greatly enhance protein iodination and H2O2 generation.** The action of thyrotropin [TSH] is ... mediated by cyclic AMP. This suggests that the effect of carbamylcholine is mediated by the two intracellular signals generated by the Ca++ phosphatidylinositol cascade: Ca++ and diacylglycerol. **The Wolff-Chaikoff effect is the inhibition by iodide of its own organification**...In dog thyroid slices, **iodide greatly inhibited H2O2 generation stimulated by thyrotropin [TSH]** and by carbamylcholine. Iodide decreased the production of intracellular signals induced by TSH. (74-75)

Note: carbamylcholine is a common drug used in ophthalmology to dilate pupils.

Iodine Depletion – Paradoxical Toxic Effects of Acute Iodine

In 2000, Dr. Bernard Corvilain again studied the effect of iodine administration on H2O2 production in animal thyroid slices, finding **iodine depletion** is a condition in which acute iodine administration **stimulates H2O2 production rather than inhibits it.** When iodine is acutely given to an iodine-deficient animal, there is stimulation of H2O2, presumably to promote efficient oxidation and organification of the iodine into thyroid hormone. This stimulation of H2O2 explains the toxic effect of acute iodine administration in iodine-depleted animals. Dr. Bernard Corvilain writes:

> In comparison with conditions in which an inhibitory effect of iodide on H2O2 generation is observed [Wolff-Chaikoff Effect], the stimulating effect was observed for lower concentrations and for a shorter incubation time with iodide. Such a dual control of H2O2 generation by iodide has the physiological interest of **promoting an efficient oxidation of iodide when the substrate is provided to a deficient gland [iodine deficient gland]** and of avoiding excessive oxidation of iodide and thus synthesis of thyroid hormones when it is in excess. **The activation of H2O2 generation may also explain the well-described toxic effect of acute administration of iodide on iodine-depleted thyroids.** (74-77)

Hydrogen Peroxide Metabolism

in 2019, Dr. Ildiko Szanto reviewed the role of hydrogen peroxide in normal thyroid metabolism in the organification of iodine and the production of thyroid hormone. Excessive hydrogen peroxide generation is not only mutagenic; it is also at the core of most other thyroid pathologies, such as goiter, nodules, and autoimmune thyroid disease, writing:

> The synthesis of thyroid hormones... utilizes hydrogen peroxide (H2O2) as an oxidative agent. Hydrogen peroxide is contained within the lumen of the thyroid follicles, which are considered as the functional units of the thyroid gland where hormone synthesis, storage, and release take place... Thyroid hormone synthesis requires the oxidative iodination of specific tyrosine residues of TG, a process termed "iodide organification." Oxidative iodination is catalyzed by the enzyme thyroid peroxidase (TPO). **This process is a key step in thyroid hormonogenesis requiring an appropriate amount of H2O2 for oxidation**...The major

source of H2O2 in the thyroid follicle is the isoform DUOX2. In contrast to DUOX2-generated physiological reactive oxygen species (ROS) production, **pathologically elevated H2O2 levels are linked to thyroid carcinogenesis resulting from enhanced mitogenic receptor signals or oncogene activation**. (78)

Regulation of H2O2 Generation by TSH and Iodine

The hydrogen peroxide generating system is called DUOX2, and as one might expect, DUOX2 is up-regulated by TSH in two ways:

1) TSH increases messenger RNA to increase the production of the DUOX2 protein.

2) TSH increases the DUOX2 enzymatic activity.

Iodo-Lactones Mediate Autoregulation

Quite the opposite of TSH, excess iodide inhibits DUOX2-mediated production of hydrogen peroxide. This is the Wolff-Chaikoff Effect, first described in 1948, i.e., iodine inhibits its own organification. This is a form of thyroid autoregulation mediated by iodolactones and iodoaldehydes formed when molecular iodine reacts with lipids. Iodolactones mediate thyroid autoregulation and play an important role as anti-cancer agents in the prevention and treatment of breast cancer. Breast cancer cells have the NIS, sodium iodide transporter, and actively take up iodine which reacts with lipids to form iodolactones, the anticancer agent. For more on this topic, see Chapters 31 and 32 on Iodine for Prevention and Treatment of Breast Cancer. (79-92)

Dr. Ildiko Szanto writes:

DUOX2-mediated H2O2 production is inhibited by excess iodine leading to decreased TPO activity and reduced incorporation of iodine into TG [thyroglobulin]. This inhibitory effect of iodine on its own organification was already described in 1948 and was named the "Wolff-Chaikoff effect" after the authors of the original paper. (78)

Graves TSH Receptor Antibodies DO NOT increase H2O2 production

In Graves' Disease, elevated antibodies to the TSH receptor (TSI and TRAb) stimulate the thyroid gland to "go into overdrive," producing massive quantities of thyroid hormones. The elevated T3 and T4 suppress the TSH, which will be quite low, suppressed in Graves' disease. One might assume this same TSH receptor stimulation increases H2O2 generation. This would be an incorrect assumption. While the TSH hormone stimulates H2O2 generation, TSH receptor antibodies in Graves' disease **do not** stimulate H2O2 production, as reported by Dr. Eric Laurent in 1991. (93)

This may explain the difference in the appearance of the thyroid gland in untreated classical Graves' disease versus toxic nodular goiter, both of which may present with thyrotoxicosis. In untreated classical Graves' disease at initial presentation, the thyroid gland is smoothly enlarged without nodularity or fibrosis. Typically, there are none of the inflammatory infiltrative changes typically found in Hashimotos' thyroiditis, and none of the nodularity found in toxic nodular goiter. In Graves' disease, the TSH is suppressed, turning off excess hydrogen peroxide generation. This explains the pristine appearance in untreated Graves' disease where the thyroid gland is smoothly and diffusely enlarged with increased radioiodine uptake on scintigraphy. Of course, over time, after many years of anti-thyroid drug treatment and repeated bouts of thyroiditis, the morphology of the Graves' thyroid gland undergoes change. And with time, the microscopic studies may show the appearance of inflammatory infiltrates, especially if there are also elevated TPO and Thyroglobulin antibodies, as seen in 60-85 percent of Graves' disease patients.

Undulating Course of Graves' Disease with Relapse and Remission

How can we explain the undulating course of Graves' disease with cycles of relapse and remission? During remission obtained with anti-thyroid drugs such as methimazole or potassium iodide, the TSH may soar to high levels, stimulating excess H2O2 production. At this stage, if the anti-thyroid drug dosage is reduced, this excess hydrogen peroxide may trigger a bout of thyroiditis. The inflammatory effect of excess H2O2 causes rupture of follicles with the release of preformed thyroid hormone and "relapse of hyperthyroidism." This is called Painless Thyroiditis (PT). The relapse of hyperthyroidism with high Free T3 and T4 will, in turn, suppress the TSH, which "turns off" H2O2 production. This allows healing, and the cycle repeats. This will be discussed in Chapter 16, Graves' Hyperthyroidism Treatment with Iodine, Part Two.

Block and Replace

TSH elevation and its stimulation of H2O2 generation may occur during over-treatment with thyroid-blocking drugs such as methimazole (MMI), KI, or lithium carbonate, which inhibit thyroid function and drive up TSH. This TSH elevation stimulates hydrogen peroxide production, which may damage the thyroid gland. "Block and Replace" would be useful to maintain a suppressed TSH, preventing thyroid stimulation and damage from excess H2O2. This is done by adding levothyroxine or NDT which suppresses TSH while maintaining the higher Anti-Thyroid Drug (ATD) dosage. This is beneficial since reducing ATD dosage may increase TSH and provoke thyroiditis. Remember, methimazole not only irreversibly blocks the TPO enzyme, but it also inhibits hydrogen peroxide generation, a benefit lost when MMI dosage is reduced. Both methimazole and PTU inhibit H2O2 generation as discussed in 2003 by Dr. Andrea Freitas Ferreira. (49)

Dr. Hidemi Ohye Explains Production of Thyroid Hormone

In 2010, Dr. Hidemi Ohye discussed the production of thyroid hormone, again explaining "thyroid-stimulating antibody found in patients with Graves' disease does not appear to stimulate H2O2 generation." Dr. Hidemi Ohye writes:

Iodide is actively transported into thyrocytes by a sodium/iodide symporter (NIS) on the basolateral membrane and to the follicular lumen by, in part, pendrin...at the apical membrane. Iodide is rapidly oxidized by TPO in the presence of H2O2, resulting in covalent binding to the tyrosyl residues of thyroglobulin (Tg) on the luminal side of the apical membrane. This step produces monoiodotyrosine (MIT) and diiodotyrosine (DIT). Then only properly spaced MIT and DIT in Tg participate in the coupling reactions to form thyroxine (T4) and triiodothyronine (T3); this reaction is also catalyzed by TPO with H2O2. The source of thyroid H2O2 is DUOX2 expressed in the apical plasma membrane coordinated with DUOXA2. Thyroid hormones are released into the circulation after digestion of Tg... Thyroid hormone formation is predominantly regulated by thyrotropin (TSH). The binding of TSH to the TSH receptor activates both Gs and Gq proteins. The former activates the growth regulation, differentiation, and thyroid hormone secretion, whereas the latter activates H2O2 generation and iodide binding to protein through the phospholipase C-dependent **inositol** phosphate Ca2þ/ diacylglycerol pathway.... methimazole and propylthiouracil [PTU] inhibit NADPH oxidase activity [inhibit H2O2 generation]... **A thyroid-stimulating antibody found in patients with Graves' disease does not appear to stimulate H2O2 generation.** (28)

Note: There are two TSH signaling pathways. The first one involves growth and thyroid hormone secretion. The second one involves H2O2 generation and organification. The inositol acts as a signal messenger for TSH generation of H2O2. This is discussed in Chapter 28 Myo-Inositol for Hashimoto's thyroiditis. The Graves' disease antibodies,

TRAb and TSI act on the first pathway, but not on the second pathway. Therefore, although Graves' antibodies stimulate TSH receptors, they **do not** simulate the generation of hydrogen peroxide.

TSH Controls H2O2 Levels

Note in the above quote, Dr. Hidemi Ohye explains how TSH controls thyroid gland growth, regulation, differentiation, and thyroid hormone secretion, as well as H2O2 generation and iodide binding to protein (organification). Higher TSH stimulates all these steps in thyroid hormone synthesis as well as thyroglobulin production, Sodium Iodide Symporter (NIS) activity, and Thyroid Peroxidase protein expression.

Iodide Excess Reduces H2O2 Generation

Dr. Hidemi Ohye goes on to explain how iodide controls H2O2 levels. While TSH stimulates greater H2O2 production, iodide excess reduces H2O2 production. This is done through a post-transcription change in the DUOX mechanism. Note: DUOX is the Dual Oxidase system that generates hydrogen peroxide. Dr. Hidemi Ohye writes:

> Iodide controls H2O2 generation in thyroid cells. Morand et al. have studied the effect of KI on H2O2 generation in porcine thyroid follicles, the most physiological thyroid culture system. They exposed follicles to 1 mmol/L KI [potassium iodide] for two days under cAMP stimulation and showed a reduction in H2O2 production without affecting DUOX mRNA levels. **Post-transcriptional change of the DUOX molecule by KI appears to be responsible for the decreased H2O2 generation.** (28)

Wolff–Chaikoff Effect Protects Against Iodine Excess

In the normal thyroid gland, the Wolff–Chaikoff effect protects thyrocytes from iodide excess by inhibiting iodide organification, leading to the discharge of iodide which cannot be organified. After two days, the autoregulatory features of the thyroid gland down-regulate iodine uptake by the NIS, preventing further uptake of iodine. So, two things are happening. One, iodide excess inhibits organification by suppressing H2O2 generation by DUOX. Two, excess iodide has an inhibitory effect on the NIS, which then suppresses the uptake and concentration of iodide, also called the "Escape from the Wolff-Chaikoff Effect." This is the same mechanism used when passing out iodine capsules after a nuclear accident. When 65 mg potassium iodide capsules are distributed to the population surrounding a nuclear accident, the "Escape from the Wolff–Chaikoff Effect" prevents the uptake of radioactive iodine into the thyroid gland, protecting the population from thyroid cancer risk.

The Defective Wolff-Chaikoff Effect

Dr. Hidemi Ohye speculates that some animals and humans have a defective Wolff-Chaikoff Effect. Instead of inhibiting hydrogen peroxide generation, excess iodine intake **INCREASES IT**! An example of this is the iodine-depleted animal or human. Dr. Hidemi Ohye also speculates these susceptible animals or humans, thyroid damage from H2O2 production due to defective anti-oxidant systems may play a role in the etiology of autoimmune thyroid disease. Damaged TPO and thyroglobulin proteins may then serve as antigens for autoimmune attacks. Selenium or magnesium deficiency may render the anti-oxidant system defective. Dr. Hidemi Ohye writes:

> The animal experiments [in iodine-depleted animals] suggest that susceptible hosts have defective Wolff–Chaikoff effect allowing them to generate H2O2 in response to increased iodide influx, **which ordinarily should not happen** as seen in the non-susceptible mouse. Thus, abnormality of thyroid H2O2 generation in response to high iodide may play a role in the development of Hashimoto's thyroiditis in susceptible individuals. Whether iodide-mediated H2O2

generation is driven by activated DUOX or NOX4 [H2O2 generating enzymes] or defective anti-oxidants [selenium deficiency] has yet to be studied. (28)(49)

Note: studies in iodine-depleted animals show exactly what is described above. Rather than inhibiting H2O2 production, refeeding iodine to an iodine-depleted animal causes an increase in H2O2 production, which damages the TPO and thyroglobulin, leading to antigenicity. This supports the hypothesis iodine deficiency is the etiology of autoimmune thyroid disease. Here, I would add the thyroid gland in Graves' disease has very high radio-iodine uptake, with a much higher iodine requirement to keep up with massive thyroid hormone production, and therefore may mimic an iodine-depleted thyroid which also has very high radio-iodine uptake.

Graves' Antibodies DO NOT Stimulate Hydrogen Peroxide!

As mentioned above, TSH stimulates all steps in thyroid hormone synthesis, including the generation of hydrogen peroxide (H2O2). In 1991, Dr. Eric Laurent studied human thyroid slices in vitro and, surprisingly, found Graves' disease antibodies **do not** stimulate hydrogen peroxide generation. This makes sense to me. If Graves antibodies did stimulate excess hydrogen peroxide, this would lead to severe thyroid damage, chronic thyroiditis, and early complete destruction of the thyroid gland, similar to myxoedematous cretinism described in Zaire, Africa. This would also lead to immune cell infiltration and rapid, complete destruction of the thyroid gland. Instead, in early untreated Graves' disease, the gland is smoothly enlarged without evidence of chronic changes. Dr. Eric Laurent writes:

The effects of thyroid-stimulating antibodies (TSAb) and of thyrotropin (TSH) were compared...The patterns of the response curves of TSAb and TSH on cyclic AMP accumulation were different, suggesting that

different mechanisms may be involved. In addition, unlike TSH, **TSAb was not able to stimulate H2O2 generation, which in human tissue mainly depends on the activation of the phosphatidylinositol-Ca2+ cascade. ... In conclusion, our results show that TSAb does not share all the metabolic actions of TSH on human thyroid tissue.** (93)

As mentioned above, under normal circumstances, hydrogen peroxide generation is inhibited by excess iodide and partially inhibited by methimazole and PTU (propylthiouracil). Hydrogen peroxide generation is stimulated by TSH but not by Graves' TSH receptor antibodies. (49) (97-98)

Dr. Guy Abraham: How to Reverse Autoimmune Thyroid Disease

Dr. Guy Abraham, inventor of the Iodoral tablet, explains iodine deficiency causes increased TSH. This stimulates excess hydrogen peroxide, which damages TPO and thyroglobulin, causing Hashimoto's thyroiditis. The mechanism of excess H2O2 production is caused by combined iodine and magnesium deficiencies resulting in low levels of **iodinated lipids and high cytosolic calcium, respectively.** The excess hydrogen peroxide damages structures in closest proximity, TPO and the substrate thyroglobulin (Tg). These damaged proteins stimulate autoimmunity, thus explaining the origin of Hashimoto's disease from iodine deficiency. In Dr. Abraham's opinion, supplementing with iodine (12.5 mg/day or above) and magnesium (1200 mg per day) should reverse autoimmune thyroiditis in both Hashimoto's and Graves' Disease. Dr. Guy Abraham writes:

We would like to propose a mechanism for the oxidative damage caused by **low levels of iodide** combined with anti-thyroid drugs: inadequate iodide supply to the thyroid gland, aggravated by goitrogens [a substance that blocks iodine uptake, worsening the iodine deficiency], activates the thyroid peroxidase (TPO) system through **elevated TSH, low levels of iodinated lipids, and high** cytosolic free calcium, **resulting in excess production of H2O2**. ...This H2O2 production is above normal due to a deficient feedback system caused by **high cytosolic calcium resulting from magnesium deficiency** and low levels of **iodinated lipids, which requires for their synthesis iodide levels two orders of magnitude greater than the RDA for iodine.** Once the low iodide supply is depleted, TPO in the presence of H2O2 and organic substrate reverts to its peroxidase function, which is the primary function of haloperoxydases, **causing oxidative damage to molecules nearest to the site of action: TPO and the substrate thyroglobulin (Tg). Oxidized TPO and Tg elicit an autoimmune reaction** with production of antibodies against these altered proteins with subsequent damage to the apical membrane of the thyroid cells, resulting in the lymphocytic infiltration and in the clinical manifestations of Hashimoto's thyroiditis... In laboratory animals prone to autoimmune thyroiditis, **the genetic defect may be in the production of H2O2 in excess of what is needed.** The iodination of tyrosine residues by TPO requires the presence of Tg, H2O2, and iodide. **The supply of H2O2 comes from the NADPH oxidase system. This system is inhibited by certain iodinated lipids and is enhanced by cytosolic-free calcium Ca++.** The equation for organification of iodide by TPO is displayed in Figure 1, together with the feedback system controlling the production of H2O2. The logical deduction from this equation is that increased cytosolic free calcium will cause an excess of H2O2. **Increased levels of iodinated lipids, on the other hand, would limit the production of H2O2.** How much iodide is required for the production of iodinated lipids? In 1976, Rabinovitch et al. reported their results regarding the effect of three levels of iodide supplementation on the production of iodinated lipids in the thyroid glands of dogs: low iodide diet, normal iodide diet, and high iodine diet. The dogs were kept on those diets for six weeks. Iodinated lipids in the plasma membrane and in the cell total lipids were observed only in the dogs receiving the high iodide diet. What about

human subjects? In 1994, Dugrillon et al. reported for the first time the presence of delta lactone [delta iodolactone] in human thyroid following the **ingestion of 15 mg iodide/day for 10 days** in the host. It was the first time this biologically active iodolipid was isolated from human thyroid glands. The amount of iodide the host received was **100 times the RDA**, but it is the amount of iodine/iodide we recommended for orthoiodosupplementation... Dugrillon et al. stated, "These results demonstrate for the first time that **delta-iodo-lactone** is present in the iodide-treated human thyroid." Magnesium deficiency, which is prevalent in the US population, results in increased levels of cytosolic-free calcium. Intracellular free calcium levels above the normal range are cytotoxic, causing calcification of mitochondria and cell death. The cell membrane possesses an ATP-dependent calcium pump that keeps intracellular levels of free ionized calcium within narrow limits. **This calcium pump is magnesium-dependent for normal function. Magnesium deficiency results in a defective calcium pump and intracellular accumulation of ionized calcium.** Inadequate iodine/iodide intake below orthoiodosupplementation results in decreased levels of **delta-iodo-lactone**. Combined magnesium and iodine/iodide deficiency based on the concept of orthoiodosupplementation are the basic factors involved in the oxidative damage caused by excess H2O2 and reactive oxygen species. If this proposed mechanism is valid, orthoiodosupplementation, combined with magnesium intake between 800-1,200 mg/day, a daily amount this author recommended 21 years ago for magnesium sufficiency, **should reverse autoimmune thyroiditis. This nutritional approach is also effective in Graves' autoimmune thyroiditis, as previously discussed**. (99-101)

To my knowledge, there are no clinical trials examining the above hypothesis using iodine and magnesium to reverse autoimmune thyroid disease, as proposed by Dr. Abraham. This would be a fertile area for further studies.

The Role of Iodinated Lipids – Iodolactones

Iodo-lipids (iodolactones) are made by the reaction of excess iodine with lipids and are thought to be involved in thyroid auto-regulation and inhibition of H2O2 production in the thyroid gland. Iodolipids are also thought to be active in extra-thyroidal tissues with NIS activity, such as normal breast tissue and cancerous breast tissue. For example, iodolactones generated by iodine intake may prevent or treat breast cancer. (79-92)

In 2001, Drs. Dunn and Dunn reviewed iodide metabolism in the thyroid, explaining iodinated lipids increase linearly with the addition of iodide and inhibit hydrogen peroxide generation:

> Iodinated lipids also occur in the thyroid, especially after high doses of iodide. One of these, 2-iodohexadecanal, increases linearly with iodine addition. **It inhibits NADPH oxidase, and lipid iodination appears to decrease H2O2 production and may thus retard Tg iodination as well.** (89-90)

In 2014, Drs. Mario Nava-Villalba and Carmen Aceves studied 6-iodolactone, finding that it is not only involved in thyroid auto-regulation, it is also involved in extra-thyroidal tissues containing NIS (sodium iodide symporter) such as mammary gland, prostate, colon, or the nervous system, writing:

> An iodinated derivative of arachidonic acid, 5-hydroxy-6-iodo-8,11,14-eicosatrienoic acid, δ-lactone (6-IL) has been implicated as **a possible intermediate in the autoregulation of the thyroid gland by iodine.** In addition to antiproliferative and apoptotic effects observed in thyrocytes, this iodolipid could also exert similar actions in cells derived from extrathyroidal tissues like **mammary gland, prostate, colon, or the nervous system**. In mammary cancer (solid tumors or tumor cell lines), 6-IL has been detected after molecular iodine (I2) supplement and is a potent activator of peroxisome proliferator-activated receptor type gamma (PPARγ). **These observations led us to propose I2 [molecular iodine] supplement as a novel coadjutant therapy which, by inducing differentiation mechanisms, decreases tumor progression and prevents chemoresistance. Some kinds of tumoral cells, in contrast to normal cells, contain high concentrations of arachidonic acid, making the I2 supplement a potential "magic bullet" that enables local, specific production of 6-IL, which then exerts antineoplastic actions with minimal deleterious effects on normal tissues.** (87-92)

H2O2 and Various Thyroid Pathologies

In 2008, Dr. Song explained various thyroid pathologies are caused by either overproduction of hydrogen peroxide or its lack of degradation due to selenium deprivation and consequent GSH [glutathione peroxidase] depletion, thus explaining the etiology of autoimmune thyroid disease, goiter, thyroid nodules, thyroid cancer, etc.

Excess H2O2 is Carcinogen and Killer

Dr. Song reminds us excess H2O2 in thyroid cells is a carcinogen and "a killer." Dr. Song then discusses the etiology of myxedematous endemic cretinism in Zaire, Africa, a form of thyroid destruction after birth associated with iodine deficiency, which stimulates elevated TSH and consequently H2O2 generation, combined with selenium deficiency (causing decreased GSH peroxidase and thioredoxin reductase activity), combined with dietary thiocyanate. Dr. Song proposes a similar mechanism for the pathophysiology of thyroiditis and proposes dietary selenium supplementation for the prevention and treatment of thyroiditis. Dr. Song writes:

> In thyrocytes of most species, including humans, TSH and its receptor activate…H2O2 generation, iodide binding to proteins [organification], thyroid hormone formation, and secretion…In all species studied, iodide at high concentrations, presumably

through an iodinated lipid, iodohexadecanal [6-iodo-lactone], inhibits H2O2 generation (the Wolff-Chaikoff effect) and adenylate cyclase...**H2O2 in various cell types, and presumably in thyroid cells, is a signal, a mitogen, a mutagen, a carcinogen, and a killer**...It is proposed that various pathologies can be explained, at least in part, by **overproduction and lack of degradation of H2O2 (tumorigenesis, myxedematous cretinism, and thyroiditis)** and by failure of the H2O2 generation or its positive control system (congenital hypothyroidism)......We have repeatedly suggested that the important generation of H2O2 in thyroid cells might account for **mutagenesis and the important generation of nodules in the thyroid**. This would also explain in part why more nodules are found in iodine-deficient areas... Myxedematous endemic cretinism [Zaire, Africa], caused by thyroid destruction after birth, has been linked to low iodine supply in early life, leading to intense stimulation [by elevated TSH] and presumably H2O2 generation, to passage from low O2 to high O2 at birth, to selenium deficiency, and thus to decreases in GSH peroxidase and thioredoxin reductase activity and to dietary thiocyanate...**Interestingly, a similar scenario has been proposed for the physiopathology of thyroiditis. Selenium dietary supplementation has therefore been proposed for prevention and treatment of thyroiditis and has indeed alleviated it. (20)**

Dr. Robyn Murphy Clears Everything Up

In 2016, Dr. Robyn Murphy agrees with Dr. Guy Abraham and Dr. Song, suggesting iodine deficiency as a causative factor in patients with autoimmune thyroid disease. Firstly, Dr. Murphy points out the observed increase in autoimmune thyroiditis after the introduction of salt iodination programs. This can be understood as refeeding iodine to an iodine-deficient population. Chronic iodine deficiency creates a loss of autoregulation in the thyroid leading to excess hydrogen peroxide generation when iodine is re-introduced. This was confirmed by Dr. Corvilan's and Dr. Cohen's in vitro studies using thyroid slices and in mice. In 1973 Dr. Bruce Belshaw administered iodine to iodine-deficient dogs, creating follicular cell necrosis. (4) (102-104)

Dr. Robyn Murphy goes on to describe the train of events in the production of thyroid hormones, explaining how iodide deficiency is causative in the etiology of autoimmune thyroid disease. Iodide intake of at least 1.5 mg per day (1,500 micrograms) is required to produce enough iodo-lactones to inhibit hydrogen peroxide generation. Dr. Murphy writes:

> In iodine deficiency, the loss of negative feedback on H2O2 production has been implicated in thyroid dysfunction and as a possible mechanism in the generation of autoantibodies [Hashimoto's Antibodies] ...The sodium-iodide symporter (NIS) transports iodide (I–) into the thyrocyte to be organified to iodine (I2) and bound to thyroglobulin (TG) by thyroid peroxidase (TPO) and hydrogen peroxide (H2O2). The iodine–thyroglobulin complexes then combine to form thyroid hormones. The nicotinamide adenine dinucleotide phosphate (NADPH) oxidase system is upregulated by intracellular calcium to generate H2O2, a reactive oxygen species (ROS). To prevent excess H2O2, iodolactones negatively inhibit NADPH oxidase, and glutathione peroxidase degrades H2O2... **Iodinated lipids provide negative feedback on NADPH oxidase to reduce H2O2 and oxidative damage to the thyrocyte**...Studies suggest that when iodine intake is above 1.5 mg daily, TPO synthesizes iodolactones. TPO facilitates the iodination of arachidonic acid and other polyunsaturated fatty acids to produce iodolactones. Research shows that measurable concentrations of δ-iodolactone are found in the thyroid tissue, prevent excess iodide uptake and the generation of H2O2 by NADPH oxidase, and regulate thyroid function. However, in iodine deficiency, iodolactones are obsolete, and the thyroid gland is susceptible to oxidative damage and loss of cell-cycle control...In chronic iodine

deficiency, compensatory mechanisms fail to maintain iodine concentration, and the thyroid is susceptible to damage. As iodine concentrations decrease, the pituitary gland secretes thyroid-stimulating hormone (TSH) to induce NIS expression. TSH remains high, and the NIS fails to shut down, predisposing the gland to excess iodine during supplementation, a phenomenon found in individuals with preexisting autoimmune thyroiditis (AIT). In addition, thyroid activity remains high, leading to hyperplasia and goiter. Researchers in cross-sectional studies reported that patients with nodular goiters often have an increase in thyroid antibodies, which is more common in iodine deficiency. These observations suggest that immune stimulation to thyroid proteins occurs during iodine deficiency and **may be a causative factor in the development of thyroid autoimmunity**...In iodine deficiency, the thyroid is susceptible to oxidative damage. **As TSH stimulates NIS and TPO activity, low levels of iodinated lipids with high cytosolic free calcium allow for excess H2O2 to be produced [Dr Abraham's same point].** Iodine alone fails to initiate immune activation; rather, experimental studies show that iodine in the presence of inflammatory cytokines [associated with increased hydrogen peroxide] augments immune function... In the presence of excess H2O2, oxidative damage to TPO [Thyroperoxidase] and TG [Thyroglobulin] leads to antigen presentation and lymphocytic infiltration, which facilitates the production of anti-TPO and anti-TG antibodies. This mechanism may account for the prevalence of AIT [autoimmune thyroiditis] upon iodine supplementation through USI [Univeral Salt Iodination] programs...The lowest concentrations of iodine are found in individuals with thyroid autoimmunity. In 13 patients with overt symptoms of hypothyroidism and AIT, an average of 2.3 mg of iodine was found in the thyroid, as compared with 10 mg in healthy subjects. On the basis of data derived from the National Health and Nutrition Examination Survey, although iodine intake in the United States continues to decrease, the prevalence of AIT continues to increase. This correlation suggests that iodine deficiency may be a causative factor in patients with AIT [autoimmune thyroiditis]. (4)

TSH Stimulates the Conversion of T4 to T3

In 1990, Dr. Kohrle found TSH receptor stimulation controls the activity of intra-thyroidal D1 Deiodinase, which converts T4 to T3. Thus, high TSH receptor stimulation, as found in severe forms of Graves' disease, increases the peripheral FreeT3/ FreeT4 ratio. A high Free T3 blood level is an indicator of a more severe form of Graves' thyrotoxicosis. Quite the opposite in inflammatory thyroiditis, the Free T4 predominates rather than the Free T3, representing a useful method to differentiate the two entities. Dr. Kohrle writes:

TSH, the major signaling factor for the thyroid follicles, controls thyrocyte function... TSH is involved in the regulation of thyroidal uptake of small molecules and nutrients, intracellular transport of thyrocyte-specific proteins, and most of the steps of thyroid hormone synthesis, storage, and release... Thyrocytes also express a highly active Type I iodothyronine 5' deiodinase [D1 Deiodinase] which is controlled by TSH-stimulated cAMP production. The thyrocyte specific 5' deiodinase isozyme has a marked influence on the amount of T3 secreted by the thyroid. This 5' deiodinase isozyme shows most of the characteristics of the type I 5' deiodinase found in liver and kidney and is also blocked by PTU, other 5' deiodinase inhibitors [propranolol and corticosteroids], and iodinated X-ray contrast agents such as iopanoic acid, which are occasionally used in thyrotoxicosis to inhibit thyroidal T3-production by this enzyme. (105)

Note: D1 deiodinase inhibitors such as PTU, corticosteroids, propranolol, and iopanoic acid are sometimes used for treating thyrotoxicosis.

Deiodinases D1, D2 and D3

D1 deiodinase is attached to the plasma membrane, is present in all tissues of the body, and converts T4 to T3 in the periphery, accounting for the majority of the circulating T3. D2 is present intracellularly at the endoplasmic reticulum near the cell nucleus and converts T4 to T3 in the thyroid and pituitary. D3 is present in all tissues and converts T4 to inactive reverse T3.

Amiodarone inhibits D1 deiodinase, blocking the peripheral conversion of T4 to T3, thus causing "tissue hypothyroidism." Amiodarone also blocks the direct effect of T3 on heart muscle cells. This effect is beneficial as an anti-arrhythmia agent. In 2007, Dr. Irwin Klein writes:

> The heart relies mainly on serum T3 because no significant myocyte intracellular deiodinase activity takes place, and it appears that T3, and not T4, is transported into the myocyte. T3 exerts its cellular actions through binding to thyroid hormone nuclear receptors (TRs). (106)

In 2019, Dr. Robin Maskey writes:

> The thyroid gland primarily secretes T4 (85%), which is converted to T3 by 5 -monodeiodination in the liver, kidney, and skeletal muscle. The heart relies mainly on serum T3 because no significant myocyte intracellular deiodinase activity takes place, and it appears that T3, and not T4, is transported into the myocyte. (107)

Peripheral conversion of T4 to T3 is inhibited by PTU, the beta blocker drug, propranolol, and corticosteroids, **but not methimazole (MMI)**. In 2022, Dr. G. Bereda writes: "PTU (but not MMI) also inhibits the peripheral conversion of T4 to T3." This was previously found by Dr. Saberi in 1975. (108-113) (152)

Explaining the Deiodinase System, D1, D2, and D3

In 2018, Dr. Antonio Bianco reviewed the three Deiodinase enzymes, D1, D2, and D3, writing:

> Types 1 and 2 deiodinases (D1 and D2) activate thyroid hormone [Convert T4 to T3] whereas the type 3 deiodinase (D3) inactivates both T4 and T3 [converts T4 to reverse T3]... Deiodinases are anchored in cell membranes... D2 produces T3 and thus increases thyroid hormone signaling whereas D3 inactivates T4 and T3, silencing thyroid hormone signaling... Residency in the ER [endoplasmic reticulum] is critical for D2's ability to contribute to thyroid hormone signaling. Physical proximity with the nucleus allows for D2-generated T3 to gain easy access to the TR [thyroid receptor]-containing nuclear compartment... Because T4-induced down-regulation of D2 is turned off in the hypothalamus, the TRH-producing neuron is wired to have increased sensitivity to T4. Therefore, tissue-specific differences in D2 ubiquitination are an inherent property of the TRH/TSH feedback mechanism... D1, on the other hand, does not contribute significantly to the local control of thyroid hormone signaling. This is explained by its localization in the plasma membrane, which facilitates rapid exit of D1-generated T3 back to the circulation. (114) Note: TRH is thyrotopin-releasing hormone, which is made by the hypothalamus, and travels to the pituitary where it stimulates the release of TSH. Note: Dr. Bianco explains the D2 in the hypothalamus is "hard-wired" to have increased sensitivity to T4, and is not downregulated by high T4 levels. This is pertinent to the levothyroxine patient receiving T4. Thus, the pituitary intracellular D2 converts T4 to T3 which suppresses TSH to low levels. Whereas in the periphery, D1 is inhibited by high T4 leading to intracellular T3 deficiency and tissue hypothyroidism in spite of the suppressed TSH. This explains why the levothyroxine-treated patient has continued peripheral hypothyroidism in spite of a suppressed TSH centally. The action of the pituitary D2 is different from the peripheral D1. (114)

In 2021, Dr. Laura Sabatino reviewed the three Deiodinase enzymes, D1, D2, and D3 (also called DIO1, DIO2, and DIO3), explaining the plasma membrane location of D1 involves maintaining plasma T3 levels, while the intracellular location of D2 near the nucleus facilitates intracellular T3 nuclear signaling. The majority of circulating T3 is derived from the D1 conversion of T4 to T3 in the periphery. On the other hand, D2 deiodinase activity is directed toward the nuclear compartment of the cell. Both D1 and D2 convert T4 to T3, their active form. On the other hand, D3 inactivates T4 by converting T4 to reverse T3. Dr. Laura Sabatino writes:

> The three enzymes have different subcellular locations; DIO1 and DIO3 are found at the plasma membrane, whereas DIO2 is found at the endoplasmic reticulum, making it very proximal to the nucleus. The DIO1 and DIO2 catalytic globular domains face the cytosol [inside the cell], whereas DIO3 molecules, including the catalytic domain, mostly protrude towards the extracellular space... The cellular location of the three deiodinases is functionally associated with their role in maintaining the equilibrium with the plasma compartment ... The presence of DIO1 in the plasma membrane is associated with its major role in rapid equilibration with plasma T3, whereas the DIO2-mediated activation of TH [thyroid hormone] is principally finalized in the nuclear compartment due to the location of DIO2 in the endoplasmic reticulum membrane, which is very proximal to the nucleus... **The majority of circulating T3 derives from T4 deiodination by DIO1 activity, which mainly occurs in the thyroid, but also in the liver and kidney**... In contrast, DIO2 is considered primarily responsible for the local production of T3 inside cells, and its presence has been detected in several locations, such as the pituitary gland and hypothalamus, cochlea, brown adipose tissue, bones, muscles, heart, and central nervous system. Although the details underlying the distinction between DIO1-generated T3 and DIO2-generated T3 are still not completely known, it is clear that DIO1-generated T3 equilibrates rapidly with the plasma in about 30 minutes, whereas DIO2-generated T3 persists longer in the cell. (115)

Preventing Conversion of T4 to T3 with Propranolol

In 1983, Dr. Van Doom studied athyreotic mice finding initiation of MMI actually increased peripheral conversion of T4 to T3. This could explain the initial paradoxical worsening of thyrotoxicosis symptoms when starting MMI, which may last a day or so. Avoiding this effect can be done with the use of propranolol, a non-selective beta blocker, which slows the heart rate in the thyrotoxic patient. Propranolol is preferred over atenolol, a selective Beta Blocker, since propranolol inhibits the D1 deiodinase, thus inhibiting the conversion of T4 to T3, reducing peripheral Free T3 levels. In 1980, Dr. How gave atenolol 100 mg twice daily for two weeks to twelve hyperthyroid humans finding no change in free T3 or reverse T3 levels, concluding atenolol does not inhibit the peripheral conversion of T4 to T3. Thus, propranolol is preferred in the treatment of thyrotoxicosis. Both drugs should be used with caution in patients with underlying heart disease, as they may worsen heart failure in the cardiomyopathy patient. The more selective atenolol may be preferred in patients with asthma or COPD since asthma may be worsened by propranolol. (109-110) (116-121)

In 2017, Dr Hossam Abubakar writes:

> Propranolol is the preferred agent for Beta-blockade in hyperthyroidism and thyroid storm due to its additional effect of blocking the peripheral conversion of inactive T4 to active form T3. (116)

Dr. Margaret Rayman Explains the Importance of Iron

TPO is a Heme Protein with Central Iron

As mentioned above, TPO thyroperoxidase is directly responsible for the organification of iodine into thyroglobulin. TPO is a heme enzyme containing a porphyrin ring with a central iron atom. Thus, thyroid hormone production is dependent on adequate iron stores. Iron supplementation to a ferritin level of 100 µg/l is suggested in 2019 by Dr. Margaret Rayman, writing:

> It is important to recognize that low iron stores may contribute to symptom persistence in patients treated for hypothyroidism...An example is afforded by a small study in twenty-five Finnish women with persistent symptoms of hypothyroidism, despite appropriate L-T4 [levothyroxine] therapy, who became symptom-free when treated with oral iron supplements for 6–12 months... all had serum ferritin <60 µg/l. Restoration of serum ferritin above 100 µg/l ameliorated the symptoms in two-thirds of the women. At least 30–50 % of hypothyroid patients with persisting symptoms despite adequate L-T4 therapy may, in fact, have covert ID [iron deficiency]...Patients with AITD or hypothyroidism should be routinely screened for ID [iron deficiency]. If either ID or serum ferritin below 70 µg/l is found, coeliac disease or autoimmune gastritis may be the cause and should be treated. (122-123)

Iron and B12 deficiency in the autoimmune thyroid patient are quite common and may be related to autoimmune gastric achlorhydria with malabsorption of iron and B12. Further discussion of autoimmune gastritis can be found in Chapter 27. Hashimoto's Thyroiditis with Normal TSH, When to Treat?

Conclusion: The Nuclear Reactor Analogy

The thyroid gland can be compared to a nuclear reactor. Under normal working conditions, the nuclear reactor generates energy safely. However, when the cooling system fails, the reactor may go into catastrophic meltdown, a "nuclear accident" with leakage of radioactivity. Similarly, when the cooling system of the thyroid, the selenium-based glutathione peroxidase anti-oxidant system, is dysfunctional, or when H2O2 generation is excessive, the thyroid gland undergoes "nuclear meltdown," causing various thyroid pathologies, autoimmune thyroid disease, thyroiditis, nodules, mutagenesis, and thyroid cancer. (124-152)

♦ References for Chapter 14

1) Portulano, Carla, et al. "The Na+/I– Symporter (NIS): Mechanism and Medical Impact." Endocrine Reviews 35.1 (2014): 106-149.

2) Harper, Mary-Ellen, and Erin L. Seifert. "Thyroid Hormone Effects on Mitochondrial Energetics." Thyroid 18.2 (2008): 145-156.

3) Cioffi, Federica, et al. "Bioenergetic Aspects of Mitochondrial Actions of Thyroid Hormones." Cells 11.6 (2022): 997.

4) Murphy, Robyn, et al. "The Role of Iodine Deficiency and Subsequent Repletion in Autoimmune Thyroid Disease and Thyroid Cancer." Journal of Restorative Medicine 5.1 (2016): 32.

5) Shahid, Muhammad A., et al. "Physiology, Thyroid Hormone." StatPearls Publishing, 2022.

6) Eleftheriadou, Anna-Maria, et al. "Re-visiting Autoimmunity to Sodium-Iodide Symporter and Pendrin in Thyroid Disease." European Journal of Endocrinology 183.6 (2020): 571-580.

7) Dohan, Orsolya, et al. "The Sodium/Iodide Symporter (NIS): Characterization, Regulation, and Medical Significance." Endocrine Reviews 24.1 (2003): 48-77.

8) Ravera, Silvia, et al. "The Sodium/Iodide Symporter (NIS): Molecular Physiology and Preclinical and Clinical Applications." Annual Review of Physiology 79 (2017): 261.

9) Riesco-Eizaguirre, et al. "The Complex Regulation of NIS Expression and Activity in Thyroid and Extrathyroidal Tissues." (2021).

10) Martín, Mariano, et al. "Implications of Na+/I-Symporter Transport to the Plasma Membrane for Thyroid Hormonogenesis and Radioiodide Therapy." Journal of the Endocrine Society 3.1 (2019): 222-234.

11) Micali, Salvatore, et al. "Sodium Iodide Symporter (NIS) in Extrathyroidal Malignancies: Focus on Breast and Urological Cancer." BMC Cancer 14.1 (2014): 1-12.

12) Shiozaki, Atsushi, et al. "Functional Analysis and Clinical Significance of Sodium Iodide Symporter Expression in Gastric Cancer." Gastric Cancer 22.3 (2019): 473-485.

13) Dwyer, R. M., et al. "Sodium Iodide Symporter-Mediated Radioiodide Imaging and Therapy of Ovarian Tumor Xenografts in Mice." Gene Therapy 13.1 (2006): 60-66.

14) Nicola, Juan Pablo, et al. "The Na+/I– Symporter Mediates Active Iodide Uptake in the Intestine." American Journal of Physiology-Cell Physiology 296.4 (2009): C654-C662.

15) Spitzweg, Christine, et al. "Expression of The Sodium Iodide Symporter in Human Kidney." Kidney International 59.3 (2001): 1013-1023.

16) De la Vieja, Antonio, et al. "Molecular Analysis of the Sodium/Iodide Symporter: Impact on Thyroid and Extrathyroid Pathophysiology." Physiological Reviews 80.3 (2000): 1083-1105.

17) Pavelka, S. "Metabolism of Bromide and Its Interference with the Metabolism of Iodine." Physiological Research 53 (2004): S81-90.

18) Rousset, Bernard, et al. "Thyroid Hormone Synthesis and Secretion, Chapter 2." Endotext [Internet] (2015).

19) Miot, Françoise, et al. "Thyroid Hormone Synthesis and Secretion." Thyroid Disease Manager (2010).

20) Song, Yue, et al. "Roles of Hydrogen Peroxide in Thyroid Physiology and Disease." The Journal of Clinical Endocrinology & Metabolism 92.10 (2007): 3764-3773.

21) Nakamura, Masao, et al. "Iodination and Oxidation of Thyroglobulin Catalyzed by Thyroid Peroxidase." Journal of Biological Chemistry 259.1 (1984): 359-364.

22) Czarnocka, Barbara. "Thyroperoxidase, Thyroglobulin, Na (+)/I (-) Symporter, Pendrin in Thyroid Autoimmunity." Frontiers in Bioscience-Landmark 16.2 (2011): 783-802.

23) Strum, Judy M., and Morris J. Karnovsky. "Cytochemical Localization of Endogenous Peroxidase in Thyroid Follicular Cells." The Journal of Cell Biology 44.3 (1970): 655-666.

24) Wu, J. Y., et al. "Mutation Analysis of Thyroid Peroxidase Gene in Chinese Patients with Total Iodide Organification Defect: Identification of Five Novel Mutations." Journal of Endocrinology 172.3 (2002): 627-635.

25) Nagasaka, Akio, and Hiroyoshi Hidaka. "Effect of Anti-Thyroid Agents 6-Propyl-2-Thiouracil And L-Methyl-2-Mercaptoimidazole on Human Thyroid Iodide Peroxidase." The Journal of Clinical Endocrinology & Metabolism 43.1 (1976): 152-158.

26) Mizukami, Y., et al. "Cytochemical Localization of Peroxidase and Hydrogen-Peroxide-Producing NAD (P) H-Oxidase in Thyroid Follicular Cells of Propylthiouracil-Treated Rats." Histochemistry 82.3 (1985): 263-268.

27) Labato, Mary Anna. "Cytochemical Localization of Hydrogen Peroxide Generating Sites in the Rat Thyroid Gland." Tissue and Cell 17.6 (1985): 889-900.

28) Ohye, Hidemi, and Masahiro Sugawara. "Dual Oxidase, Hydrogen Peroxide, and Thyroid Diseases." Experimental Biology and Medicine 235.4 (2010): 424-433.

29) Saygili, Emre Sedar, et al. "Is Only Thyroid Peroxidase Antibody Sufficient for Diagnosing Chronic Lymphocytic Thyroiditis?" The Medical Bulletin of Sisli Etfal Hospital 52.2: 97-102.

30) Betterle, C., et al. "Thyroid Autoantibodies: A Good Marker for the Study of Symptomless Autoimmune Thyroiditis." European Journal of Endocrinology 114.3 (1987): 321-327.

31) Rotondi, Mario, et al. "Serum Negative Autoimmune Thyroiditis Displays a Milder Clinical Picture Compared with Classic Hashimoto's Thyroiditis." European Journal of Endocrinology 171.1 (2014): 31-36.

32) Baker Jr, James R., et al. "Seronegative Hashimoto Thyroiditis with Thyroid Autoantibody Production Localized to The Thyroid." Annals of Internal Medicine 108.1 (1988): 26-30.

33) Eleftheriadou, Anna-Maria, et al. "Re-visiting Autoimmunity to Sodium-Iodide Symporter and Pendrin in Thyroid Disease." European Journal of Endocrinology 183.6 (2020): 571-580.

34) Kalderon, Albert E., and Hendrik A. Bogaars. "Immune Complex Deposits in Graves' Disease and Hashimoto's Thyroiditis." The American Journal of Medicine 63.5 (1977): 729-734.

35) Matsuta, Morimasa. "Immunohistochemical and Electron Microscopic Studies on Hashimoto's Thyroiditis." Pathology International 32.1 (1982): 41-56.

36) Fujiwara, Hiroshi, et al. "Immune Complex Deposits in Thyroid Glands of Patients with Graves' Disease: II. Anti-Thyroglobulin and Anti-Microsome Activities of Gamma-Globulin Eluted from Thyroid Homogenates." Clinical Immunology and Immunopathology 19.1 (1981): 109-117.

37) Betterle, Corrado, and Renato Zanchetta. "The Immunofluorescence Techniques in the Diagnosis of Endocrine Autoimmune Diseases." Autoimmunity Highlights 3.2 (2012): 67-78.

38) Masini-Repiso, Ana M., et al. "Ultrastructural Localization of Thyroid Peroxidase, Hydrogen Peroxide-Generating Sites, and Monoamine Oxidase in Benign and Malignant Thyroid Diseases." Human Pathology 35.4 (2004): 436-446.

39) Takeuchi, Keisuke, et al. "Significance of Iodide-Perchlorate Discharge Test for Detection of Iodine Organification Defect of the Thyroid." The Journal of Clinical Endocrinology & Metabolism 31.2 (1970): 144-146.

40) Buchanan, W. Watson, et al. "Iodine Metabolism in Hashimoto's Thyroiditis." The Journal of Clinical Endocrinology & Metabolism 21.7 (1961): 806-816.

41) Suzuki, Hoji, and Keimei Mashimo. "Significance of the Iodide-Perchlorate Discharge Test in Patients With 131I-Treated and Untreated Hyperthyroidism." The Journal of Clinical Endocrinology & Metabolism 34.2 (1972): 332-338.

42) Andersen, B. Friis. "Iodide Perchlorate Discharge Test in Lithium-Treated Patients." European Journal of Endocrinology 73.1 (1973): 35-42.

43) Morgans, M. E., and W. R. Trotter. "Defective Organic Binding of Iodine by the Thyroid in Hashimoto's Thyroiditis." The Lancet 269.6968 (1957): 553-555.

44) Hilditch, T. E., et al. "Defects in Intrathyroidal Binding of Iodine and the Perchlorate Discharge Test." European Journal of Endocrinology 100.2 (1982): 237-244.

45) Gray, H. W., et al. "Intravenous Perchlorate Test in the Diagnosis of Hashimoto's Disease." The Lancet 303.7853 (1974): 335-338.

46) Tajiri, Junichi, et al. "Studies of Hypothyroidism in Patients with High Iodine Intake." The Journal of Clinical Endocrinology & Metabolism 63.2 (1986): 412-417.

47) Ross, Douglas S. "Thionamides in the Treatment of Graves' Disease." UpToDate 9 (2001): 1.

48) Ross, Douglas S. "Graves' Hyperthyroidism in Nonpregnant Adults: Overview of Treatment." UpToDate (2020).

49) Freitas Ferreira, Andrea C., et al. "Thyroid Ca2+/NADPH-Dependent H2O2 Generation Is Partially Inhibited by Propylthiouracil and Methimazole." European Journal of Biochemistry 270.11 (2003): 2363-2368.

50) Van Doom, J., et al. "The Effect of Propylthiouracil and Methimazole on the Peripheral Conversion of Thyroxine to 3, 5, 3'-Triiodothyronine in Athyreotic Thyroxine-Maintained Rats." European Journal of Endocrinology 103.4 (1983): 509-5

51) Sugawara, M., et al. "Methimazole and Propylthiouracil Increase Cellular Thyroid Peroxidase Activity and Thyroid Peroxidase mRNA in Cultured Porcine Thyroid Follicles." Thyroid: Official Journal of the American Thyroid Association 9.5 (1999): 513-518.

52) Tötterman, Thomas H., et al. "Induction of Circulating Activated Suppressor-Like T Cells by Methimazole Therapy for Graves' Disease." New England Journal of Medicine 316.1 (1987): 15-22.

53) Kim, Ho, et al. "Methimazole as an Antioxidant and Immunomodulator in Thyroid Cells: Mechanisms Involving Interferon-Gamma Signaling and H2O2 Scavenging." Molecular Pharmacology 60.5 (2001): 972-980.

54) Liu, Wing-Keung, et al. "Immunomodulatory Effect of Methimazole on Inbred Mice." Immunobiology 180.1 (1989): 23-32.

55) Wing, Tsui Kai. The Immunomodulatory Effect of Methimazole on Inbred Mice. Diss. The Chinese University of Hong Kong, 1992.

56) Volpé, Robert. "The Immunomodulatory Effects of Anti-Thyroid Drugs Are Mediated Via Actions on Thyroid Cells, Affecting Thyrocyte-Immunocyte Signaling a Review." Current Pharmaceutical Design 7.6 (2001): 451-460.

57) Crescioli, C., et al. "Methimazole Inhibits CXC Chemokine Ligand 10 Secretion in Human Thyrocytes." Journal of Endocrinology 195.1 (2007): 145-155.

58) McDonald, David O., and Simon HS Pearce. "Thyroid Peroxidase Forms Thionamide-Sensitive Homodimers: Relevance for Immunomodulation of Thyroid Autoimmunity." Journal of Molecular Medicine 87 (2009): 971-980.

59) Laurberg, Peter. "Remission of Graves' Disease During Anti-Thyroid Drug Therapy. Time To Reconsider the Mechanism?" European Journal of Endocrinology 155.6 (2006): 783-786.

60) Wolff, Jirj, et al. "The Temporary Nature of the Inhibitory Action of Excess Iodide on Organic Iodine Synthesis in the Normal Thyroid." Endocrinology 45.5 (1949): 504-513.

61) Eng, Peter HK, et al. "Escape from the Acute Wolff-Chaikoff Effect Is Associated with a Decrease in Thyroid Sodium/Iodide Symporter Messenger Ribonucleic Acid and Protein." Endocrinology 140.8 (1999): 3404-3410.

62) Leung, Angela M., and Lewis E. Braverman. "Iodine-Induced Thyroid Dysfunction." Current Opinion in Endocrinology, Diabetes, And Obesity 19.5 (2012): 414.

63) Leoni, Suzana G., et al. "Regulation of Thyroid Oxidative State by Thioredoxin Reductase Has a Crucial Role in Thyroid Responses to Iodide Excess." Molecular Endocrinology 25.11 (2011): 1924.

64) Katahira, Masahito, et al. "Clinical Significance of Thyroglobulin Antibodies and Thyroid Peroxidase Antibodies in Graves' Disease: A Cross-Sectional Study." Hormones (2023): 1-9.

65) Okamura, Ken, et al. "Painless Thyroiditis Mimicking Relapse of Hyperthyroidism During or After Potassium Iodide or Thionamide Therapy for Graves' Disease Resulting in Remission." Endocrine Journal (2022): EJ22-0207.

66) Landex, N. L., et al. "Methimazole Increases H2O2 Toxicity in Human Thyroid Epithelial Cells." Acta Histochemical 108.6 (2006): 431-439.

67) Roy, Gouriprasanna, and Govindasamy Mugesh. "Selenium Analogs of Anti-Thyroid Drugs—Recent Developments." Chemistry & Biodiversity 5.3 (2008): 414-439.

68) Schmutzler, Cornelia, et al. "Selenoproteins of the Thyroid Gland: Expression, Localization and Possible Function of Glutathione Peroxidase 3." (2007): 1053-1059.

69) Schweizer, Ulrich, et al. "Peroxides and Peroxide-Degrading Enzymes in the Thyroid." Anti-Oxidants & Redox Signaling 10.9 (2008): 1577-1592.

70) Ige, A. O., et al. "Oral Magnesium Potentiates Glutathione Activity in Experimental Diabetic Rats." Int. J. Diabetes Res 5.2 (2016): 21-25.

71) Zhang, Qian, et al. "Effects of Oral Selenium and Magnesium Co-Supplementation on Lipid Metabolism, Antioxidative Status, Histopathological Lesions, and Related Gene Expression in Rats Fed a High-Fat Diet." Lipids in Health and Disease 17.1 (2018): 1-12.

72) Zhu, Zongjian, et al. "Selenium Concentration and Glutathione Peroxidase Activity in Selenium and Magnesium Deficient Rats." Biological trace element research 37 (1993): 209-217.

73) Markou, K., et al. "Iodine-Induced Hypothyroidism." Thyroid 11.5 (2001): 501-510.

74) Corvilain, Bernard, et al. "Stimulation by Iodide of H2O2 Generation in Thyroid Slices from Several Species." American Journal of Physiology-Endocrinology and Metabolism 278.4 (2000): E692-E699.

75) Corvilain, Bernard, et al. "Inhibition by Iodide of Iodide Binding to Proteins: The "Wolff-Chaikoff" Effect Is Caused by Inhibition of H2O2 Generation." Biochemical and Biophysical Research Communications 154.3 (1988): 1287-1292.

76) Poncin, Sylvie, et al. "Oxidative Stress in the Thyroid Gland: From Harmlessness to Hazard Depending on the Iodine Content." Endocrinology 149.1 (2008): 424-433.

77) Sun, Rong, et al. "Protection of Vitamin C on Oxidative Damage Caused by Long-Term Excess Iodine Exposure in Wistar Rats." Nutrients 14.24 (2022): 5245.

78) Szanto, Ildiko, et al. "H2O2 Metabolism in Normal Thyroid Cells and in Thyroid Tumorigenesis: Focus on NADPH Oxidases." Anti-Oxidants 8.5 (2019): 126.

79) Elliyanti, Aisyah, et al. "An Iodine Treatments Effect on Cell Proliferation Rates of Breast Cancer Cell Lines; In Vitro Study." Open Access Macedonian Journal of Medical Sciences 8.B (2020): 1064-1070.

80) Zuckier, Lionel S., et al. "The Endogenous Mammary Gland Na+/I− Symporter May Mediate Effective Radioiodide Therapy in Breast Cancer." Journal of Nuclear Medicine 42.6 (2001): 987-987.

81) Ravera, Silvia, et al. "The Sodium/Iodide Symporter (NIS): Molecular Physiology and Preclinical and Clinical Applications." Annual Review of Physiology 79 (2017): 261.

82) Tazebay, Uygar H., et al. "The Mammary Gland Iodide Transporter Is Expressed During Lactation and In Breast Cancer." Nature Medicine 6.8 (2000): 871-878.

83) Zuckier, Lionel S., et al. "The Endogenous Mammary Gland Na+/I– Symporter May Mediate Effective Radioiodide Therapy in Breast Cancer." Journal of Nuclear Medicine 42.6 (2001): 987-987.

84) Serrano-Nascimento, Caroline, et al. "The Acute Inhibitory Effect of Iodide Excess on Sodium/Iodide Symporter Expression and Activity Involves the PI3K/Akt Signaling Pathway." Endocrinology 155.3 (2014): 1145-1156.

85) Yao, Chen, et al. "Effect of Sodium/Iodide Symporter (NIS)-Mediated Radioiodine Therapy on Estrogen Receptor-Negative Breast Cancer." Oncology Reports 34.1 (2015): 59-66.

86) Elliyanti, Aisyah, et al. "Analysis Natrium Iodide Symporter Expression in Breast Cancer Subtypes for Radioiodine Therapy Response." Nuclear Medicine and Molecular Imaging 54.1 (2020): 35-42.

87) Nava-Villalba, Mario, and Carmen Aceves. "6-Iodolactone, Key Mediator of Antitumoral Properties of Iodine." Prostaglandins & other lipid mediators 112 (2014): 27-33.

88) Aceves, Carmen, et al. "Molecular Iodine Has Extrathyroidal Effects as an Anti-Oxidant, Differentiator, And Immunomodulator." International Journal of Molecular Sciences 22.3 (2021): 1228.

89) Dunn, John T., and Ann D. Dunn. "Update On Intrathyroidal Iodine Metabolism." Thyroid 11.5 (2001): 407-414.

90) Rossich, Luciano E., et al. "Effects Of 2-Iodohexadecanal in the Physiology of Thyroid Cells." Molecular and Cellular Endocrinology 437 (2016): 292-301.

91) Solis-S, Juan C., et al. "Inhibition of Intrathyroidal Dehalogenation by Iodide." Journal Of Endocrinology 208.1 (2011): 89.

92) Dugrillon, A. "Iodolactones and Iodoaldehydes—Mediators of Iodine in Thyroid Autoregulation." Experimental and clinical endocrinology & diabetes 104.S 04 (1996): 41-45.

93) Laurent, Eric, et al. "Unlike Thyrotropin, Thyroid-Stimulating Antibodies Do Not Activate Phospholipase C In Human Thyroid Slices." The Journal of Clinical Investigation 87.5 (1991): 1634-1642.

94) Roy, Gouriprasanna, and G. Mugesh. "Thyroid Hormone Synthesis and Anti-Thyroid Drugs: A Bioinorganic Chemistry Approach." Journal of Chemical Sciences 118.6 (2006): 619-625.

95) Manna, Debasish, et al. "Anti-Thyroid Drugs and Their Analogs: Synthesis, Structure, and Mechanism of Action." Accounts of Chemical Research 46.11 (2013): 2706-2715.

96) deleted

97) Morand, Stanislas, et al. "Effect of Iodide on Nicotinamide Adenine Dinucleotide Phosphate Oxidase Activity and Duox2 Protein Expression in Isolated Porcine Thyroid Follicles." Endocrinology 144.4 (2003): 1241-1248.

98) Cardoso, Luciene C., et al. "Ca2+/Nicotinamide Adenine Dinucleotide Phosphate-Dependent H2O2 Generation Is Inhibited by Iodide in Human Thyroids." The Journal of Clinical Endocrinology & Metabolism 86.9 (2001): 4339-4343.

99) Abraham, Guy E. "The Safe and Effective Implementation of Orthoiodosupplementation in Medical Practice." The Original Internist 11.1 (2004): 17-36.

100) Suzuki, Hiroshi, Hiroshi Sano, and Hisashi Fukuzaki. "Decreased Cytosolic Free Calcium Concentration in Lymphocytes of Magnesium-Supplemented DOCA-Salt Hypertensive Rats." Clinical and Experimental Hypertension. Part A: Theory and Practice 11.3 (1989): 487-500.

101) Yang, Ying, et al. "Magnesium Deficiency Enhances Hydrogen Peroxide Production and Oxidative Damage in Chick Embryo Hepatocyte In Vitro." Biometals 19.1 (2006): 71-81.

102) Corvilain, Bernard, et al. "Stimulation by Iodide of H2O2 Generation in Thyroid Slices from Several Species." American Journal of Physiology-Endocrinology and Metabolism 278.4 (2000): E692-E699.

103) Cohen, S. B., and A. P. Weetman. "The Effect of Iodide Depletion and Supplementation in the Buffalo Strain Rat." Journal of Endocrinological Investigation 11 (1988): 625-627.

104) Belshaw, Bruce E., and David V. Becker. "Necrosis of Follicular Cells and Discharge of Thyroidal Iodine-Induced by Administering Iodide to Iodine-Deficient Dogs." The Journal of Clinical Endocrinology & Metabolism 36.3 (1973): 466-474.

105) Köhrle, J. "Thyrotropin (TSH) Action on Thyroid Hormone Deiodination and Secretion: One Aspect of Thyrotropin Regulation of Thyroid Cell Biology." Hormone and Metabolic Research. Supplement Series 23 (1990): 18-28.

106) Klein, Irwin, and Sara Danzi. "Thyroid Disease and the Heart." Circulation 116.15 (2007): 1725-1735.

107) Maskey, Robin. "Thyroid and Heart." Journal of Diabetes and Endocrinology Association of Nepal 3.2 (2019): 1-2.

108) Bereda, G. "Hyperthyroidism: Definition, Causes, Pathophysiology and Management." Journal of Biomedical and Biological Sciences 1.2 (2022): 1-11.

109) Van Doom, J., et al. "The Effect of Propylthiouracil and Methimazole on the Peripheral Conversion of Thyroxine to 3, 5, 3'-Triiodothyronine in Athyreotic Thyroxine-Maintained Rats." European Journal of Endocrinology 103.4 (1983): 509-5

110) Bianco, Antonio C., et al. "Biochemistry, Cellular and Molecular Biology, and Physiological Roles of the Iodothyronine Selenodeiodinases." Endocrine Reviews 23.1 (2002): 38-89.

111) Sharma, Anu, and Marius N. Stan. "Thyrotoxicosis: Diagnosis and Management." Mayo Clinic Proceedings. Vol. 94. No. 6. Elsevier, 2019.

112) Pandey, Rahul, et al. "Thyroid Storm: Clinical Manifestation, Pathophysiology, and Treatment." Goiter-Causes and Treatment. IntechOpen, 2019.

113) Chopra, Inder J., et al. "Opposite Effects of Dexamethasone on Serum Concentrations Of 3, 3', 5'-Triiodothyronine (Reverse T3) and 3, 3', 5'-Triiodothyronine (T3)." The Journal of Clinical Endocrinology & Metabolism 41.5 (1975): 911-920.

114) Bianco, Antonio C., and Rodrigo R. da Conceicao. "The Deiodinase Trio and Thyroid Hormone Signaling." Thyroid Hormone Nuclear Receptor: Methods and Protocols (2018): 67-83.

115) Sabatino, Laura, et al. "Deiodinases and the Three Types of Thyroid Hormone Deiodination Reactions." Endocrinology and Metabolism 36.5 (2021): 952-964.

116) Abubakar, Hossam, et al. "Propranolol-Induced Circulatory Collapse in a Patient with Thyroid Crisis and Underlying Thyrocardiac Disease: A Word of Caution." Journal of Investigative Medicine High Impact Case Reports 5.4 (2017): 2324709617747903.

117) Kravets, Igor. "Hyperthyroidism: Diagnosis and Treatment." American Family Physician 93.5 (2016): 363-370.

118) Heyma, Paul, et al. "D-Propranolol And DL-Propranolol Both Decrease Conversion of L-Thyroxine to L-Triiodothyronine." Br Med J 281.6232 (1980): 24-25.

119) Perrild, H., et al. "Different Effects of Propranolol, Alprenolol, Sotalol, Atenolol and Metoprolol on Serum T3 and Serum Rt3 in Hyperthyroidism." Clinical Endocrinology 18.2 (1983): 139-142.

120) Lotti, G., et al. "Reduction of Plasma Triiodothyronine (T3) Induced by Propranolol." Clinical endocrinology 6.6 (1977): 405-410.

121) How, J., et al. "The Effect of Atenolol on Serum Thyroid Hormones in Hyperthyroid Patients." Clinical Endocrinology 13.3 (1980): 299-302.

122) Rayman, Margaret P. "Multiple Nutritional Factors and Thyroid Disease, with Particular Reference to Autoimmune Thyroid Disease." Proceedings of the Nutrition Society 78.1 (2019): 34-44.

123) Fayadat, Laurence, et al. "Role of Heme in Intracellular Trafficking of Thyroperoxidase and Involvement of H2O2 Generated at the Apical Surface of Thyroid Cells in Autocatalytic Covalent Heme Binding." Journal of Biological Chemistry 274.15 (1999): 10533-10538.

124) Benvenga, Salvatore, et al. "Thyroid Gland: Anatomy and Physiology." Encyclopedia of Endocrine Diseases 4 (2018): 382-390.

125) Ghaddhab, Chiraz, et al. "Factors Contributing to the Resistance of the Thyrocyte to Hydrogen Peroxide." Molecular and Cellular Endocrinology 481 (2019): 62-70.

126) Fortunato, Rodrigo Soares, et al. "Functional Consequences of Dual Oxidase-Thyroperoxidase Interaction at The Plasma Membrane." The Journal of Clinical Endocrinology & Metabolism 95.12 (2010): 5403-5411.

127) Lanzolla, Giulia, et al. "Selenium in the Treatment of Graves' Hyperthyroidism and Eye Disease." Frontiers in Endocrinology 11 (2021): 608428.

128) Ruggeri, Rosaria M., et al. "Selenium Exerts Protective Effects Against Oxidative Stress and Cell Damage in Human Thyrocytes and Fibroblasts." Endocrine 68.1 (2020): 151-162.

129) Schomburg, Lutz, and Josef Köhrle. "On the Importance of Selenium and Iodine Metabolism for Thyroid Hormone Biosynthesis and Human Health." Molecular Nutrition & Food Research 52.11 (2008): 1235-1246.

130) Brix, Klaudia, et al. "Thyroglobulin Storage, Processing and Degradation for Thyroid Hormone Liberation." the Thyroid and Its Diseases. Springer, Cham, 2019. 25-48.

131) Fallahi, Poupak, et al. "Myo-inositol in Autoimmune Thyroiditis, and Hypothyroidism." Reviews in Endocrine and Metabolic Disorders 19.4 (2018): 349-354.

132) Ferrari, Silvia Martina, et al. "The Protective Effect of Myoinositol on Human Thyrocytes." Reviews in Endocrine and Metabolic Disorders 19.4 (2018): 355-362.

133) Benvenga, Salvatore, et al. "The Role of Inositol in Thyroid Physiology and in Subclinical Hypothyroidism Management." Frontiers in Endocrinology (2021): 458.

134) Lane, Laura C., et al. "Graves' Disease: Moving Forwards." Archives of Disease in Childhood 108.4 (2023): 276-281.

135) Ihnatowicz, Paulina, et al. "Supplementation in Autoimmune Thyroid Hashimoto's Disease. Vitamin D and Selenium." J. Food Nutr. Res 7 (2019): 584-591.

136) Tsatsoulis, Agathocles. "The Role of Iodine Vs Selenium on the Rising Trend of Autoimmune Thyroiditis in Iodine Sufficient Countries-an Opinion Article." Open Access J Thy Res 2.1 (2018): 12-14.

137) Rostami, Rahim, et al. "Serum Selenium Status and Its Interrelationship with Serum Biomarkers of Thyroid Function and Anti-Oxidant Defense in Hashimoto's Thyroiditis." Anti-oxidants 9.11 (2020): 1070.

138) Tian, Xun, et al. "Selenium Supplementation May Decrease Thyroid Peroxidase Antibody Titer Via Reducing Oxidative Stress in Euthyroid Patients with Autoimmune Thyroiditis." International Journal of Endocrinology 2020 (2020).

139) Vasiliu, Ioana, et al. "Experimentally Induced Autoimmune Thyroiditis in Wistar Rats: Possible Protective Role of Selenium." Endocrine Abstracts. Vol. 70. Bioscientifica, 2020.

140) Dashdamirova, Gulnara, et al. "Pathogenic Mechanisms of Autoimmune Thyroid Disease." Int J Med Sci Health Res 6 (2022): 26-33

141) Moncayo, Roy, et al. "Global View on The Pathogenesis of Benign Thyroid Disease Based on Historical, Experimental, Biochemical and Genetic Data, Identifying the Role of Magnesium, Selenium, Coenzyme Q10, and Iron in the Context of the Unfolded Protein Response and Protein Quality Control of Thyroglobulin." Journal of Translational Genetics and Genomics 4.4 (2020): 356-383.

142) Xu, Bin, et al. "A Pilot Study on the Beneficial Effects of Additional Selenium Supplementation to Methimazole for Treating Patients with Graves' Disease." Turkish Journal of Medical Sciences 49.3 (2019): 715-722.

143) Zhang, Xiao-Hong, et al. "Clinical Effect of Methimazole Combined with Selenium in the Treatment of Toxic Diffuse Goiter in Children." World Journal of Clinical Cases 10.4 (2022): 1190.

144) Gallo, Daniela, et al. "Add-on Effect of Selenium and Vitamin D Combined Supplementation in Early Control of Graves' Disease Hyperthyroidism During Methimazole Treatment." Frontiers in Endocrinology 13 (2022).

145) Barbaro, Daniele, et al. "Iodine and Myo-inositol: a Novel Promising Combination for Iodine Deficiency." Frontiers in Endocrinology 10 (2019): 457.

146) Rus-Hrincu, Florentina, et al. "DUOX2, a New Player on the Scene of Thyroid Hormones." Practica Medicala 14.3 (2019): 67.

147) Eng, Peter HK, et al. "Escape from the Acute Wolff-Chaikoff Effect Is Associated with a Decrease in Thyroid Sodium/Iodide Symporter Messenger Ribonucleic Acid and Protein." Endocrinology 140.8 (1999): 3404-3410.

148) Bogusławska, Joanna, et al. "Cellular and Molecular Basis of Thyroid Autoimmunity." European Thyroid Journal 11.1 (2022).

149) Alhubaish, Emad S., et al. "The Clinical Implications of Anti-Thyroid Peroxidase Antibodies in Graves' Disease in Basrah." Cureus 15.3 (2023).

150) Wahab, Furat, et al. "The Presence of Thyroid Peroxidase Antibodies in Graves'." Endocrine Abstracts. Vol. 31. Bioscientifica, 2013.

151) Yoshihara, Aya, et al. "Inhibitory Effects of Methimazole and Propylthiouracil on Iodotyrosine Deiodinase 1 in Thyrocytes." Endocrine Journal 66.4 (2019): 349-357.

152) Saberi, M., et al. "Reduction in Extrathyroidal Triiodothyronine Production by Propylthiouracil in Man." The Journal of Clinical Investigation 55.2 (1975): 218-223.

Chapter 15

Graves' Hyperthyroidism Remission with Iodine Part One

Case Report

CAROL IS A 56-YEAR-OLD REAL estate agent who noticed a feeling of nervousness, warmth, and rapid heart rate, which worsened over a few days. Carol called a friend who drove her to the Emergency Room, where the doctors gave her propranolol, a Beta Blocker drug that slowed her heart rate, and she felt more comfortable. Lab testing showed elevated Free T3, Free T4, and suppressed TSH confirming thyrotoxicosis. Carol was sent home with an appointment to see an endocrinologist a week later.

The Endocrinologist

The endocrinologist saw Carol and ran a thyroid lab panel showing a suppressed TSH of .001 mU/L. Other lab tests showed a Free T3 of 1200 pg/dL (normally less than 420) and a Free T4 of 4.4 ng/dl (normally less than 1.8), both markedly elevated. Her Thyroid Stimulating Immune-Globulin (TSI) and TRAb test were very elevated, indicating Graves' Hyperthyroidism. This is an autoimmune disease in which antibodies attack and stimulate the TSH receptors, causing thyrotoxicosis and excessive thyroid hormone production. Carol's endocrinologist started her on a thyroid-blocking drug, methimazole 30 mg daily.

Carol Goes to a Health Ranch in Arizona

Unhappy with conventional treatment, Carol traveled to a Health Ranch in Arizona specializing in organic raw vegetarian meals and fresh vegetable juices. She went to daily yoga classes, meditation, and sauna treatments. The doctor at the Health Ranch started Carol on a vitamin supplement program for her thyroid condition, including a potassium iodide capsule containing 65 mg of iodide.

Carol Starts to Feel Better!!

At the Health Ranch, Carol started feeling much better, almost normal, and her repeat lab panel showed the TSH had returned to normal, 3.2 mU/L. The other thyroid labs, the Free T3 and Free T4, had also normalized. However, the TSI and TRAb antibodies remained quite elevated with little change.

Carol returned home and visited the endocrinology office. Her endocrinologist reviewed the labs and then stopped the methimazole thyroid-blocking drug. He said it was no longer needed. However, the Graves' antibodies, the TRAb and TSI thyroid stimulating antibodies, were still very elevated, so the endocrinologist recommended a thyroidectomy, a surgical procedure to remove the thyroid gland. Carol was unhappy with this recommendation. She was not keen on thyroid surgery and came to see me in the office for a second opinion.

Coming for a Second Opinion

This case illustrates the beneficial effect of potassium iodide for Graves' disease, showing complete remission with a daily 65 mg potassium iodine tablet given at a health resort as part of a vitamin program. Was it the methimazole, the potassium iodide or both that caused the complete remission?

Symptoms of Graves' Thyrotoxicosis

Typical symptoms of thyrotoxicosis include Weight loss, Nervousness, Rapid Heart Rate, Palpitations, Feeling Hot, Sweating, Loose bowel movements, Poor stamina, Restlessness, Breathlessness, Tremulousness, Poor concentration, and Loss of appetite.

Signs of Graves Thyrotoxicosis

Typical signs of thyrotoxicosis include Weight Loss, Tachycardia, Sweating, Fine Tremors, Atrial Fibrillation, Apathy (older people), Goiter (enlarged thyroid), Exophthalmos (eye signs) *, Pretibial dermopathy*, Finger clubbing*

*Features specific to Graves' disease (1)

The History of Iodine Use for Hyperthyroidism- Exophthalmos Goiter

1811- Discovery of Iodine by Courtois. In 1811, Bernard Courtois, a French chemist, accidentally discovered a purple substance that he named iodine. (2)

1835 Graves' disease owes its name to the Irish physician, Robert James Graves first to describe the condition. (121)

1863 – Dr. Trousseau Accidentally Discovers Iodine Treats Thyrotoxicosis of Graves' Disease.

In 1863, Dr. Trousseau was called to visit a young woman with tachycardia (rapid heart rate) caused by Graves' disease. Dr. Trousseau intended to write a prescription for a tincture of digitalis to slow the heart rate but instead wrote for a tincture of iodine by mistake. Upon initial examination, the woman's heart rate was 140 to 150 times per minute (normal = 80 bpm). When Trousseau returned the next day, the lady's heart rate had slowed back to normal. It was then he realized his mistake and discovered overnight the patient had taken 75-100 mg of iodine. He canceled the iodine and again prescribed a tincture of Digitalis.

The next day, Trousseau again examined the patient and found the pulse had again gone up to 150 beats per minute. Trousseau realized the iodine induced a beneficial slowing of the heart rate and remission of hyperthyroid symptoms. Trousseau then returned to the use of iodine, placing the patient back on her original iodine prescription. (3)

How Does Iodine Work in Graves' Disease? What is the Mechanism of Inhibition?

It has been more than 150 years since Trousseau's accidental discovery of the inhibitory effect of iodine on hyperthyroidism in Graves' disease. The question you might ask is: How does it work? What is the mechanism of inhibition?

In 1988, Dr. Bernard Corvilain performed an in-vitro study using dog thyroid slices, finding iodide excess inhibits hydrogen peroxide generation in the thyroid follicle, thus inhibiting organification of iodine to the thyroglobulin molecule, a critical step in thyroid hormone production. (4)

In 1981, Dr. Chiraseveenuprapund studied the hydrogen peroxide generating system in bovine thyroid slices under conditions of iodine excess, finding that iodide inhibited its own organification. However, this inhibition of organification was prevented by high TSH, which stimulates the generation of hydrogen peroxide. Typically, Graves' disease patients in thyrotoxicosis will have a suppressed, very low TSH, near zero. However, the condition of high TSH in Graves' disease patients may arise after overtreatment with potassium iodide or thyroid-blocking drugs such as methimazole. Dr. Chiraseveenuprapund writes:

> In bovine thyroid slices, the inhibition of organic binding of iodide by excess iodide in the range 5–10 µg/ml was **prevented by incubating the slices in the presence of TSH**...TSH and hydrogen peroxide enhanced the synthesis of both iodothyronine and iodothyronines [organification of thryglobulin]. ... These findings suggest that the inhibition of organic binding of iodine in the presence of excess iodide **may be due to a diminished generation or a decreased availability of hydrogen peroxide in the thyroid.** (5)

Excess Iodine Inhibits the Release of Thyroid Hormones

In addition, iodine excess inhibits the release of thyroxine (T4) from the thyroid gland, first demonstrated in 1970 by Dr. Wartofsky, who showed a reduction in T4 levels after iodine treatment. The iodine-induced inhibition of T4 release is independent of treatment with other thyroid-blocking drugs, such as methimazole. (6)

Iodine Excess Inhibits Thyroglobulin Hydrolysis

In 1985, Dr. Bagchi used thyroid glands cultured in vitro to study the inhibition of thyroid hormone release by iodine, finding inhibition of thyroglobulin hydrolysis, a key step in thyroid hormone release, which is stimulated by the TSH hormone. Dr. Bagchi writes:

> **Thyrotrophin (TSH) administered in vivo acutely stimulated the rate of thyroglobulin hydrolysis. Adding NaI (sodium iodide) to the culture medium acutely inhibited basal and TSH-stimulated thyroglobulin hydrolysis.** The effect of iodide was demonstrable after 2 h, maximal after 6 h, and was not reversible upon removal of iodide. (7)

Escape from the Wolff-Chaikoff Effect

Thus, by inhibiting both the organic binding of iodine as well as thyroid hormone release, thyroid hormone levels decline promptly after administration of large doses of potassium iodide (KI) (50-100 mg), accounting for its success in treating Graves' thyrotoxicosis. Here I should mention that the inhibitory effect of KI works best in Graves' and Hashimoto's autoimmune thyroid disease patients in whom thyroid auto-regulation has been lost. Fortunately, in healthy normal patients, the inhibitory effect of KI is only temporary. The resumption of normal thyroid function is called the "Escape from the Wolff-Chaikoff Effect". Thyroid auto-regulation compensates for the increased intra-thyroidal iodide by decreasing the activity of the NIS (sodium iodide symporter), the active transport of iodine into the thyroid cells. This type of autoregulation is mediated by the formation of iodo-lactones induced by high intracellular iodide levels, as discussed in 1996 by Dr. Dugrillon. (8)

In normal healthy patients exposed to excess iodine, the autoregulatory reduction in NIS (sodium iodide symporter) activity reduces iodine uptake and reduces the concentration of iodine in the thyroid gland. TSH and serum thyroid hormone levels eventually return to normal, a phenomenon called "Escape from the Wolf Chaikoff Effect," which usually takes 26-50 hours in laboratory animals. (9-11)

Autoregulation Lost in Autoimmune Thyroid Disease

In 2022, Dr. Jeronimo F. Torti found the effect of high doses of potassium iodide on thyroid function varies, depending on whether the patient is euthyroid or has an underlying autoimmune disease. Within 2-4 weeks of continuous exposure to potassium iodide, the normal euthyroid patient's thyroid function will return to normal baseline thyroid function, a phenomenon known as the "Escape from the Wolf-Chaikoff Effect." However, in patients with underlying autoimmune disease, autoregulation has been lost, and inhibition of thyroid function by potassium iodide persists, resulting in worsening hypothyroidism in patients with Hashimoto's thyroiditis or improvement in hyperthyroidism in Graves' disease. Dr. Jeronimo F. Torti explains patients with "Graves' hyperthyroidism are more sensitive than normal subjects to the inhibitory effect of pharmacologic doses of iodine, making iodine treatment effective in some patients." In 2022, Dr. Jeronimo F. Torti writes:

> In euthyroid patients, iodine has two effects at two different times. The most rapid (hours to days) effect, at pharmacologic doses of KI [potassium iodide], decreases thyroglobulin proteolysis, thereby decreasing thyroid hormone secretion.

The resulting slight reductions of T4 and T3 concentrations in serum cause transient increases of thyrotropin (TSH) concentrations in serum. Secondly, **KI inhibits thyroid hormone synthesis**. The administration of KI leads to temporary **inhibition of iodine organification** in the thyroid gland, thereby decreasing thyroid hormone biosynthesis, a phenomenon called the Wolff-Chaikoff effect. However, **within two to four weeks** of continual exposure to excess iodine, organification, and thyroid hormone, biosynthesis resumes normally, called escape from the Wolff-Chaikoff effect. This phenomenon is produced by lower iodide uptake during the escape from the acute Wolff–Chaikoff effect. It results from a decrease in Na+/I– symporter (NIS) expression, **except in abnormal autoregulation of the iodine in autoimmune thyroid disease.** The [inhibition of] iodine organification persists and can result in or **exacerbate hypothyroidism in patients with Hashimoto's thyroiditis or ameliorate hyperthyroidism in Graves' disease.** Thus, patients with Graves' hyperthyroidism are more sensitive than normal subjects to the inhibitory effect of pharmacologic doses of iodine, making iodine treatment effective in some patients. Also, pharmacologic amounts of iodine may acutely ameliorate hyperthyroidism by **blocking thyroid hormone release.** Furthermore, it is used in preparation for thyroidectomy because **it decreases the vascularity of the thyroid gland.** Therefore, this decreases the risk of post-thyroidectomy hemorrhaging. KI should be administered at least one hour after administering thioamides to prevent new hormone synthesis since the new iodine substrate [when both methimazole (MMI) and potassium iodide (KI) may be given in preparation for thyroidectomy, the MMI is given an hour before the KI. The MMI blocks any production of thyroid hormone from the new iodide bolus]. (12)

As mentioned above, in patients with autoimmune thyroid disease, Graves' disease, or Hashimoto's disease, the auto-regulatory function has been lost, and the inhibitory function of potassium iodide continues without escape from the acute Wolff–Chaikoff effect. Also, autoregulation may be lost in post-thyroiditis and post-radioiodine ablation patients. (13-14)

Early Use Iodine for Treatment of Graves' Disease.

In the 1920s, Drs. Plummer, Starr, Lahey, and Charles Don reported success with high-dose iodine (Lugol's solution) in treating Graves' disease. Note: Lugol's solution is 5 percent iodine and 10 percent potassium iodide. The formula was invented in 1829 by Dr. Jean Lugol. (15-19)

In the 1930s and 1940s, the successful use of iodine to treat Graves' hyperthyroidism was reported by Drs. Thompson and Redisch. (20-21)

Iodine Contra-Indicated for Toxic Nodular Goiter and Autonomous Nodule

In 1940, Dr. Redisch reported the importance of distinguishing Graves' hyperthyroidism from toxic nodular goiter. Both may cause thyrotoxicosis. However, while iodine may be used to treat Graves' disease, iodine is contra-indicated in Toxic Nodular Goiter. This is also true for the solitary autonomous nodule discussed in Chapter 19. Dr. Redisch writes:

> Iodine should never be given to patients with old nodular goiters become toxic. (21)

The patient with multinodular goiter typically presents with a visibly palpable irregular and nodular neck mass on examination. Ultrasound and radionuclide imaging clearly shows the multiple nodules with irregular radio-iodine uptake from "hot" autonomous nodule (or nodules) superimposed on a background of suppressed normal tissue. The toxic nodular goiter has one or more autonomous nodules that harbor a mutation in the TSH receptor. These autonomous nodules convert iodine into thyroid hormone rapidly and uncontrollably, outside of normal TSH control. When such a patient consumes iodine, it worsens their hyperthyroidism, and they become thyrotoxic. For this reason, toxic nodular goiter is an absolute contraindication to the use of potassium iodide (KI). This topic is discussed more completely in Chapter 19. Iodine Induced Hyperthyroidism - the Autonomous Thyroid Nodule. (22-25)

The Autonomous Thyroid Nodule

The clinical history usually includes some form of iodine exposure in patients with thyrotoxicosis caused by the autonomous thyroid nodule. Perhaps the patient recently obtained iodized salt or iodine supplements from the health food store. Ultrasound thyroid imaging usually shows a dominant thyroid nodule or multiple nodules. Radionuclide imaging of the thyroid using Iodine-123 or Technetium 99M usually shows the "Hot Nodule" causing the thyrotoxicosis against a background of suppressed thyroid tissue with reduced activity. The toxic nodule may be solitary or multiple, i.e., the toxic nodular goiter. (26-28)

Potassium Iodide Inhibition of Organification and Inhibition of Release

As mentioned above, iodide Inhibits its own organification, as well as inhibits release of thyroid hormone from the thyroid gland. Inhibition of organification is done by inhibition of hydrogen peroxide production. In 1948, Drs. Wolff and Chaikoff published a report which concludes iodide inhibits organification, thus bringing about remission in Graves' disease, writing:

> we do believe that our findings justify the conclusion that an **interference in the organic binding of iodine** by the gland is an integral part of the mechanism by which **iodine brings about a remission in Graves' disease**. (29)

Inhibition of Release

The second mechanism of iodide, namely, the inhibition of hormone release, was proposed in 1970 by Dr. Wartofsky and later confirmed in 1985 by Dr. Bagchi, finding iodide inhibits hydrolysis of thyroglobulin, thus decreasing the secretion of thyroid hormone by the thyroid gland. Hydrolysis of thyroglobulin is the major step in the release of thyroid hormone. (6-7)

Microscopic Appearance of Thyroid in Graves' Disease

On microscopic evaluation of the thyroid gland in Graves' disease, one sees hyperplasia of thyroid cells lining the follicular spaces. The thyroid follicles are the central spherical areas for the collection and storage of thyroglobulin, the precursor to thyroid hormone. See the cover image of this book for a view of follicle architecture under the microscope.

Upregulated D1 and D2 Deiodinase in Graves' Disease

In order to release thyroid hormone into circulation, the thyrocyte cells take in the thyroglobulin by pinocytosis and liberate the free thyroid hormone through a process of enzymatic digestion called hydrolysis to yield thyroxine, T4, which is then released into the bloodstream. The D1 and D2 deiodinase enzyme is present in the thyroid gland, for conversion of T4 to T3. In Graves' hyperthyroidism, both D1 and D2 intra-thyroid deiodinases are upregulated, accounting for greater amounts of T3 secreted into circulation by the thyroid gland in Graves' disease. As such, the T3/T4 ratio may be useful as a prognostic indicator of the severity of Graves' disease. Higher T3 indicates more severe disease. For more discussion on this topic, see Chapter 14 on the Production of Thyroid Hormone. (30-32)

Diffusely Enlarged Hyperactive Thyroid Gland

The thyroid cells lining the follicles are the worker cells that secrete thyroglobulin into the follicles. In Graves' disease, thyroid cells lining the follicles are enlarged and more numerous, the result of TSH receptor stimulation from

TSI and TRAB antibodies. Although high TSH (thyroid stimulating hormone) will cause an increase in hydrogen peroxide generation, the TSI and TRAB antibodies in Graves' Disease **DO NOT** increase hydrogen peroxide generation, since a different signaling cascade is used. As a result, stimulation of H202 generation is performed solely by TSH, which is typically suppressed near zero in severe Graves' disease patients. In Graves' disease, TSH receptors are stimulated by the TSI and TRAB antibodies resulting in thyroid growth and enlargement. The follicles contain greater amounts of colloid, and the entire gland is usually diffusely enlarged. At initial clinical presentation, the thyroid gland in Graves' disease is diffusely enlarged with diffuse epithelial hyperplasia and hypervascularity. Over many years, the smooth diffuse enlargement and pristine histology may change after repeated bouts of thyroiditis. (33)

Graves' Disease After Treatment

Once under treatment, the histology of the thyroid gland in Graves' disease undergoes changes. For example, in 1986, Dr. Hirota studied thyroid histology after long-term methimazole treatment and repeated bouts of thyroiditis, finding diffuse epithelial hyperplasia was no longer seen, as this was replaced with chronic lymphocytic thyroiditis. (34)

After I-131, radioactive iodine ablation therapy for Graves' Disease, the histology pattern changes to multiple adenomatous nodules, some with cystic changes, with various degrees of chronic thyroiditis. (35)

After treatment with potassium iodide (KI) in Graves' Disease, follicular cells revert back to their normal shape, and some of the hyperplastic features regress. In 2009, Dr Thompson writes:

> Potassium iodide causes involution as follicular cells revert to their normal cuboidal or flattened appearance, alternating with areas that have retained some of the features of hyperplasia. (36)

Is it Graves' Disease or Autonomous Nodule?

The most reliable way to differentiate Graves' disease from Toxic Nodular Goiter is the serum antibody tests for TRAb and TSI antibodies. With only rare exceptions, Graves' disease will show elevated TRAb, while autonomous nodules will not. The ultrasound scan usually reveals the nodule or multiple nodules. The radionuclide scan will show the autonomous nodule as "hot' with greater activity than the surrounding thyroid tissue. In 2021, Dr. Carolina Perdomo evaluated the use of thyroid scintigraphy (radio nuclide imaging) finding it useful in the diagnosis of Graves' disease when the first generation TRAb and TSI antibodies test is negative. This problem of antibody negative Graves' disease vanishes when switching to the updated second-generation TRAb assays. Second-generation TRAb assays are more sensitive than first-generation and should be used for routine clinical practice with a sensitivity of 97-99 percent. (37-41)

Use of Radioactive Iodine Uptake to Differentiate Hashitoxicosis from Graves' Disease.

What is Hashitoxicosis? This is thyrotoxicosis in the patient with Hashimoto's thyroiditis. Hashitoxicosis may be easily confused with the thyrotoxicosis of Graves' disease. Hashitoxicosis can be differentiated from Graves' thyrotoxicosis by doing a radionuclide uptake scan with I-123 or technetium 99M showing low radioiodine uptake. The 4 hr. and 24 hr. radioactive iodine uptake are both high in Graves' disease (over 50%) and very low, less than 5%, in Hashitoxicosis (Painless Thyroiditis in Hashimoto's), as reported in 2016 by Dr. Ashley Schaffer who writes:

> Interestingly, anti-TPO Ab and anti-TG Ab can be detected in up to 70% of patients with GD [Graves' disease], in addition to TBII and TSIG antibodies at the time of diagnosis... The recurrence of thyrotoxicosis, associated with presence of HT [Hashimoto's] antibodies when GD antibodies remained

negative, and mild course associated with absence of clinical symptoms and signs were all suggestive of Hashitoxicosis and not GD. **Furthermore, repeat I123 uptake and scans revealed uptake indicative of an inflammatory thyroiditis associated with HT and not increased uptake diagnostic for GD.** (42)

The low radio-iodine uptake of Hashitoxicosis is similar to that seen in subacute thyroiditis, which is less than 1 percent, as discussed in 1998 by Dr. Douglas Ross writing:

> mechanism of thyrotoxicosis in subacute thyroiditis is inflammation of thyroid follicles with release of preformed hormone into the circulation. In this group of disorders, the 24-hour radioiodine uptake is almost always less than 1%. (43-46)

In 1975 and 1980, Drs. Savoie and Skare reported low radio-iodine uptake in cases of iodine-induced thyrotoxicosis in apparently normal thyroid glands. The low radio-iodine uptake indicates thyroiditis. However, the authors were unable to explain the mechanism or cause. I would speculate these cases of thyroiditis in "normal thyroid glands" are related to selenium/iodine deficiency. These thyroid glands are unable to neutralize the excess hydrogen peroxide induced by an acute iodine load. In the future, measuring selenium and iodine levels in these types of cases might be useful. (122-123)

Ultrasound Imaging

In toxic nodular goiter, ultrasound imaging will show a typical appearance of multiple thyroid nodules. If a radionuclide scan is done, one of the nodules may stand out as a "hot nodule" against a background of variably reduced uptake. This is the autonomous nodule. In untreated Graves' disease, however, the radionuclide thyroid scan will typically show a smooth, diffusely enlarged thyroid gland with diffusely increased radiotracer uptake. Occasionally, in long-standing Graves' disease

after many years of medical treatment and episodes of thyroiditis, the gland becomes nodular. However, at initial presentation in the untreated Graves' disease patient, palpation of the thyroid gland typically reveals a diffuse, smoothly enlarged gland. A similar pattern is also demonstrated with medical imaging. On the other hand, in the patient with Toxic Multi-Nodular Goiter, the thyroid gland is usually irregular and bumpy with either solitary or multiple nodules on palpation, confirmed with ultrasound or radionuclide imaging. (26-28)

Graves' Disease TSI and TRAb Antibodies

As mentioned above, Graves' disease is an autoimmune thyroid disorder with anti-thyroid antibodies specific for the TSH Receptor. The two antibody tests for Graves' disease are the TSI, Thyroid Stimulatory Immune Globulin, and the TRAb, Thyroid Receptor Antibody test. The newer second generation TRAb test is specific for Graves' disease with 97-97 percent sensitivity. The TRAb antibodies come in three varieties, stimulatory, inhibitory, and neutral. Unfortunately, the TRAb test cannot distinguish between these three types. However, if the thyroid gland is smoothly enlarged without nodularity and the TSI and TRAb are elevated, this is a reliable way to confirm the diagnosis of Graves' disease and exclude Toxic Nodular Goiter. Persistent elevation of TRAb antibody in the Graves's disease patient is associated with a 50% chance for relapse, even though the patient has been able to taper off methimazole, and achieve a euthyroid state. (47-50)

In 2004, Dr. Wallaschofski from Germany writes the TRAb test should be performed on all patients to differentiate Graves' disease from Toxic Multinodular Goiter, writing:

> the h-TBII (TRAb antibody test) should be performed in all patients with hyperthyroidism to differentiate Graves' disease from non-autoimmune hyperthyroidism, such as toxic multinodular goiter. (51)

Graves' Orbitopathy

In some patients, these same Graves' anti-bodies (TSI and TRAb) attack the extra-ocular muscles and peri-orbital fat. This causes inflammation and enlargement of the muscles behind the eye, which control eye movement, pushing the eye forward, causing the characteristic exophthalmos, a medical term for "the eyes bulging out." There may be proptosis and lid retraction with a reddened, inflamed conjunctiva resembling dry eye syndrome. If severe, the optic nerve can be compromised at the orbital apex resulting in loss of vision. Studies show the fibroblast cells in the peri-orbital fat contain TSH Receptors in Graves Orbitopathy. Other areas of the body may contain TSH receptors in the fat and connective tissue, explaining pretibial myxedema and thyroid acropachy, a useful sign upon physical examination. In 2006, Dr. Tani writes:

> autoimmunity against TSH-r [TSH Receptor], expressed in fat and connective tissue, could explain the development of pretibial myxedema, acropachy and the OCT [Orbital Connective Tissue] component of TAO [thyroid-associated ophthalmopathy]. (52-56)

Modern Treatment of Hyperthyroidism

Prior to 1980, Lugol's iodine and potassium iodide were the treatment of Graves' disease. After 1980, these were replaced by anti-thyroid drugs, the thionamides such as PTU (propylthiouracil) and methimazole (Tapazole). Lugol's iodine and potassium iodide are still in use today as a short-term treatment of Graves' disease in preparation for thyroidectomy. In the past, this was done in the hospital setting, and more recently as an outpatient. The standard dosage is 50 mg of potassium iodide three times a day for 10 days prior to thyroidectomy. The iodine is given with Beta Blocker (propranolol) to control heart rate. Methimazole or PTU may also be added as needed. In 2009, Dr. Sinem Kiyici reported the use of Lugol's iodine in combination with anti-thyroid drugs for preparation of the hyperthyroid patient for thyroidectomy. Note: this is for short-term use only. Long-term use of Lugol's solution is avoided here because of the chance for a rebound or escape from the suppressive effects of iodine. Dr. Sinem Kiyici writes:

> Lugol [iodine] treatment with and without antithyroid drugs is a safe and effective choice in the rapid preparation of patients with hyperthyroidism to thyroidectomy when surgery cannot be delayed. (57-59)

Long-term Use of Iodine for Graves' Disease

In Japan, the use of potassium iodide for long-term treatment of Graves' disease is widely accepted by thyroid specialists; however, in the United States, long-term use of iodine for Graves' disease is not accepted by conventional endocrinologists for fear of iodine escape, also called "rebound effect." (60-62)

Thyroid Ablation with Radioactive Iodine or Surgery

Thyroid ablation is considered a definitive treatment and consists of two techniques. The first technique is a thyroidectomy. The second is radioactive iodine. Both forms of thyroid ablation leave the patient hypothyroid, requiring life-long thyroid hormone replacement, usually with levothyroxine.

Radio ablation of the thyroid gland is performed by giving the patient a radioactive iodine (I-131) capsule by mouth. The thyroid gland takes up and concentrates the radioactive iodine, causing radiation damage to the thyroid gland. Afterward, the patient is usually in a hypothyroid state requiring lifelong levothyroxine treatment. Because of convenience and ease of use with rare adverse side effects, radioactive iodine (I-131) has been the popular choice for hyperthyroid patients. About 80% of patients achieve "remission" with a single dose of Iodine-131. The remaining 20% of treatment failures require a second dose of I-131.

Treatment failure is most associated with very high levels of TRAb antibodies (an indicator of the severity of the autoimmune disease) and larger goiters. These may opt for thyroidectomy rather than radio ablation. Pretreatment with lithium carbonate increases Iodine-131 retention in the thyroid gland and is thought to make radioactive iodine more effective. (63-68)

Radioactive Iodine May Worsen Graves' Orbitopathy

In 2013 Clinical Thyroidology, Dr. Jerome M. Hershman cited studies from Italy showing radioactive iodine may worsen thyroid eye disease. For this reason, patients with thyroid eye disease may choose thyroidectomy rather than radio ablation. Selenium supplementation has been found beneficial for thyroid eye disease. A new intravenous drug has recently been approved to treat Graves' orbitopathy, the IGF Receptor blocker drug, Teprotumumab. (69-72)

Surgical Treatment for Graves' Disease

Many Graves' disease patients will decide on thyroidectomy because it provides rapid and definitive control of hyperthyroidism. Of course, thyroidectomy renders patients hypothyroid requiring lifelong thyroid hormone replacement. Thyroidectomy is not without risk for post-operative complications. The procedure may cause parathyroid glands to be removed or damaged, resulting in hypocalcemia, requiring treatment with calcium tablets. A second post-operative complication is an unintended injury to the recurrent laryngeal nerve causing temporary or permanent hoarseness. In 2019, Dr. Calogero Cipolla from Palermo, Italy, did a single-center retrospective review of 594 cases of total thyroidectomy for Graves' Disease, writing:

> Temporary and permanent hypocalcemia developed in 241 (40.6%) and 3 patients (0.5%), respectively. Temporary and permanent recurrent laryngeal nerve

palsy were recorded in 31 (5.2%) and 1 patient (0.16%) respectively.... This high-volume surgeon experience demonstrates that total thyroidectomy is a safe and effective treatment for Graves' disease. It is associated with a very low incidence rate of postoperative complications, most of which are transitory; therefore, it offers a rapid and definitive control of hyperthyroidism and its related symptoms. (73)

Iodine Alone in Treatment of Graves' Disease

In 2000, Dr. Jamieson reported on the successful treatment of Graves' disease in pregnancy with Lugol's iodine. (74)

In 2013, Dr. Gangadharan reported on the use of iodine as first-line therapy in a child with Graves' disease. Thionamide drugs were contraindicated because of neutropenia. (75)

However, others have concluded iodine alone is not an ideal treatment for long-term control of hyperthyroidism. In 1975, Dr. Charles Emerson studied serum hormone levels during iodine treatment of 9 patients with hyperthyroidism. Thyroid hormone levels fell initially in all 9 patients. However, after 11 days or so, levels began to rise again in 6 of the 9. In the remaining 3, thyroid hormone levels remained suppressed. Dr. Emerson writes:

> These data support the concept that iodide alone is not an ideal agent for the treatment of hyperthyroidism. (76)

In 1992, Dr. George Phillppou studied 21 hyperthyroid patients given 150 mg of potassium iodide daily, compared to 12 healthy controls. For the first three weeks, the 21 patients had a good response with a decline in thyroid hormone levels. However, after 21 days, the Free T3 and Free T4 levels started increasing again in some cases. Dr. Phillppou concludes:

> Iodides in hyperthyroidism have a variable and unpredictable intensity and duration of antithyroid effect. Their antithyroid effect is smaller in normal controls. (77)

Long Term Use of Iodide Alone or Combined with Methimazole

In 2014, Dr. Ken Okamura in Japan treated 1388 patients with thionamides (methimazole) for Graves' hyperthyroidism. However, 44 patients of the 1388 discontinued methimazole because of adverse side effects. These patients were then switched to KI (potassium iodide) long-term at a dosage of 10-400 mg/d and followed for 8 to 28 years (median 17.6 years). (78)

Twenty-five or 65 percent of these 44 patients were well-controlled with iodide alone. Of these, about 40% went into remission after an average of 7.4 years. The other 15 of the 44 patients (30%) could not be controlled with iodide alone, even at high dosages (100-750 mg/d). However, 7 of the 15 were controlled with a combination of iodide and low-dose methimazole for a few years and then with iodide alone, resulting in remission after 7 years (2-11 years). The other seven were treated with radioactive iodine (I-131) uneventfully after a period of iodine restriction. Dr. Okamura felt that the effect of the suppressive effects of methimazole and iodine were additive. Dr. Okamura writes:

our clinical study suggested that the effects of thionamides [methimazole] and excess iodide are additive when a large amount of iodide required for the Wolff-Chaikoff effect is administered concomitantly... prompt re-evaluation of the treatment was required when escape occurred or thyrotoxicosis remained for more than 3 months requiring more than 200 mg KI. Note: The Wolff-Chaikoff effect refers to the suppressive effect of iodine on thyroid function. (78)

Block and Replace

For the five patients who became hypothyroid, with elevated TSH on iodine-alone, Dr. Okamura used the "Block and Replace" technique, a combination of potassium iodide with levothyroxine (50-75 mcg/d) to maintain a euthyroid state. In 1991, Dr. Hashizume reported that "Block and Replace" with the addition of levothyroxine reduces the TSI (Graves' antibody) and increases the chance of remission. In my opinion, Block and Replace is justified in Graves' disease patients who have an undulating course with frequent biochemical relapse. Block and Replace reduces the TSH, thus preventing TSH generation of hydrogen peroxide, a trigger for thyroiditis. It would be prudent to give the patient selenium and magnesium to maintain the good antioxidant capacity needed for the neutralization of excess hydrogen peroxide. In Block and Replace anti-thyroid drug dosage is not reduced. TSH is kept low by the addition of thyroid medication which inhibits the pituitary release of TSH. If KI is used, keeping the dosage high maintains the Wolff-Chaikoff Effect and inhibits thyroid hormone release. If methimazole is used, keeping the dosage high maintains inhibition of TPO and blocks organification. (79)

Switching from Methimazole to Iodide for Pregnant Patients

In 2015, Dr. Yoshihara from Japan substituted potassium iodide (KI) for methimazole (MMI) in 240 pregnant women to control hyperthyroidism in the first trimester. This was done to avoid the risk of fetal malformations associated with MMI. About 90% of the patients responded well to the KI. However, about 9% escaped from the suppressive effect of KI alone and required a higher dose of MMI (worsened group).

The mean age of the 240 pregnant women was 33 years. Of the 240 patients, 55% went into remission, and KI could be completely tapered during the pregnancy. The other 45% were still taking thyroid-blocking medication at delivery. Of these, roughly half were taking potassium iodide (KI) alone, and half were taking an anti-thyroid drug (MMI) with or without KI. Higher TRAb values predicted the continuation of anti-thyroid medication. Dr. Yoshihara writes:

Treatment of Graves' Disease (GD) with Potassium Iodide (KI) is widely accepted by Japanese thyroid specialists, and its efficacy has been reported ...It was difficult to control the maternal thyrotoxicosis of 22 of the 107 patients [9% of the total 240 pts.] with KI alone, and a higher dose of MMI compared with the dose at the time of conception was required (worsened group). Multivariate analysis revealed that the **TRAb value at the time of the switch from MMI to KI was the only factor that predicted the continuation of the thyroid suppression medication, but none of the parameters was a predictor of the worsened group**...Conclusions: It must be kept in mind that **a certain proportion of GD patients escape from the antithyroid effect of iodide** and that careful follow-up is necessary after switching a pregnant patient's medication to KI. Note: TRAb is a Thyroid Receptor Antibody, a general measure of the severity of Graves' Disease. (60)

Not Recommended Outside of Japan

In 2020, Dr. Elizabeth Pearce reviewed Dr. Yoshihara's 2015 study concluding KI for Graves' Disease should not be recommended outside of Japan because of the 9.2 percent worsened group with "Escape" from the anti-thyroid effect of KI. Dr. Elizabeth Pearce writes:

The switch from MMI to KI treatment occurred at a median of 6 weeks of gestation (range 4–12). The mean initial KI dose was 20 mg daily. Of the 133 (55%) patients who were able to taper off of all medication during pregnancy, four patients still needed levothyroxine therapy by the time of delivery. Women who were able to discontinue therapy required lower MMI doses prior to the switch to KI, had lower TRAb titers, higher serum TSH levels, and were on lower KI doses as compared with women who needed treatment for hyperthyroidism throughout gestation... **Worsened hyperthyroidism occurred in 22 patients (9.2%) following the switch to KI, requiring higher MMI doses by the**

third trimester than before the medication switch...incidence of birth defects was lower in children of the mothers who were switched to KI...The current American Thyroid Association guideline for the management of thyroid disease in pregnancy cautions, with regard to KI treatment for Graves' disease, that **"at present, such therapy cannot be recommended outside Japan until more evidence on safety and efficacy is available** ."I do not think that the results of the current study are likely to alter that guidance. (62)

Selenium Status and Escape from Iodine

Although there was a 91 percent success rate with switching patients from MMI to KI for treatment of Graves' hyperthyroidism, there was a 9.2 % escape rate in which hyperthyroidism worsened, requiring higher doses of MMI for control. There was no obvious explanation for why this occurs in some patients and not others. A few possible explanations will be offered below.

Same Success Rate as in 1920s and 1930s

By the way, this 90 percent success rate in Dr. Yoshihara's 2015 study was similar to the success rate in a 1924 study by Dr. Paul Starr at the Massachusetts General Hospital, treating 25 patients with Graves' Disease (exophthalmic goiter) with KI alone, at the dosage of 90 mg per day. (17)

A similar 88% success rate was obtained in 1930 by Dr. Thompson, who treated 24 Graves' Disease patients with Lugol's Solution. Dr. Thompson writes:

Twenty-four patients with exophthalmic goiter (14 mild and 10 severe or moderately severe cases) have been treated in this clinic with iodine [Lugol's] alone, either continuously or intermittently for periods ranging from one and one-half months to three years. The period of treatment was a year or more in 13 instances. With three exceptions (all unsatisfactory responses to iodine), the patients pursued their daily work throughout the period of observation, thus eliminating the effect of rest. (20)

Predicting Escape from KI

Although Dr. Yoshihara had no parameter to predict iodine escape, it may be possible to suggest a mechanism based on understanding the production of thyroid hormone and its pathophysiology. Firstly, it is known that in normal humans and animal studies, toxic effects of excess iodine may cause thyroiditis, an inflammatory condition known to cause hyperthyroidism from rupture of follicles with release of preformed thyroid hormone. Thus, one possible explanation for escape or resistance to KI is this represents an episode of iodine-induced thyroiditis.

In normal people consuming dietary excess iodine, there is an initial inhibition of thyroid function with elevation of TSH. However, a few weeks later, the thyroid autoregulatory ability normalizes the TSH and thyroid hormone levels through downregulation of the Sodium/Iodide Symporter, the active transport mechanism. The reduced iodide uptake normalizes intra-thyroid iodide content. Once TSH is normalized, this reduces the TSH-stimulated generation of excess hydrogen peroxide, with no further risk of thyroiditis, even if the patient is at high risk of selenium and magnesium deficiency. (11)

Autoimmune thyroid disease patients have no autoregulatory ability. The suppressive effect of high-dose potassium iodide on thyroid function continues indefinitely, producing a high TSH. In this group, there may be intermittent episodes of thyroiditis. If the patient has underlying Hashimoto's thyroiditis, these episodes of thyroiditis cause a type of thyrotoxicosis with low radio-iodine uptake, called Hashitoxicosis. A reliable way to differentiate Graves' thyrotoxicosis from Hashitoxicosis is the radio-iodine uptake scan which shows high iodine uptake in Graves' disease, while iodine uptake is low in Hashitoxicosis. (43-46)

TSH Receptor Antibodies Do Not Stimulate Hydrogen Peroxide

High radio-iodine uptake in Graves' disease means NIS function is hyper-stimulated by TSH receptor antibodies. However, unlike TSH, which stimulates hydrogen peroxide ($H2O2$) generation, TSH receptor antibodies do not stimulate $H2O2$ by activating phospho lipase C, thus explaining the smooth diffuse enlargement of the thyroid gland with lack of thyroiditis in the early onset presentation of untreated Graves' disease patients. However, with treatment with KI or thyroid-blocking drugs, thyroid function may be completely inhibited, resulting in elevated TSH. This high TSH may trigger excess $H2O2$ generation, leading to recurring bouts of thyroiditis. This is more completely discussed in Chapter 14 Production of Thyroid Hormone. (80-82)

NIS Auto-Antibodies and Iodine Escape

In 2010, Dr. Anna-Maria Eleftheriadou found that about 12 percent of Graves' Disease patients have auto-antibodies to NIS, the sodium iodide symporter, the active transport for iodide. A second explanation for KI "resistance or escape" in Graves' disease is the presence of NIS antibodies in about 12 percent of Graves' disease patients. The NIS is embedded in the basolateral membrane of the thyrocyte and mediates the active transport of iodine into the thyroid cell, concentrating iodine 100 times that of plasma. However, NIS antibodies are the monkey wrench in the machinery, inhibiting iodine uptake and concentration, thus explaining the iodine "Escape" or "Resistance" in a subset of Graves' disease patients treated with KI. (83-85)

Immune Complex Deposits at Basolateral Membrane of Follicles

In 1977, Dr. Kalderon identified immune complex deposits at the follicular basal lamina of the follicles in the thyroid glands of patients with Hashimotos' and Graves' autoimmune thyroid disease. Note: this is the same location as the NIS, the sodium iodide symporter. Dr. Kalderon also identified this same finding in a hereditary model of autoimmune thyroid disease in obese chickens. One might speculate deposition of immune complexes in this location could interfere with the NIS function and impact thyroid autoregulation. (86-87)

Selenium/Magnesium Levels in Graves' Disease

Selenium/magnesium levels could be the defining factor in these intermittent bouts of thyroiditis. According to studies in which animals are fed excess iodine by Drs. Jian Xu, Christine Thomson, and Ioana Vasiliu, excess iodine causes selenium depletion and selenium deficiency. In addition, selenium alleviates the toxic effects of excess iodine. One of the toxic effects is increased accumulation of colloids in the follicles, causing goiter. Such iodine-induced changes in thyroid morphology were described in Graves' disease patients after potassium iodide pre-thyroidectomy by Dr. FW Rienhoff in 1925 and Dr. Joseph DeCourcy in 1927. (88-93)

To reiterate, under conditions of iodine excess, in both humans and mice, there is an enlargement of the follicles with increased colloid formation (thyroglobulin), which forms a goiter.

Selenium Alleviates Toxic Effects of Iodine

In 2011, Dr. Christine Thomson studied the effect of excess iodine intake on thyroid hormones and selenium status in older New Zealanders, agreeing with Dr. Jian Xu, who found selenium alleviates the toxic effects of iodine in humans as well as mice. Dr. Thomson advised co-administration of selenium along with iodine, writing:

> Our results agree with those of Xu et al., who showed in mice that decreased activities of GPx [Glutathione Peroxidase] resulting from excessive iodine intake could be restored through supplementing with selenium. These observations indicate that when high iodate [iodine] supplements are used to eliminate iodine deficiency, it would appear important to co-administer selenium to ensure adequate selenium intake. (93-100)

Myxoedematous Cretinism in Zaire, Africa

Myxoedematous cretinism is a form of thyroid destruction first described in Zaire, Africa. In myxoedematous endemic cretinism, iodine deficiency and resulting hypothyroidism caused severe elevation of TSH with marked stimulation of the TSH receptors, causing upregulation of all steps in thyroid hormone synthesis. One of these upregulated steps is the production of hydrogen peroxide. In the selenium-deficient population of Zaire, the selenium-based antioxidant system is dysfunctional, and excess hydrogen peroxide cannot be neutralized. Thus, hydrogen peroxide accumulates in the follicles at the apical villous membrane causing oxidative damage to thyrocytes (cells lining the follicles), thyroiditis, inflammatory changes with apoptosis, and necrosis. This type of thyroiditis leads to the release of preformed thyroid hormone, a form of thyrotoxicosis with low radio-iodine uptake. Treatment with thyroid-blocking drugs that block the TPO enzyme, such as methimazole, is usually ineffective since thyrotoxicosis is caused by the rupture of follicles with the release of preformed thyroid hormone and is not caused by the usual TPO organification machinery. One might suggest the mechanism of thyroiditis in myxoedematous cretinism resembles that of thyroiditis of Hashitoxicosis. Indeed, a similar mechanism has been described for the etiology of autoimmune thyroid disease, in which excess hydrogen peroxide causes oxidative damage to Thyroglobulin and TPO. These damaged proteins are then recognized by the immune system as foreign proteins, causing the immune system to produce antibodies against Thyroglobulin and TPO (thyroid peroxidase). In 2007, Dr. Yue Song studied the role of hydrogen peroxide in thyroid physiology and disease, writing:

> It is proposed that various pathologies can be explained, at least in part, by overproduction and lack of degradation of H2O2 (tumorigenesis, myxedematous cretinism, and thyroiditis) and by failure of the H2O2 generation or its positive control system (congenital hypothyroidism). (81)

The Selenium/Magnesium Deficient Patient

Let us consider the case of the methimazole-treated Graves' disease patient. If the methimazole dosage is high enough to suppress Free T3 and Free T4 below the reference range, feedback to the HPA (hypothalamic-pituitary axis) will eventually cause a very high TSH. As mentioned in the chapter on the production of thyroid hormone, high TSH stimulates the generation of hydrogen peroxide, thyroglobulin production, and organification. The increased thyroglobulin (also called colloid) fills the follicles, causing thyroid enlargement and goiter.

The treating physician will see the elevated TSH and low Free T4 and will be tempted to reduce the dosage of MMI. In the 2015 study by Dr. Yoshihara, in a subset of Graves' disease patients with elevated TSH after starting iodine, rather than reducing the MMI dosage, these patients were treated with "Block and Replace." The thyroid is blocked with MMI and replaced with levothyroxine. The added levothyroxine serves to bring down the TSH and raise the FreeT4. "Block and Replace" suppresses the TSH, thus turning off hydrogen peroxide generation and reducing the risk of thyroiditis. However, for those not treated with "Block and Replace," lowering the MMI while the TSH is still elevated allows the generation of hydrogen peroxide and subsequent thyroiditis. This may trigger massive oxidative damage leading to inflammation, apoptosis, and necrosis of thyrocytes. The inflammatory process may stimulate thyroid autoimmunity as well as spill preformed thyroid hormone from the follicles into the bloodstream. Although we

are discussing a scenario in the Graves' disease patient, this mechanism of thyroiditis bears a similarity with Hashitoxicosis, an inflammatory process associated with decreased radio-iodine uptake. Indeed, 70% of Graves' disease patients will also have anti-TPO and anti-thyroglobulin antibodies, indicating coexisting Graves' and Hashimoto's thyroiditis, suggesting these are not separate disease entities but merely two variations of the same disease. In 2016, Dr. Ashley Schaffer made this same observation, writing:

> We believe this report is important as not only is it the first to report thyrotoxicosis due to GD [Graves' Disease], then due to Hashitoxicosis, and then due to GD in the same individuals, but also the **cooccurrence of these 2 autoimmune processes highlights the concept that these are not separate processes but parts of the same autoimmune spectrum.** (42)

Painless Thyroiditis Causing Unexpected Relapsing Hyperthyroidism

This thyroiditis mechanism was confirmed in 2022 by Dr. Ken Okamura, who reviewed 100 Graves' disease patients who presented with unexpected relapsing hyperthyroidism while decreasing the dosage of anti-thyroid drug methimazole (MMI), PTU, or potassium iodide.

Dr. Ken Okamura reports when the dosage of antithyroid medication (MMI or KI) is tapered (decreased), this may provoke an episode of painless thyroiditis (PT) which mimics a relapse of Graves' hyperthyroidism. This is not a relapse of Graves' hyperthyroidism. Rather, this is painless thyroiditis (PT), a form of thyroiditis that causes thyrotoxicosis with low radio-iodine uptake, a destructive inflammatory process within the thyroid gland representing a form of "self-ablation." Dr. Ken Okamura writes:

> The golden-standard factor to consider for the differential diagnosis is the **thyroidal radioactive iodine uptake (RAIU), which is high in GD [Graves' Disease] and almost null**

in typical **PT [painless thyroiditis] cases.** PT is also suggested when thyroid-stimulating hormone (TSH) receptor antibody (TRAb), measured by the TSH Binding Inhibitor Immunoglobulin (TBII) or thyroid-stimulating antibody activity (TSAb), is negative and **thyrotoxicosis resolves spontaneously without antithyroid drugs (ATDs) followed by an episode of transient hypothyroidism...** Autoregulatory mechanisms in the thyroid gland are well known, and thyroid hormone synthesis was thought to be regulated by organified iodine compound X, probably an iodoaldehyde and/or iodolactone, which requires active thyroid peroxidase (TPO) to be synthesized, although the mechanisms underlying the effects of compound X remain elusive . It is therefore plausible that a **decreased ATD dosage might increase TPO activity and thereby increase the production of compound X [iodolactones] , which suppresses the thyroid function, including that of sodium-iodide symporter (NIS), resulting in a decreased iodine uptake possibly accompanying Tg proteolysis and thyroid hormone release.** From a therapeutic perspective, it is very important to keep in mind that **PT can occur during ATD treatment of GD, especially when the dosage is reduced [and TSH goes high]...** PT was frequently observed during KI treatment. In Group A, 19 (54.3%) patients were treated by KI alone or KI and MMI before the episode of PT. Given the effect of excess iodine on the morphological changes in the thyroid, KI treatment may precipitate the "iodide thyroiditis" reported by Edmunds in 1955. In the same year as Gluck reported convincing cases with PT, Savoie reported 10 cases of iodine-induced thyrotoxicosis in apparently normal thyroid glands, ranging from 1 to 40 months after exposure to excess iodine. **They all showed a typical clinical course of PT with a low RAIU followed by hypothyroidism.** (82)

Painless Thyroiditis (PT) When Switching from Methimazole to Iodine

In 2021, Dr. Keiichi Kamijo studied potassium iodide-induced painless thyroiditis (PT) in 11 Graves' Disease patients finding 10 of the 11 patients also harbored Hashimoto's antibodies (TPO or Thyroglobulin Abs), suggesting a resemblance with Hashitoxicosis. Physicians should be alerted to induction of Painless Thyroiditis in patients discontinuing ATD (anti-thyroid drug such as MMI) and switching to potassium iodide (KI). Dr. Keiichi Kamijo writes:

> Painless thyroiditis (PT) is characterized by transient hyperthyroidism with a low Tc-99m uptake... We herein describe 11 cases of **PT that occurred during treatment with potassium iodide (KI) for Graves' disease (GD)**...the administration of stable iodine to hyperthyroid patients produces clinical benefits by inhibiting the release of thyroid hormone and its synthesis due to a decrease in TPO mRNA...The pathogenesis of KI-induced PT is unclear but may be related to this cytotoxic effect of KI. In addition, because **10 of the 11 patients in our current study with KI-induced PT were positive for TgAb and/or TPOAb,** an autoimmune mechanism may be involved in this process. **Finally, we emphasize that clinicians who manage GD patients who received KI after discontinuing ATD [anti-thyroid drug, methimazole] due to side effects should be alert for KI-induce PT.** (44)

Myxedematous Cretinism Combined Iodine / Selenium Deficiency

In 2017, Dr. Mara Ventura proposed combined iodine and selenium deficiency as a mechanism for Myxedematous Cretinism, a form of destruction of the thyroid gland in young children in Zaire, Africa. Dr. Mara Ventura proposed that combined iodine/selenium deficiency causes thyroid failure and increased TSH, which stimulates thyroid hormone production, creating excess hydrogen peroxide, which cannot be neutralized, leading to thyroiditis and fibrosis. Dr. Mara Ventura writes:

> In fact, it was found that selenium deficiency decreases the synthesis of thyroid hormones, as it decreases the function of

selenoproteins, in particular iodothyronine deiodinases (DIOs), which are responsible for the conversion of T4 to T3. This decreased production of thyroid hormones leads to the stimulation of the hypothalamic-pituitary axis due to the lack of negative feedback control, increasing TSH production. TSH stimulates the DIOs [deiodinases] to convert T4 to T3, with consequent production of hydrogen peroxide, which is not adequately removed by less active glutathione peroxidases (GPx) and accumulates itself in the thyroid tissue causing thyrocyte damage with subsequent fibrosis. (101)

In 1993, Dr. Bernard Contempre reproduced this mechanism of thyroid destruction in selenium-deficient mice fed perchlorate for a month. Note: perchlorate is a thyroid-blocking drug that prevents iodine uptake, thus worsening iodine deficiency. After perchlorate withdrawal, the mice were fed iodine. The selenium-deficient mice had markedly reduced glutathione peroxidase levels (a selenium-protein antioxidant). The perchlorate-treated mice developed goiters and were hypothyroid, with elevated TSH. After iodide refeeding, thyroid hormone levels markedly increased, and necrotic thyrocyte cells were observed in numbers three times greater in the selenium-deficient mice. Dr. Bernard Contempre writes:

These experimental data demonstrate the detrimental role of selenium deficiency in one experimental case of thyroid disease. Such reduction of cell defenses could contribute to the thyroid failure of African myxedematous cretins. (102-103)

Magnesium Deficiency Worsens Selenium Deficiency

In 2006, Dr. Cornelia V. Gilroy studied magnesium levels in hyperthyroid cats, finding hyperthyroidism increases renal excretion of magnesium and causes magnesium deficiency, which correlates with the severity of hyperthyroidism. Dr. Cornelia V. Gilroy writes:

Hyperthyroidism can increase the renal excretion of magnesium and thus cause hypomagnesemia in various species...the severity of hyperthyroidism may contribute to a decrease in the ionized magnesium concentration. (104)

Magnesium deficiency worsens the defect in selenium deficiency, while oral supplementation with magnesium potentiates the glutathione peroxidase antioxidant system. Thus, magnesium supplementation is recommended for Graves' disease patients. Perhaps selenium/magnesium deficiency could explain the 9% percent worsened group in the 2015 Yoshihara study. Could insufficient levels of selenium/magnesium predict escape from the suppressive effects of iodine? Unfortunately, Dr. Ai Yoshihara's study did not measure selenium or magnesium levels. Future studies, which include measuring selenium and magnesium levels, might be useful. (60) (104-111)

Current Status of KI for Graves' Disease

In 2017, Dr. Jan Calissendorf reviewed the current status of iodine (KI or Lugol's) for the treatment of Graves' disease, discussing the iodide escape phenomenon, writing:

Iodide has been shown to decrease thyroid hormone levels and reduce blood flow within the thyroid gland. An escape phenomenon has been feared as the iodide effect has been claimed to only be temporary.... Antithyroid drugs [methimazole] are often chosen since these are mostly well-tolerated and can induce cure in around 50% after 12–18 months of treatment. These pharmacologic compounds, propylthiouracil, methimazole, or carbimazole, block the thyroid hormone synthesis by inhibiting thyroid peroxidase... In the short-term, LS [Lugol's Solution] reduces the thyroid hormones, T4 and T3, by increasing iodine uptake and inhibiting the enzyme thyroid peroxidase, thus attenuating oxidation and organification of thyroid hormones. Moreover, the release of thyroid hormones is also blocked...

Wolff-Chaikoff is the effect of iodide in **normal mice**, which leads to an increase of intrathyroidal iodine concentration within 24–48 h and a subsequent decrease of thyroid hormone synthesis. In healthy subjects, there is an adaption to iodine excess by an **autoregulatory mechanism** within the thyroid, which serves as a defense against fluctuations in the supply of iodine and permits escape from the paradoxical inhibition of hormone synthesis that a very large quantity of iodine induces. **Defective or absent autoregulation** can occur in predisposed patients, as in those with euthyroid Hashimoto's thyroiditis and in GD [Graves' Disease]-patients treated with radioiodine or subtotal thyroidectomy. Thus, these are more prone to develop hypothyroidism secondary to an iodine overload...**The escape from the acute Wolff-Chaikoff effect is associated with a decrease in thyroid sodium/iodide symporter, causing a reduction in intrathyroidal iodide concentration.** There is also a form of escape following iodide therapy in GD, which has been described as common [thyroiditis?]. Thus, in treating patients with hyperthyroidism with LS [Lugol's Solution], an exacerbation of thyroid hormone levels could be a consequence after a period of blocking the thyroid, as the gland has become loaded with iodine substrate for hormone synthesis...However, in the investigation by Takata et al., a combination of iodide solution was used together with methimazole for up to 8 weeks. Iodide was discontinued when patients showed normal free T4. Eleven patients (25%) escaped from the Wolff-Chaikoff effect, and 3 derived no benefit at all. Moreover, in another study, including patients with mild GD who received primary treatment with LS (50–100 mg daily), control of hyperthyroidism after 12 months was comparable with that seen in patients receiving low-dose methimazole treatment...How often and how early escape occurs is not clear, but in an observational study from Japan long-term treatment with LS alone or in combination with antithyroid drugs has been used, with 29/44 (66%) being well-controlled on 100 mg LS daily alone for

7 years. In another study of 21 patients with hyperthyroidism given iodide daily, hormone levels started to increase again after 3 weeks in some, but others remained euthyroid even after 6 weeks. (13) (112-113)

Iodine Plus Magnesium Pretreatment for Graves' Disease

Dr. Guy Abraham, the inventor of the Iodoral tablet, recommends iodine alone for the treatment of Graves' hyperthyroidism. However, Dr. Abraham advocates magnesium as a pretreatment prior to using iodine. In 2004, Dr. Guy Abraham reported a 40-year-old female with Graves' disease, undetectable TSH <0.01 μU/ml, and elevated Free T4 = 5.0 ng/dL. (Normal ranges: free T4 = 0.8 - 1.8 ng/dL, TSH =0.3-3.0 μU/ml.) Dr. Guy Abraham writes:

> A complete nutritional program in our experience improved further the response to orthoiodosupplementation [using Lugol's or Iodoral] in Graves' disease and other thyroid disorders.... 40-year-old female patient with severe hyperthyroidism... She was a classic case of Graves' disease with exophthalmia... She was placed on the nutritional program, including 1,200 mg of magnesium/day for one month prior to iodine supplementation, followed by the same program with the addition of 12.5 mg elemental iodine (1 tablet Iodoral®) daily afterward... Following one month on this program, she slept better and was better organized with improved social activities. Her palpitation decreased markedly with normal pulse rates. Serum TSH became normal at 2.3 μU/ml; Total T4, Total T3, and Free T4 were all within the normal range at 8.0 μg/dL, 195 ng/dL, and 1.2 ng/dL. (2)

Complete Nutritional Supplement Protocol:

Note that Dr. Abraham's iodine dosage of 12.5 mg per day was considerably lower than the 50-100 mg used in Japan by Dr. Ken Okamura and Dr. Ai Yoshihara. Although Dr. Abraham **did not** mention selenium supplementation, it is obvious from the above discussion selenium is at the heart of the issue and is not to be ignored. Our supplement program includes selenium 200-400 mcg/day, magnesium 500-1200 md/day, unrefined sea salt 1/2 tsp. or more per day, vitamin C 3,000-10,000 mg per day, and Omega-3 fatty acids. The unrefined sea salt is to allow for bromine detoxification. For more on this topic, see Chapter 29 on Bromine Detoxification with Unrefined Sea Salt. (60-61) (78) (82) (114-116)

Iodine Escape Rate with Selenium and Magnesium Supplementation

What is the "iodine escape rate" when using selenium and magnesium in the above supplement protocol? Unfortunately, we do not have studies to answer this question. Dr. Abraham's work gives value to magnesium supplementation. Can the iodine escape and/or episodes of thyroiditis be eliminated by the supplement protocol proposed by Dr. Guy Abraham? Another question concerns the protective effect of Block and Replace to keep the TSH suppressed. Would Block and Replace prevent episodes of painless thyroiditis? We await confirmatory studies. In the meantime, it might be prudent to incorporate testing and supplementation for selenium and magnesium and use Block and Replace when the opportunity arises. The topic of selenium is covered more completely in Chapters 20-22. (2) (124)

Medical Iodophobia

In 2004, Dr. Guy Abraham coined the term "Medical iodophobia," meaning fear of using iodine as a medical treatment for iodine deficiency. Dr. Guy Abraham writes:

> Medical iodophobia is the unwarranted fear of using and recommending inorganic, non-radioactive iodine/iodide within the range known from the collective experience of three generations of clinicians to be the safest and most effective amounts for treating symptoms and signs of iodine/iodide deficiency (12.5-37.5 mg). (2)(124)

Dr. Abraham also recognizes this "iodophobia" began in the 1940s with the introduction of thyroid-blocking drugs, the thionamides, which he calls goitrogens, which replaced iodine as a treatment for Graves' disease. Perhaps drug industry capture of the field of endocrinology may be playing a role here. Additional reasons could very well be the complexity and nuances involved in the use of iodine, requiring an extensive medical history, pretesting for selenium, magnesium, and vitamin C levels, and pretreatment with supplements for good results. The average physician may not have knowledge of various thyroid disorders in which iodine is contraindicated, such as hyperthyroidism from toxic multinodular goiter or autonomous nodule.

Iodine for Dermatologists

For example, in 2000, Dr. Warren Heymann reviewed the knowledge required of dermatologists before prescribing potassium iodide (KI). Dr. Warren Heymann is mostly concerned with KI suppression of thyroid function, the Wolf-Chaikoff Effect (WCE) causing elevation of the TSH, reversible with discontinuation of the KI. Dr. Warren Heymann writes:

> For dermatologists who use KI [potassium iodide], knowledge of the WCE [Wolf-Chaikoff Effect], the inhibition of thyroid function by iodine, is imperative. Before KI is prescribed, it would be prudent for the physician to inquire about any history of thyroid disease, autoimmune or otherwise. It is also essential to determine whether a patient is taking other medications, such as amiodarone, that could affect thyroid function. Unless there is a suspicion of underlying thyroid disease, baseline thyroid function studies (i.e., TSH, T4, antithyroglobulin, and anti microsomal antibodies) are not indicated. Fortunately, with the dermatoses for which KI is currently indicated, it is likely that any therapeutic effect will be apparent within a few weeks. This is within the time frame that thyroid autoregulatory processes will

ordinarily allow for escape from the WCE [Wolff-Chaifoff Effect]. If therapy with KI is continued for more than 1 month, however, a screening TSH would be prudent to ensure that iodide-induced hypothyroidism does not ensue. If iodide-induced hypothyroidism is detected, these changes are reversible by discontinuing the administration of KI. In a study of 7 patients with iodide-induced hypothyroidism, serum T4, T3, and TSH concentrations returned to normal within 1 month of iodide withdrawal. (125)

The above description of the complexity of KI use in clinical practice may dissuade the average clinician from using potassium iodide (KI).

If KI is used in Graves' thyrotoxicosis, the patient must be followed more closely than is usually done in today's busy medical office based on the insurance business model. Such patients require more frequent laboratory testing and follow-up and even direct access to the physician's cell phone number, a practice not usually done by mainstream medical practitioners. Clinicians wishing to simplify their practice may choose to avoid KI altogether.

Can Graves' Disease be Cured?

In 2019, Dr. Wilmar Wiersinga from Amsterdam asked, "Can Graves' disease be cured?" If we exclude thyroid ablation as not a "cure" and only include permanent remission while on medical therapy as a "cure," then only about 30 percent of Graves' disease patients achieve such a permanent remission on medical therapy. Remission requires Graves' antibodies (TSI and TRAB) to return to normal levels, as well as normalization of TSH, Free T3, and Free T4 levels. Regarding remission after long-term treatment with antithyroid drugs [methimazole], Dr. Wiersinga writes:

> Graves' hyperthyroidism is not really cured as long as TSH receptor antibodies [TRAb] are present, and I quite agree with this line of thinking. (69-70)

Natural Course of Graves' Disease

The chance of developing Graves' disease during one's lifetime is about 3% for women and 0.5% for men. About two-thirds (60-70 percent) of patients exhibit an undulating course with alternating episodes of hyperthyroid and euthyroid states. In other words, most patients have relapsing and remitting courses over many years. Note: euthyroid means normal thyroid lab tests. For patients with more severe undulating courses, the "Block and Replace" strategy may be justified.

Conclusion

Ignoring the use of potassium iodide (KI) in Graves' disease is an error of modern endocrinology. Early studies suggested that KI alone could control thyrotoxicosis long-term in Graves' disease patients. However, later studies found that about 9-12 percent of cases escape from the suppressive effects of iodine for unknown reasons, with worsening thyrotoxicosis. This escape phenomenon is avoided by using KI as Short-Term treatment, as is commonly done in preparation of the thyrotoxic patient for thyroidectomy. Another option is KI in combination with another drug, such as methimazole or lithium carbonate, discussed below in Chapters 16 and 17. Supplementation with magnesium and selenium ameliorates the toxic effects of iodine excess and may hold value for the autoimmune thyroid patient. (117-120)

♦ **References for Chapter 15**

1) Vaidya, Bijay, and Simon HS Pearce. "Diagnosis and Management of Thyrotoxicosis." BMJ 349 (2014).

2) Abraham, Guy E. "The Safe and Effective Implementation of Orthoiodosupplementation in Medical Practice." The Original Internist 11.1 (2004): 17-36.

3) Trousseau, Armand. "Lectures on Clinical Medicine, Trans. by P." V. Bazire, London, New Sydenham Society (1868).

4) Corvilain, Bernard, et al. "Inhibition by Iodide of Iodide Binding to Proteins: The "Wolff-Chaikoff" Effect Is Caused by Inhibition of H2O2 Generation." Biochemical and biophysical research communications 154.3 (1988): 1287-1292.

5) Chiraseveenuprapund, P., and I. N. Rosenberg. "Effects Of Hydrogen Peroxide-Generating Systems on the Wolff-Chaikoff Effect." Endocrinology 109.6 (1981): 2095-2101.

6) Wartofsky L, et al. "Inhibition by Iodine of the Release of Thyroxine from the Thyroid Glands of Patients with Thyrotoxicosis." J Clin Invest, 1970; 49:78-86.

7) Bagchi, N., et al. "Studies on the Mechanism of Acute Inhibition of Thyroglobulin Hydrolysis by Iodine." Acta Endocrinologica 108.4 (1985): 511-517.

8) Dugrillon, A. "Iodolactones and Iodoaldehydes—Mediators of Iodine in Thyroid Autoregulation." Experimental and Clinical Endocrinology and Diabetes 104.S 04 (1996): 41-45.

9) Eng, Peter HK, et al. "Escape from the Acute Wolff-Chaikoff Effect Is Associated with a Decrease in Thyroid Sodium/Iodide Symporter Messenger Ribonucleic Acid and Protein." Endocrinology 140.8 (1999): 3404-3410.

10) Park, Young Joo, et al. "Iodide Itself Regulates Iodide Uptake in Thyrocyte by Regulating Sodium-iodide Symporter (NIS) Activity as Well as NIS Expression." International Journal of Thyroidology 1.1 (2008): 39-47.

11) Bizhanova, Aigerim, and Peter Kopp. "The Sodium-Iodide Symporter NIS and Pendrin in Iodide Homeostasis of the Thyroid." Endocrinology 150.3 (2009): 1084-1090.

12) Torti, Jeronimo F., and Ricardo Correa. "Potassium Iodide." StatPearls [Internet]. StatPearls Publishing, 2022.

13) Calissendorff, Jan, and Henrik Falhammar. "Lugol's Solution and Other Iodide Preparations: Perspectives and Research Directions in Graves' Disease." Endocrine 58.3 (2017): 467-473.

14) Vagenakis, Apostolos G., and Lewis E. Braverman. "Adverse Effects of Iodides on Thyroid Function." The Medical Clinics of North America 59.5 (1975): 1075-1088.

15) Plummer HS and Boothby WM. "The Value of Iodine in Exophthalmic Goiter." J Iowa Med Soc, 1924; 14:65.

16) Plummer, WA. "Iodine in the Treatment of Goiter." Med Cl North America, 1925; 8:1145-1151.

17) Starr, Paul, et al. "The Effect of Iodin in Exophthalmic Goiter." Archives of Internal Medicine 34.3 (1924): 355-364.

18) Lahey, Frank H. "The Use of Iodine in Goiter." The Boston Medical and Surgical Journal 193.11 (1925): 487-490.

19) Don, Charles SD. "The Treatment of Exophthalmic Goitre." British Medical Journal 1.3572 (1929): 1108.

20) Thompson WO, et al. "Prolonged Treatment of Exophthalmic Goiter by Iodine Alone." Arch Int Med, 1930; 45:481-502.

21) Redisch W and Perloff WH. "The Medical Treatment of Hyperthyroidism." Endocrinology, 1940; 26:221-228.

22) Cerqueira, Charlotte, et al. "Iodine Fortification and Hyperthyroidism." Handbook of Food Fortification and Health. Humana Press, New York, NY, 2013. 243-254.

23) Stanbury, John Burton, et al. "Iodine-Induced Hyperthyroidism: Occurrence and Epidemiology." Thyroid 8.1 (1998): 83-100.

24) Corvilain, Bernard, et al. "Autonomy in Endemic Goiter." Thyroid 8.1 (1998): 107-113.

25) Müssig, Karsten, et al. "Iodine-Induced Thyrotoxicosis After Ingestion of Kelp-Containing Tea." Journal Of General Internal Medicine 21.6 (2006): C11-C14.

26) Boi, Francesco, et al. "The Usefulness of Conventional and Echo Colour Doppler Sonography in the Differential Diagnosis of Toxic Multinodular Goitres." European Journal of Endocrinology 143.3 (2000): 339-346.

27) Mariani, Giuliano, et al. "The Role of Nuclear Medicine in The Clinical Management of Benign Thyroid Disorders, Part 1: Hyperthyroidism." Journal of Nuclear Medicine 62.3 (2021): 304-312.

28) Mariani, Giuliano, et al. "The Role of Nuclear Medicine in The Clinical Management of Benign Thyroid Disorders, Part 2: Nodular Goiter, Hypothyroidism, And Subacute Thyroiditis." Journal of Nuclear Medicine 62.7 (2021): 886-895.

29) Wolff, J., and I. L. Chaikoff. "Plasma Inorganic Iodide as a Homeostatic Regulator of Thyroid Function." Journal of Biological Chemistry 174 (1948): 555-564.

30) Minasyan, Mari, et al. "FT3: FT4 Ratio in Graves' Disease: Correlation with TRAb Level, Goiter Size and Age of Onset." Folia Medica Cracoviensia 60.2 (2020).

31) Ito, Mitsuru, et al. "Type 1 and Type 2 Iodothyronine Deiodinases in the Thyroid Gland of Patients with 3, 5, 3'-Triiodothyronine-Predominant Graves' Disease." European Journal of Endocrinology 164.1 (2011): 95-100.

32) Grmek, Jernej, et al. "Usefulness of Free Thyroxine to Free Triiodothyronine Ratio for Diagnostics of Various Types of Hyperthyroidism." Slovenian Medical Journal 84.5 (2015).

33) Livolsi, Virginia A., and Zubair W. Baloch. "The Pathology of Hyperthyroidism." Frontiers in Endocrinology 9 (2018): 737.

34) Hirota, Yoshihiko, et al. "Thyroid Function and Histology in Forty-Five Patients with Hyperthyroid Graves' Disease in Clinical Remission More Than Ten Years After Thionamide Drug Treatment." The Journal of Clinical Endocrinology & Metabolism 62.1 (1986): 165-169.

35) Mizukami, Yuji, et al. "Histologic Changes in Graves' Thyroid Gland After I-131 Therapy for Hyperthyroidism." Pathology International 42.6 (1992): 419-426.

36) Thompson, Lester. "Diffuse Hyperplasia of the Thyroid Gland (Graves' Disease)." Ear, Nose & Throat Journal 86.11 (2007): 666-667.

37) Perdomo, Carolina M., et al. "Evaluation of the Role of Thyroid Scintigraphy in the Differential Diagnosis of Thyrotoxicosis." Clinical Endocrinology 94.3 (2021): 466-472.

38) Boi, Francesco, et al. "The Usefulness of Conventional and Echo Colour Doppler Sonography in the Differential Diagnosis of Toxic Multinodular Goitres." European Journal of Endocrinology 143.3 (2000): 339-346.

39) Summaria, V., et al. "Diagnostic Imaging in Thyrotoxicosis." Rays 24.2 (1999): 273-300.

40) Giovanella, Luca, Luca Ceriani, and Silvana Garancini. "Clinical Applications of the 2nd Generation Assay for Anti-TSH Receptor Antibodies in Graves' Disease. Evaluation in Patients with Negative 1st Generation Test." (2001): 25-28.

41) Tozzoli, R., et al. "TSH Receptor Autoantibody Immunoassay in Patients with Graves' Disease: Improvement of Diagnostic Accuracy Over Different Generations of Methods. Systematic Review and Meta-Analysis." Autoimmunity Reviews 12.2 (2012): 107-113.

42) Shaffer, Ashley, et al. "Recurrent Thyrotoxicosis due to Both Graves' Disease and Hashimoto's Thyroiditis in the Same Three Patients." Case Reports in Endocrinology 2016 (2016).

43) Ross, Douglas S. "Syndromes of Thyrotoxicosis with Low Radioactive Iodine Uptake." Endocrinology And Metabolism Clinics of North America 27.1 (1998): 169-185.

44) Kamijo, Keiichi. "Clinical Studies on Potassium Iodide-Induced Painless Thyroiditis in 11 Graves' Disease Patients." Internal Medicine (2021): 6411-20.

45) Gluck, Franklin B., et al. "Chronic Lymphocytic Thyroiditis, Thyrotoxicosis, and Low Radioactive Iodine Uptake: Report of Four Cases." New England Journal of Medicine 293.13 (1975): 624-628.

46) Baral, Neelam, Leonard Wartofsky, and Meeta Sharma. "SUN-560 Thyrotoxic Hashimoto's Disease: Is It Graves' Thyrotoxicosis or Hashitoxicosis?" Journal of the Endocrine Society 3. Supplement_1 (2019): SUN-560.

47) Pedersen, Inge Bülow, et al. "TSH-Receptor Antibody Measurement for Differentiation of Hyperthyroidism into Graves' Disease and Multinodular Toxic Goiter: A Comparison of Two Competitive Binding Assays." Clinical Endocrinology 55.3 (2001): 381-390.

48) Kamath, C., et al. "The Role of Thyrotrophin Receptor Antibody Assays in Graves' Disease." Journal of Thyroid Research 2012 (2012).

49) Michalek, Krzysztof, et al. "TSH Receptor Autoantibodies." Autoimmunity Reviews 9.2 (2009): 113-116.

50) Macchia, Enrico, et al. "Assays of TSH-Receptor Antibodies In 576 Patients with Various Thyroid Disorders: Their Incidence, Significance and Clinical Usefulness." Autoimmunity 3.2 (1989): 103-112.

51) Wallaschofski, H., et al. "TSH-Receptor Autoantibodies-Differentiation of Hyperthyroidism Between Graves' Disease and Toxic Multinodular Goiter." Experimental And Clinical Endocrinology & Diabetes 112.04 (2004): 171-174.

52) Bothun, Erick D., et al. "Update on Thyroid Eye Disease and Management." Clinical Ophthalmology (Auckland, NZ) 3 (2009): 543.

53) Yang, Dawn D., et al. "Medical Management of Thyroid Eye Disease." Saudi Journal of Ophthalmology 25.1 (2011): 3-13.

54) Boschi, Antonella, et al. "Quantification of Cells Expressing the Thyrotropin Receptor in Extraocular Muscles in Thyroid-Associated Orbitopathy." British Journal of Ophthalmology 89.6 (2005): 724-729.

55) Tani, Junichi, and Jack R. Wall. "Autoimmunity Against Eye-Muscle Antigens May Explain Thyroid-Associated Ophthalmopathy." CMAJ 175.3 (2006): 239-239.

56) Lahooti, Hooshang, et al. "Pathogenesis of Thyroid-Associated Ophthalmopathy: Does Autoimmunity Against Calsequestrin and Collagen XIII Play a Role?" Clinical Ophthalmology (Auckland, NZ) 4 (2010): 417.

57) Feek, Colin M., et al. "Combination of Potassium Iodide and Propranolol in Preparation of Patients with Graves' Disease for Thyroid Surgery." New England Journal of Medicine 302.16 (1980): 883-885.

58) Kaur, Sukhvender, et al. "Effect of Preoperative Iodine in Patients with Graves' Disease Controlled with Antithyroid Drugs and Thyroxine." Annals of the Royal College of Surgeons of England 70.3 (1988): 123.

59) Kiyici, Sinem, et al. "Rapid Preparation of Patients with Hyperthyroidism for Thyroidectomy." Endocrine Abstracts. Vol. 20. Bioscientifica, 2009.

60) Yoshihara, Ai, et al. "Substituting Potassium Iodide for Methimazole as the Treatment for Graves' Disease During the First Trimester May Reduce the Incidence of Congenital Anomalies: A Retrospective Study at a Single Medical Institution in Japan." Thyroid 25.10 (2015): 1155-1161

61) Okamura, Ken, et al. "Iodide-Sensitive Graves' Hyperthyroidism and the Strategy for Resistant or Escaped Patients During Potassium Iodide Treatment." Endocrine Journal (2022): EJ21-0436.

62) Pearce, Elizabeth N. "Substituting Potassium Iodide for Methimazole in First-Trimester Pregnant Women with Graves' Disease May Unpredictably Worsen Hyperthyroidism." Clinical Thyroidology 32.3 (2020): 117-119.

63) Tay, Wei Lin, et al. "High Thyroid Stimulating Receptor Antibody Titer and Large Goiter Size at First-Time Radioactive Iodine Treatment Are Associated with Treatment Failure in Graves' Disease." Ann Acad Med Singap 48.6 (2019): 181-187.

64) Ma, Emily Z., et al. "Total Thyroidectomy Is More Cost-Effective than Radioactive Iodine as an Alternative to Antithyroid Medication for Graves' Disease." Surgery 173.1 (2023): 193-200.

65) Liu, Xiaodong, et al. "Attaining Biochemical Euthyroidism Early After Total Thyroidectomy in Graves' Disease May Lower Long-Term Morbidity Risk." BJS open 6.4 (2022): zrac079.

66) Bartalena, Luigi, et al. "Management of Graves' Hyperthyroidism: Present and Future." Expert Review of Endocrinology & Metabolism 17.2 (2022): 153-166.

67) Sekulić, Vladan, et al. "Short Term Treatment with Lithium Carbonate as Adjunct to Radioiodine Treatment for Long-Lasting Graves' Hyperthyroidism." Hell J Nucl Med 18.3 (2015): 186-8.

68) Kessler, Lynn, et al. "Lithium as an Adjunct to Radioactive Iodine for the Treatment of Hyperthyroidism: A Systematic Review and Meta-Analysis." Endocrine Practice 20.7 (2014): 737-745.

69) Hershman, Jerome M. "A Survey of Management of Uncomplicated Graves' Disease Shows that Use of Methimazole Is Increasing and Use of Radioactive Iodine Is Decreasing." Children 95.3260 (2010).

70) Wiersinga, Wilmar M. "Graves' Disease: Can It Be Cured?" Endocrinology and Metabolism 34.1 (2019): 29-38.

71) Dharmasena, Aruna. "Selenium Supplementation in Thyroid-Associated Ophthalmopathy: An Update." International Journal of Ophthalmology 7.2 (2014): 365.

72) Douglas, Raymond S., et al. "OR11-4 Teprotumumab Markedly Improves Disease-Related Quality of Life: Lessons from Two Randomized, Placebo-Controlled Trials." Journal of the Endocrine Society 6. Supplement_1 (2022): A799-A800.

73) Cipolla, Calogero, et al. "The Value of Total Thyroidectomy as the Definitive Treatment for Graves' Disease: A Single Center Experience Of 594 Cases." Journal of Clinical & translational endocrinology 16 (2019): 100183.

74) Jamieson, A., and C. G. Semple. "Successful Treatment of Graves' Disease in Pregnancy with Lugol's Iodine." Scottish Medical Journal 45.1 (2000): 20-21.

75) Gangadharan, Arundoss, et al. "The Use of Iodine as First-Line Therapy in Graves' Disease Complicated with Neutropenia at First Presentation in a Pediatric Patient." British Journal of Medicine and Medical Research 3.2 (2013): 324.

76) Emerson, Charles H., et al. "Serum Thyroxine and Triiodothyronine Concentrations During Iodide Treatment of Hyperthyroidism." The Journal of Clinical Endocrinology & Metabolism 40.1 (1975): 33-36.

77) Phillppou, George, et al. "The Effect of Iodide on Serum Thyroid Hormone Levels in Normal Persons, In Hyperthyroid Patients, and in Hypothyroid Patients on Thyroxine Replacement." Clinical endocrinology 36.6 (1992): 573-578.

78) Okamura, Ken, et al. "Remission After Potassium Iodide Therapy in Patients with Graves' Hyperthyroidism Exhibiting Thionamide-Associated Side Effects." The Journal of Clinical Endocrinology & Metabolism 99.11 (2014): 3995-4002.

79) Hashizume, Kiyoshi, et al. "Administration of Thyroxine in Treated Graves' Disease: Effects on the Level of Antibodies to Thyroid-Stimulating Hormone Receptors and on the Risk of Recurrence of Hyperthyroidism." New England Journal of Medicine 324.14 (1991): 947-953.

80) Laurent, Eric, et al. "Unlike Thyrotropin, Thyroid-Stimulating Antibodies Do Not Activate Phospholipase C In Human Thyroid Slices." The Journal of clinical investigation 87.5 (1991): 1634-1642.

81) Song, Yue, et al. "Roles of Hydrogen Peroxide in Thyroid Physiology and Disease." The Journal of Clinical Endocrinology & Metabolism 92.10 (2007): 3764-3773.

82) Okamura, Ken, et al. "Painless Thyroiditis Mimicking Relapse of Hyperthyroidism During or After Potassium Iodide or Thionamide Therapy for Graves' Disease Resulting in Remission." Endocrine Journal (2022): EJ22-0207.

83) Eleftheriadou, Anna-Maria, et al. "Re-Visiting Autoimmunity to Sodium-Iodide Symporter and Pendrin in Thyroid Disease." European Journal of Endocrinology 183.6 (2020): 571-580.

84) Czarnocka, Barbara. "Thyroperoxidase, Thyroglobulin, Na (+)/I (-) Symporter, Pendrin in Thyroid Autoimmunity." Frontiers in Bioscience-Landmark 16.2 (2011): 783-802.

85) Seissler, Jochen, et al. "Low Frequency of Autoantibodies to the Human Na+/I– Symporter in Patients with Autoimmune Thyroid Disease." The Journal of Clinical Endocrinology & Metabolism 85.12 (2000): 4630-4634.

86) Kalderon, A. E., and H. A. Bogaars. "Immune Complex Deposits in Graves' Disease and Hashimoto's Thyroiditis." The American Journal of Medicine 63.5 (1977): 729-734.

87) Kalderon, A. E., et al. "Electron-Dense Deposits in The Follicular Basal Lamina of Obese Strain Chickens with Spontaneous Hereditary Autoimmune Thyroiditis. An Electron Microscopic Study." Laboratory Investigation; a Journal of Technical Methods and Pathology 37.5 (1977): 487-496.

88) Xu, Jian, et al. "Supplemental Selenium Alleviates the Toxic Effects of Excessive Iodine on the Thyroid." Biological Trace Element Research 141.1 (2011): 110-118.

89) Vasiliu, Ioana, et al. "Protective Role of Selenium on Thyroid Morphology in Iodine-Induced Autoimmune Thyroiditis in Wistar Rats." Experimental and Therapeutic Medicine 20.4 (2020): 3425-3437.

90) Vasiliu, Ioana, et al. "Experimentally Induced Autoimmune Thyroiditis in Wistar Rats: Possible Protective Role of Selenium." Endocrine Abstracts. Vol. 70. Bioscientifica, 2020.

91) Rienhoff, F. W. "The Histological Changes Brought About in Cases of Exophthalmic Goiter." Bull. Johns Hopkins Hosp. 37 (1925): 285.

92) DeCourcy, Joseph L. "The Use of Lugol's Solution in Exophthalmic Goitre: An Explanation for the Beneficial Results of Pre-Operative Medication." Annals of Surgery 86.6 (1927): 871.

93) Thomson, Christine D., et al. "Minimal Impact of Excess Iodate Intake on Thyroid Hormones and Selenium Status in Older New Zealanders." European Journal of Endocrinology 165.5 (2011): 745.

94) Wang, Weiwei, et al. "Effects of Selenium Supplementation on Spontaneous Autoimmune Thyroiditis In NOD. H-2h4 Mice." Thyroid 25.10 (2015): 1137-1144.

95) Zheng, Huijuan, et al. "Effects of Selenium Supplementation on Graves' Disease: A Systematic Review and Meta-Analysis." Evidence-Based Complementary and Alternative Medicine 2018 (2018).

96) Ruggeri, Rosaria M., et al. "Selenium Exerts Protective Effects Against Oxidative Stress and Cell Damage in Human Thyrocytes and Fibroblasts." Endocrine 68.1 (2020): 151-162.

97) Pekar, Joanna, et al. "Effect of Selenium Supplementation in Thyroid Gland Diseases." J. Elementol 22 (2017): 91-103.

98) Duntas, Leonidas H. "Selenium and the Thyroid: A Close-Knit Connection." The Journal of Clinical Endocrinology & Metabolism 95.12 (2010): 5180-5188.

99) Rayman, Margaret P. "Multiple Nutritional Factors and Thyroid Disease, With Particular Reference to Autoimmune Thyroid Disease." Proceedings of the Nutrition Society 78.1 (2019): 34-44.

100) McGregor, Brock. "The Role of Selenium in Thyroid Autoimmunity: A Review." Journal of Restorative Medicine 4.1 (2015): 83.

101) Ventura, Mara, et al. "Selenium and Thyroid Disease: From Pathophysiology to Treatment." International Journal of Endocrinology 2017 (2017).

102) Contempre, Bernard, et al. "Selenium Deficiency Aggravates the Necrotizing Effects of a High Iodide Dose in Iodine-Deficient Rats." Endocrinology 132.4 (1993): 1866-1868.

103) Goyens, Philippe, et al. "Selenium Deficiency as a Possible Factor in The Pathogenesis of Myxoedematous Endemic Cretinism." European Journal of Endocrinology 114.4 (1987): 497-502.

104) Gilroy, Cornelia V., et al. "Evaluation of Ionized and Total Serum Magnesium Concentrations in Hyperthyroid Cats." Canadian Journal of Veterinary Research 70.2 (2006): 137.

105) Ige, A.O., et al. "Oral Magnesium Potentiates Glutathione Activity in Experimental Diabetic Rats." Int. J. Diabetes Res 5.2 (2016): 21-25.

106) Zhu, Zongjian, et al. "Selenium Concentration and Glutathione Peroxidase Activity in Selenium and Magnesium Deficient Rats." Biological Trace Element Research 37.2 (1993): 209-217.

107) Jiménez, Alicia, et al. "Changes in Bioavailability and Tissue Distribution of Selenium Caused by Magnesium Deficiency in Rats." Journal of the American College of Nutrition 16.2 (1997): 175-180.

108) Moncayo, Roy, et al. "The Role of Selenium, Vitamin C, and Zinc in Benign Thyroid Diseases and of Selenium in Malignant Thyroid Diseases: Low Selenium Levels Are Found in Subacute and Silent Thyroiditis and in Papillary and Follicular Carcinoma." BMC Endocrine Disorders 8.1 (2008): 1-12.

109) Shibutani, Yuhei, et al. "Plasma and Erythrocyte Magnesium Concentrations in Thyroid Disease: Relation to Thyroid Function and the Duration of Illness." Japanese Journal of Medicine 28.4 (1989): 496-502.

110) Ford, Henry C., et al. "Disturbances of Calcium and Magnesium Metabolism Occur in Most Hyperthyroid Patients." Clinical biochemistry 22.5 (1989): 373-376.

111) Ko, Young Hee, et al. "Chemical Mechanism of ATP Synthase: Magnesium Plays a Pivotal Role in the Formation of the Transition State Where ATP Is Synthesized from ADP and Inorganic Phosphate." Journal of Biological Chemistry 274.41 (1999): 28853-28856.

112) Takata, Kazuna, et al. "Benefit of Short-Term Iodide Supplementation to Antithyroid Drug Treatment of Thyrotoxicosis Due to Graves' Disease." Clinical Endocrinology 72.6 (2010): 845-850.

113) Uchida, Toyoyoshi, et al. "Therapeutic Effectiveness of Potassium Iodine in Drug-Naïve Patients with Graves' Disease: A Single-Center Experience." Endocrine 47 (2014): 506-511.

114) Nichol, R. W. "Bromism: The Sodium Chloride Treatment." British Medical Journal 1.3405 (1926): 636.

115) Bechet, Paul E. "The Intravenous Administration of Sodium Chloride in Bromoderma." Journal of the American Medical Association 87.5 (1926): 320-321.

116) Togawa, Go, et al. "Effects of Chloride in the Diet on Serum Bromide Concentrations in Dogs." International Journal of Applied Research in Veterinary Medicine 16.3 (2018): 197-202.

117) Ehlers, Margret, et al. "Graves, Disease in Clinical Perspective." Frontiers in Bioscience-Landmark 24.1 (2019): 33-45.

118) Girgis, Christian M., et al." Current Concepts in Graves' Disease." Therapeutic Advances in Endocrinology and Metabolism 2.3 (2011): 135-144.

119) Fujita, Naoya, et al. "Serum Diiodotyrosine–A Biomarker to Differentiate Destructive Thyroiditis from Graves' Disease." European Journal of Endocrinology 186.2 (2022): 245-253.

120) Brito, Juan P., et al. "Patterns of Use, Efficacy, and Safety of Treatment Options for Patients with Graves' Disease: A Nationwide Population-Based Study." Thyroid 30.3 (2020): 357-364.

121) Coco, Grace, et al. "Analysis of Graves' Disease from the Origins to the Recent Historical Evolution." Medicina 5.3 (2021): e2021030

122) Savoie, J. C., et al. "Iodine-Induced Thyrotoxicosis in Apparently Normal Thyroid Glands." The Journal of Clinical Endocrinology & Metabolism 41.4 (1975): 685-691.

123) Skare, Ståle, and Harald MM Frey. "Iodine-Induced Thyrotoxicosis in Apparently Normal Thyroid Glands." European Journal of Endocrinology 94.3 (1980): 332-336.

124) Abraham, Guy E. "Facts About Iodine and Autoimmune Thyroiditis." The Original Internist 15.2 (2008): 75-76.

125) Heymann, Warren R. "Potassium Iodide and the Wolff-Chaikoff Effect: Relevance for the Dermatologist." Journal of the American Academy of Dermatology 42.3 (2000): 490-492.

Chapter 16

Iodine Treatment of Graves' Disease, Part Two

THE MAIN OBJECTION TO THE use of iodine for first-line therapy of Graves' disease is resistance or escape from the suppressive effects of iodine, leading to more difficulty in treating thyrotoxicosis in about 9-12 percent of patients. This was described in a 2015 study by Dr. Ai Yoshihara, switching pregnant women from methimazole to potassium iodide treatment for Graves' disease. Although 90 percent successful, about 9-12 percent of patients escaped from the suppressive effects of potassium iodide and worsened hyperthyroidism. This was unpredictable, with no obvious parameters to predict which patients would respond well and which would worsen. (1-3)

Dr. Ken Okamura 504 Graves' Patients Treated with Potassium Iodide (KI) Alone

In 2022, Dr. Ken Okamura provided us with a protocol for treating Graves' disease with KI as first-line therapy, including the management of iodine escape or iodine resistance. Proclaiming that "iodide in higher doses is an established and time-honored treatment of Graves' disease" and is safer than thyroid-blocking drugs such as methimazole, Dr. Ken Okamura recruited 504 untreated Graves' disease patients and began treatment with 100 mg of potassium iodide daily, seeking to avoid thionamide drugs, methimazole and PTU, which carry potentially severe adverse side effects. In Japan, one person dies annually from thionamide drug-induced suppression of the white blood cells (agranulocytosis). Dr. Ken Okamura writes:

> iodide in higher doses is an established and time-honored treatment of GD [Graves' disease]…However, both MMI [methimazole] and PTU [propylthiouracil] were still associated with severe notorious

or unfamiliar side effects. In Japan, one GD patient on average dies due to thionamide-induced agranulocytosis every year…The possibility of KI therapy was therefore suggested in general untreated GD from the beginning…many patients have mild or even asymptomatic GD that may be sensitive to excess iodine. (4)

Note: Especially good candidates for KI treatment are females with mild untreated Graves' disease. These patients have the best response. Males with severe Graves' disease are usually poor candidates for KI. Also, Graves' disease patients after many years of long term methimazole treatment have chronic changes in thyroid histology and are no longer good candidates for KI treatment. This is discussed below.

Block and Replace to Avoid Relapse of Hyperthyroidism

A subset of 92 of the 504 Graves' patients, 18.3% were overly sensitive to potassium iodide. The KI suppressive effects worked too well, rendering them hypothyroid with high TSH and low Free T4.

Before KI treatment, these 92 patients were thyrotoxic with high Free T3 and T4 levels and a suppressed, very low, TSH. After KI treatment, the serum thyroid hormone levels plummeted to very low levels. The TSH rocketed up to very high levels. In the first half of the study, in 41 such patients with high TSH after iodine treatment, the KI dosage was tapered down. However, 71% of these then relapsed into hyperthyroidism after tapering the KI dosage. Dr. Ken Okamura found the relapse into hyperthyroidism upon tapering the KI can be avoided with Block and Replace, also called "combination therapy". In the second half of the study, for 39 "overly sensitive to KI" patients with high TSH and low Free T4, the KI was no longer tapered down. Instead, the next 39 patients were treated with Block and Replace by adding levothyroxine to reduce the TSH. **Using Block and Replace, none of the next 39 patients had a relapse of hyperthyroidism!** This is a justifiable use of Block and Replace. Note: Block and Replace is the addition of levothyroxine to replace the missing thyroid hormone, thus suppressing the TSH and raising the Free T4. The usual dose of levothyroxine is 100 mcg daily. Dr. Ken Okamura writes:

> in the latter half of this study, the patients were treated with the combination of 100 mg KI and LT4 [levothyroxine] when the serum fT4 level became low and the TSH level became detectable (combined fixed dose KI and LT4 therapy). In this combined therapy (n = 39) [Block and Replace], compared with tapering therapy (n = 41), **a relapse of hyperthyroidism was not observed** (0% vs. 71%, p < 0.0001) and the degree of TSH elevation was reduced (e.g. 10.7 [6.6–23.3] µU/mL vs. 27.3 [8.6–68.3] µU/mL), although the difference was not significant (p = 0.0561). ... **It was very important to keep the serum iodide level above the threshold for the WC [Wolf- Chaikoff] effect, avoiding the tapering method usually performed in MMI therapy.** The KI dosage could be reduced later when TBII [TRAb] became negative, or patients had nearly achieved remission. (4)

Relapse of hyperthyroidism was 71 percent when the iodine dosage was tapered down and zero in the Block and Replace group in which the addition of levothyroxine reduced the TSH from about 27µU/mL to 10µU/mL. Lesson Number One: Do not taper the potassium iodide dosage when T4 goes too low, and TSH goes too high. Instead, use Block and Replace with levothyroxine or NDT natural desiccated thyroid.

The History of Block and Replace

In 1983, Dr. Romaldini from Sao Paolo, Brazil was perhaps the earliest to try Block and Replace in 113 patients with Graves' disease, randomly divided into two groups. 65 patients (Group A) were treated with high dose ATD, either MMI (40-100 mg/d) or PTU (500-1200 mg/d). When thyroid function became overly suppressed with high TSH, then 50-75 micrograms T3 daily was added to suppress the TSH. This T3 is generic Cytomel, called liothyronine. 48 patients (Group B) were treated with a lower dose of ATD without the added T3. Dr. Romaldini found Group A with TSH suppression from added T3 had a higher remission rate (75% vs. 41%) and higher frequency of negative Graves's TSH receptor antibody levels (71 vs 29%) compared to Group B at the end of the treatment period which ranged from 17-80 months. Dr. Romaldini writes:

> Remission occurred in 75.4% of patients from group A and in 41.6% of patients from group B (P less than 0.001)... The frequency of negative tests of thyroid-stimulating antibodies was higher in group A patients (71%) than in group B (29%) at the end of therapy. (5)

In 1991, Dr. Kiyoshi Hashizume was another early pioneer in using levothyroxine to suppress TSH in Graves' disease, also called Block and Replace. Dr. Hashizume thought that TSH stimulation of the thyroid gland was reason for continued elevation of TSH receptor antibody levels in this disease. Dr. Hashizume had previously published studies on TSH stimulation causing the release of TSH receptor antigens from membranes. This effect was inhibited by hydrocortisone and propranolol. There may be merit to this hypothesis which adds to the growing tide of evidence for the benefits of TSH suppression. In my opinion, the main benefit of TSH suppression is turning off the generation of excess hydrogen peroxide, a damaging oxidant implicated in most if not all thyroid pathologies as described by Dr. Song in 2007. This was discussed in Chapter 14 on the Production of Thyroid Hormones. Dr. Kiyoshi Hashizume writes:

> One factor that might contribute to the persistent production of antibodies to TSH receptors is stimulation of the release of thyroid antigens by TSH during antithyroid drug therapy. We therefore studied **the effect of the suppression of TSH secretion by thyroxine on the levels of antibodies to TSH receptors after thyroid hormone secretion had been normalized by methimazole.** (6-8)

In 2005, Dr. Luigi Bartalena from Italy made discouraging comments on the use of Block and Replace by Drs. Romaldini and Hashizume, mentioned above. Dr. Bartalena stated that the addition of levothyroxine to methimazole in Graves' disease (Block and Replace) is not useful because several follow-up studies could not replicate the original findings, writing:

> A third therapeutic regimen of antithyroid drug therapy was proposed several years ago in Japan [Hashizume, 1991]. After restoring euthyroidism with MMI [methimazole] alone, patients were randomized to continue for 12 months with either MMI alone or MMI and L-T4 [levothyroxine]; the latter group then continued treatment with L-T4 for an additional 36 months. Relapses in the L-T4-treated group were significantly lower than in the group not receiving L-T4 (2 versus 35%) [Hashizume, 1991]. Unfortunately, this study has not been reproduced by several studies thereafter, in which either L-T4 or L-T3 were used after thionamide withdrawal...The reason for this discrepancy remains unclear but the number of negative studies suggests that the addition of L-T4, as originally proposed by the Japanese group [Hashizume, 1991], is not useful. (9)

Hey, Not So Fast!

In 2006, about one year after Dr. Bartalena's disparaging remarks about Block and Replace, Dr. Salman Razvi reviewed the topic and dis-

agrees. Dr. Razvi concluded Block and Replace remains an excellent approach to managing Graves' disease. And so, the debate rages on. (10)

Iodine Escape – Add Methimazole

Back to Dr. Ken Okamura's 2022 study, 202 patients were considered to have "escaped" or resistant to the KI. These were treated with a combination of potassium iodide (KI) 100 mg/per day and methimazole 5-15 mg per day with good results. Once starting the combination of methimazole with KI, it was about 7 weeks until FreeT4 normalization.

Potassium Iodide Did Not Interfere with Radioiodine Ablative Treatment

During Dr. Ken Okamura's 2022 study, 126 (25.0%) patients were treated by ablative therapy, 104 patients with radioactive iodine (RAI), and 22 patients with thyroidectomy, usually 2-3 years after starting medical therapy. Patients treated with RAI had the 100 mg/day potassium iodide withheld for 4-7 days and then had 60% radioiodine uptake prior to RAI ablative therapy. This uptake is similar to untreated Graves' disease, so Dr. Ken Okamura felt the KI treatment did not interfere with RAI, writing:

> After RAI treatment in Groups B and C [iodine escaped or resistant], 86% of the patients achieved a euthyroid- or hypothyroid status with a decrease in thyroid volume. It was then concluded that KI therapy did not interfere with the efficacy of RAI. (4)

Note: Although the use of KI will decrease radioiodine uptake in normal healthy individuals, for Graves' disease patients this was not an issue and did not interfere with ablative therapy with radioactive iodine I-131. The reasons for this were discussed in 2017 by Dr. Sanjana Ballal. Radioiodine uptake (24-h RAIU) values in normal healthy individuals will decrease after iodine supplementation with the introduction of iodized salt programs. Since the uptake values in healthy people are now lower, this requires adjustment of the lab reference range lower. However not in Graves's disease patients who have very high radioiodine uptake regardless of iodine supplementation. Dr. Sanjana Ballal writes:

> Milakovic et al from Sweden reported the effect of long-term iodine supplementation on thyroid 131 I uptake. **There was a significant decrease in the uptake in euthyroid individuals but not in hyperthyroid individuals as compared to observations 50 years ago.** In our study also there was a significant decrease in the 24-h RAIU [24-hour radioiodine uptake] values in the healthy euthyroid individuals **but not in Graves' disease patients.** (11)

Note: as we will see below, if the Graves' disease patient has Painless Thyroiditis, then the radioiodine uptake will be very low, rendering useless I-131 radioiodine thyroid ablation which is not effective for this Painless Thyroiditis.

Features Predicting Escape, Goiter Size, Free T3 Levels, and TSH

Escape or iodine resistance was more frequent in patients with larger thyroid goiters and with higher Free T3 levels (greater than 10 pg/ml). Dr. Ken Okamura thought this high Free T3 was a marker of strong TSH receptor stimulation from Graves' antibodies, with a high turnover of both thyroglobulin and iodide. The third factor was TSH level, as there was no escape in patients who responded early to iodine with normalization of TSH and T4 levels. Escape from iodine was seen only in those patients with continued TSH suppression after iodine treatment. Dr. Ken Okamura comments on the similarity between Graves's disease and an iodine deficiency state, as both have T3 predominant synthesis/secretion indicating intense stimulation, writing:

> T3 predominant synthesis and secretion is a good marker of the thyroid gland being

strongly stimulated with high turnover of both Tg [thyroglobulin] and iodide, as found in cases of iodine deficiency. (4)

High TSH receptor stimulation upregulates the intrathyroidal D1 deiodinase, which converts T4 to T3, rendering a higher T3/T4 ratio a good marker of severity in Graves' disease. Severe iodine deficiency also results in high TSH levels, which in turn induces higher T3 production. Such similarity in greater T3 production for both Graves' disease and iodine deficiency was also noted in 2019 by Dr. Antonio Bianco, who writes:

> The molar ratio of T4 to T3 in the thyroglobulin molecule is sensitive to TSH receptor stimulation. Thyroidal stimulation by TSH increases T3 formation within thyroglobulin, thus lowering the thyroidal T4/T3 molar ratio and increasing the relative secretion of T3. **Iodine deficiency and Graves' disease are two extreme examples of this phenomenon, in which the molar ratio of T4 to T3 in the thyroglobulin can drop to 5:1.** (12-15)

Timing of Adding Methimazole – 60-Day Window

Dr. Ken Okamura feels the 60-day window for achieving euthyroid status is essential. If the patient fails to achieve euthyroid status (normal Free T4) or "escapes" within 60 days, then methimazole (MMI) 5-15 mg/day should be added to the potassium iodide 100 mg/day. The addition of MMI to potassium iodide overcomes iodide resistance or escape. In the event, the patient is still resistant to medical therapy, radioactive iodine therapy is effective. Note: iodine escape means the patient initially achieves normal Free T4, then later relapses with high Free T4. Dr. Ken Okamura writes:

> When treating GD [Graves' Disease] with KI [potassium iodide], the timing for adding MMI [methimazole] is important. If patients fail to achieve euthyroid status within 60 days or escape occurs, it may be better

to begin combined KI and MMI therapy... The important conclusion from this study was that KI resistance or escape from the KI effect could be overcome either by combined KI and MMI therapy...or RAI [radioactive iodine] therapy...In conclusion, the serum fT4 levels declined in all patients with GD [Graves' Disease] following KI therapy. Among GD patients treated with 100 mg KI, 34% were KI-sensitive with detectable TSH and a good prognosis, 50% were KI-sensitive with TSH suppression, and 16% were KI-resistant. KI was immediately excreted into urine without serious side effects. Escape was only observed in TSH-suppressed patients. KI-resistant and escaped patients were able to be treated with a combination of KI and a small dosage MMI, or RAI, as usual. We can minimize the use of thionamide with serious side effects by adopting the "KI or RAI" strategy for the treatment of GD without impending serious symptoms. (4)

Note: Graves's disease patients with exophthalmos usually prefer surgical thyroidectomy rather than RAI (radioactive iodine), which may worsen thyroid eye disease.

Eighty Percent Remission Rate for Responders

Dr. Ken Okamura found that patients who show a good early response to iodine with normalization of TSH (34% of total), will ultimately achieve an 80% remission rate. If the patient does not achieve euthyroid status within 60 days, then additional MMI is indicated, as these patients would otherwise have a high rate of escape from potassium iodide (33-83%). This combined group has a 50% chance of remission. Dr. Ken Okamura writes:

Regarding the strategy for GD treatment, depending on the early response to 100 mg KI, KI treatment could be continued in Group A [responders]. Nearly 80% remission or spontaneous hypothyroidism could be expected. If the serum fT4 and fT3 levels do not normalize within 60 days, the

patients may belong to Group B or C [poor responders, resistant or escaped]. Combined KI and MMI therapy is then recommended, as a 33%–82% chance of escape is expected later.... (4)

Dr. Nami Suzuki KI Potassium Iodide Treatment for Mild Graves' Disease

As discussed previously, many authors of KI for GD studies had no explanation and no criteria for determining which patients were at risk for becoming non-responders or resistant to KI therapy. Credit and thanks go to Dr. Namu Suzuki for her work in unraveling this non-responder criterion. In 2020, Dr. Nami Suzuki studied the use of potassium iodide for mild newly diagnosed Graves' disease, defined as FreeT4 < 5.0 ng/dl, in 122 patients (13 males, 109 females), concluding this is a safer and more effective option for about 60% of females with Graves' disease. Dr. Nami Suzuki found that males had a 3.6-fold greater risk of non-responder status than females. The initial Free T4 of 2.76 ng/dl or less could be used to predict which patients are most likely to respond to KI treatment. Another factor affecting the efficacy of KI is prior methimazole treatment which causes degeneration of thyroid tissue. A long history of methimazole treatment predicts non-responder to potassium iodide therapy.

In terms of details of the study, all patients were newly diagnosed and never treated with methimazole. KI dosage was started at 50 mg/day and increased to 100 mg for non-responders, defined as not reaching a FreeT4 of 1.6 ng/dl (upper range of normal). After about 6 months of treatment, about 60 percent were responders, and 40 percent were non-responders. Non-responders were most likely male, with FreeT4 remaining above 2.8 ng/dl. For responders with TSH within the normal range (0.2–4.5 µU/mL), the KI dose was tapered down by 10 mg/day. Medication was stopped when TSH and TRAb normalized for 6 months on 10 mg KI every other day. There were no adverse side effects from KI treatment.

Note: this tapering method differs from Dr. Ken Okamura's study above, in which better results were obtained with "Block and Replace."

Non-Responders Are Switched to Methimazole

51 of the 122 patients were KI non-responders and were switched from KI to ATDs (Anti-Thyroid Drugs, methimazole). 5 of the 51 patients (about 10 percent) had adverse side effects from ATDs. Two patients developed agranulocytosis (low white count) due to methimazole (MMI), one patient developed liver injury due to propylthiouracil (PTU), and two patients developed drug eruption (skin rash) from MMI. (16)

Note: switching non-responders to methimazole was also done in the Okamura study above. Dr. Okamura felt that a trial of 60 days of KI was sufficient to determine if a patient is a non-responder, at which time non-responders are switched to MMI. Dr. Nami Suzuki's treatment duration required to judge non-responsiveness to KI was considerably longer, 5.9 months. Another difference was the use of Block and Replace in Dr. Okamura's study, while Dr. Suzuki used KI tapering. (4) (16)

Increase in Thyroid Volume with KI

Dr. Nami Suzuki reported a significant increase in thyroid volume in both responders and non-responders, with a greater volume increase after one year in the non-responder group. This represents increased colloid formation and enlargement of thyroid follicles after KI administration. Dr. Suzuki writes:

> Excessive iodine intake is well known to reduce thyroid hormone secretion and production, as excess iodine inhibits iodine organification in the thyroid gland. This phenomenon is known as the Wolff-Chaikoff effect. A detailed animal experiment showed that excess iodine reduces the expression of thyroid peroxidase (TPO) mRNA and expressions of sodium/iodine symporter (NIS) mRNA and protein...The

effect of excess iodine supplementation has been used as a treatment for GD [Graves' Disease] for decades, especially during thyroid crisis, in combined use with anti-thyroid drugs (ATDs) for patients with severe hyperthyroidism and as a surgical preparation. However, that effect is not believed to last long, with the loss of effect termed "escape from the Wolff-Chaikoff effect." Although almost seven decades have passed since ATDs were first used in the treatment of GD, potassium iodide (KI) has seen preferential use for patients with GD in Japan who display adverse reactions to ATDs...This study enrolled patients newly diagnosed with mild GD, defined as free thyroxine (FT4) <5.0 ng/dL, between July 2014 and June 2016. KI was started at a dose of 50 mg/day, and if FT4 values did not decrease after initiation of treatment, doses were increased to 100 mg/day. Patients for whom thyroid hormone levels could not be controlled with KI at 100 mg/day were regarded as non-responders. Of the 122 patients (13 males, 109 females) included in this study, 71 (58.2%) responded to KI therapy. The remaining 51 patients (41.8%) were non-responders. The median duration required to judge non-responsiveness was 5.9 months. Multiple logistic regression analysis performed on parameters measured at the initial visit **indicated FT4 ...and male sex... were significantly associated with KI responsiveness**. Receiver operating characteristic (ROC) curve analysis of the relationship between FT4 and KI responsiveness indicated an **FT4 cut-off of 2.76 ng/dL was optimal for differentiating between responders and non-responders**. KI therapy was effective and safe for about 60% of patients with mild GD. (16)

Dr. Nami Suzuki writes KI therapy is safer than ATD's and is effective in about 60 percent of females with mild Graves' Disease, defined as initial Free T4 less than 2.76 ng/dl (FT4 <5.0). Males with severe GD defined as FreeT4 >2.76 ng/dl are more likely to be non-responders. Compared to female non-responders, males were 3.6-fold more likely to be non-responders. In prior unfavorable KI (potassium iodide) studies, patients had been previously treated with ATD's (methimazole, MMI) associated with degenerative changes in thyroid tissue. This factor may have impacted the efficacy of KI. Dr. Nami Suzuki writes:

> the present study confirmed that **KI therapy is effective for GD in patients with FT4 values <5.0 ng/dL...**subjects in previous studies had also been treated with ATDs as a first-line treatment. **ATDs are known to induce morphological changes in thyroid tissue, such as increased cellularity and diminished amounts of colloid.** Considering this fact, thyroid tissues from subjects analyzed in previous reports were likely to have been affected by ATDs, and **such degeneration might have impacted the efficacy of KI...**KI monotherapy appears potentially safer as a treatment for patients with GD...In the present study, **males displayed a 3.6-fold higher risk of KI non-responsiveness than females...KI therapy appears to offer an effective and potentially safer therapy for about 60% of female patients with mild GD and thus could represent a third drug option for these patients.** (16)

In 2017, Dr. Akira Honda treated 24 Graves' disease patients who had adverse effects and could not tolerate thioamides (methimazole). These 24 patients were switched to potassium iodide. Responders maintained euthyroid function for six months, while non-responders did not. Dr. Honda was in agreement with Dr. Suzuki, finding the efficacy of KI therapy was inversely correlated with thyrotoxicosis severity. (17)

Escape from Iodine or Painless Thyroiditis?

A second paper by Dr. Ken Okamura in 2022 makes the bold assertion that many patients under treatment for Graves' disease who relapse into hyperthyroidism do not have a relapse of their Graves' disease. They have an inflammatory process called painless thyroiditis (PT). This may be true for both forms of

therapy, potassium iodide, and methimazole. As mentioned above, this relapse into hyperthyroidism is usually associated with decreasing or tapering the drug dosage. This gives more support to the use of Block and Replace instead of tapering down the dosage of the iodine or methimazole thyroid-blocking drug.

Dr. Okamura reviewed 100 patients who presented unexpected relapsing hyperthyroidism while decreasing dosage under treatment for Graves' disease with potassium iodide, methimazole, or PTU. All had radio-iodine uptake scans. Many of these scans showed under 5 percent uptake, indicating thyroiditis (PT) as the cause of the thyrotoxicosis rather than worsening Graves' disease. In this regard, PT may resemble Hashitoxicosis, a type of thyrotoxicosis with very low radio-iodine uptake. Remember, 70 percent of Graves' patients are also positive for Hashimoto's antibodies, indicating frequent co-existence of the two disease entities. Dr. Okamura writes:

> Graves' Disease (GD) and Hashimoto's thyroiditis are recognized as being pathologically interrelated, as GD may occur in patients whose thyroid glands histologically show either Hashimoto's thyroiditis alone or a mixture of both parenchymatous hypertrophy of GD and extensive lymphocytic infiltration. **These two conditions may represent a single disease entity with a wide range of manifestations.** (18)

A Single Entity with Different Manifestations

In agreement with Dr. Okamura's statement that Hashimoto's and Graves' disease are a single entity, Drs. Baral and Wartofsy in a 2019 case report of a patient with long-standing Hashimotos' thyroiditis (HT) who transformed into Graves' Disease (GD). The authors commented patients with Hashimotos' thyroiditis might transform into Graves' Disease at any point, writing:

> Hashimoto's Thyroiditis (HT) and Graves' Disease (GD) reflect two extremes in

the spectrum of autoimmune thyroid diseases.... Patients with autoimmune thyroid disease have both thyroid hormone receptor stimulating and thyroid hormone receptor blocking antibodies and clinical manifestations depend upon the level of these antibodies and the state of the thyroid gland. Because patients with HT can transform to GD at any point due to a change of blocking to stimulating antibodies, clinicians should be aware of the potential for this transformation. (19-23)

Mechanism of Thyroiditis

What is the mechanism causing thyroiditis upon reduction in dosage of anti-thyroid medication? Dr. Okamura reminds us that excess iodine can cause a "toxic effect," i.e. thyroiditis. Animal studies show that selenium supplementation ameliorates the toxic effects of iodine excess. Production of thyroid hormone requires the oxidation of iodide to iodine by the TPO enzyme using hydrogen peroxide as a substrate. TSH stimulation of the thyroid gland increases all steps in thyroid hormone synthesis, including hydrogen peroxide generation. I suggest the mechanism here involves increased hydrogen peroxide generation in the face of insufficient selenium-based antioxidant ability caused by underlying selenium and magnesium deficiency. The excess hydrogen peroxide causes oxidative damage to adjacent structures, which are thyroglobulin, TPO, and thyrocytes, leading to inflammation, rupture of follicles, and release of preformed thyroid hormone. (25-40)

Dr. Okamura writes:

PT [painless thyroiditis] was frequently observed during KI treatment. In Group A [low radio-iodine uptake], 19 (54.3%) patients were treated by KI alone or KI and MMI before the episode of PT. Given the effect of excess iodide on the morphological changes in the thyroid, KI treatment may precipitate the "iodide thyroiditis" reported by Edmunds in 1955. In the same year as Gluck reported convincing cases with PT,

Savoie reported 10 cases of iodine-induced thyrotoxicosis in apparently normal thyroid glands, ranging from 1 to 40 months after exposure to excess iodine. They all showed a typical clinical course of PT with a low RAIU followed by hypothyroidism... **From a therapeutic perspective, it is very important to keep in mind that PT [painless thyroiditis] can occur during ATD [anti-thyroid drug] treatment of GD [Graves' Disease], especially when the dosage is reduced**...The diagnosis can be confirmed by the suppressed RAIU [radio iodine uptake] (<5%/5 h) in the thyrotoxic state, which remains a valuable factor for differentiating PT from relapse of GD. (18)(41-45)

Anti-Thyroid Drugs Contraindicated in Painless Thyroiditis

In 1975, Dr. Franklin Gluck reported four cases of Painless Thyroiditis (PT) with low radio-iodine uptake, in which thyroid-blocking drugs are ineffective and contraindicated, writing:

Thus, this form of thyrotoxicosis differs from the usual form found in Graves' disease in that histologic features of Graves' disease are absent, the radioactive iodine uptake is low, and specific anti-thyroid therapy is contraindicated. (42)

Differentiating Painless Thyroiditis from Graves' Disease

In 2006, Dr. Afsana Begum explained how to differentiate Painless Thyroiditis (PT) from Graves' Disease (GD), noting in PT, there is a disproportionate increase in T4 compared to T3, and the radio-iodine uptake is almost always less than 3 percent:

Painless thyroiditis is more difficult to distinguish from Graves' disease, but it is imperative for the clinician to distinguish between these two diseases since important therapeutic differences exist. The ESR (sedimentation rate) and white blood cell count are normal. T4 and triiodothyronine (T3) levels are initially elevated, with a disproportionate increase in T4 compared with T3. RAIU (radio-iodine uptake) is decreased in the hyperthyroid phase of the disease and is almost always less than 3 percent. This situation contrasts markedly with the elevated RAIU found in patients with Graves' disease. (46)

Histopathology Studies

In 2015, Dr. Zhaowei Meng studied the histopathology differences in new patients presenting with thyrotoxicosis when the diagnosis could be either Graves' disease (GD) or Painless Thyroiditis (PT), writing:

> For GD, the follicular epithelial cells were tall and more crowded than those of a normal thyroid gland. Some small papillae were formed, which projected into the follicular lumen and encroached on the colloid. The colloid within the follicular lumen was pale, with scalloped margins. Lymphoid infiltrates were present in the interstitium (Fig 4A) …For PT [Painless Thyroiditis], the most prominent and specific histopathological feature was the massive lymphocytic infiltration with hyperplastic germinal centers within the thyroid parenchyma. **Thyroid follicles were disrupted and collapsed**. (Fig 4B) It was evident that the tissue cellularity in PT was much higher than that in GD… (47)

What Was the Selenium Level?

Returning to the 2015 Yoshihara study of pregnant Graves' patients showing a 9-10 percent iodine escape rate when converting from methimazole to iodine, one wonders how many of these iodine escape cases are related to thyroiditis, an inflammatory process similar to Hashitoxicosis. A radionuclide uptake study would have resolved the issue. It would also be useful to know the selenium and magnesium status of these patients. One would ask the obvious question: Would the escape rate be decreased if patients had been given selenium and magnesium supplements? (24-40)

Why Not Use Block and Replace?

Another question is, "Why not use Block and Replace strategy as was done in the 2015 Yoshihara study?" Painless thyroiditis (PT) and hyperthyroidism with low RAI uptake usually occur when the dosage of thyroid blocking drug is reduced and TSH goes high. The high TSH stimulates excess hydrogen peroxide (H202). The damaging effect of H202 on thyrocytes is thought to be the trigger for thyroiditis. In Block and Replace strategy, instead of reducing dosage of thyroid blocking drug (iodine or methimazole), a replacement dose of thyroid hormone (Levothyroxine) is added. Thyroid hormone medication will suppress the TSH and alleviate the TSH stimulation for hydrogen peroxide generation. Block and Replace is a logical treatment to avoid episodes of hyperthyroidism from PT (painless thyroiditis) and prevent alternating extremes of thyroid function, the undulating course, with alternating relapse and remission seen in many patients with Graves' disease.

One also wonders if the duration of the disease is a factor in determining the success rate of iodine therapy. If patients are treated early, upon the first presentation of Graves' disease, would these patients have a higher success rate? Alternatively, if patients have many years of methimazole treatment with an undulating course prior to switching to potassium iodide (KI) therapy, would this be a factor in decreasing the success rate for KI therapy, as suggested above by Dr. Nami Suzuki? (16)

Co-Existence of Graves' and Hashimoto's Antibodies

Another factor to be considered is the co-existence of Hashimoto's' antibodies in 70 percent of Graves' disease patients. Would this be a factor in determining the success rate with potassium iodide, as discussed by Dr. Okamura? Here is a quote from Dr. Kamijo in which elevated anti-thyroglobulin antibodies were associated with episodes of PT (Painless Thyroiditis). One is tempted to suggest Dr.

Kamijo is describing Hashitoxicosis in patients with Graves' Antibodies:

> Kamijo reported 11 patients with PT [Painless Thyroiditis] following KI [potassium iodide] treatment for GD [Graves' Disease]. Anti-Tg antibody [Anti-thyroglobulin antibody] was positive in 10 of the 11 patients [54]. The role of anti-thyroid antibody and iodine in the clinical course of GD or PT should be re-evaluated in the future. (18) (48)

> Note: elevated TPO antibodies were also present.

In 2021, Dr. Kamijo found 10 of 11 Graves' disease patients who developed iodine-induced PT after switching from MMI [methimazole] to KI [potassium iodide] had elevated anti-thyroid antibodies (TPO or Thyroglobulin Antibodies), suggesting an autoimmune etiology, as well as a direct toxic effect of the excess iodide, writing:

> KI has a cytotoxic effect on only human thyroid follicles that is abolished by MMI [methimazole]. Furthermore, Xu et al. (20) showed a cytotoxic effect due to KI by demonstrating that excess iodine contributes to autophagy suppression and apoptosis of thyroid follicular cells using a cell line of human thyroid follicular epithelial cells. The pathogenesis of KI-induced PT is unclear but may be related to this cytotoxic effect of KI. In addition, because 10 of the 11 patients in our current study with KI-induced PT were positive for TgAb and/or TPOAb, an autoimmune mechanism may be involved in this process...Finally, we emphasize that clinicians who manage GD patients who received KI after discontinuing ATD due to side effects should be alert for KI-induce PT. (48) (61)

Conclusion

Another error in Modern Thyroid Endocrinology is ignoring the use of KI (potassium iodide) in treatment of Graves' disease. Ki is safer than thyroid-blocking drugs (methi-

mazole) and can achieve good response in 60 percent of females with mild Graves' disease. Dr. Okamura makes a brilliant case for the first-line use of potassium iodide (KI) for Graves' disease. Firstly, KI is safer than thyroid blocking drugs. Secondly, early responders enjoy a high complete remission rate. For those patients who escape or are resistant to iodine, Dr. Okamura presents a clear and well-thought-out protocol for adding a second drug, methimazole, to the KI or, if that fails, radio-iodine ablation. One wonders what would have been the escape rate if all patients had been given selenium, magnesium and, vitamin D, Vitamin C and tested for H. Pylori and Anti-Gliadin antibodies. Another consideration is using Block and Replace to prevent relapse of hyperthyroidism, as described in Dr. Ken Okamura's study. (4-10)

Regarding "escape" from the inhibitory effects of iodine in Graves' disease patients, Dr. Okamura proposes many of these cases are not relapses of Graves' hyperthyroidism. Instead, they are hyperthyroidism from Painless Thyroiditis (PI) an inflammatory condition with low radio-iodine uptake. This frequently occurs when switching from MMI to KI or when tapering drug dosage and is thought to be related to the toxic effect of excess iodine or elevated anti-thyroid antibodies (autoimmune factors). Our state of knowledge is still incomplete, and we have many more questions than answers. One can only hope future knowledge will eventually lead to improved treatment. (49-60)

♦ **References for Chapter 16**

1) Yoshihara, Ai, et al. "Substituting Potassium Iodide for Methimazole as the Treatment for Graves' Disease During the First Trimester May Reduce the Incidence of Congenital Anomalies: A Retrospective Study at a Single Medical Institution in Japan." Thyroid 25.10 (2015): 1155-1161

2) Yoshihara, Ai, et al. "Characteristics of Patients with Graves' Disease Whose Thyroid Hormone Levels Increase After Substituting Potassium Iodide for Methimazole in the First Trimester of Pregnancy." Thyroid: Official Journal of the American Thyroid Association 30.3 (2020): 451-456.

3) Pearce, Elizabeth N. "Substituting Potassium Iodide for Methimazole in First-Trimester Pregnant Women with Graves' Disease May Unpredictably Worsen Hyperthyroidism." Clinical Thyroidology 32.3 (2020): 117-119.

4) Okamura, Ken, et al. "Iodide-Sensitive Graves' Hyperthyroidism and the Strategy for Resistant or Escaped Patients During Potassium Iodide Treatment." Endocrine Journal (2022): EJ21-0436.

5) Romaldini, J. H., et al. "Comparison of Effects of High and Low Dosage Regimens of Antithyroid Drugs in the Management of Graves' Hyperthyroidism." The Journal of Clinical Endocrinology and Metabolism 57.3 (1983): 563-570.

6) Hashizume, Kiyoshi, et al. "Administration of Thyroxine in Treated Graves' Disease: Effects on the Level of Antibodies to Thyroid-Stimulating Hormone Receptors and on the Risk of Recurrence of Hyperthyroidism." New England Journal of Medicine 324.14 (1991): 947-953.

7) Hashizume, K., and L. J. DeGroot. "Release Of Thyrotropin Receptor from Thyroid Plasma Membranes: Effect of Hydrocortisone, Propranolol, And Adenosine 3', 5'-Monophosphate." Endocrinology 106.5 (1980): 1463-1468.

8) Song, Yue, et al. "Roles of Hydrogen Peroxide in Thyroid Physiology and Disease." The Journal of Clinical Endocrinology & Metabolism 92.10 (2007): 3764-3773.

9) Bartalena, Luigi, et al. "An Update on The Pharmacological Management of Hyperthyroidism Due to Graves' Disease." Expert Opinion on Pharmacotherapy 6.6 (2005): 851-861.

10) Razvi, Salman, et al. "What is the Evidence Behind the Evidence-Base? The Premature Death of Block-Replace Antithyroid Drug Regimens for Graves' Disease." European Journal of Endocrinology 154.6 (2006): 783-786.

11) Ballal, Sanjana, et al. "Re-Establishment of Normal Radioactive Iodine Uptake Reference Range in the Era of Universal Salt Iodization in the Indian Population." The Indian Journal of Medical Research 145.3 (2017): 358.

12) Bianco, Antonio C., et al. "Paradigms of Dynamic Control of Thyroid Hormone Signaling." Endocrine Reviews 40.4 (2019): 1000-1047.

13) Chen, Xinxin, et al. "Diagnostic Values of Free Triiodothyronine and Free Thyroxine and the Ratio of Free Triiodothyronine to Free Thyroxine in Thyrotoxicosis." International Journal of Endocrinology 2018 (2018).

14) Köhrle, J. "Thyrotropin (TSH) Action on Thyroid Hormone Deiodination and Secretion: One Aspect of Thyrotropin Regulation of Thyroid Cell Biology." Hormone and Metabolic research. Supplement Series 23 (1990): 18-28.

15) Sriphrapradang, Chutintorn, and Adikan Bhasipol. "Differentiating Graves' Disease from Subacute Thyroiditis Using Ratio of Serum Free Triiodothyronine to Free Thyroxine." Annals of Medicine and Surgery 10 (2016): 69-72.

16) Suzuki, Nami, et al. "Therapeutic Efficacy and Limitations of Potassium Iodide for Patients Newly Diagnosed with Graves' Disease." Endocrine Journal 67.6 (2020): 631-638.

17) Honda, Akira, et al. "Relationship Between the Effectiveness of Inorganic Iodine and Severity of Graves Thyrotoxicosis: A Retrospective Study." Endocrine Practice: Official Journal of the American College of Endocrinology and the American Association of Clinical Endocrinologists 23.12 (2017): 1408-1413.

18) Okamura, Ken, et al. "Painless Thyroiditis Mimicking Relapse of Hyperthyroidism During or After Potassium Iodide or Thionamide Therapy for Graves' Disease Resulting in Remission." Endocrine Journal (2022): EJ22-0207.

19) Baral, Neelam, Leonard Wartofsky, and Meeta Sharma. "SUN-560 Thyrotoxic Hashimoto's Disease: Is It Graves' Thyrotoxicosis or" Hashitoxicosis"?" Journal of the Endocrine Society 3. Supplement_1 (2019): SUN-560.

20) Penaherrera, Carlos A., and Valentina Rodriguez. "SAT-482 Simultaneous Hashimoto/Graves' Disease or Prolonged Hashitoxicosis? A Diagnostic Challenge with Therapeutic Implications." Journal of the Endocrine Society 4. Supplement_1 (2020): SAT-482.

21) Takasu, N., et al. "Graves' Disease Following Hypothyroidism Due to Hashimoto's Disease: Studies of Eight Cases." Clinical endocrinology 33.6 (1990): 687-698.

22) Aye, Thant, et al. "A Challenging Case of Oscillating Hashimoto's Thyroiditis and Hyperthyroidism." Endocrine Abstracts. Vol. 86. Bioscientifica, 2022.

23) Schaffer, Ashley, et al. "Recurrent Thyrotoxicosis due to Both Graves' Disease and Hashimoto's Thyroiditis in the Same Three Patients." Case Reports in Endocrinology 2016 (2016).

24) Vasiliu, Ioana, et al. "Protective Role of Selenium on Thyroid Morphology in Iodine-Induced Autoimmune Thyroiditis in Wistar Rats." Experimental And Therapeutic Medicine 20.4 (2020): 3425-3437.

25) Xu, Jian, et al. "Selenium Supplement Alleviated the Toxic Effects of Excessive Iodine in Mice." Biological Trace Element Research 111.1 (2006): 229-238.

26) Xu, Jian, et al. "Intervention of Selenium on Injured Thyroid Hormone Metabolism by Excessive Iodine." Journal of Hygiene Research 38.4 (2009): 398-400.

27) Xu, Jian, et al. "Supplemental Selenium Alleviates the Toxic Effects of Excessive Iodine on the Thyroid." Biological Trace Element Research 141.1 (2011): 110-118.

28) Wang, Weiwei, et al. "Effects of Selenium Supplementation on Spontaneous Autoimmune Thyroiditis In NOD. H-2h4 Mice." Thyroid 25.10 (2015): 1137-1144.

29) Duntas, L. H. "The Role of Iodine and Selenium in Autoimmune Thyroiditis." Hormone and Metabolic Research 47.10 (2015): 721-726.

30) Vanderpas, Jean B., et al. "Iodine and Selenium Deficiency Associated with Cretinism in Northern Zaire." The American Journal of Clinical Nutrition 52.6 (1990): 1087-1093.

31) Vanderpas, Jean-Baptiste, et al. "Iodine and Selenium Deficiency in Northern Zaire." The American Journal of Clinical Nutrition 56.5 (1992): 957-958.

32) Contempre, Bernard, et al. "Effects of Selenium Deficiency on Thyroid Necrosis, Fibrosis and Proliferation: A Possible Role in Myxoedematous Cretinism." European Journal of Endocrinology 133.1 (1995): 99-109.

33) Contempre, Bernard, et al. "Selenium Deficiency Aggravates the Necrotizing Effects of a High Iodide Dose in Iodine-Deficient Rats." Endocrinology 132.4 (1993): 1866-1868.

34) Davcheva, Delyana M., et al. "Serum Selenium Concentration in Patients with Autoimmune Thyroid Disease." Folia Medica 64.3 (2022): 443-449.

35) Bogusławska, Joanna, et al. "Cellular and Molecular Basis of Thyroid Autoimmunity." European Thyroid Journal 11.1 (2022).

36) Negro, Roberto. "Selenium and Thyroid Autoimmunity." Biologics: Targets and Therapy 2.2 (2008): 265-273.

37) Kimura, T., et al. "Thyrotropin-Induced Hydrogen Peroxide Production In FRTL-5 Thyroid Cells Is Mediated Not by Adenosine 3', 5'-Monophosphate, But by Ca2+ Signaling Followed by Phospholipase-A2 Activation and Potentiated by an Adenosine Derivative." Endocrinology 136.1 (1995): 116-123.

38) Tsatsoulis, Agathocles. "The Role of Iodine Vs Selenium on the Rising Trend of Autoimmune Thyroiditis in Iodine Sufficient Countries-An Opinion Article." Open Access J Thy Res 2.1 (2018): 12-14.

39) Vasiliu, Ioana, et al. "Protective Role of Selenium on Thyroid Morphology in Iodine-Induced Autoimmune Thyroiditis in Wistar Rats." Experimental and Therapeutic Medicine 20.4 (2020): 3425-3437.

40) Giammanco, Marco, and Manfredi M. Giammanco. "Selenium: A Cure for Autoimmune Thyroiditis." Endocrine, Metabolic & Immune Disorders-Drug Targets 21.8 (2021): 1377-1378.

41) Edmunds, H. Tudor. "Acute Thyroiditis from Potassium Iodide." British Medical Journal 1.4909 (1955): 354.

42) Gluck, Franklin B., et al. "Chronic Lymphocytic Thyroiditis, Thyrotoxicosis, and Low Radioactive Iodine Uptake: Report of Four Cases." New England Journal of Medicine 293.13 (1975): 624-628.

43) Savoie, J. C., et al. "Iodine-Induced Thyrotoxicosis in Apparently Normal Thyroid Glands." The Journal of Clinical Endocrinology & Metabolism 41.4 (1975): 685-691.

44) Skare, Ståle, and Harald MM Frey. "Iodine-Induced Thyrotoxicosis in Apparently Normal Thyroid Glands." European Journal of Endocrinology 94.3 (1980): 332-336.

45) Shilo, S., and H. J. Hirsch. "Iodine-Induced Hyperthyroidism in a Patient with a Normal Thyroid Gland." Postgraduate Medical Journal 62.729 (1986): 661.

46) Begum, Afsana, et al. "Thyroiditis, a Review." Journal of Medicine 7.2 (2006): 58-63.

47) Meng, Zhaowei, et al. "Differentiation Between Graves' Disease and Painless Thyroiditis by Diffusion-Weighted Imaging, Thyroid Iodine Uptake, Thyroid Scintigraphy and Serum Parameters." Experimental and Therapeutic Medicine 9.6 (2015): 2165-2172.

48) Kamijo, Keiichi. "Clinical Studies on Potassium Iodide-induced Painless Thyroiditis in 11 Graves' Disease Patients." Internal Medicine 60.11 (2021): 1675-1680.

49) Calvi, Laura, and Gilbert H. Daniels. "Acute Thyrotoxicosis Secondary to Destructive Thyroiditis Associated with Cardiac Catheterization Contrast Dye." Thyroid: Official Journal of the American Thyroid Association 21.4 (2011): 443-449.

50) Bogazzi, Fausto, et al. "Glucocorticoids Are Preferable to Thioamides as First-Line Treatment for Amiodarone-Induced Thyrotoxicosis Due to Destructive Thyroiditis: A Matched Retrospective Cohort Study." The Journal of Clinical Endocrinology & Metabolism 94.10 (2009): 3757-3762.

51) Medić, Filip, et al. "Amiodarone and Thyroid Dysfunction." Acta Clinica Croatica 61.2 (2022): 327-341.

52) Mushref, Malek, et al. "Amiodarone Induced Thyrotoxicosis: A Case of Refractory Disease Treated with Thyroidectomy." Journal of the Endocrine Society 5. Supplement_1 (2021): A920-A920.

53) Henzen, C., et al. "Iodine-Induced Hyperthyroidism (Iodine-Induced Basedow's Disease): A Current Disease Picture." Schweizerische Medizinische Wochenschrift 129.17 (1999): 658-664.

54) Hiraiwa, Tetsuya, et al. "High Diagnostic Value of a Radio-Iodine Uptake Test With and Without Iodine Restriction in Graves' Disease and Silent Thyroiditis." Thyroid: Official Journal of the American Thyroid Association 14.7 (2004): 531-535.

55) Yang, Ji Wei, and Jacques How. "Lugol's Solution-Induced Painless Thyroiditis." Endocrinology, Diabetes & Metabolism Case Reports 2017 (2017).

56) Leustean, Letitia, et al. "Jod-Basedow Effect Due to Prolonged Use of Lugol Solution-Case Report." The Medical-Surgical Journal 118.4 (2014): 1013-1017.

57) Uchida, Toyoyoshi, et al. "Therapeutic Effectiveness of Potassium Iodine in Drug-Naïve Patients with Graves' Disease: A Single-Center Experience." Endocrine 47 (2014): 506-511.

58) Suwansaksri, Nattakarn, et al. "Nonthionamide Drugs for the Treatment of Hyperthyroidism: From Present to Future." International Journal of Endocrinology 2018 (2018).

59) Mao, Xiao-Ming, et al. "Prevention of Relapse of Graves' Disease by Treatment with an Intrathyroid Injection of Dexamethasone." The Journal of Clinical Endocrinology & Metabolism 94.12 (2009): 4984-4991.

60) Roti, E., et al. "Effects of Chronic Iodine Administration on Thyroid Status in Euthyroid Subjects Previously Treated with Anti-Thyroid Drugs for Graves' Hyperthyroidism." The Journal of Clinical Endocrinology & Metabolism 76.4 (1993): 928-932.

61) Freitas Ferreira, Andrea C., et al. "Thyroid Ca2+/NADPH-Dependent H2O2 Generation is Partially Inhibited by Propylthiouracil and Methimazole." European Journal of Biochemistry 270.11 (2003): 2363-2368.

Chapter 17

Combined Use of Lithium and Potassium Iodide for Graves' Disease

Use of Lithium Carbonate for Manic Depression

LITHIUM CARBONATE HAS BEEN USED as a psychiatric drug to treat manic depression for well over a century. Like iodide, lithium is actively concentrated within the thyroid cells to achieve a concentration three to four times higher than that of plasma. The active transport for iodide, the Sodium/Iodide Symporter (NIS), is also the active transport for lithium. (1-2)

Lithium Blocks Thyroid Hormone Synthesis and Release

Lithium improves the retention of iodine in the thyroid while blocking hormone synthesis and release. These properties make lithium ideal as an adjunct to radioactive iodine therapy with I-131. Lithium increases radio-iodine uptake even after iodine administration. In 2020, Dr. Czarnywojtek writes:

> the thyroid shows an increased ability to accumulate iodine during lithium carbonate treatment regardless of the degree of prolonged iodine retention in the thyroid gland...[lithium salts] inhibit the formation of colloid in thyrocytes, change the structure of thyroglobulin, weaken the iodination of tyrosines, and disrupt their coupling... An additional benefit is the use of adjuvant lithium therapy to increase the iodine uptake of the thyroid gland, which allows to obtain satisfactory results in treatment with radioactive iodine and potentially facilitates the treatment of thyrotoxicosis. In addition, because of the numerous side effects of lithium and its narrow therapeutic index, its concentration in the blood must be constantly monitored. (2)

As mentioned above, lithium increases the retention of iodine in the thyroid, a useful feature when combined with KI in the treatment of Graves' thyrotoxicosis, thus preventing the escape from the inhibitory effects of KI.

Jonathan Wright MD – Success with Lithium/Iodine Combination

Jonathan Wright, MD, a legendary pioneer in natural medicine, found success with the combination of lithium and Lugol's Iodine Solution for the long-term treatment of Graves'. Note: Lugol's Iodine Solution contains 5% iodine and 10% potassium iodide.

Dr. Wright writes:

> I have my patients use five drops of Lugol's iodine three times a day for two or three days. (90-100 mg/day) Then I have them add 300 milligrams of lithium carbonate three times a day in addition to the Lugol's Solution ...In 1972, Dr. R Temple at the Mayo Clinic published the first clinical investigation of lithium treatment for Graves' disease. Using high-dose lithium for 10 individuals, they reported that thyroid hormone levels fell by 20-30 percent within five days. Twenty-six years later, in a review of more than 10 successful trials of lithium therapy for Graves' disease, the authors wrote:

> a small number of studies have documented [lithium's] use in the treatment of patients with Graves' disease... Its efficacy and utility as an alternative anti-thyroid [treatment] are not widely recognized... lithium normalizes [thyroid hormone] levels in one to two weeks...toxicity precludes its use as a first-line or long-term therapeutic agent... (Temple, R., 1972) ...

> But if they had just added flaxseed oil and vitamin E to their treatment, they would

have basically eliminated the risk of toxicity. In fact, every individual (except one) whom I've [Dr. Wright] treated with iodine-iodide (in the form of Lugol's Solution) and high-dose lithium has had blood tests for thyroid hormone return to normal within two weeks. Their tests then stay normal as long as they use Lugol's solution and high-dose lithium. (3-4)

Comparing Iodine and Lithium for Thyrotoxicosis

In 1980, Dr. T. M. Boehm and Wartofsky at Walter Reed Army Hospital compared the relative efficacy of potassium iodide and lithium in 17 patients with thyrotoxicosis. Half the patients also received methimazole (MMI). Further studies using radiolabeled Iodine-125 provided an index of thyroid hormone release from the thyroid gland. I-131 Radiolabeled T4 was used as a marker of the T4 disposal or degradation by the liver. The slope of the ratio of I-125/I-131 in the serum indicated the percent inhibition of T4 release from the thyroid gland. (5)

The potassium iodide (KI) and lithium treatments induced a similar reduction in T4 thyroidal release. The combination of KI and lithium showed an additive inhibition on T4 release only if KI was started first and then lithium was added a few days later. This explains why Dr. Wright's protocol starts the KI first. Treatment with lithium caused a similar reduction in T4 thyroidal release with or without MMI. The MMI had no additive effect when combined with lithium. However, when MMI was combined with KI, there was a more profound reduction indicating an additive effect of KI with MMI. This additive effect of combining KI with methimazole was used to advantage by Dr. Okamura in his 2022 study treating 504 Graves' disease patients with potassium iodide alone. The problem of KI-resistant or "escaped" patients was solved by adding methimazole 5-15 mg per day in combination with the potassium iodide 100 mg per day, resulting in good control of the hyperthyroidism. (5-6)

Methimazole Mechanism of Action

Compared to KI or lithium, methimazole has a different mechanism of action, irreversibly blocking the TPO enzyme responsible for iodination of thyroglobulin, thus blocking hormone synthesis. In 2005, Dr. Cooper wrote:

MMI [methimazole] inhibits thyroid hormone synthesis by preventing the iodination of tyrosine residues in thyroglobulin by thyroid peroxidase. (7)

Kinetic Studies of Lithium in Graves' Disease

In 1972, Dr. R.M. Temple studied the use of lithium to treat thyrotoxicosis, performing I-131 kinetic studies in seven thyrotoxic women with lithium levels of 1 mEq/L. Dr. Temple found lithium treatment "inhibited hormonal and nonhormonal thyroid iodine release," while MMI did not inhibit release. Dr. Temple felt that lithium and potassium iodide have a similar mechanism of action, and for prolonged therapy, lithium must be combined with a second drug, MMI. Dr. Temple writes:

Neither inhibition of release nor hormone disappearance seemed affected by methimazole [MMI]...For prolonged therapy, therefore, a thiocarbamide drug [methimazole or propylthiouracil] must be used in conjunction with lithium. The similarity of inhibition of iodine release from the thyroid produced by lithium and iodides is discussed. (4)

Lithium Alone for Long-Term Control of Graves' Thyrotoxicosis

In 1974, Dr. J. Lazarus used lithium as the sole therapy for six months in eleven thyrotoxic Graves' disease patients. All had long-standing severe disease (mean duration five and a half years) with characteristic relapsing, remitting course. Eight of the eleven were clinically euthyroid, with normal hormone levels after two weeks of lithium treatment. They remained so for the six months of the study. Dr. J. Lazarus comments that there was "no iodide type escape phenomenon even after 6 months." This is an obvious advantage over KI alone, limited to short-term use because of the iodine escape phenomenon in 10-12 percent of treated patients. Dr. J. Lazarus writes:

> This study has shown that an adequate dosage of lithium is effective in rapidly producing a euthyroid state in a thyrotoxic patient. Lithium administration maintained the euthyroid state for the duration of therapy but clearly had no significant effect on Graves' disease [the autoimmune component] in this group of patients. However, **all these patients had long-standing severe disease (mean duration of five and a half years) characterized by several relapses and remissions. In the present study, there was no iodide-type escape phenomenon even after 6 months...** It [lithium] seems to be as effective as iodide in blocking hormone release ... Its use is therefore indicated in cases of hyperthyroidism in which it is necessary to reduce hormone levels very rapidly, especially if the patient is sensitive to iodides...Also, **lithium could be administered for longer than 2 weeks with no danger of an escape phenomenon as seen with iodides**...This study has shown that the therapeutic effect depends on the serum level, which is readily and easily measured. In general, side effects are few and rapidly disappear once the patient is stabilized on therapy. Nevertheless, lithium does have toxic effects and should not be administered when renal function is impaired or serum electrolytes are abnormal. (8)

Comparing Lithium to Methimazole – No Significant Difference

In 1976, Dr. Kristensen compared lithium to methimazole in 24 patients with newly diagnosed Graves' thyrotoxicosis. 13 were treated with methimazole (MMI) alone 40 mg/d and 11 with lithium carbonate alone, rendering a serum level of 0.5 to 1.3 mEq/L. Dr. Kristensen found a similar reduction in Free T4 levels for both treatment modalities. However, the lithi-um-treated patients had more side effects. He writes:

> The lithium treatment brought about a fall in serum-thyroxine iodine (T4I) of 27.0% and in the free-thyroxine index (FTI) of 38.1% after 10 days. A comparison of the two patient groups with regard to the fall in FTI after 3 and 10 days showed **no statistically significant difference...** 8 of the 11 patients subjected to lithium treatment had side effects, so the general condition, which was already affected by the hyperthyroidism, was worsened. **It is concluded that lithium cannot be considered superior to thiocarbamides [methimazole] for the rapid control of thyrotoxicosis. (9)**

How to Avoid Lithium Side Effects

Most of the lithium side effects can be prevented with Vitamin E, Flax Seed Oil, Vitamin B6 (pyridoxine, P-5-P version), and zinc. In 2004, Dr. Jonathan Wright recommended the use of these supplements to prevent and alleviate lithium toxicity, writing:

> An initial dosage of flaxseed oil, one tablespoon (15ccs) three times daily, along with 800 IU of vitamin E (mixed tocopherols). Later dosage is reduced to flaxseed oil to one tablespoon daily along with 400 IU of vitamin E. (10-19)

Lithium Induced Hand Tremor

A common adverse effect of lithium is hand tremors, alleviated with the addition of Vitamin B6. Make sure to use the P-5-P version of B6. Lithium toxicity may be avoided with the use of Flax Seed Oil Essential Fatty Acids, Vitamin E, and Vitamin C. (10-19)

Long-Term Adverse Effects of Chronic Lithium for Bipolar Patients

Over the years, the psychiatric community has used lithium carbonate for the long-term management of bipolar disorder (also called manic depressive disorder). After many years of use, many patients have a gradual decline in renal function with proteinuria, forcing them to stop the drug. In 2023, Dr. Elise Boivin writes long-term lithium carbonate therapy is nephrotoxic and causes a dose-related gradual decline in renal function, and is associated with hypercalcemia and hyperparathyroidism. These adverse effects have dampened enthusiasm for lithium for long-term use. Could the above supplement cocktail alleviate the long-term adverse effects of lithium on renal function? Possibly, however further studies are needed. In the meantime, it would be prudent for the patient on long-term lithium carbonate to take advantage of the protective effects of the above supplement protocol. (20-22)

Autoimmune Thyroid Disease – Greater Sensitivity to Inhibitory Effect of Lithium and Iodine

In 1976, Dr. Kenneth Burman studied six euthyroid Graves' disease patients, all euthyroid for 11 months following treatment with radioactive iodine, and one patient euthyroid following medical treatment with methimazole. The seven euthyroid Graves' disease patients were given lithium carbonate 300 mg three times daily, which maintained the serum lithium level between 0.5 and 1.0 mEq/L. Dr. Burman comments that in normal healthy controls, lithium does not usually induce hypothyroidism. However, in the seven euthyroid Graves' patients, lithium did cause hypothyroidism with a reduction in Free T3 and Free T4 in all seven.

Dr. Burman writes people with autoimmune thyroid disease are more sensitive to the inhibitory effects of either agent, lithium, or iodide, as their mechanism of action appears similar, producing hypothyroidism. Healthy normal controls are resistant to this effect and can compensate using the autoregulatory properties of the normal thyroid. In Dr. Burman's opinion, the beneficial effect of lithium may be due to its ability to increase the intrathyroidal iodine content, and this increased iodine then inhibits both thyroid hormone synthesis and

release. If this is true, this would explain why the lithium/KI combination is so effective in controlling thyrotoxicosis. Dr. Burman writes:

> Recently it has become apparent that subjects with a history of thyroid abnormalities such as diffuse toxic goiter [Graves' disease] or Hashimoto's thyroiditis may be extremely sensitive to the antithyroid effects of iodine even though they may be euthyroid prior to the administration of this drug...Lithium decreases hormonal synthesis and thyroidal secretion but does not affect iodine uptake [i.e., allows iodine uptake]. Consequently, **intrathyroidal iodine content may increase during lithium administration, and excessive quantities of intrathyroidal iodine may inhibit both thyroid hormone synthesis and release**. The normal thyroid gland, however, will gradually overcome the inhibitory effects of iodine upon thyroid hormone synthesis and restore normal synthetic ability despite intrathyroidal iodine concentrations that remain elevated. Patients with diffuse toxic goiter [Graves' disease] may be unable to re-establish normal autoregulation of thyroidal iodine economy, possibly due to a defect in organic binding. As a result, there may be enhanced sensitivity for the development of hypothyroidism during treatment with either lithium or iodine... these observations support the thesis that the inhibitory effects of lithium and iodine upon thyroid hormone synthesis or secretion may involve a similar mechanism of action since **increased thyroidal iodine content may be a consequence of therapy with either agent**. (23)

Note the above comment, lithium increases intrathyroidal iodine content. This is advantageous for radioiodine ablation in Graves' disease patients in which accumulation of radioactive iodine within the thyroid is desired for more effective treatment. This also explains the advantage of combined lithium and potassium iodide treatment of Graves' disease. The lithium makes the iodide accumulate and remain within the thyroid gland, providing more effective inhibition of both organification and thyroid hormone release. In addition, this combination of lithium and KI prevents the iodine escape phenomenon with relapse of thyrotoxicosis, also named the Jod-Basedow Phenomenon. (24)

Lithium for Radiographic Contrast and Amiodarone Thyrotoxicosis

In 1984, Dr. C. Wunsch studied the short-term combination of lithium and methimazole in hyperthyroidism induced by iodine-containing radiographic contrast material finding lithium effective treatment without severe side effects. (25-28)

Lithium for Methimazole Failures

In 1998, Dr. Benbassat used lithium effectively to treat four patients in whom methimazole had failed to control hyperthyroidism. Dr. Benbassat writes:

> We describe four patients treated with lithium for the control of hyperthyroidism. Conventional therapy with propylthiouracil and/or methimazole was tried initially, but the patients were either unresponsive or developed side effects during the drug administration. Within several days of reaching therapeutic levels of lithium, a euthyroid state was achieved in three of the four cases. **Our observations support the use of lithium as an alternative anti-thyroid drug in the treatment of hyperthyroidism in certain defined indications, a clinical use that is not widely known.** (29)

Lithium in Preparation for Radio Ablation or Thyroidectomy

In 2006, Drs. YW Ng and Shek from Hong Kong used lithium in 13 thyrotoxic patients in preparation for radio ablation or thyroidectomy for Graves' disease. Contrary to Dr. J. Lazarus above, Dr. Shek reports one of the 13 patients "escaped" from the effects of lithium. After deliberation, one might quibble over whether this was really a true escape or merely a slower delayed response to the drug. Dr. J. Lazarus writing:

> A satisfactory response, defined as a fall by 40% or more in free thyroxine levels and clinical improvement, was achieved in eight patients within 1 to 2 weeks of lithium therapy. In four others, the response occurred in 3 to 5 weeks. The response was slow and inadequate in one patient due to 'escape.' The median dosage of lithium was 750 mg daily, with a range of 500 to 1500 mg daily. The median serum lithium level was 0.63 mmol/L. Lithium toxicity was observed in one patient...A relatively low dose of lithium offers a safe and effective alternative means of controlling thyrotoxicosis in patients who cannot tolerate or do not respond to thioamides [methimazole]. (30-32)

Lithium in Preparation for Radioablation

In 2008, Dr. Fulya Akin used lithium to prepare five Graves' disease patients and one toxic nodular goiter for radioablation with I-131. Lithium was used as the second-line because of adverse reactions or the ineffectiveness of thioamides (methimazole). Dr. Fulya Akin writes:

> This report shows that lithium carbonate can be safely used preoperatively or prior to radioiodide therapy in circumstances where anti-thyroid medications are contraindicated and are ineffective in obtaining euthyroid status. When administered (800–1,200 mg daily) to patients suffering from Graves' thyrotoxicosis, the serum T4 and T3 levels have been shown to decrease by as much as 35% and most patients become clinically euthyroid within two weeks of treatment. (33-40)

Note: As discussed in 2019 by Dr. Wei Lin Tay, larger goiter size and higher TSH Receptor antibody levels (TRAb and TSI) indicating more severe disease predicts treatment failure upon first radioiodine ablation for Graves' disease or Multinodular goiter. These patients may prefer surgical ablation with thyroidectomy rather than radioactive iodine. (40)

Lithium in Preparation for Thyroidectomy

In 2018, Dr. G. Nair preferred thionamide drugs rather than SSKI (Super Saturated Potassium Iodide) to prepare 162 thyrotoxic patients for thyroidectomy. However, in six patients who could not tolerate thioamides, Dr. Nair switched to lithium in preparation for thyroidectomy. Lithium was combined with dexamethasone and propranolol (Beta Blocker). Dr. Nair writes:

> Lithium is concentrated by the follicular cells…and inhibits iodotyrosine coupling, alters thyroglobulin structure, and thereby inhibits thyroid hormone secretion. We used a combination of lithium carbonate and dexamethasone in refractory HT [hyperthyroidism] as a preoperative regimen…. Lithium carbonate was used in combination with dexamethasone and propranolol in six patients. Indications for lithium salts were drug reactions (n = 3) and failure to control toxicity with 60 mg of carbimazole for 2 months (n = 3)…The entire cohort underwent total thyroidectomy… We used a combination of lithium carbonate and dexamethasone in selected patients of the series and found effective biochemical and clinical control of toxicity. None of the patients experienced drug-related side effects…The rate of complications did not differ in six patients who received lithium salts from the other subgroups. (41-42)

Note: Dexamethasone inhibits D1 deiodinase conversion of T4 to T3, resulting in a reduction in Free T3 levels within 24 hours, a benefit in treating Graves' thyrotoxicosis. Also, D3 deiodinase is upregulated with an increase in reverse T3. In addition to propranolol's slowing of the heart rate due to beta-adrenergic blockade, propranolol also inhibits the D1 deiodinase conversion of T4 to T3 and increases reverse T3. (43-47)

Case Report, Graves' Disease Treated with Lithium, and Iodine (SSKI) Combination

In 2022, Dr. Pranjali P. Sharma reported a case of Graves' Disease managed with a combination of lithium and Super Saturated Potassium Iodide (SSKI) in a 26-year-old male in the blast phase of CML (chronic myeloid leukemia). Methimazole was contraindicated because of low white blood cell count. Dr. Pranjali P. Sharma writes:

> A 26-year-old man, admitted with acute blast crisis secondary to chronic myeloid leukemia (CML), reported palpitations, 40-lb weight loss, heat intolerance, and fatigue. An examination revealed sinus tachycardia, elevated body temperature, and thyromegaly. Laboratory evaluation confirmed hyperthyroidism (TSH <0.005 mU/L, FT4 5.57 ng/dl, TT3 629 ng/dl) secondary to GD (TRAb >40 IU/l, TSIg 178%). Thionamides and surgery were contraindicated due to pancytopenia from a blast crisis… after 2 weeks of inpatient hospital stay, **oral lithium carbonate 300 mg 3 times a day, with SSKI 50 mg/drop 1 drop 3 times a day**, was introduced. Lithium levels were monitored every 2–3 days. Two weeks into treatment, FT4 and TT3 dropped to 4.51 ng/dl and 359 ng/dl, respectively… At hospital discharge 1 month later, thyroid tests showed improvement (TSH 0.007 mcIU/l, FT4 0.82 ng/dl, TT3 122 ng/dl) with stable Lithium level (within 0.5–0.8 mmol/l)…So far, he [the patient] remains on **oral Lithium carbonate 300 mg 3 times a day and SSKI 50 mg/drop 1 drop 3 times a day, without adverse effects**. Most recent laboratory test results continue to show an undetectable TSH, but FT4 and TT3 are within normal range (1.42 ng/dl and 98 ng/dl, respectively). The ultimate plan for this patient is a total thyroidectomy when his cell counts improve…Conclusions: Lithium inhibits…tyrosine iodination, thyroglobulin structure changes, peripheral deiodinase blockage, and prevents TSH and Tg [thyroglobulin] stimulation. Our case shows that a low therapeutic level of lithium, in combination with oral iodine, can suppress

thyroid overactivity without adverse effects. We suggest that low-dose Lithium carbonate is a safe and effective adjunctive anti-thyroid medication to be considered if primary therapies for hyperthyroidism are unavailable...Methimazole and propylthiouracil (PTU) are the most common ATDs [anti-thyroid drugs] used in the United States. Relatively mild adverse effects from ATDs include pruritus, rash, urticaria, arthralgias, arthritis, nausea, vomiting, or abnormal taste, occurring in up to 13% of patients. **Serious adverse effects include agranulocytosis, hepatotoxicity, and vasculitis.** Agranulocytosis is more likely to occur with any dose of PTU than with low-dose methimazole and can be life-threatening while it is dose-dependent with methimazole. It usually occurs within the first 2–3 months of therapy; however, the overall incidence is relatively low, at 0.1–0.5%. (48)

Lithium and Iodine Combination Treatment

Because of "iodine escape" in 10-12 percent of cases, potassium iodide (KI) alone was deemed inadequate for long-term control of Graves' disease. Perhaps a combination of KI with a second drug could be effective? In 2022, Dr. Okamura successfully used methimazole (MMI) combined with KI. (6)

Another combination is KI with lithium, effective for long-term treatment of Graves' disease, with a subset of such treated patients achieving full remission, and can safely taper off all drugs. Lithium carbonate dosage for Graves' disease is usually 300 mg three times a day. Lithium blood levels are checked serially to maintain lithium levels in the therapeutic range, between 0.5 and 1.0 mEq/L, avoiding lithium toxicity which occurs above 1.0 mEq/L.

Conclusion

Another error in modern endocrinology is ignoring the use of lithium for the treatment of Graves' thyrotoxicosis or as preparation for either radioactive I-131 ablation or thyroidec-

tomy. The lithium/KI combination is a promising treatment, yet ignored by conventional mainstream endocrinology. (49-57)

♦ **References for Chapter 17**

1) Amdisen, A. "Lithium Treatment of Mania and Depression Over One Hundred Years." Current Trends in Lithium and Rubidium Therapy. Springer, Dordrecht, 1984. 11-26.

2) Czarnywojtek, A., et al. "Effect of Lithium Carbonate on the Function of the Thyroid Gland: Mechanism of Action and Clinical Implications." J Physiol Pharmacol 71.2 (2020): 191-199.

3) Wright, Jonathan, "Reversing Hyperthyroidism by Jonathan Wright MD," Nutrition & Healing Newsletter Sept 8, 2011.

4) Temple, R. M. J. J., et al. "The Use of Lithium in the Treatment of Thyrotoxicosis." The Journal of Clinical Investigation 51.10 (1972): 2746-2756.

5) Boehm, Timothy M., et al. "Lithium and Iodine Combination Therapy for Thyrotoxicosis." European Journal of Endocrinology 94.2 (1980): 174-183.

6) Okamura, Ken, et al. "Iodide-Sensitive Graves' Hyperthyroidism and the Strategy for Resistant or Escaped Patients During Potassium Iodide Treatment." Endocrine Journal (2022): EJ21-0436.

7) Cooper, David S. "Anti-Thyroid Drugs." New England Journal of Medicine 352.9 (2005): 905-917.

8) Lazarus, J. H., et al. "Treatment of Thyrotoxicosis with Lithium Carbonate." The Lancet 304.7890 (1974): 11 60-1163.

9) Kristensen, O. H., et al. "Lithium Carbonate in the Treatment of Thyrotoxicosis: A Controlled Trial." The Lancet 307.7960 (1976): 603-605.

10) Wright, Jonathan V. "Lithium, Part 1: Protect and Renew Your Brain." Townsend Letter for Doctors and Patients 247-248 (2004): 78-82.

11) Wright, Jonathan V. "Lithium, Part 2: Other Effects." Townsend Letter for Doctors and Patients 249 (2004): 59-62.

12) Miodownik, Chanoch, et al. "Lithium-Induced Tremor Treated with Vitamin B6: A Preliminary Case Series." The International Journal of Psychiatry in Medicine 32.1 (2002): 103-108.

13) Umar, Musa U., et al. "High Dose Pyridoxine for the Treatment of Tardive Dyskinesia: Clinical Case and Review of Literature." Therapeutic Advances in Psychopharmacology 6.2 (2016): 152-156.

14) Reda, Fatma A., et al. "Lithium Carbonate in the Treatment of Tardive Dyskinesia." The American Journal of Psychiatry (1975).

15) Ibrahim, Ahmed Th, et al. "The Protective Effects of Vitamin E and Zinc Supplementation Against Lithium-Induced Brain Toxicity of Male Albino Rats." Environment and Pollution 4.1 (2015): 9.

16) Omar, H. E., et al. "The Protective Effects of Zinc and Vitamin E Supplementation Against Kidney Toxicity by Lithium in Rats." European Journal of Biological Research 6.1 (2016): 21-27.

17) Bondok, Adel A., et al. "Lithium Carbonate-Induced Nephrotoxicity in Albino Rats and the Possible Protective Effect of Vitamin E: Histological and Immunohistochemical Study." The Egyptian Journal of Anatomy 41.1 (2018): 105-118.

18) Gupta, Neena, et al. "Lithium-Induced Chronic Kidney Disease in a Pediatric Patient." Case Reports in Pediatrics 2019 (2019).

19) GA, Modawe, and N. M. ElBagir. "Lithium Carbonate Therapy Causes Nephrotoxicity and its Alleviation with Ascorbic Acid in Wistar Albino Rats."

20) Boivin, Elise, et al. "Long-Term Lithium Therapy and Risk of Chronic Kidney Disease, Hyperparathyroidism and Hypercalcemia: A Cohort Study." International Journal of Bipolar Disorders 11.1 (2023): 4.

21) Yazıcı, M. Kâzım, et al. "Renal Effects of Long-Term Lithium Therapy, Revisited." Human Psychopharmacology: Clinical and Experimental 37.2 (2022): e2812.

22) Gitlin, Michael. "Lithium Side Effects and Toxicity: Prevalence and Management Strategies." International Journal of Bipolar Disorders 4.1 (2016): 1-10.

23) Burman, Kenneth D., et al. "Sensitivity to Lithium in Treated Graves' Disease: Effects on Serum T4, T3 and Reverse T3." The Journal of Clinical Endocrinology & Metabolism 43.3 (1976): 606-613.

24) Rose, Hannah R., and Hassam Zulfiqar. "Jod Basedow Syndrome." StatPearls Publishing, 2022.

25) Wünsch, C., and H. J. Heberling. "Results of Lithium Treatment in Severe Hyperthyroidism." Deutsche Zeitschrift fur Verdauungs-und Stoffwechselkrankheiten 44.1 (1984): 26-31.

26) Dickstein, G., et al. "Lithium Treatment in Amiodarone-Induced Thyrotoxicosis." The American Journal of Medicine 102.5 (1997): 454-458.

27) Boeving, Anke, et al. "Use of Lithium Carbonate for the Treatment of Amiodarone-Induced Thyrotoxicosis." Arquivos Brasileiros de Endocrinologia & Metabologia 49 (2005): 991-995.

28) Claxton, Scott, et al. "Refractory Amiodarone-Associated Thyrotoxicosis: An Indication for Thyroidectomy." Australian and New Zealand Journal of Surgery 70.3 (2000): 174-178.

29) Benbassat, Carlos A., and Mark E. Molitch. "The Use of Lithium in the Treatment of Hyperthyroidism." The Endocrinologist 8.5 (1998): 383-388.

30) Shek, C. C., et al." Use of Lithium in the Treatment of Thyrotoxicosis." Hong Kong Med J 12.4 (2006): 254-9.

31) Ng, Y. W., et al. "Use of Lithium in The Treatment of Thyrotoxicosis." Hong Kong Medical Journal 12.4 (2006): 254.

32) Suwansaksri, Nattakarnet al. "Nonthionamide Drugs for The Treatment of Hyperthyroidism: From Present to Future." International Journal of Endocrinology 2018 (2018).

33) Akin, Fulya, et al. "The Use of Lithium Carbonate in the Preparation for Definitive Therapy in Hyperthyroid Patients." Medical Principles and Practice 17.2 (2008): 167-170.

34) Abd-ElGawad, Mohamed, et al. "Lithium Carbonate as Add-On Therapy to Radio-Iodine in the Treatment of Hyperthyroidism: A Systematic Review and Meta-Analysis." BMC Endocrine Disorders 21.1 (2021): 1-11.

35) Thakkar, Aditi, and Constance Lee Chen. "A Case for Lithium Pretreatment Prior to Radioactive Iodine Ablation in Graves' Disease." Journal of the Endocrine Society 5. Suppl 1 (2021): A906.

36) Kumar, Sanny B., et al. "Dose Optimization of Lithium to Increase the Uptake and Retention Of I-131 In Rat Thyroid." Radiation and Environmental Biophysics 58.2 (2019): 257-262.

37) Dharan, Shalini Sree, et al. "A Prospective Clinical Trial on The Efficacy of Lithium as Adjuvant Therapy to Radio-Iodine in the Treatment of Hyperthyroidism (RAILIT Study)." Endocrine Abstracts. Vol. 65. Bioscientifica, 2019.

38) Martin, Niamh M., et al. "Adjuvant Lithium Improves the Efficacy of Radioactive Iodine Treatment in Graves' and Toxic Nodular Disease." Clinical Endocrinology 77.4 (2012): 621-627.

39) Bogazzi, Fausto, et al. "Impact of Lithium on Efficacy of Radioactive Iodine Therapy for Graves' Disease: A Cohort Study on Cure Rate, Time to Cure, and Frequency of Increased Serum Thyroxine After Anti-Thyroid Drug Withdrawal." The Journal of Clinical Endocrinology & Metabolism 95.1 (2010): 201-208.

40) Tay, Wei Lin, et al. "High Thyroid Stimulating Receptor Antibody Titer and Large Goiter Size at First-Time Radioactive Iodine Treatment Are Associated with Treatment Failure in Graves' Disease." Ann Acad Med Singap 48.6 (2019): 181-187.

41) Nair, Gopalakrishnan C., et al. "Preoperative Preparation of Hyperthyroidism for Thyroidectomy—Role of Supersaturated Iodine and Lithium Carbonate." Indian Journal of Endocrinology and Metabolism 22.3 (2018): 392.

42) Kauschansky, A., and M. Genel. "Preoperative Treatment of Intractable Hyperthyroidism with Acute Lithium Administration." European Journal of Pediatric Surgery 6.05 (1996): 301-302.

43) Suwansaksri, Nattakarn et al. "Nonthionamide Drugs for the Treatment of Hyperthyroidism: From Present to Future." International Journal of Endocrinology 2018 (2018).

44) Chopra, Inder J., et al. "Opposite Effects of Dexamethasone on Serum Concentrations Of 3, 3′, 5′-Triiodothyronine (Reverse T3) And 3, 3′, 5′-Triiodothyronine (T3)." The Journal of Clinical Endocrinology & Metabolism 41.5 (1975): 911-920.

45) Williams, D. E., et al. "Acute Effects of Corticosteroids on Thyroid Activity in Graves' Disease." The Journal of Clinical Endocrinology and Metabolism 41.2 (1975): 354-361.

46) Heyma, Paul, et al. "D-Propranolol and DL-Propranolol Both Decrease Conversion of L-Thyroxine to L-Triiodothyronine." Br Med J 281.6232 (1980): 24-25.

47) Perrild, H., et al. "Different Effects of Propranolol, Alprenolol, Sotalol, Atenolol and Metoprolol on Serum T3 and Serum Rt3 in Hyperthyroidism." Clinical Endocrinology 18.2 (1983): 139-142.

48) Sharma, Pranjali P. "Use of Lithium in Hyperthyroidism Secondary to Graves' Disease: A Case Report." The American Journal of Case Reports 23 (2022): e935789-1.

49) Mori, Yusaku, et al. "Very Rare Case of Graves' Disease with Resistance to Methimazole: A Case Report and Literature Review." The Journal of International Medical Research 49.3 (2021).

50) Fantin, Esther H., and Luri Martin Goemann. "Successful Management of Hyperthyroidism with Lithium and Radio-iodine in a Patient with Previous Methimazole-Induced Agranulocytosis." Journal of the Endocrine Society 5. Supplement_1 (2021): A958-A958.

51) Ahmed, Fahad Wali, et al. "Meta-Analysis of Randomized Controlled Trials Comparing the Efficacy of Radioactive Iodine Monotherapy Versus Radioactive Iodine Therapy and Adjunctive Lithium for The Treatment of Hyperthyroidism." Endocrine Research 46.4 (2021): 160-169.

52) Dickstein, G., et al. "Lithium Treatment in Amiodarone-Induced Thyrotoxicosis." The American Journal of Medicine 102.5 (1997): 454-458.

53) Eigenmann, F., and H. Bürgi. "Lithium Acetate, A Useful and Well Tolerated Thyrostatic for Selected Cases of Hyperthyroidism." Schweizerische Medizinische Wochenschrift 108.47 (1978): 1850-1853.

54) Turner, J. G., et al. "An Evaluation of Lithium as an Adjunct to Carbimazole Treatment in Acute Thyrotoxicosis." European Journal of Endocrinology 83.1 (1976): 86-92.

55) Eulry, F., et al. "Do Lithium Salts Have a Place in the Treatment of Severe Hyperthyroidism? (Author's Transl)." La Nouvelle Presse Medicale 6.33 (1977): 2955-2958.

56) Jonderko, G., and C. Marcisz. "Short-Term Use of Lithium Carbonate in the Treatment of Thyrotoxicosis." Zeitschrift fur die Gesamte Innere Medizin und Ihre Grenzgebiete 34.15 (1979): 408-411.

57) Hedley, J. M., et al. "Low Dose Lithium-Carbimazole in the Treatment of Thyrotoxicosis." Australian and New Zealand Journal of Medicine 8.6 (1978): 628-630.

Chapter 18

Addressing the Auto Immune Component of Thyroid Disease

The Role of H. Pylori, Gluten Free Diet, Vitamin D3, Selenium, Excess Iodine, etc.

ONE OF THE ERRORS OF modern endocrinology is to ignore the autoimmune component of Hashimoto's and Graves' Disease. The typical mainstream endocrinologist is concerned solely with managing thyroid function, believing there is no known cause or treatment for the autoimmune component. In 2010, Dr. Jerome M. Hershman made this exact point in Clinical Thyroidology, expressing the hope a "rational therapy" for the autoimmune origin of thyroid disease can be found. Dr. Jerome M. Hershman writes:

> It is difficult to predict how patients with Graves' disease will be treated 20 years from now, but I hope that we will have some rational therapy that is directed at the autoimmune origin and that makes our entire current armamentarium obsolete. (1)

The reality is that we do know the causes, origins, and "rational therapy" of autoimmune thyroid disease. This information is widely available in the medical literature.

Vitamin D3 and Autoimmune Disease

I give credit and thanks to Abram Hoffer, MD, who alerted me to the importance of Vitamin D3 in preventing autoimmune disease. In Toronto, Canada in April 2007, my wife and I attended Dr. Abram Hoffer's lifetime achievement award black-tie gala dinner. This was also his 90th birthday celebration. After the gala dinner, all guests received a copy of Dr. Hoffer's book, "Adventures in Psychiatry." The next day was the start of the annual meeting of Orthomolecular Medical Society. During the daytime meeting program, a Canadian nurse

sitting next to me confided that Dr. Hoffer had cured her son of multiple sclerosis (M.S.) with large doses of Vitamin D3. Dr. Hoffer did a neurologic exam on the young man, made the diagnosis of Multiple Sclerosis, and then advised him to take large doses of Vitamin D. The young man did so, and his neurologic symptoms soon resolved. Dr. Hoffer cured this young man's autoimmune disease with Vitamin D3, a vitamin that plays a role in preventing and treating most, if not all autoimmune diseases. (2-6)

Vitamin D3 Reduces Autoimmune Disease by 22 percent.

In 2022, Dr. Jill Hahn did a 5.3-year randomized clinical trial giving either placebo or 2,000 iu of vitamin D3/day to 25,871 people over age 50. The Vitamin D group had a 22 percent reduction in various autoimmune diseases, such as rheumatoid arthritis, psoriasis, autoimmune thyroid disease, etc. Dr. Hahn concludes:

> Vitamin D supplementation for five years, with or without omega-3 fatty acids, reduced autoimmune disease by 22%. (7)

Vitamin D as a Public Health Measure

Vitamin D is not only important for a functioning immune system but also as a public health measure. Vitamin D deficiency is associated with an increased risk for various autoimmune diseases, cancer, and increased mortality from viral infection. For example, in a 2021 study by Dr. Lorenz Borsche, mortality from infection with the SARS Cov-2 virus was reduced to zero when the vitamin 25 hydroxy D3 level was raised above 50 ng/mL! Studies in 2021 by Dr. Casey Johnson and in 2023 by Dr. Kye-Yeung Park showed Vitamin D level is inversely associated with all-cause mortality and cancer incidence. (8-12)

In 2020, Dr. William Grant reviewed the health benefits of Vitamin D, finding concentrations above 30 ng/ml reduce all-cause mortality, the risk of acute upper respiratory infections, cancer, type 2 diabetes mellitus, and improve outcomes of pregnancy and newborns, writing:

> Over the past two decades, many studies reported the benefits of higher 25-hydroxyvitamin D [25(OH)D] concentrations for nonskeletal effects. Researchers found significant benefits in reducing risk of acute respiratory tract infections, many types of cancer, type 2 diabetes mellitus, premature death, and adverse pregnancy and birth outcomes. In addition, 25(OH)D concentrations are low for various reasons in several categories of people, including the obese, those with dark skin living at higher latitudes, the elderly, and those who do not eat much eggs, fish, meat, or vitamin D fortified milk. Measuring 25(OH) D concentrations is one way to both increase the awareness of vitamin D's importance in maintaining good health and to encourage vitamin D supplementation or increased solar ultraviolet-B exposure to sustain well-being throughout life by reducing disease incidence. Although 20 ng/ml seems adequate to reduce risk of skeletal problems and acute respiratory tract infections, **concentrations above 30 ng/ml have been associated with reduced risk of cancer, type 2 diabetes mellitus, and adverse pregnancy and birth outcomes.** Thus, judicious testing of 25(OH)D concentrations could reduce disease incidence and make treatment expenditures more cost-effective. (13)

For these reasons, we routinely measure serum vitamin D3 levels and supplement to a target level over 50 ng/mL. I once had a conversation with a pediatric surgeon who felt it was dangerous to advise the public to take vitamin D supplements. This is a preposterous position and accomplishes only one thing, a sicker population with increasing expenditures on health care and greater profits for the medical system.

Since vitamin D is considered safe and is available over the counter without a prescription, vitamin D supplementation can be considered a public health measure. The general public should take advantage of vitamin D supplementation to improve health. However, it is advisable to work with a knowledgeable physician who can monitor serum vitamin D levels once or twice a year, and adjust dosage based on levels. The laboratory reference range for Vitamin D is 30-100 ng/mL (Quest Lab). (13-15)

Vitamin D and Autoimmune Thyroid Disease

In 2022, Dr. Dorina Galuşca reviewed Vitamin D in autoimmune thyroid disorders, writing:

> In Hashimoto's disease, vitamin D deficiency appears to be correlated with a higher titer of anti-TPO antibodies and with thyroid volume, and supplementation was associated with reduction of antibodies in some studies. In other studies, supplementation appeared to reduce TSH levels. In Graves' disease, there was a significant correlation regarding vitamin D levels and thyroid volume respective to the degree of exophthalmos... Vitamin D deficiency is highly prevalent in endocrine disorders, and its supplementation appears to have numerous beneficial effects. (16-22)

Wheat Gluten and Leaky Gut

I give credit and thanks to Dr. Jonathan Wright for alerting me to the link between gluten sensitivity and autoimmune disease. Here is a quote from Dr. Jonathan Wright's newsletter, Nutrition & Healing newsletter; Vol. 8 Issue 12, February 2012:

> In 1989, my wife Holly and I visited the office of Christopher Reading in Dee Why, a suburb of Sydney, Australia. He showed us documentation of over 500 individuals who came to see him with a diagnosis of Lupus [erythematosus] ... How did over 500 individuals eliminate all signs and symptoms of Lupus – and all patent medicines given for it, too – over 20 years ago? **Reading had**

them totally eliminate all gluten, all milk and dairy products, and often other foods to which they were found to be allergic. The other major part of Reading's treatment included repeated massive (but safe) doses of vitamins and minerals given intravenously. (23)

Gluten, Autoimmune Disease, and Alessio Fasano MD

How does wheat consumption cause auto-immune disease? This mystery was finally explained by the groundbreaking work on cholera by Dr. Alessio Fasano, a pediatric gastroenterologist at the University of Pennsylvania who discovered Zonulin, the hormone that controls the tight junctions in the gut epithelium. The tight junctions are normally closed. However, in certain sensitive people, wheat consumption stimulates excess Zonulin secretion, opening the tight junctions for prolonged periods of time, thus increasing gut permeability and creating what is known as a "leaky gut," the leakage of bacteria and partially digested food particles from the gut lumen into the bloodstream. These leaked particles may have amino acid sequences that mimic those of our own tissues and organs, triggering an autoimmune attack in a mechanism called "molecular mimicry." If our immune system attacks the thyroid, we may find an elevation of the anti-TPO and anti-thyroglobulin antibodies. This is called Hashimoto's autoimmune thyroiditis. If we have an elevation of the TSI and TRAb antibodies, this is Graves' Disease, a hyperthyroid state. Note: a competing mechanism was described in Chapter 14 on the Production of Thyroid Hormones, in which excess hydrogen peroxide damages TPO and thyroglobulin, rendering them antigenic, thus leading to autoimmune disease. (24-34) Note: TPO Ab is the thyroperoxidase antibody.

Anti-Gliadin Antibody Test

We routinely test all patients for wheat gluten sensitivity using the serum anti-gliadin antibody test done by all commercial labs. If negative, we suggest doing the more sensitive and accurate stool test for the same anti-gliadin antibody using an out-of-network lab called Enterolabs. Typically, mainstream primary care doctors and gastroenterologists will not use the anti-gliadin antibody stool test, and instead run the celiac disease blood tests. These are the TTG (tissue transglutaminase antibody plus IgA) and EMA (anti-endomysial antibody). About 1-2 percent of the population will screen positive with these tests. If positive, the gastroenterologist will confirm the diagnosis with an endoscopic small bowel biopsy. If the symptomatic patient tests negative for the TTG and EMA, then the primary care doctor will declare them negative and the diagnosis of non-celiac gluten sensitivity could be missed. To avoid missing these cases, we use the more sensitive serum and stool anti-gliadin antibody test.

Compared to non-celiac gluten sensitivity, Celiac disease is a more severe reaction to wheat, a form of auto-immune disease in which the immune system attacks the duodenal and small bowel lining causing villous atrophy and malabsorption, as well as protean symptoms related to the gastrointestinal and nervous systems. There is increased gut permeability and a high correlation with other auto-immune diseases. There is a genetic predisposition, and genetic testing is usually positive for a variant of the HLA-DQ2 or HLA-DQ8 allele. The diagnosis of Celiac disease is usually when the child fails to thrive. However, about 40 percent of cases are found in adults who somehow escape the diagnosis their entire lives because of atypical presentation. The tip-off may be chronic iron deficiency anemia, perhaps the most frequent marker for malabsorption of iron from celiac disease or non-celiac gluten sensitivity. Another frequently missed presentation is the patient with atypical stress fractures from metabolic bone disease from calcium malabsorption. This may be the only symptom. There may be an overlap of symptoms and clinical presentation between non-celiac gluten sensitivity, and classic celiac disease. However, both are treated the same with a strict one hundred percent gluten-free diet with curative results. In my opinion, a gluten-free diet is advised for all patients with autoimmune thyroid disease, even with negative testing. The testing is not perfect and we do see some occasional false negatives. To follow this, a larger panel of food sensitivity testing is advised since many auto-immune thyroid patients have additional food sensitivities for egg, dairy, and soy proteins. (35-44)

Iodine, Selenium, and Autoimmune Thyroid Disease

As mentioned in the previous chapter, sele-nium deficiency has been implicated in the eti-ology of autoimmune thyroid disease. Selenium is the only mineral in which our DNA codes for selenium insertion into a protein (using sele-nocysteine). In 2002, Dr. Vadim N. Gladyshev at the University of Nebraska unraveled the mystery by decoding the selenium insertion sequence (SECIS) in our DNA code. Upstream SECIS code determines the function of the UGA termination code by switching it from STOP to INSERT SELENOCYSTEINE into the amino acid sequence of the protein. The SECIS does this by changing the function of the STOP Codon, UGA, into a new function, "insert selenocyste-ine" instead of STOP.

In 2002, Dr. Vadim N. Gladyshev writes:

Selenium is ...inserted into protein as the amino acid selenocysteine (Sec). The elucidation of how Sec is incorporated into protein has progressed at a rapid pace in the last decade and has revealed some surprising results. In fact, unraveling this mystery has altered our understanding of the genetic code, as the code has now been expanded to include Sec as the 21st naturally occurring amino acid. We now know that UGA serves as both a termination codon and a Sec codon. (45-46)

Selenoprotein Families

Selenium, as the amino acid selenocysteine, is incorporated into seleno-proteins involved in anti-oxidant function, immune function, wound healing, and cancer prevention. Adequate selenium intake is required for a functioning anti-oxidant system. The thyroid gland has the highest concentration of selenium in the body, incorporated into glutathione peroxi-dases (GPx) and thioredoxin reductases (TrxR). These are anti-oxidants used in the neutraliza-tion of hydrogen peroxide generated in the pro-duction of thyroid hormones. Another family of seleno-proteins is the iodothyronine deio-dinase enzyme system (all three D1, D2, and D3). Note: D1 and D2 convert T4 to T3 (the active form), while D3 converts T4 to reverse T3 (the inactive form). (47-51)

Selenium deficiency is implicated in various thyroid and systemic diseases, such as auto-immune thyroid disease, muscle degenera-tion (White Marble Disease in Oregon Cattle), cardiomyopathy (Keshan's Disease), cancer, infection, etc. All of these are directly related to deficiency of the seleno-protein anti-oxidant system, leading to cellular oxidative damage from reactive oxygen species (ROS) arising from cellular energy production (mitochon-drial oxidative phosphorylation). Or, in the case of the thyroid gland, deficiency of the sele-no-protein anti-oxidant system means failure to neutralize excess hydrogen peroxide, leading to inflammation and damage to thyroid cells and proteins. (52-63)

Low Selenium in Hashimoto's and Graves' Disease

In 2020, Dr. Kristian Hillert Winther reviewed selenium in thyroid disorders, writ-ing low selenium status is linked to autoim-mune thyroiditis:

Epidemiological studies have linked an increased risk of autoimmune thyroiditis, Graves' disease, and goiter to low selenium status. Trials of selenium supplementation in patients with chronic autoimmune thyroiditis have generally resulted in reduced thyroid autoantibody titer without apparent improvements in the clinical course of the disease. In Graves' disease, selenium supplementation might lead to faster remission of hyperthyroidism and improved quality of life and eye involvement in patients with mild thyroid eye disease. Despite recommendations only extending to patients with Graves' ophthalmopathy, selenium supplementation is widely used by clinicians for other thyroid phenotypes. (64)

Selenium in Iodine Escape Phenomenon

In view of the above, one might wonder if selenium deficiency might explain the "iodine escape phenomenon" when using iodine for the treatment of Graves' thyrotoxicosis. In Japan, treatment of Graves' disease with potassium iodide alone (KI) is widely accepted by thyroid specialists. In 2015, Dr. Yoshihara switched 260 women with Graves' disease (GD) from methimazole to potassium iodide to control hyperthyroidism in the first trimester of pregnancy. For 88%, this switch was successful. However, 12% (22 patients, Worsened Group) remained hyperthyroid, requiring a higher dose of methimazole for control. This suggests an "escape from the anti-thyroid effect of iodide." In a follow-up paper in 2020, Dr. Yoshihara reviewed this data, finding that higher TRAb levels predicted the continuation of thyroid suppressive medication. However, Dr. Yoshihara had no parameter to predict iodine escape (worsened group), writing:

It was difficult to control the maternal thyrotoxicosis of 22 of the 107 patients with KI [potassium iodide] alone, and a higher dose of MMI [methimazole] compared with the dose at the time of conception was required (worsened group).....It must be kept in mind that a certain proportion of GD [Graves' disease] patients **escape from the anti-thyroid effect of iodide**, and that careful follow-up is necessary after switching a pregnant patient's medication to KI. (65-66)

One wonders if the parameter to explain the 11-12 percent "escape phenomenon" is selenium and magnesium deficiency in this subgroup, unable to "alleviate the toxic effects of iodine." Unfortunately, selenium levels were not measured in this study, so this remains speculation. Perhaps this question could be answered in future studies, which include measurement of selenium and magnesium levels in Graves' disease patients before and during treatment with potassium iodide. A second factor to consider is the use of Block and Replace. Dr. Ken Okamura's 2022 study showed the efficacy of Block and Replace in preventing relapse of hyperthyroidism in Graves' disease patients who are resistant or escape during treatment with potassium iodide. Note: In Dr. Ken Okamura's 2022 article, he used the term "combined therapy" in place of the term Block and Replace which has an identical meaning, this was discussed more fully in Chapters 15 and 16, Graves' Hyperthyroidism Treatment with Iodine, Parts One and Two. (67-69)

NIS Auto-Antibodies and Iodine Escape

In 2010, Dr. Anna-Maria Eleftheriadou found that about 12 percent of Graves' disease patients have auto-antibodies to the NIS, the sodium iodide symporter active transport for iodine. A second speculative explanation for iodine "resistance or escape" in Graves' disease is the presence of NIS antibodies in about 12 percent of Graves' disease patients. The NIS (sodium iodide symporter) is embedded in the basolateral membrane of the thyrocyte and mediates the active transport of iodine into the thyroid cell, concentrating iodine 100 times that of plasma in Graves' disease. NIS antibodies inhibit iodine uptake and concentration, thus a possible explanation for iodine "escape" or "resistance" in a subset of Graves' disease patients treated with potassium iodide to control hyperthyroidism. If the NIS is inhibited by antibody deposition, this will interfere with iodide concentration within the thyrocyte with the failure of the Wolff-Chaikoff Effect. (70-72)

Immune Complex Deposits at Basolateral Membrane of Follicles

In 1977, Dr. Kalderon identified immune complex deposits at the follicular basal lamina of the follicles in the thyroid glands of patients with Hashimotos' and Graves' autoimmune thyroid disease. Note this is the location of the NIS sodium iodide symporter. Dr. Kalderon also identified this same finding in a hereditary model of autoimmune thyroid disease in obese chickens. Perhaps these immune complexes of Dr. Kalderon are the same NIS antibodies discovered by Dr. Anna-Maria Eleftheriadou (above). Deposition of immune complexes at the basolateral membrane interferes with NIS function which concentrates iodine, and thyroid autoregulation. This could be an explanation for "iodine escape" in 12 percent of patients. Currently, the laboratory test for anti-NIS antibodies is research only and not available for clinical use at commercial laboratories. (73-74)

Dr. Daniela Gallo – Adding Selenium and Vitamin D

Observational studies show newly diagnosed Graves' disease patients have low selenium and vitamin D3 levels. In 2022, Dr. Daniela Gallo did a randomized clinical trial in 42 patients, half treated with methimazole and half treated with methimazole combined with selenium (Se) and Vitamin D3. Dr. Daniela Gallo found the combination of selenium and Vitamin D3 improved the efficacy of the methimazole and improved quality of life, writing:

> Low Se [selenium] levels might exacerbate oxidative stress by compromising the anti-oxidant machinery's response to reactive oxygen species, and low Vitamin D levels might hamper the anti-inflammatory immune response... Our results suggest that reaching optimal Se and Vit D levels increases the early efficacy of MMI [methimazole] treatment when Se and Vit D levels are sub-optimal. (75)

Dr. Christine Hotz, Selenium, and Iodine in Laboratory Mice

In 1997, Dr. Christine S. Hotz studied the effect of dietary iodine and selenium on thyroid function and anti-oxidant status in laboratory mice. Dr. Hotz found the combination of low selenium and high iodine intake causes low anti-oxidant status leading to thyroidal damage, writing:

> Activity of thyroidal GSH-Px [Glutathione-peroxidase, selenoprotein anti-oxidant] was lowest in rats fed a diet containing high iodine and low selenium. The results suggest that high iodine intake when selenium is deficient, may permit thyroid tissue damage as a result of low thyroidal GSH-Px activity during thyroid stimulation. (76)

Dr. Jian Xu, Iodine and Selenium in Mice

In 2006 and 2011, Dr. Jian Xu studied mice given excess iodine, comparing them to laboratory mice fed both excess iodine and selenium combined. Dr. Jian Xu found selenium supplementation in mice alleviates the toxic effects of iodine excess. Dr. Jian Xu found in mice fed iodine excess, there is the exhaustion of glutathione peroxidase, the seleno-protein anti-oxidant system. This impairment of the anti-oxidant system results in excess accumulation of hydrogen peroxide (H_2O_2), which inhibits thyroperoxidase (TPO) activity. Excess iodine also increases the iodine content in the thyroid gland and alters thyroid gland histology with enlargement of colloid-containing follicles leading to goiter. Excess iodine also reduces deiodinase type I (D1) activity by 30-40% in the liver, kidneys, and thyroid, causing higher plasma T4 and lower T3. However, the activity of D1 is restored to normal when selenium is added. Excess iodine also inhibits TPO, thyroperoxidase activity. However, selenium refeeding restores TPO activity by restoring the seleno-protein glutathione peroxidase, which neutralizes excess H_2O_2. Since excess hydrogen peroxide (H_2O_2) inhibits TPO, this neutralization restores TPO activity. One might then conclude from Dr. Xu's study in mice similarity to humans. In other words, treating the selenium-deficient Graves' disease patient with excess iodide to control hyperthyroidism will increase H202 causing oxidative damage and thyroiditis. Thus, selenium deficiency could explain the "escape or resistance" to potassium iodide treatment of Graves' disease. Note: selenium levels must be maintained for good glutathione peroxidase (GSHPx) activity. Colloid is thyroglobulin, the precursor protein to thyroid hormone. D1, Deiodinase Type I converts T4 to T3 in the periphery. In 2006, Dr. Jian Xu writes:

> The experimental results show that...**hepatic selenium and the activity of GSHPx [glutathione peroxidase]** in EI [excess iodine] group **decrease** compared with those in NI [normal iodine] group. **So, the H2O2 from thyroid hormone biosynthesis could not be converted effectively neutralized [by GSHPx]; therefore, the thyroid hormone biosynthesis will be damaged**. There was no significant difference in hepatic selenium and GSHPx between the NI [normal iodine] and IS [iodine/selenium combination] groups, which means that **the oxidative/anti-oxidative balance has been maintained in IS groups [iodine and selenium given]** ...The activity of TPO [thyroperoxidase] was inhibited by excessive iodine significantly [Note: this is the Wolff-Chaikoff effect]. Compared with the effect of iodine alone, iodine in combination with selenium increased the activity of TPO, indicating that **selenium supplement alleviated the damage of TPO resulting from iodide excess**... [in the excess iodine group] the excessive H2O2 in thyroid would depress the activity of TPO. Supplemental selenium could increase GSHPx activity and correct the unbalanced oxidative/anti-oxidative system. It is the ultimate reason for TPO activity recovery. Supplemental selenium could decrease the level of TPO antibody and the damage of thyroid in the patients with Graves' disease... **We could draw the conclusion that supplemental selenium could alleviate the toxic effect of excessive iodine on the thyroid.** (77-78)

Note: Inhibition of TPO (inhibition of organification) by excess iodine is the Wolff-Chaikoff Effect.

In 2020, Dr. Ioana Vasiliu confirmed the 2006 and 2011 studies of Dr. Jian Xu. Dr. Ioana Vasiliu again studied the protective role of selenium in iodide-induced autoimmune thyroiditis in laboratory mice. When the mice were fed excessive amounts of iodide, moderate to severe thyroiditis was observed in 83% of males and 50% of female rats. When mice were fed the combination of selenium and iodide, none developed moderate to severe thyroiditis. Dr. Ioana Vasiliu writes:

> Excess iodine may induce and exacerbate autoimmune thyroiditis (AIT) in humans and animals...Thus, the administration of Se [selenium] was proven to have protective effects against thyroiditis cytology in both male and female Wistar rats. (79-80)

Iodide Depletion - Toxic Effects of Iodide

In 2000, Dr. Bernard Corvilain studied animal models showing, under normal conditions, excess iodide will inhibit H202 generation, the Wolff-Chaikoff Effect. However, the opposite is found in iodide-depleted animals. In these animals, instead of inhibiting hydrogen peroxide generation, acute iodide exposure activates H2O2 generation. This is thought to promote efficient oxidation and organification of the iodide and may explain the toxic effects of acute administration of iodide on iodine-depleted thyroids. This could represent another explanation for "iodine escape or iodine resistance" in the iodine-treated Graves' disease patient who is also severely iodine deficient at the start of treatment.

For this reason, it is prudent to test for iodine deficiency with the spot urine for iodine, a test available at all commercial laboratories. In the iodine-depleted animal or humans, the administration of iodine has the paradoxical effect of increasing hydrogen dioxide generation. This excess hydrogen peroxide may trigger thyroiditis. In 2000, Dr. Bernard Corvilain writes:

In comparison with conditions in which an inhibitory effect of iodide on H2O2 generation is observed, the stimulating effect was observed for lower concentrations and for a shorter incubation time with iodide. Such a dual control of H2O2 generation by iodide has the physiological interest of promoting an efficient oxidation of iodide when the substrate is provided to a deficient gland and of avoiding excessive oxidation of iodide and thus synthesis of thyroid hormones when it is in excess. The activation of H2O2 generation may also explain the well-described toxic effect of acute administration of iodide on iodine-depleted thyroids. (81)

Graves' Disease Mimics Iodine-Depleted State

Although Graves' disease (GD) patients may have normal dietary iodine intake, their thyroid gland behaves as if it is iodine depleted, similar to the iodine-depleted animals in the above study by Dr. Bernard Corvilain. Remember, in GD, TSI and TRAb antibodies stimulate the thyroid gland to increase the production of thyroid hormone, thus inducing thyrotoxicosis. This hyperthyroidism requires massive amounts of iodine to manufacture the high levels of thyroid hormones found in the blood. This explains why the thyroid gland in Graves' disease mimics iodine depletion even though dietary iodine intake may be within normal limits. Enlargement of the thyroid gland with increased 5-hour radio-iodine uptake related to TSH receptor stimulation is common to both iodine deficiency and Graves' disease. In iodine deficiency, high TSH stimulates the thyroid and increases radioiodine uptake. In Graves' disease, TSH Receptor antibodies stimulate the thyroid and increase radioiodine uptake. Both the iodine deficient gland and the hyperactive thyroid gland in Graves' disease are "starved" of iodine. One might then consider the experiments of Dr. Bernard Corvilain using dog thyroid slices, showing administer-ing iodide to iodide-depleted thyroid glands increases H2O2 production leading to thyroiditis; this also applies to the Graves' disease thyroid gland, which acts and behaves as if iodine depleted, a condition caused by massive TSH Receptor stimulation. Thus, we have arrived at a possible mechanism for iodine-induced thyroiditis from excess H2O2 generation in the selenium-depleted Graves' disease patient treated with potassium iodide monotherapy. (81-84)

Antibodies to Selenium Transport Proteins

In 2021, Dr. Qian Sun found that Hashimoto's patients have antibodies to the blood selenium transport protein called SELENOP. These antibodies inhibit selenium uptake by the thyroid and lead to low glutathione peroxidase anti-oxidant status. One might speculate this same defect in Graves' disease. Dr. Qian Sun writes:

Using a newly established quantitative immunoassay, SELENOP autoantibodies were particularly prevalent in Hashimoto's thyroiditis as compared with healthy control subjects (6.6% versus 0.3%)....
GPX3 [anti-oxidant status] activity was low and correlated inversely to SELENOP autoantibody concentrations. In renal cells in culture, **antibodies to SELENOP inhibited Se [selenium] uptake.** Our results indicate an impairment of SELENOP-dependent Se transport by natural SELENOP autoantibodies, suggesting that the characterization of health risks from Se deficiency may need to include autoimmunity to SELENOP as an additional biomarker of Se status. (85)

Note: the SELENOP antibody test is a research test and not commercially available as of this writing.

Magnesium Deficiency

Magnesium (Mg) deficiency worsens the anti-oxidant status of selenium deficiency. In 1993, Dr. Zongjian Zhu studied selenium and magnesium-deficient mice, finding that combined magnesium and selenium deficiency made the anti-oxidant status worse than selenium deficiency alone, writing:

> Magnesium deficiency had an influence on the distribution of Se [selenium], which was increased in muscle and decreased in other tissues. The changes in GSHPx [glutathione peroxidase] matched those in Se. The levels of Se and GSHPx in most tissues were lower in Se-Mg-deficient rats than in Se-deficient rats. **Thus, selenium and Mg deficiencies would make oxidant lesions more serious than Se deficiency**. (68)

We routinely test for RBC magnesium in all patients in our office. The above studies highlight the importance of routine testing for serum selenium (Se), RBC magnesium, Vitamin D3, and spot urinary iodine levels in every autoimmune thyroid patient, as suggested in 2017 by Dr. Liontiris, who also advises a Gluten-Free Diet. Dr. Liontiris writes:

> Serum levels of iodine, selenium, and vitamin D in HT [Hashimoto's thyroiditis] patients are necessary, and careful supplementation in case of deficiency of these agents is recommended. Due to the increasing coexistence of HT with CD [celiac disease] and other autoimmune diseases, a low-gluten diet is important. (86-87)

TPO is a Heme Protein with Central Iron

As previously mentioned, thyroid peroxidase (TPO) is directly responsible for organification of iodine into thyroglobulin using H2O2 as a substrate. TPO is a heme protein, meaning it contains a heme chemical structure, a porphyrin ring with a central iron atom. Thus, thyroid hormone production is dependent on adequate iron stores. In autoimmune thyroid patients, there may be co-existing autoimmune gastritis or gluten sensitivity with iron malabsorption, both associated with iron deficiency. Iron supplementation to a ferritin level of 100 µg/l is suggested by Dr. Margaret Rayman, who writes in 2019:

> It is important to recognize that low iron stores may contribute to symptom persistence in patients treated for hypothyroidism... An example is afforded by a small study in twenty-five Finnish women with persistent symptoms of hypothyroidism, despite appropriate L-T4 [levothyroxine] therapy, who became symptom-free when treated with oral iron supplements for 6–12 months... all had serum ferritin <60 µg/l. Restoration of serum ferritin above 100 µg/l ameliorated the symptoms in two-thirds of the women. At least 30–50 % of hypothyroid patients with persisting symptoms despite adequate L-T4 therapy may, in fact, have covert ID [iron deficiency] ...Patients with AITD or hypothyroidism should be routinely screened for ID [iron deficiency]. If either ID or serum ferritin below 70 µg/l is found, coeliac disease or autoimmune gastritis may be the cause and should be treated. (88-92)

Dr. Margaret Rayman is quite correct about the benefits of iron supplementation when ferritin is low. Many auto-immune thyroid patients have malabsorption of iron secondary to auto-immune atrophic gastritis. The simple use of iron supplements should be more widely adopted. However, I would not dogmatically adhere to the ferritin level of 100 mcg/L, as discussed by Dr. Rayman. Perhaps good outcomes may be achieved with lower ferritin levels. Hopefully, future studies will shed more light on this.

Graves' Disease is an Autoimmune Disease

What is the etiology of Graves' disease? Gluten sensitivity and leaky gut have been implicated in the etiology of Graves' disease, and all other autoimmune diseases for that matter. This statement is based on the pioneering work of Alessio Fasano, MD, a pediatric gastroenterologist at Mass. General in Boston. A gluten-free diet is recommended by Dr. Liontiris for all autoimmune thyroid patients. (41)(86)

Wheat, Leaky Gut, and Molecular Mimicry

Underlying gluten sensitivity is a common cause of leaky gut and autoimmune disease. The mechanism of molecular mimicry has been proposed with the leakage of bacteria into the bloodstream, which invokes an immune response. Various infectious organisms have been implicated in molecular mimicry. One is Yersinia, a bacteria implicated in Graves' Disease. Antibodies to Yersinia cross-react with the TSH receptor, producing hyperthyroidism by stimulating the TSH receptors in the thyroid gland. Similarly, thyroid eye disease (TED) is the result of an autoimmune attack on TSH receptors or other antigens in the extra-ocular muscles, peri-orbital adipose, and connective tissue. (93)

Helicobacter Pylori and Its Eradication

In 2005, Drs. Robin Warren and Barry Marshall were awarded the Nobel Prize in Physiology or Medicine for their 1982 discovery of Helicobacter Pylori, a bacterial infection in the stomach wall thought to cause gastritis, gastric ulcers, and gastric cancer. H. Pylori is treatable with a protocol known as Triple Therapy consisting of a PPI proton pump inhibitor antacid (omeprazole) and two antibiotics over a ten-day course. The infection can be diagnosed easily with a breath test developed in 1991 by Dr. Barry Marshal. Infection with H. Pylori bacteria is associated with Graves' disease and other autoimmune conditions. Triple therapy may be more effective when combined with probiotics and bismuth. (94-114)

H. Pylori Eradication Reduces Thyroid Antibodies

A 2004 study by Dr. Giovanni Bertalot found a significant decrease in anti-thyroid antibodies after eradication of H. Pylori. (115)

In 2017, Dr. Yi Hou performed a meta-analysis correlating H. Pylori infection with auto-immune thyroid disease and found five studies in the Chinese medical literature showing H. Pylori eradication reduces anti-thyroid antibody levels for both Hashimoto's thyroiditis and Graves' disease. Dr. Yi Hou writes:

> Five studies reported the influence of eradication therapy on thyroid autoantibodies. Patients with AITD who had H. pylori infection were selected from each study and were randomly allocated to observation and control groups. Only patients in the observation group were treated with eradication therapy...We also observed that pharmaceutical eradication of H. pylori infection reduced levels of thyroid autoantibodies in patients with GD and HT...Antibody levels differed significantly before and after eradication therapy in the observation group, but did not differ in the control group, suggesting that H. pylori infection was associated with the development of Hashimoto's thyroiditis... The rate of hyperthyroidism remission in the observation group was significantly higher than in the control group, suggesting that H. pylori infection was associated with Graves' disease. (116)

I think it is safe to say we have enough evidence of benefit for the autoimmune thyroid patient to justify routine H. Pylori Breath Testing, and eradication with Triple Therapy if positive. One might expand this to all patients regardless of their immune status, simply to improve their quality of life. (117)

Use of Probiotics for Graves' Disease

The connection between the gut microbiome and autoimmune thyroid disease was touched upon in the above discussion of wheat gluten sensitivity and leaky gut. Therefore, it is not surprising that restoring the microbiome with probiotics can be enormously beneficial in Graves' disease patients. (118-123)

In 2021, Dr. Huo studied the effect of a probiotic Bifidobacterium longum supplied in addition to the usual methimazole treatment in 9 Graves' disease (GD) patients. As expected, methimazole alone (MMI) controlled hyperthyroidism, effectively reducing Free T3 and Free

T4 thyroid hormone levels but had no effect on the autoimmune disease measured by the TRAb antibodies. However, when probiotics were administered in combination with methimazole, Dr. Huo found a dramatic reduction in TRAb antibodies, indicating improvement in the autoimmune component of the disease. Dr. Huo writes:

> Unsurprisingly, MI [methimazole] intake significantly improved several thyroid indexes but not the most important thyrotropin receptor antibody (TRAb), which is an indicator of the GD [Graves' Disease] recurrence rate...**the clinical thyroid indexes of patients with GD in the probiotic supplied with MI treatment group continued to improve. Dramatically, the concentration of TRAb recovered to a healthy level.** (118)

Autoimmune Thyroid Disease and GI Health

In 2022, Dr. Michael Ruscio made the bold statement that treating the GI (gastro-intestinal) tract directly reduces autoimmunity, and the health of the GI tract may be a root cause in the pathogenesis of autoimmunity. Dr. Michael Ruscio feels dysbiosis [altered microbiome], and intestinal permeability are directly related to thyroid autoimmunity in both Hashimoto's and Graves' disease. Dr. Michael Ruscio writes:

> The connection between GI health and autoimmunity may be mediated by increased intestinal permeability caused by various forms of GI imbalances (i.e., SIBO, dysbiosis, pathogens). One study found that increased GI permeability is found at higher rates in those with thyroid dysfunction and is associated with more thyroid symptoms...A small pilot study found that children with Hashimoto's disease have increased markers of leaky GI when compared to controls. In this study, higher serum zonulin was associated with higher levothyroxine dose. In other words, more intestinal permeability was associated with more thyroid dysfunction...Similarly, higher GI permeability levels among Graves'

patients were associated with higher antibody levels, lower TSH, higher fT4/fT3, and more symptoms. **This suggests that dysbiosis and intestinal permeability have a direct interaction and impact on thyroid autoimmunity (both Hashimoto's and Graves' disease)** and can contribute to the autoimmune phenomenon as a whole. **GI therapies directly reduce autoimmunity, suggesting that GI health may be a root cause behind the pathogenesis of autoimmunity.** For example, a small study found an average of a 2000-point decrease in TPO antibodies after H. pylori eradication. Probiotics have multiple lines of evidence showing that they lower inflammation and autoimmunity. (123)

Use of Berberine for Autoimmune Thyroid Disease

Berberine is a botanical used for hundreds of years to prevent or reverse "leaky gut" and to alter the gut microbiome in beneficial ways, increasing beneficial bacteria and decreasing pathogenic bacteria. Numerous studies in animals and humans have shown the benefits of berberine for improving intestinal barrier function (tight junctions) and the gut microbiome. (124-131)

Berberine for Graves' Disease

In 2021, Dr. Zhe Han studied the use of berberine in Graves' Disease (GD). Eight patients were given methimazole (MMI) alone, and ten patients were given both MMI and berberine over six months. Dr. Zhe Han notes berberine had a beneficial effect on the gut microbiome, increasing beneficial Lactococcus lactis while decreasing pathogenic bacteria, writing:

> The results showed that the addition of berberine [to the MMI] restored the patients' TSH and FT3 [Free T3] indices to normal levels, whereas MMI alone restored only FT3. In addition, TRAb [TSH Receptor Antibodies] was closer to the healthy threshold at the end of treatment with the drug combination. MMI alone failed to

modulate the gut microbiota of the patients. However, the combination of berberine with methimazole **significantly altered the microbiota structure of the patients, increasing the abundance of the beneficial bacteria Lactococcus lactis while decreasing the abundance of the pathogenic bacteria …** In conclusion, methimazole combined with berberine has better efficacy in patients with GD. (124)

In 2022, Dr. Diao found the use of berberine and probiotics beneficial for Graves' Orbitopathy, the exophthalmos eye disease associated with Graves'. (125)

A new drug for Graves Orbitopathy

A new drug for Graves Orbitopathy, the IGF-IR inhibitor teprotumumab, is given by intravenous infusions. At 24 weeks in a controlled trial, the percentage of patients responding with improvement in proptosis was higher (83%) with teprotumumab than with placebo (10%). Note: IGF-IR is an insulin-like growth factor I receptor. There is an overlap in activity between the TSH and IGF-1 (a marker for Growth Hormone level). (132-134)

Low Dose Naltrexone (LDN)

Naltrexone is an oral opiate antagonist initially developed in the 1970s to treat opiate addiction. Although available as 50 mg. tablets, Naltrexone capsules are available from compounding pharmacies at lower doses, usually 3-4.5 mg taken orally at night before sleep, providing benefits for various autoimmune diseases, neuropathic pain, and cancer. Although clinical trials for autoimmune thyroid disease are lacking, anecdotal reports have suggested a possible benefit in Hashimoto's' and Graves' Disease and Graves' Orbitopathy. Other than its obvious withdrawal effects in opiate addicts, LDN has virtually no adverse side effects, a factor that has liberalized its use. (135-140)

Vitamin C is Protective of the Toxic Effects of Excess Iodine

in 2022, Dr. Rong Sun studied Vitamin C in an animal model, finding that Vitamin C counteracts the oxidative damage caused by excess iodine intake, writing:

> **additional supplements of vitamin C are a better method to counteract the oxidative damage caused by excess iodine exposure.** Vitamin C represents one of the most prominent anti-oxidants both in plasma as well as intracellular regions; enables the quenching and scavenging of free radicals; and is required in the body for collagen formation in the bones, blood vessels, and muscles…In this study, it could be found that vitamin C can increase the activity of anti-oxidant enzymes, which decreased in the HI [Hi Iodine] group and had a protective effect on oxidative stress caused by excessive iodine… **Long-term chronic excessive iodine exposure caused oxidative damage in rats,** such as decreasing the activity of anti-oxidant enzymes and increasing the content of lipid peroxides, and there was a difference between females and males. **Vitamin C had a certain protective effect against oxidative damage induced by excess iodine exposure;** a high-dose intake of vitamin C reduced the content of MDA [Malondialdehyde, a lipid peroxide], while a low-dose intake of it promoted oxidative damage. (141)

In 2019, Dr. Karimi studied patients with autoimmune thyroid disease, finding administration of Vitamin C, 500 mg/day over 3 months reduced anti-thyroid antibody (TPO-Ab) levels to the same degree as selenium 200 mcg/d supplementation. (142-143)

For the above reasons, we routinely measure serum vitamin C levels and supplement to the upper half of the normal range (0.2-2.1 mg/dL).

Combination of Anti-Oxidants Beneficial in Graves' Disease

A 2005 study by Dr. Vesna Bacic-Vrca from Croatia evaluated the effects of supplementation with a combination of anti-oxidants (vitamins C and E, beta-carotene, and selenium) in a group of patients with Graves' disease (GD) treated with methimazole. The results show that patients receiving anti-oxidant supplementation and methimazole therapy achieve euthyroidism faster than those treated with methimazole alone. (144)

How to Address Underlying Autoimmune Cause of Thyroid Disease

1. Gluten sensitivity testing with anti-gliadin antibody and genetic testing. If positive, a Gluten-Free Diet is advisable.

2. Testing and supplementation for serum selenium, Vitamin C, Vitamin D3, magnesium RBC and spot urine for iodine.

3. Extended Food Reactivity testing and dietary modification to eliminate reactive foods.

4. Triple Therapy eradication if the H. Pylori Breath Test is positive.

5. Healing the Gut with Probiotics, Berberine, Gluten Free Diet, etc.

6. Low Dose Naltrexone, an immune modulator, has been useful in some autoimmune disease patients.

7. Iron and Ferritin testing and supplementation when found low.

8. Myo-Inositol supplementation improves TSH and Antibody levels in Hashimoto's Thyroiditis. This is discussed in Chapter 28 on Myo-inositol for Hashimoto's Thyroiditis.

Conclusion

One of the errors of modern endocrinology is to ignore the autoimmune component of Hashimotos' and Graves' disease. Treating the autoimmune component has a beneficial impact on the course of the disease.

♦ References Chapter 18

1) Hershman, Jerome M. "A Survey of Management of Uncomplicated Graves' Disease Shows That Use of Methimazole is Increasing and Use of Radioactive Iodine Is Decreasing." Children 95.3260 (2010).

2) Hoffer, A. "Adventures in Psychiatry: The Scientific Memoirs of Dr." Abram Hoffer (2005)

3) Hayes, Colleen E. "Vitamin D: a Natural Inhibitor of Multiple Sclerosis." Proceedings of the Nutrition Society 59.4 (2000): 531-535.

4) Mowry, Ellen M., et al. "Vitamin D Status Predicts New Brain Magnetic Resonance Imaging Activity in Multiple Sclerosis." Annals of Neurology 72.2 (2012): 234-240.

5) Pierrot-Deseilligny, Charles, and Jean-Claude Souberbielle. "Vitamin D and Multiple Sclerosis: An Update." Multiple Sclerosis and Related Disorders 14 (2017): 35-45.

6) Sîrbe, Claudia, et al. "An Update on The Effects of Vitamin D on the Immune System and Autoimmune Diseases." International Journal of Molecular Sciences 23.17 (2022): 9784.

7) Hahn, Jill, et al. "Vitamin D and Marine Omega 3 Fatty Acid Supplementation and Incident Autoimmune Disease: VITAL Randomized Controlled Trial." BMJ 376 (2022).

8) Borsche, Lorenz, et al. "COVID-19 Mortality Risk Correlates Inversely with Vitamin D3 Status, and a Mortality Rate Close to Zero Could Theoretically Be Achieved at 50 ng/ml 25 (OH) D3: Results of a Systematic Review and Meta-Analysis." Nutrients 13.10 (2021): 3596.

9) Johnson, Casey R., et al. "Serum 25-Hydroxyvitamin D and Subsequent Cancer Incidence and Mortality: A Population-Based Retrospective Cohort Study." Mayo Clinic Proceedings. Vol. 96. No. 8. Elsevier, 2021.

10) Park, Kye-Yeung, et al. "Serum 25-Hydroxyvitamin D Concentrations Are Inversely Associated with All-Cause Mortality Among Koreans: A Nationwide Cohort Study." Nutrition Research 113 (2023): 49-58.

11) Keum, N., et al. "Cancer Mortality Reduced 40 Percent by 2000 IU Vitamin D daily if Normal Weight–Meta-Analysis June 2022." Br J Cancer (2022).

12) Niedermaier, Tobias, et al. "Vitamin D Food Fortification in European Countries: The Underused Potential to Prevent Cancer Deaths." European Journal of Epidemiology (2022): 1-12.

13) Grant, William B., et al. "Targeted 25-Hydroxyvitamin D Concentration Measurements and Vitamin D3 Supplementation Can Have Important Patient and Public Health Benefits." European Journal of Clinical Nutrition 74.3 (2020): 366-376.

14) Palacios, Cristina, and Lilliana Gonzalez. "Is Vitamin D Deficiency a Major Global Public Health Problem?" The Journal of Steroid Biochemistry and Molecular Biology 144 (2014): 138-145.

15) Wilson, Louise R., et al. "Vitamin D Deficiency as a Public Health Issue: Using Vitamin D2 or Vitamin D3 In Future Fortification Strategies." Proceedings of the nutrition society 76.3 (2017): 392-399.

16) Galușca, Dorina, et al. "Vitamin D Implications and Effect of Supplementation in Endocrine Disorders: Autoimmune Thyroid Disorders (Hashimoto's Disease and Graves' Disease), Diabetes Mellitus and Obesity." Medicina 58.2 (2022): 194.

17) Vieira, Inês Henriques, et al. "Vitamin D and Autoimmune Thyroid Disease—Cause, Consequence, or a Vicious Cycle?" Nutrients 12.9 (2020): 2791.

18) Miteva, Mariya Zh, et al. "Vitamin D and Autoimmune Thyroid Diseases - A Review." Folia Medica 62.2 (2020): 223-229.

19) Płazińska, Maria Teresa, et al. "Vitamin D Deficiency and Thyroid Autoantibody Fluctuations in Patients with Graves' Disease–A Mere Coincidence or A Real Relationship?" Advances in Medical Sciences 65.1 (2020): 39-45.

20) Pratita, Winra, et sl. "Efficacy of Vitamin-D Supplement on Thyroid Profile in Children with Graves' Disease." Open Access Macedonian Journal of Medical Sciences 8. B (2020): 798-801.

21) Heisel, Curtis J., et al. "Serum Vitamin D Deficiency is an Independent Risk Factor for Thyroid Eye Disease." Ophthalmic Plastic and Reconstructive Surgery 36.1 (2020): 17-20.

22) Gallo, Daniela, et al. "Add-on Effect of Selenium and Vitamin D Combined Supplementation in Early Control of Graves' Disease Hyperthyroidism During Methimazole Treatment." Frontiers In Endocrinology 13 (2022).

23) Wright, Jonathan V, "The Root Cause of Your Autoimmune Disease – and Why Treating It Can Be Easier Than You Think", Nutrition & Healing Newsletter; Vol. 8 Issue 12, February 2012. https://www.faim.org/the-root-cause-of-your-autoimmune-disease-and-why-treating-it-can-be-easier-than-you-think

24) Fasano, Alessio. "All Disease Begins in the (Leaky) Gut: Role of Zonulin-Mediated Gut Permeability in the Pathogenesis of Some Chronic Inflammatory Diseases." F1000Research 9 (2020).

25) Lammers, Karen M., et al. "Gliadin Induces an Increase in Intestinal Permeability and Zonulin Release by Binding to the Chemokine Receptor CXCR3." Gastroenterology 135.1 (2008): 194-204.

26) Fasano, Alessio. "Zonulin, Regulation of Tight Junctions, and Autoimmune Diseases." Annals of the New York Academy of Sciences 1258.1 (2012): 25-33.

27) Fasano, Alessio. "Intestinal Permeability and its Regulation by Zonulin: Diagnostic and Therapeutic Implications." Clinical Gastroenterology and Hepatology 10.10 (2012): 1096-1100.

28) Fasano, Alessio. "Zonulin and its Regulation of Intestinal Barrier Function: The Biological Door to Inflammation, Autoimmunity, and Cancer." Physiological reviews (2011).

29) Fasano, Alessio. "Leaky Gut and Autoimmune Diseases." Clinical Reviews in Allergy and Immunology 42 (2012): 71-78.

32) Sturgeon, Craig, and Alessio Fasano. "Zonulin, a Regulator of Epithelial and Endothelial Barrier Functions, And Its Involvement in Chronic Inflammatory Diseases." Tissue Barriers 4.4 (2016): e1251384.

33) Benvenga, Salvatore, and Fabrizio Guarneri. "Molecular Mimicry and Autoimmune Thyroid Disease." Reviews in Endocrine and Metabolic Disorders 17.4 (2016): 485-498.

34) Rojas, Manuel, et al. "Molecular Mimicry and Autoimmunity." Journal of Autoimmunity 95 (2018): 100-123.

35) Leonard, Maureen M., et al. "Celiac Disease and Nonceliac Gluten Sensitivity: A Review." JAMA 318.7 (2017): 647-656.

36) Freeman, Hugh J. "Adult Celiac Disease and its Malignant Complications." Gut and Liver 3.4 (2009): 237.

37) Nejad, Mohammad Rostami, et al. "Atypical Presentation Is Dominant and Typical for Coeliac Disease." Journal of Gastrointestinal & Liver Diseases 18.3 (2009).

38) Collin, P., et al. "Coeliac Disease in Later Life Must Not Be Missed." Alimentary Pharmacology & Therapeutics 47.5 (2018): 563-572.

39) Talarico, Valentina, et al. "Iron Deficiency Anemia in Celiac Disease." Nutrients 13.5 (2021): 1695.

40) Rastogi, Ashu, et al. "Celiac Disease: A Missed Cause of Metabolic Bone Disease." Indian Journal of Endocrinology and Metabolism 16.5 (2012): 780.

41) Pinto-Sanchez, María Inés, et al. "Gluten-Free Diet Reduces Symptoms, Particularly Diarrhea, in Patients with Irritable Bowel Syndrome and Antigliadin IgG." Clinical Gastroenterology and Hepatology 19.11 (2021): 2343-2352.

42) Ch'ng, Chin Lye, et al. "Prospective Screening for Coeliac Disease in Patients with Graves' Hyperthyroidism Using Anti-Gliadin and Tissue Transglutaminase Antibodies." Clinical Endocrinology 62.3 (2005): 303-306.

43) Coucke, Francis. "Food Intolerance in Patients with Manifest Autoimmunity. Observational Study." Autoimmunity Reviews 17.11 (2018): 1078-1080.

44) Mansueto, Pasquale, et al. "Autoimmunity Features in Patients with Non-Celiac Wheat Sensitivity." Official Journal of the American College of Gastroenterology| ACG 116.5 (2021): 1015-1023.

45) Hatfield, Dolph L., and Vadim N. Gladyshev. "How Selenium Has Altered Our Understanding of the Genetic Code." Molecular and Cellular Biology 22.11 (2002): 3565-3576.

46) Korotkov, Konstantin V., et al. "Mammalian Selenoprotein in Which Selenocysteine (Sec) Incorporation Is Supported by a New Form of Sec Insertion Sequence Element." Molecular and Cellular Biology 22.5 (2002): 1402-1411.

47) Gladyshev, Vadim N., and Dolph L. Hatfield. "Selenocysteine-Containing Proteins in Mammals." Journal of Biomedical Science 6.3 (1999): 151-160.

48) Rayman, Margaret P., and Leonidas H. Duntas. "Selenium Deficiency and Thyroid Disease." The Thyroid and its Diseases: A Comprehensive Guide for the Clinician (2019): 109-126.

49) Al-Taie, Oliver H., et al. "Selenium Supplementation Enhances Low Selenium Levels and Stimulates Glutathione Peroxidase Activity in Peripheral Blood and Distal Colon Mucosa in Past and Present Carriers of Colon Adenomas." Nutrition And Cancer 46.2 (2003): 125-130.

50) Beckett, Geoffrey J., et al. "Inhibition of Type I and Type II Iodothyronine Deiodinase Activity in Rat Liver, Kidney and Brain Produced by Selenium Deficiency." Biochemical Journal 259.3 (1989): 887-892.

51) Köhrle, Josef. "Selenium and the Thyroid." Current Opinion in Endocrinology & Diabetes and Obesity 22.5 (2015): 392-401.

52) Tsuji, Petra A., et al. "Historical Roles of Selenium and Selenoproteins in Health and Development: The Good, the Bad and the Ugly." International Journal of Molecular Sciences 23.1 (2021): 5

53) Hariharan, Sneha, and Selvakumar Dharmaraj. "Selenium and Selenoproteins: Its Role in Regulation of Inflammation." Inflammopharmacology 28.3 (2020): 667-695.

54) Radomska, Dominika, et al. "Selenium as a Bioactive Micronutrient in the Human Diet and its Cancer Chemopreventive Activity." Nutrients 13.5 (2021): 1649.

55) Wu, Qian, et al. "Increased Incidence of Hashimoto Thyroiditis in Selenium Deficiency: A Prospective 6-Year Cohort Study." The Journal of Clinical Endocrinology & Metabolism 107.9 (2022): e3603-e3611.

56) Davcheva, Delyana M., et al. "Serum Selenium Concentration in Patients with Autoimmune Thyroid Disease." Folia Medica 64.3 (2022): 443-449.

57) Kryczyk-Kozioł, Jadwiga, et al. "Positive Effects of Selenium Supplementation in Women with Newly Diagnosed Hashimoto's Thyroiditis in an Area with Low Selenium Status." International Journal of Clinical Practice 75.9 (2021): e14484.

58) Wang, Lan-Feng, et al. "The Effects of Selenium Supplementation on Antibody Titers in Patients with Hashimoto's Thyroiditis." Endokrynologia Polska 72.6 (2021): 666-667.

59) Davcheva, Delyana M., et al. "Serum Selenium Concentration in Patients with Autoimmune Thyroid Disease." Folia Medica 64.3 (2022): 443-449.

60) Karimi, F., and G. R. Omrani. "Effects of Selenium and Vitamin C on the Serum Level of Anti-Thyroid Peroxidase Antibody in Patients with Autoimmune Thyroiditis." (2019): 481-487.

61) Krysiak, Robert, et al. "Selenomethionine Potentiates the Impact of Vitamin D on Thyroid Autoimmunity in Euthyroid Women with Hashimoto's Thyroiditis and Low Vitamin D Status." Pharmacological Reports 71.2 (2019): 367-373.

62) Pace, Cinzia, et al. "Role of Selenium and Myo-Inositol Supplementation on Autoimmune Thyroiditis Progression." Endocrine Journal (2020): EJ20-0062.

63) Rayman, Margaret P. "The Importance of Selenium to Human Health." The Lancet 356.9225 (2000): 233-241.

64) Winther, Kristian Hillert, et al. "Selenium in Thyroid Disorders—Essential Knowledge for Clinicians." Nature Reviews Endocrinology 16.3 (2020): 165-176.

65) Yoshihara, Ai, et al. "Characteristics of Patients with Graves' Disease Whose Thyroid Hormone Levels Increase After Substituting Potassium Iodide for Methimazole in the First Trimester of Pregnancy." Thyroid 30.3 (2020): 451-456.

66) Yoshihara, Ai, et al. "Substituting Potassium Iodide for Methimazole as the Treatment for Graves' Disease During the First Trimester May Reduce the Incidence of Congenital Anomalies: A Retrospective Study at a Single Medical Institution in Japan." Thyroid 25.10 (2015): 1155-1161.

67) Okamura, Ken, et al. "Iodide-Sensitive Graves' Hyperthyroidism and the Strategy for Resistant or Escaped Patients During Potassium Iodide Treatment." Endocrine Journal (2022): EJ21-0436.

68) Zhu, Zongjian, et al. "Selenium Concentration and Glutathione Peroxidase Activity in Selenium and Magnesium Deficient Rats." Biological trace element research 37.2 (1993): 209-217.

69) Moncayo, Roy, et al. "Global View on The Pathogenesis of Benign Thyroid Disease Based on Historical, Experimental, Biochemical and Genetic Data, Identifying the Role of Magnesium, Selenium, Coenzyme Q10, and Iron in the Context of the Unfolded Protein Response and Protein Quality Control of Thyroglobulin." Journal of Translational Genetics and Genomics 4.4 (2020): 356-383.

70) Eleftheriadou, Anna-Maria, et al. "Re-Visiting Autoimmunity to Sodium-Iodide Symporter and Pendrin in Thyroid Disease." European Journal of Endocrinology 183.6 (2020): 571-580.

71) Czarnocka, Barbara. "Thyroperoxidase, Thyroglobulin, Na (+)/I (-) Symporter, Pendrin in Thyroid Autoimmunity." Frontiers in Bioscience-Landmark 16.2 (2011): 783-802.

72) Seissler, Jochen, et al. "Low Frequency of Autoantibodies to The Human Na+/I− Symporter in Patients with Autoimmune Thyroid Disease." The Journal of Clinical Endocrinology & Metabolism 85.12 (2000): 4630-4634.

73) Kalderon, A. E., and H. A. Bogaars. "Immune Complex Deposits in Graves' Disease and Hashimoto's Thyroiditis." The American Journal of Medicine 63.5 (1977): 729-734.

74) Kalderon, A. E., et al. "Electron-Dense Deposits in The Follicular Basal Lamina of Obese Strain Chickens with Spontaneous Hereditary Autoimmune Thyroiditis. An Electron Microscopic Study." Laboratory Investigation; a Journal of Technical Methods and Pathology 37.5 (1977): 487-496.

75) Gallo, Daniela, et al. "Add-on Effect of Selenium and Vitamin D Combined Supplementation in Early Control of Graves' Disease Hyperthyroidism During Methimazole Treatment." Frontiers In Endocrinology 13 (2022).

76) Hotz, Christine S., et al. "Dietary Iodine and Selenium Interact to Affect Thyroid Hormone Metabolism of Rats." The Journal of Nutrition 127.6 (1997): 1214-1218.

77) Xu, Jian, et al. "Supplemental Selenium Alleviates the Toxic Effects of Excessive Iodine on the Thyroid." Biological Trace Element Research 141.1 (2011): 110-118.

78) Xu, Jian, et al. "Selenium Supplement Alleviated the Toxic Effects of Excessive Iodine in Mice." Biological Trace Element Research 111 (2006): 229-238.

79) Vasiliu, Ioana, et al. "Protective Role of Selenium on Thyroid Morphology in Iodine-Induced Autoimmune Thyroiditis in Wistar Rats." Experimental and Therapeutic Medicine 20.4 (2020): 3425-3437.

80) Vasiliu, Ioana, et al. "Experimentally Induced Autoimmune Thyroiditis in Wistar Rats: Possible Protective Role of Selenium." Endocrine Abstracts. Vol. 70. Bioscientifica, 2020.

81) Corvilain, Bernard, et al. "Stimulation by Iodide of H2O2 Generation in Thyroid Slices from Several Species." American Journal of Physiology-Endocrinology and Metabolism 278.4 (2000): E692-E699.

82) Mikura, Kentaro, et al. "Radioiodine Uptake After Monotherapy with Potassium Iodide in Patients with Graves' Disease." Endocrine Journal (2023): EJ22-0505.

83) Al-Muqbel, Kusai M., and Reema M. Tashtoush. "Patterns of Thyroid Radioiodine Uptake: Jordanian Experience." Journal of Nuclear Medicine Technology 38.1 (2010): 32-36.

84) Ballal, Sanjana, et al. "Re-Establishment of Normal Radioactive Iodine Uptake Reference Range in the Era of Universal Salt Iodization in the Indian Population." The Indian Journal of Medical Research 145.3 (2017): 358.

85) Sun, Qian, et al. "Natural Autoimmunity to Selenoprotein P Impairs Selenium Transport in Hashimoto's Thyroiditis." International Journal of Molecular Sciences 22.23 (2021): 13088.

86) Liontiris, Michael I., and Elias E. Mazokopakis. "A Concise Review of Hashimoto Thyroiditis (HT) and the Importance of Iodine, Selenium, Vitamin D and Gluten on the Autoimmunity and Dietary Management of HT Patients. Points That Need More Investigation." Hell J Nucl Med 20.1 (2017): 51-56.

87) Wang, Kunling, et al. "Severely Low Serum Magnesium Is Associated with Increased Risks of Positive Anti-Thyroglobulin Antibody and Hypothyroidism: A Cross-Sectional Study." Scientific Reports 8.1 (2018): 1-9.

88) Rayman, Margaret P. "Multiple Nutritional Factors and Thyroid Disease, with Particular Reference to Autoimmune Thyroid Disease." Proceedings of the Nutrition Society 78.1 (2019): 34-44.

89) Fayadat, Laurence, et al. "Role of Heme in Intracellular Trafficking of Thyroperoxidase and Involvement of H2O2 Generated at the Apical Surface of Thyroid Cells in Autocatalytic Covalent Heme Binding." Journal of Biological Chemistry 274.15 (1999): 10533-10538.

90) Lahner, Edith, et al. "Thyro-Entero-Gastric Autoimmunity: Pathophysiology and Implications for Patient Management." Best Practice & Research Clinical Endocrinology & Metabolism 34.1 (2020): 101373.

91) Massironi, Sara, et al. "The Changing Face of Chronic Autoimmune Atrophic Gastritis: An Updated Comprehensive Perspective." Autoimmunity Reviews 18.3 (2019): 215-222.

92) Gianoukakis, Andrew G., et al. "Graves' Disease Patients with Iron Deficiency Anemia: Serologic Evidence of Co-Existent Autoimmune Gastritis." American Journal of Blood Research 11.3 (2021): 238.

93) Zangiabadian, Moein, et al. "Associations of Yersinia Enterocolitica Infection with Autoimmune Thyroid Diseases: A Systematic Review and Meta-Analysis." Endocrine, Metabolic & Immune Disorders-Drug Targets 21.4 (2021): 682-687.

94) Marshall, Barry J., et al. "A 20-Minute Breath Test for Helicobacter Pylori." American Journal of Gastroenterology (Springer Nature) 86.4 (1991).

95) Hellström, Per M. "This Year's Nobel Prize to Gastroenterology: Robin Warren and Barry Marshall Awarded for Their Discovery of Helicobacter Pylori as a Pathogen in the Gastrointestinal Tract." World Journal of Gastroenterology: WJG 12.19 (2006): 3126.

96) Marshall, Barry. "A Brief History of the Discovery of Helicobacter Pylori." Helicobacter Pylori. Springer, Tokyo, 2016. 3-15.

97) Marshall, Barry J. "One Hundred Years of Discovery and Rediscovery of Helicobacter Pylori and its Association with Peptic Ulcer Disease." Helicobacter Pylori: Physiology and Genetics (2001): 19-24.

98) Thiyagarajan, Santhanamari, et al. "Helicobacter Pylori-Induced Autoimmune Thyroiditis: Is the Pathogenic Link Concluded or Still a Hypothesis?" Reviews in Medical Microbiology 29.2 (2018): 64-72.

99) Youssefi, Masoud, et al. "Helicobacter Pylori Infection and Autoimmune Diseases; Is There an Association with Systemic Lupus Erythematosus, Rheumatoid Arthritis, Autoimmune Atrophy Gastritis and Autoimmune Pancreatitis? A Systematic Review and Meta-Analysis Study." Journal of Microbiology, Immunology, and Infection 54.3 (2021): 359-369.

100) Figura, Natale, et al. "Helicobacter Pylori Infection and Autoimmune Thyroid Diseases: The Role of Virulent Strains." Antibiotics 9.1 (2019): 12.

101) Abdalla, Taghrid Mohamed, et al. "The Association Between Helicobacter Pylori and Graves' Disease." Afro-Egyptian Journal of Infectious and Endemic Diseases 8.4 (2018): 196-201.

102) Raafat, Mohammed Nabil, et al. "Correlation Between Autoimmune Thyroid Diseases and Helicobacter Pylori Infection." The Egyptian Journal of Hospital Medicine 76.7 (2019): 4499-4505.

103) Oudah, Marwah Ali. "Relationship Between H. Pylori Patients and Autoimmune Thyroid Disease." Indian Journal of Forensic Medicine & Toxicology 14.3 (2020).

104) Thiyagarajan, Santhanamari, et al. "Helicobacter Pylori-Induced Autoimmune Thyroiditis: Is the Pathogenic Link Concluded or Still a Hypothesis?" Reviews in Medical Microbiology 29.2 (2018): 64-72.

105) Elmahalawy, Mostafa Haseeb, et al. "Study of Chronic Atrophic Gastritis in Patients with Autoimmune Thyroid Disease." Al-Azhar International Medical Journal (2021).

106) Bassi, Vincenzo, et al. "Autoimmune Thyroid Diseases and Helicobacter Pylori." Open Journal of Thyroid Research 1.1 (2017): 001-003.

107) Wang, Li, et al. "Helicobacter Pylori and Autoimmune Diseases: Involving Multiple Systems." Frontiers in Immunology 13 (2022).

108) Shmuely, Haim, et al. "Helicobacter Pylori Infection in Women with Hashimoto Thyroiditis: A Case-Control Study." Medicine 95.29 (2016).

109) Choi, Yun Mi, et al. "Association Between Thyroid Autoimmunity and Helicobacter Pylori Infection." The Korean Journal of Internal Medicine 32.2 (2017): 309.

110) De Luis, Daniel A., et al. "Helicobacter Pylori Infection Is Markedly Increased in Patients with Autoimmune Atrophic Thyroiditis." Journal of Clinical Gastroenterology 26.4 (1998): 259-263.

111) Figura, N. et al. "The Infection by Helicobacter Pylori Strains Expressing CAGA Is Highly Prevalent in Women with Autoimmune Thyroid Disorders." Journal of Physiology and Pharmacology 50.5 (1999): 817-826.

112) Choi, I. J., et al. "Efficacy of Low-Dose Clarithromycin Triple Therapy and Tinidazole-Containing Triple Therapy for Helicobacter Pylori Eradication." Alimentary pharmacology & therapeutics 16.1 (2002): 145-151.

113) McNicholl, Adrian G., et al. "Combination of Bismuth and Standard Triple Therapy Eradicates Helicobacter Pylori Infection in More Than 90% Of Patients." Clinical Gastroenterology and Hepatology 18.1 (2020): 89-98.

114) Fang, Hao-Ran, et al. "Efficacy of Lactobacillus-Supplemented Triple Therapy for Helicobacter Pylori Infection in Children: A Meta-Analysis of Randomized Controlled Trials." European Journal of Pediatrics 178.1 (2019): 7-16.

115) Bertalot, Giovanni, et al. "Decrease in Thyroid Autoantibodies After Eradication of Helicobacter Pylori Infection." Clinical Endocrinology 61.5 (2004): 650-652.

116) Hou, Yi, et al. "Meta-Analysis of the Correlation Between Helicobacter Pylori Infection and Autoimmune Thyroid Diseases." Oncotarget 8.70 (2017): 115691.

117) Taguchi, Hiroki, et al. "Helicobacter Pylori Eradication Improves the Quality of Life Regardless of the Treatment Outcome: A Multicenter Prospective Cohort Study." Medicine 96.52 (2017).

118) Huo, Dongxue, et al. "Probiotic Bifidobacterium Longum Supplied with Methimazole Improved the Thyroid Function of Graves' Disease Patients Through the Gut-Thyroid Axis." Communications Biology 4 (2021).

119) Virili, Camilla, et al. "Gut Microbiome and Thyroid Autoimmunity." Best Practice & Research Clinical Endocrinology & Metabolism 35.3 (2021): 101506.

120) Hou, Jueyu, et al. "The Role of the Microbiota in Graves' Disease and Graves' Orbitopathy." Frontiers in Cellular and Infection Microbiology (2021): 1301.

121) Jiang, Wen, et al. "Gut Microbiota May Play a Significant Role in the Pathogenesis of Graves' Disease." Thyroid 31.5 (2021): 810.

123) Ruscio, Michael, et al. "The Relationship Between Gastrointestinal Health, Micronutrient Concentrations, and Autoimmunity: A Focus on the Thyroid." Nutrients 14.17 (2022): 3572.

124) Han, Zhe, et al. "The Potential Prebiotic Berberine Combined with Methimazole Improved the Therapeutic Effect of Graves' Disease Patients Through Regulating the Intestinal Microbiome." Frontiers in Immunology 12 (2021).

125) Diao, J., et al. "Potential Therapeutic Activity of Berberine in Thyroid-Associated Ophthalmopathy: Inhibitory Effects on Tissue Remodeling in Orbital Fibroblasts." Investigative Ophthalmology & Visual Science 63.10 (2022): 6-6.

126) Cheng, Hao, et al. "Interactions Between Gut Microbiota and Berberine, A Necessary Procedure to Understand the Mechanisms of Berberine." Journal of Pharmaceutical Analysis (2021).

127) Yang, Shengjie, et al. "Multi-Pharmacology of Berberine in Atherosclerosis and Metabolic Diseases: Potential Contribution of Gut Microbiota." Frontiers in Pharmacology 12 (2021): 1774.

128) Tang, Min, Daixiu Yuan, and Peng Liao. "Berberine Improves Intestinal Barrier Function and Reduces Inflammation, Immunosuppression, and Oxidative Stress by Regulating the NF-Kb/MAPK Signaling Pathway in Deoxynivalenol-Challenged Piglets." Environmental Pollution 289 (2021): 117865.

129) Li, Yanning, et al. "Berberine Reduces Gut-Vascular Barrier Permeability Via Modulation of Apom/S1P Pathway in a Model of Polymicrobial Sepsis." Life Sciences 261 (2020): 118460.

130) Hou, Qiuke, et al. "Berberine Improves Intestinal Epithelial Tight Junctions by Upregulating A20 Expression In IBS-D Mice." Biomedicine & Pharmacotherapy 118 (2019): 109206.

131) Wang, Yuzhen, et al. "Berberine Ameliorates Intestinal Mucosal Barrier Dysfunction in Nonalcoholic Fatty Liver Disease (NAFLD) Rats." Journal of King Saud University-Science 32.5 (2020): 2534-2539.

132) Douglas, Raymond S., et al. "Teprotumumab Efficacy, Safety, And Durability in Longer-Duration Thyroid Eye Disease and Re-Treatment: OPTIC-X Study." Ophthalmology 129.4 (2022): 438-449.

133) Douglas, Raymond S., et al. "Teprotumumab for the Treatment of Active Thyroid Eye Disease." New England Journal of Medicine 382.4 (2020): 341-352.

134) Kahaly, George J., et al. "Teprotumumab for Patients with Active Thyroid Eye Disease: A Pooled Data Analysis, Subgroup Analyses, And Off-Treatment Follow-Up Results from Two Randomized, Double-Masked, Placebo-Controlled, Multicentre Trials." The Lancet Diabetes & Endocrinology 9.6 (2021): 360-372.

135) McDermott, Michael T. "Low-Dose Naltrexone Treatment of Hashimoto's Thyroiditis." Management of Patients with Pseudo-Endocrine Disorders. Springer, Cham, 2019. 317-326.

136) Kim, Yoon Hang John. "Case Report: Reversing Hypothyroidism with Low Dose Naltrexone (LDN)." Multiple sclerosis 3: 4.

137) Wentz, Izabella. "Low Dose Naltrexone and Hashimoto's" (2023) https://focusonallergies-com.ngontinh24.com/article/low-dose-naltrexone-and-hashimoto-s-dr-izabella-wentz

138) Moore, Elaine A., and Lisa Marie Moore. Advances in Graves' Disease and Other Hyperthyroid Disorders. McFarland, 2013.

139) Li, Zijian, et al. "Low-Dose Naltrexone (LDN): A Promising Treatment in Immune-Related Diseases and Cancer Therapy." International Immunopharmacology 61 (2018): 178-184.

140) Toljan, Karlo, and Bruce Vrooman. "Low-Dose Naltrexone (LDN)—Review of Therapeutic Utilization." Medical Sciences 6.4 (2018): 82.

141) Sun, Rong, et al. "Protection of Vitamin C on Oxidative Damage Caused by Long-Term Excess Iodine Exposure in Wistar Rats." Nutrients 14.24 (2022): 5245.

142) Karimi, F., and G. R. Omrani. "Effects of Selenium and Vitamin C on the Serum Level of Anti-Thyroid Peroxidase Antibody in Patients with Autoimmune Thyroiditis." Journal of Endocrinological Investigation 42.4 (2019): 481-487.

143) Abdul-Majeed, Abdullah F., et al. "Effect of Vitamin C as Anti-Oxidant on Stressed Quail Induced by Hydrogen Peroxide." Euphrates Journal of Agriculture Science 13.4 (2021).

144) Bacic-Vrca, Vesna, et al. "The Effect of Anti-Oxidant Supplementation on Superoxide Dismutase Activity, Cu and Zn Levels, and Total Anti-Oxidant Status in Erythrocytes of Patients with Graves' Disease." Clinical Chemistry and Laboratory Medicine (CCLM) 43.4 (2005): 383-388.

Chapter 19

Iodine Induced Hyperthyroidism – the Autonomous Thyroid Nodule

BRENDA IS A 26-YEAR-OLD NURSE seen at my office for menstrual irregularities, and upon evaluation and testing was found to have a spot urine test of 32 mcg/L, indicating severe iodine deficiency. Although Brenda had been in the U.S. for twenty years, she was born and grew up in one of the Caribbean islands. Because of the severe iodine deficiency, Brenda began iodine supplementation with iodized salt. About a week later, Brenda experienced an episode of tachycardia, a severe rapid heart rate, with a sustained pulse rate of 220 beats per minute. The tachycardia resolved spontaneously shortly after arriving at the local emergency room. The doctors had no explanation for the tachycardia, and Brenda was sent home with a Beta-Blocker Drug called propranolol to slow the heart rate should the tachycardia return.

What Caused Brenda's Tachycardia? The Autonomous Nodule.

Brenda's tachycardia was a symptom of hyperthyroidism from an autonomous thyroid nodule. When Brenda began the iodized salt, the autonomous nodule converted the new iodine into excess thyroid hormone. This is an example of hyperthyroidism associated with dietary iodine intake. The autonomous thyroid nodule manufactures thyroid hormone uncontrollably depending on iodine availability, outside of the normal control mechanism of TSH (thyroid stimulating hormone). When these patients ingest dietary iodine, they become thyrotoxic, and new lab studies will typically reveal a very low TSH, high Free T3, and high Free T4. Despite the very low TSH, the autonomous nodule continues to take up iodine and produce large amounts of thyroid hormone. Yet, because the TSH is so low from the thyroid hormone from the autonomous nodule,

the surrounding normal thyroid tissue has very little iodine uptake. The nodule appears hot, with high iodine uptake, while the background is "cold" with very little uptake. Thus, explaining the "hot nodule" appearance of the autonomous nodule on the I-123 radio-nuclide scan (also called scintigram).

The Sonogram and Radio-Nuclide Thyroid Scan

Brenda was advised to stop the dietary iodine and sent for diagnostic imaging. Sure enough, Brenda's thyroid sonogram showed the nodule, which was "hot" on the I-123 radio-nuclide scan indicating an autonomous nodule. (1-7)

Thyroxine Suppression Test

In some cases, the nodule may not be hot enough to be visible on the radionuclide scan. A Thyroxine Suppression Test is sometimes used to improve visibility. The I-123 (radioisotope iodine 123) scan is repeated after giving levothyroxine, which suppresses I-123 uptake in the remaining normal thyroid tissue yet does not affect the autonomous nodule, making the hot nodule stand out from the suppressed background thyroid tissue. (1-7)

Mutational Events Lead to Autonomy of Function

In 1998, Dr. John Stanbury concluded the most common cause of iodine-induced hyperthyroidism is mutational events leading to an autonomous nodule, writing:

> The biological basis for IIH (iodine-induced hyperthyroidism) appears most often to be **mutational events** in thyroid cells that lead to **autonomy of function**. When the mass of cells with such an event becomes

sufficient, and the iodine supply is increased, the **subject may become thyrotoxic**. These changes may occur in localized foci within the gland or in the process of nodule formation. (7)

What is an Autonomous Nodule?

Medical research since 1998 has shown that autonomous thyroid nodules are made up of clones of cells with a mutated TSH receptor. TSH is Thyroid Stimulating Hormone. Mutations in the TSH Receptor (TSHR) typically occur due to iodine deficiency in individuals who grow up in areas with low iodine levels during childhood. Mutations in the gene for the TSH receptor make these nodules independent of TSH control. Thus, based on the availability of iodine, the autonomous nodule makes thyroid hormone uncontrollably. (8-13)

What is the Etiology of Autonomous Nodules? H202 is Mutagenic

What causes the autonomous nodule? Remember, iodine is needed to produce thyroid hormones, and iodine deficiency impairs this process, rendering the patient hypothyroid. The pituitary responds to low thyroid hormone levels by secreting more TSH, resulting in high TSH blood levels. The TSH travels in the bloodstream to the thyroid gland and where it stimulates all steps in thyroid hormone production, including the generation of hydrogen peroxide. If the patient happens to have a selenium deficiency, the selenium-based anti-oxidant system will be deficient, with impaired degradation of hydrogen peroxide. This excess hydrogen peroxide is toxic, highly oxidative, and mutagenic to thyroid cells. Oxidative damage to thyroid cells leads to mutations in the DNA, including mutations to the DNA for the TSH receptor. Such a mutation within a clone of thyroid cells creates the autonomous nodule. Note: this is the same mechanism for carcinogenesis. In 2007, Dr. Knut Krohn writes:

We reconstruct a line of events that could explain the predominant neoplastic character (i.e., originating from a single mutated cell) of thyroid nodular lesions. This process might be triggered by the **oxidative** nature of thyroid hormone synthesis or additional oxidative stress **caused by iodine deficiency** or smoking. If the anti-oxidant defense is not effective, this **oxidative stress can cause DNA damage** followed by an increase in the spontaneous mutation rate, which is a platform for tumor genesis. **The hallmark of thyroid physiology—H2O2 [hydrogen peroxide] production during hormone synthesis—is therefore very likely to be the ultimate cause of frequent mutagenesis in the thyroid gland**. DNA damage and mutagenesis could provide the basis for the frequent **nodular transformation of endemic goiters**. (14-16)

Universal Salt Iodination (USI)

In 1924, based on the work of Drs. David Marine and David Cowie, the United States, began a program of iodine supplementation with iodized salt. This was done as a public health measure to reduce the health risks associated with iodine deficiency in the population. Health risks in newborns and young children include impaired growth, delayed neurodevelopment, impaired cognitive function in newborns, and goiter in young children. In 2020, Dr. Michael B Zimmerman writes:

Iodine deficiency has multiple adverse effects in humans due to inadequate thyroid hormone production... Iodine deficiency during pregnancy and infancy may impair growth and neurodevelopment of the offspring and increase infant mortality. Deficiency during childhood reduces somatic growth and cognitive and motor function... In most countries, the best strategy to control iodine deficiency in populations is carefully monitored iodization of salt. (17-20)

The Autonomous Nodule Originates in an Iodine Deficient Region

In 2015, Dr. Michael Zimmermann writes iodine deficiency is the underlying cause of most thyroid disorders, including autonomous nodules, toxic nodular goiter, benign nodules, benign goiter, and thyroid cancer. The iodine deficiency causes hypothyroidism which leads to elevated TSH, which, in turn, stimulates thyroid growth, goiter, and excess hydrogen peroxide production. If hydrogen peroxide production exceeds the capacity of the selenoprotein anti-oxidant system, this leads to oxidizing damage and mutagenicity. Occasionally, this leads to mutations in the TSH receptor, creating an autonomous nodule. A similar pathology, the toxic nodular goiter, contains multiple thyroid nodules, one or more of which is an autonomous nodule. When iodized salt is introduced into such a population, the individuals with autonomous thyroid nodules become thyrotoxic. Dr. Michael Zimmermann writes:

> iodine status is also a key determinant of thyroid disorders in adults. Severe iodine deficiency causes goiter and hypothyroidism **...increased thyroid activity [from elevated TSH] can compensate for low iodine intake and maintain euthyroidism** in most individuals but at a price: **chronic thyroid stimulation [from elevated TSH] results in an increase in the prevalence of toxic nodular goiter and hyperthyroidism** [from autonomous nodule] in populations. **This high prevalence of nodular autonomy usually results in a further increase in the prevalence of hyperthyroidism if iodine intake is subsequently increased by salt iodization...** Thus, optimization of population iodine intake is an important component of preventive health care to reduce the prevalence of thyroid disorders. (17-20)

Iodized Salt Eliminates Autonomous Nodules

With the elimination of iodine deficiency after the introduction of iodized salt in 1924, autonomous nodules became quite rare in the United States. Most cases we see now are patients migrating from iodine-deficient geographic regions outside the United States. These people may harbor autonomous nodules, presenting with features of transient hyperthyroidism when supplemented with dietary iodine. In the near future, the medical system may see an increase in autonomous nodules as migration increases from areas of endemic iodine deficiency and goiter outside the U.S. (21-28)

Hyperthyroidism After Iodized Salt Fortification

Even small amounts of dietary iodine found in iodized salt can cause transient hyperthyroidism in patients with autonomous nodules. Public records show a transient increase in mortality from thyrotoxicosis in 1926-1928 after the introduction of iodized salt. This was thought to be due to the presence of pre-existing autonomous nodules in the population that became thyrotoxic after the introduction of iodized salt. Likewise, in various other countries, iodized salt and iodized bread programs were introduced, and again a transient increase in thyrotoxicosis was reported shortly afterward. These cases were thought to be autonomous nodules responding to dietary iodine supplements. Note: some of these cases were toxic nodular goiters with one or more autonomous nodules. (29-36)

Thyrotoxicosis Caused by Iodine-Containing Medications

In addition to iodized salt programs, thyrotoxicosis in the autonomous nodule patient may be caused by various iodine-containing drugs such as amiodarone (Type I Thyrotoxicosis) and iodinated radiographic contrast material. Again, this is due to the rare patient harboring an autonomous nodule or toxic nodular goiter which responds to the iodine load by going into a thyroid storm (thyrotoxicosis). (37-38)

Iodine-Induced Thyrotoxicosis in Normal Thyroid Gland?

In a number of case reports appearing in the medical literature discussing iodine as the cause of hyperthyroidism in normal thyroid glands, one wonders if these so-called "normal thyroid glands" harbored autonomous nodules or diffuse areas of autonomous tissue that may not be visible on imaging and are simply missed. Another possible etiology for iodine-induced thyrotoxicosis in the so-called "normal thyroid gland" is Painless Thyroiditis. This is an inflammatory condition with the release of preformed thyroid hormone from ruptured follicles characterized by low radio-iodine uptake, as discussed below. (39-40)

Marine-Lenhart Syndrome

As mentioned previously in Chapters 15 and 16, potassium iodide is commonly used in Japan as a thyroid-blocking drug for the treatment of Graves' thyrotoxicosis. However, about 10-12 percent of such cases do not respond or are made worse by iodine. Could some of these cases be explained by autonomous functioning thyroid tissue? This is the Marine-Lenhart Syndrome (MLS), defined as Graves' disease with thyroid nodular lesions and clinical characteristics of both Graves' disease and Plummer's disease (toxic nodular goiter). In 2021, Dr. Hirosuke Danno found a 0.26 percent prevalence of MLS among Graves' Disease patients in Japan. This is not a high enough prevalence to explain the 10-12 percent rate of iodine escape found in 2015 by Dr. Yoshihara when switching pregnant Graves' disease patients from methimazole to iodine. However, the co-existence of Plummers with Graves' is something to keep in mind when presented with a Graves' disease patient with atypical imaging and clinical features. The imaging and clinical exam may reveal multiple nodules instead of the usual diffuse smooth enlargement indicating the possible coexistence of toxic nodular goiter (Plummer's Disease) with Graves' disease. Obviously, potassium iodide administration is contraindicated and will only make symptoms worse in these atypical cases. (41-45)

Expression of NIS in Autonomous Nodules

In 1999, Dr. Meller demonstrated overexpression of the Na+/I- symporter (NIS) in autonomous nodules, providing an explanation for enhanced uptake and clearance of iodine on radionuclide scan. As mentioned above, this high radio-iodine uptake of the autonomous nodule explains the utility of radionuclide imaging with 99mTc-pertechnetate or I-123, sometimes requiring levothyroxine suppression to enhance visualization. (1-7)

Toxic Multinodular Goiter and Medical Iodophobia

Toxic multinodular goiter is clinically similar to the autonomous nodule. Both are caused by chronic iodine deficiency, usually by growing up in an iodine-deficient country or region. A nodular goiter becomes "toxic" when one of the nodules within the thyroid is transformed into an autonomous nodule. Typically, this will cause thyrotoxicosis whenever the patient consumes dietary iodine. Palpation and imaging of the toxic nodular goiter typically reveal multiple nodules within an enlarged thyroid gland (multinodular goiter). Several case reports in the medical literature report thyrotoxicosis after iodine consumption. Typically, these cases describe a multinodular goiter that harbors at least one autonomous nodule followed by thyrotoxicosis after some form of iodine exposure. In 2018, Dr. Jayme Taylor reported a case of thyrotoxicosis in a patient with multiple thyroid nodules after taking an iodine supplement. Although this was clearly a routine case of iodine exposure in a patient with toxic nodular goiter, it provided the authors an opportunity to blame and disparage iodine supplements, revealing a mainstream bias against the use of iodine, called "medical iodophobia," a term coined in 2004 by Dr. Guy Abraham as the fear of using iodine supplements to treat iodine deficiency. In 2013, Dr. Brotfain reported a case of thyrotoxicosis in a patient with toxic multi-nodular goiter. In this case, the source of iodine exposure was an iodine-containing antiseptic solution in the operating room and ICU. (46-50)

Treatment of Toxic Adenoma and Toxic Multinodular Goiter

Treatment of thyrotoxicosis caused by autonomous thyroid nodule or toxic nodular goiter consists firstly of removing the source of iodine exposure, and then one of the following:

1) **Thyroid Blocking Drugs:** also called medical treatment. The most used drug is methimazole, 15-30 mg per day. Lithium carbonate 300 mg TID has also been found useful as a thyroid-blocking drug and may be given prior to radioactive iodine (I-131) therapy to enhance the retention of iodine in the autonomous nodule within the thyroid gland. To slow the heart rate, the Beta Blocker, propranolol 40-160 mg/day, is commonly prescribed for relief of tachycardia. Propranolol is the preferred Beta Blocker since it also independently inhibits the D1 deiodinase, which converts T4 to T3 in the periphery, an added benefit in treating thyrotoxicosis. Inhibition of D1 deiodinase by propranolol is independent of Beta Blockade and is useful in reducing Free T3 levels in thyrotoxic patients. (51-57)

2) **Thyroid Ablation with Radiation:** Radioactive Iodine (I-131) therapy for autonomous nodules is a form of radiation therapy that ablates the nodule and is quite successful for this entity. As mentioned above, autonomous nodules have upregulated activity of the Sodium Iodide Symporter, the active transport for iodine, so they exhibit good iodine uptake and soak up most of the radioactive iodine, sparing the remaining normal gland from radiation exposure. (58-61) (125)

3) **Surgical Ablation:** the surgical removal of the autonomous nodule with a unilateral thyroid lobectomy procedure. Large multinodular goiters with compressive symptoms are best treated with total thyroidectomy. (62-64)

4) **Percutaneous Injection:** Percutaneous ethanol injection into the autonomous thyroid nodule under ultrasound control. This is feasible when the nodule is single and relatively small in size. (65-67)

5) **Radiofrequency Ablation and Ultrasound Guided Laser Thermal Ablation:** are two of the newer methods for treating autonomous nodules. (122-125)

The Medical Myth of Iodine-Induced Toxic Effects on Healthy Humans

Normal healthy people may consume large amounts of iodine from food, dietary supplements, or medications without adverse effects. This is due to the normal autoregulatory function of the thyroid, called the "Escape from the Wolff-Chaikoff Effect." The thyroid gland compensates for the high dietary iodine intake by downregulating the NIS sodium iodide symporter and inhibiting organification. Let us review several facts:

1) From 1890 to 1930, physicians commonly prescribed high-dose iodine in the form of Lugol's Solution for many medical disorders. (68-69)

2) The Japanese diet is very high in iodine arising from Kombu seaweed consumption. Estimates of daily iodine intake in the Japanese diet range from one to twelve milligrams per day depending on the type and quantity of Kombu seaweed ingested. (70-73)

3) Iodine-containing medications such as SSKI, amiodarone, and radiographic contrast agents are routinely prescribed by physicians. These compounds are freely used even though iodine-induced thyrotoxicosis may occur in patients harboring autonomous thyroid tissue. (74-77)

4) Government protocol provides 130 mg of potassium iodide to prevent thyroid cancer in the surrounding vicinity of a nuclear reactor accident. (78-81)

As you can see from above, large segments of the population have been routinely exposed to high doses of iodine from various sources over the past 100 years without concern for adverse effects.

Iodine Toxic Effects in the Iodine Deficient State – Painless Thyroiditis

However, iodine may induce toxic effects under conditions of iodine deficiency. These toxic effects are mediated by excess hydrogen peroxide generation, incompletely neutralized by a dysfunctional seleno-protein anti-oxidant system. This can lead to inflammation and thyroiditis, which is very similar to painless thyroiditis (PT). This mechanism was described in 2000 by Dr. Bernard Corvilain, who found that acute iodine administration to **iodine-depleted** dogs and mice increased hydrogen peroxide generation rather than inhibited it. This toxicity was aggravated by selenium deficiency, causing insufficient glutathione peroxidase for neutralization of the hydrogen peroxide.

Dr. Ken Okamura and Painless Thyroiditis

I would suggest this same mechanism could be at play in the Painless Thyroiditis cases described by Dr. Okamura in his Graves' disease patients. Although Dr. Okamura's patients were not iodine deficient, thyroid gland hyper-stimulation in Graves' disease resembles an iodine deficiency state with hyperfunction and high radio-iodine uptake. Similarly, studies in man and animals show acute iodine depletion causes thyroid hyper-stimulation and increased radio-iodine uptake, both features shared by Graves' disease. Chronic excessive dietary iodine intake has the opposite effect, showing decreased radio-iodine uptake. This is the escape from the Wolff-Chaikoff Effect, thought to be related to the down-regulation of the NIS iodine transporter, which compensates for the iodine excess.

In human and animal studies, chronic iodine deficiency severely reduces the output of thyroid hormones producing low levels of Free T3 and Free T4. The pituitary gland responds to this hypothyroid state by secreting massive amounts of TSH (thyroid stimulating hormone). TSH stimulates all steps in thyroid hormone production, including upregulation of NIS and increased hydrogen peroxide generation. As mentioned in a previous Chapter 14 on the Production of Thyroid Hormones, the untreated Graves' disease patient is spared the damaging stimulation of excess hydrogen peroxide generation because, unlike TSH itself, TSH receptor antibodies do not stimulate hydrogen peroxide generation. (82-88)

In 2000, Dr. Bernard Corvilain writes:

> the increase in H2O2 [hydrogen peroxide] synthesis induced by iodide in **iodine-depleted thyroid** may have a toxic role in the cell. **Necrosis of follicular cells** was already described after the administration of iodide to iodine-deficient dogs but not to control dogs. **A necrotizing effect of iodide** was also described in iodine-deficient rats and mice. The **toxicity of iodide was aggravated in cases of selenium deficiency, a circumstance in which defenses against H2O2 are reduced due to a decreased activity of glutathione peroxidase**. Our data are in keeping with the hypothesis that some of these toxic effects induced by iodide in iodide-deficient thyroids may be partly related to the **toxicity of H2O2.** (89-92)

Painless Thyroiditis – Iodine-induced Hyperthyroidism in Normal Thyroid Gland

Painless Thyroiditis is an inflammatory condition with rupture of the follicles with release of preformed thyroid hormone, causing thyrotoxicosis. Painless Thyroiditis resembles Hashitoxicosis as they both have very low radio-iodine uptake, usually less than one percent, which differentiates both entities from Graves' thyrotoxicosis with very high radio-iodine uptake. Thyroid blocking drugs, useful in Graves' disease, are not effective in Painless Thyroiditis and Hashitoxicosis as they cannot prevent the release of preformed thyroid hormone from ruptured follicles.

Severe Recurrent Painless Thyroiditis Case Report

in 2013, Dr. Hiroaki Ishii reported a case of recurrent Painless Thyroiditis that was so severe it required thyroidectomy. Initially, the doctors thought the patient's diagnosis was TRAb-negative Graves' disease, and the patient was treated with methimazole for a short time. The diagnosis was then changed to Painless Thyroiditis when a low radio-iodine uptake was found on scintigraphy. Dr. Hiroaki Ishii writes:

> The treatment of painless thyroiditis is typically limited to observation, given the transient and mild nature of the thyroid dysfunction. **Beta-Adrenergic blockade (propranolol) is effective for the treatment of symptoms related to thyrotoxicosis. Neither antithyroid medication nor potassium iodide is effective in preventing hormone release from the affected gland.** At the beginning of management of this case, we treated with anti-thyroid drugs for a few weeks due to an initial diagnosis of Graves' disease, although TRAb was negative...The diagnosis of painless thyroiditis was based on the presence of thyrotoxicosis with low radioactive iodine uptake and negative TSH receptor antibodies. (83)

> Note: Methimazole and high dose potassium iodide are ineffective in preventing the release of preformed thyroid hormone from ruptured follicles. Propranolol is effective for PT because of two different mechanisms. Firstly, propranolol is effective as a Beta Blocker, slowing the heart rate. Secondly, propranolol inhibits the D1 deiodinase, inhibiting the peripheral conversion of T4 to T3, the active form of thyroid hormone. (93)

Case Report Iodine Deficient Male – Iodine Induced Hyperthyroidism

Graves' Disease, Autonomous Nodule or Painless Thyroiditis?

In 2020, Dr. Itivrita Goyal reported a case of iodine-induced thyrotoxicosis in a young male who initially presented as severely hypothyroid (low thyroid) with severe iodine deficiency. This scenario replicates the iodine-depleted animal studies mentioned above by Dr. Bernard Corvilain. In Dr. Itivrita Goyal's case report, the initial clinical presentation was that of iodine deficiency with hypothyroidism and elevated TSH. The patient had a diffusely enlarged thyroid without nodules, the TSH was elevated, 24.4 mIU/L, and the free thyroxine level (FT4) was below <0.4 ng/dL. In other words, the lab pattern showed severe hypothyroidism. Thinking the patient was hypothyroid, the primary care physician ordered levothyroxine, but the patient never took it. (92)

Very High Radio-Iodine Uptake

Dr. Goyal's young male patient's radio-iodine uptake was very high at **91 percent uptake**. In my opinion, a smooth, diffusely enlarged thyroid gland without nodules, and increased uptake of 91 percent is suggestive of Graves' disease. The patient was given a multivitamin containing the RDA [recommended daily allowance] for iodine. Following this rather modest increase in iodine intake from the multivitamin, the patient became hyperthyroid. Perhaps this patient had Graves' disease from the onset, which became apparent after iodine repletion. However, the TRAb and TSI antibody tests were not done, so we do not have confirmation of Graves' disease. However, rarely a Graves' disease patient will have negative TRAb and TSI antibodies.

Thyroid Nodule on Ultrasound

Later in this patient's clinical course, a second thyroid ultrasound was done. This time showing a nodule which raises the question of autonomous functioning nodule as the etiology of hyperthyroidism after iodine repletion. However, the radionuclide thyroid scan uptake was 91 percent, with smooth, diffuse increased uptake pattern without a "hot" nodule visible. Again, this clinical pattern is more suggestive of Graves' disease, which was made obvious upon iodine repletion. This scenario of Graves' disease unmasked by iodine repletion was described in 1998 by Dr. Stanbury, who writes:

IIH [Iodine Induced Hyperthyroidism] may also occur with an increase in iodine intake in those whose hyperthyroidism (Graves' disease) is not expressed because of iodine deficiency. (84)

Indeed, this patient's clinical features resembled Graves' disease, with a radio-iodine scan showing very high iodine uptake and a diffusely enlarged thyroid gland with increased blood flow (on ultrasound exam). Upon giving the patient iodine (150 mcg/day), the patient attained a euthyroid state for 6 months and then became thyrotoxic. Was the thyrotoxicosis secondary to underlying Graves' Disease? The authors raise this same question, writing:

Ultrasound (U.S.) of the neck showed an enlarged thyroid gland without nodules. Laboratory workup revealed thyroid-stimulating hormone (TSH) was increased to 24.4 mIU/L (reference range is 0.4 to 5.0 mIU/L), free thyroxine level (FT4) was <0.4 ng/dL (reference range is 0.8 to 1.8 ng/dL), slightly increased thyroid peroxidase antibody of 43 I.U./mL (reference range is <35 I.U./mL), and negative thyroglobulin antibody. He was started on levothyroxine supplementation by his primary care physician but never took it. Three months later, his TSH was 6.1 mIU/L, thyroid peroxidase antibody was negative, and total triiodothyronine was within normal limits. FT4 test was not ordered at this time...**The nontoxic goiter associated with primary hypothyroidism was thought to be secondary to severe iodine deficiency, given the patient's low intake of dietary iodine for many years**...Urine testing showed a very low spot urine iodine level of 4 µg/L (reference range is 28 to 544 µg/L)... The patient was started on a multivitamin supplement containing 150 µg of iodine daily and was advised to consume iodine-rich foods. On follow-up in the clinic 3 months later, the spot urine iodine levels

had improved to 91 µg/L (performed by LabCorp; reference range is 28 to 544 µg/L). Thyroid function tests had normalized with TSH within normal range (0.655 mIU/L) and FT4 normalized to 1.24 ng/dL...He was evaluated in the clinic 6 months later with repeat thyroid function tests and U.S. of the thyroid gland. **He complained of weight loss, palpitations, and pedal edema**. Laboratory data suggested primary hyperthyroidism with TSH <0.002 mIU/L, FT4 elevated to 2.8 ng/dL (reference range is 0.7 to 1.9 ng/dL), and total triiodothyronine elevated to 326 ng/dL (reference range is 80 to 180 ng/dL). At this time, 24-hour urine iodine level was normal at 145 µg/24 hours (performed by Quest Diagnostics, Secaucus, NJ; reference range is 70 to 500 µg/24 hours). **The U.S. showed enlargement of both thyroid lobes with increased blood flow and a 1.2 cm nodule in the posteroinferior aspect of the left lobe. Hyperthyroidism was likely secondary to increased uptake of iodine or an underlying autoimmune state leading to increased hormone production and secretion.** [Autonomous Nodule vs. Graves' Disease?]. (92)

The authors were not sure of the diagnosis, either autonomous nodule or Graves' disease to explain the thyrotoxicosis. In my opinion, Graves' disease was most likely. This illustrates the diagnostic difficulties and challenges of thyroid endocrinology found in case reports in the medical literature. Note: both an iodine deficiency state and Graves' disease will demonstrate high radioiodine uptake.

Amiodarone Induced Thyrotoxicosis

In 2008, Dr. Erik Mittra reported iodine-induced thyrotoxicosis is most commonly caused by autonomous nodule and toxic nodular goiter and less commonly caused by amiodarone, a cardiology drug used to treat arrhythmias. The chemical structure of amiodarone is remarkably similar to thyroxine and contains a hefty dose of iodine, 7.5 mg released into circulation with each 200 mg tablet. The effects of amiodarone are due either to the excess iodine released by the drug or due to the toxic effect of the drug itself. Dr. Erik Mittra writes:

> the iodine content is 75 mg in a 200-mg tablet of amiodarone and 18.7 mg/ml in the intravenous solution. Approximately 10% of the iodine content of oral amiodarone is released into the circulatory system. (94)

I am including this discussion of amiodarone because it encapsulates the main concepts of how the thyroid gland may react to excess iodine. Amiodarone is widely used by cardiologists to treat arrhythmias, such as atrial fibrillation, even though adverse effects such as hypothyroidism or hyperthyroidism may be induced by the drug. The drug is used freely without concern for adverse side effects.

Amiodarone Induced Thyroid Side Effects

In 2019, Dr. Richard Trohman estimated the incidence of amiodarone-induced hypothyroidism (5–10%) and hyperthyroidism (0.9–10%), writing:

> Older estimates have suggested that the overall incidence of amiodarone-induced thyroid dysfunction ranges from 2 to 24%. More recent reviews of the literature noted that hypothyroidism occurs in 5–10% and hyperthyroidism afflicts approximately 0.9–10% of amiodarone recipients. These differences may reflect the evolution of more conservative dosing regimens employed over time. A meta-analysis suggested that when lower amiodarone doses (152–330 mg daily) were used, the incidence of thyroid dysfunction was 3.7%. (95)

Here I wish to point out that mainstream medicine uses amiodarone freely without concern for inducing thyrotoxicosis in 0.9-10% of recipients. When the patient goes into amiodarone-induced thyrotoxicosis, the cardiologist calls the endocrinologist to manage the patient. Amiodarone thyrotoxicosis may be difficult to treat because of the long half-life of the drug. Potassium iodide treatment of Graves' disease is handled quite differently. Here, concern for resistance to iodide or worsening thyrotoxicosis has prevented its use in the US, even though it is considered a standard treatment in Japan. One might ask, shouldn't this same concern apply to amiodarone? Obviously not.

Amiodarone Induced Hypothyroidism

Regarding amiodarone-induced hypothyroidism, this is merely the effect of free iodine released by the amiodarone drug. Iodine has an inhibitory effect on thyroid function. Patients with autoimmune thyroid disease have a loss of autoregulation and cannot escape from the "Wolff-Chaikoff Effect", thus iodine excess causes hypothyroidism in patients with auto-immune thyroid disease. This was discussed in previous chapters.

Amiodarone-Induced Thyrotoxicosis – Two Types

Amiodarone-induced thyrotoxicosis consists of two types. Type One is due to autonomous thyroid tissue within either a single nodule or a multi-nodular goiter which uncontrollably converts iodine into thyroid hormone.

Type Two Destructive Thyroiditis

Type Two is a form of destructive thyroiditis with rupture of follicles and release of preformed thyroid hormone, a mechanism identical to Painless Thyroiditis with low radio-iodine uptake. The pathophysiology of thyroid inflammation also bears a similarity to Hashitoxicosis. The amiodarone molecule carries its own toxic effect upon the thyroid, which accounts for thyroiditis in the type II version. This is a form of severe destructive inflammatory thyroiditis, much greater than iodine's relatively milder toxic effect. Amiodarone is fat soluble with a long half-life, making treatment much more challenging in the thyrotoxic patient. Dr. Mittra writes:

> Iodine-induced thyrotoxicosis is also called Jod Basedow disease. Jod Basedow is derived from Jod, the German for iodine,

and Basedow from Von Basedow, who described in German what the English-speaking medical world knows as Graves' disease. Iodine-induced thyrotoxicosis is usually not Graves' or Basedow's disease but **toxic nodular goiter** [autonomous nodules]. It is more likely to occur in regions of iodine deficiency in people with nodular goiters who are then exposed to an excess of iodine. **The autoregulatory controls of the thyroid must fail for this to occur.** Usually, an increase in plasma inorganic iodine causes reduced trapping of iodine, organification (Wolff–Chaikoff effect), and reduced release of preformed thyroid hormones. Thus, an autonomously functioning nodular goiter is at most risk. The source of iodine is usually apparent, such as the addition of iodine to salt. There are many reports of this occurring in regions of low iodine intake soon after iodine is added to the diet. The extensive review by Stanbury et al. discusses the history, etiology, and epidemiology of this. This is rare in the population born and raised in the United States but is found in immigrants from regions of low dietary iodine who come to the United States ...**In regions of iodine deficiency, amiodarone is more likely to cause thyrotoxicosis, and in iodine-sufficient regions, hypothyroidism is more likely. This difference is attributed to nodular goiter [toxic goiter] being more prevalent in iodine-deficient regions.** The excess iodine from amiodarone provides the raw material for the **nodules to produce excess thyroid hormones.** This has been designated type 1 amiodarone–induced thyrotoxicosis. It contrasts with **type 2, which is attributable to the destruction of follicles producing a thyroiditis-like picture.** Type 2 is more common in the United States. Some patients have an overlap of these patterns. In the United States, **most patients have a low uptake of 123-I [radio-iodine].** In contrast, in **regions of low iodine intake, the uptake values in type 1 amiodarone–induced thyrotoxicosis can be normal or high**...Ultrasound with color flow Doppler shows increased vascularity in type 1 and reduced vascularity in type 2 AIT. Treatment is difficult because amiodarone

is often the most effective antiarrhythmic in the patient, and there is reluctance to stop it. In addition, because of the long half-life, its effects persist for months to years. **The low uptake of radio-iodine makes 131-I useless [as radioactive-iodine thyroid ablation treatment].** Antithyroid medication such as methimazole 30–40 mg daily has been effective, and the patient should be educated about side effects, including skin rash and agranulocytosis [methimazole is effective for Type One, but not Type Two]. Potassium perchlorate has been used as a competitive inhibitor of trapping iodine by the sodium–iodide symporter. Reports from Europe indicate a combination of methimazole and potassium perchlorate is successful. Potassium perchlorate is not available in the United States. **Corticosteroids such as prednisone at 30–60 mg/d are effective in the destructive type 2 syndrome.** Thyroidectomy can be undertaken when antithyroid therapy is ineffective, but these patients are often poor operative candidates because of the underlying cardiac disease. (94-97)

Direct Toxic Effect on Thyroid Gland

In 2019, Dr. Richard Trohman studied thyroid physiology, pathophysiology, diagnosis, and management of amiodarone thyrotoxicosis, writing that the drug has a direct toxic effect on the thyroid distinct from iodine:

Amiodarone has direct, dose-dependent cytotoxic effects on the thyroid in animal models. These findings have been confirmed in human post-operative pathologic specimens. DEA [amiodorane metabolite] is even more cytotoxic for thyroid cells than the parent drug. **Although iodide excess may induce apoptosis, amiodarone administration is associated with ultrastructural changes indicative of thyroid cytotoxicity distinct from those induced by excess iodine alone.** These changes include marked distortion of thyroid architecture, apoptosis, necrosis, inclusion bodies, lipofuscinogenesis, macrophage infiltration, and markedly dilated endoplasmic reticulum

(E.R.)...Amiodarone-induced hyperthyroidism is a much more complex entity than AIH [Amiodorone Induced Hypothyroidism]. There are two main forms of amiodarone-induced thyrotoxicosis (AIT). Type I AIT usually occurs in abnormal thyroid glands and is the result of excessive iodine-induced hormone synthesis and release. Autoregulatory mechanisms modulate the thyroid gland's iodine handling according to its iodine content. Disruption of these autoregulatory mechanisms is suggested by the **high glandular iodine content** associated with AIT compared with euthyroid amiodarone recipients and by **return of iodine content to normal during resolution of thyrotoxicosis**. Toxic nodular goiter and Graves' disease are the most common causes of Type I AIT in patients with preexisting or "latent" thyroid disease...Type II AIT is a **destructive thyroiditis** leading to the release of preformed (stored) thyroid hormones from damaged thyroid follicular cells. Type II AIT typically occurs in patients without underlying thyroid disease... **Type II AIT persists for 1–3 months until thyroid hormone stores are depleted but resolves more quickly after glucocorticoid therapy**. (95-100)

In 2007, Dr. Kazuko Yamazaki studied the effect of amiodarone on cultured thyroid follicles in-vitro, finding no cytotoxic effect at therapeutic concentrations. However, at supraphysiologic concentrations, there were cytotoxic effects, thought to be due to "exceeding endogenous anti-oxidant capacity," i.e., referring to the selenoprotein glutathione peroxidase, writing:

> When thyroid follicles obtained from a patient with Graves' disease who had been treated with amiodarone were cultured in amiodarone-free medium, **TSH-induced thyroid function was intact, suggesting that amiodarone at a maintenance dose did not elicit any cytotoxic effect on thyrocytes...** Conclusion: These in vitro and ex vivo findings suggest that **patients taking maintenance doses of amiodarone usually remain euthyroid, probably due to escape from the Wolff-Chaikoff effect mediated by decreased expression of NIS mRNA** [sodium iodide symporter messenger RNA]. Further, amiodarone is not cytotoxic for thyrocytes at therapeutic concentrations but **elicits cytotoxicity through oxidant activity at supraphysiological concentrations.** We speculate that when **amiodarone-induced prooxidant activity somehow exceeds the endogenous anti-oxidant capacity**, the thyroid follicles will be destroyed, and amiodarone-induced destructive thyrotoxicosis may develop. (100)

Note: the anti-oxidant capacity above refers to the seleno-protein anti-oxidant system, glutathione peroxidase. Notice this is the same mechanism for destructive thyroiditis seen in endemic myxedematous cretinism in Zaire, Africa, Hashitoxicosis, and Painless Thyroiditis. (101)

Pathogenesis of Amiodarone Induced Thyrotoxicosis

In 2009, Dr. Silvia Eskes and Wilmar M. Wiersinga described the pathogenesis of AIT [Amiodarone Induced Thyrotoxicosis] type 2 as like that of subacute thyroiditis (SAT), in which thyrotoxicosis is due to the release of preformed thyroid hormone from damaged thyroid follicles, writing:

> The pathogenesis of AIT [Amiodarone Induced thyrotoxicosis] type 2 is similar to that of subacute thyroiditis (SAT), in which thyrotoxicosis is due to the release of preformed thyroid hormone into the bloodstream from damaged thyroid follicular epithelium. AM [Amiodarone] and DEA have (independently from iodine) a direct cytotoxic effect on cultured human thyrocytes. AM disrupts the architecture of the thyroid at a cellular and subcellular level in an experimental animal model changes akin to the severe follicular damage and disruption observed in thyroids of **SAT [subacute thyroiditis] and AIT type 2, whereas AM-treated euthyroid**

patients show minimal or no thyroid follicular damage. The ultrastructural changes include an increased number of secondary lysosomes, exhibiting marked lipofuscinogenesis and dilation of the endoplasmic reticulum, with sparing of the mitochondria. Similar changes have been observed in other tissues damaged during AM treatment, and disruption of subcellular organelle function seems to explain the toxic effects of AM. Toxicity increases with exposure time to AM in clinical studies and, at times, is related to the cumulative dose of AM. **Other similarities of AIT type 2 with SAT, supporting the view of AIT type 2 as drug-induced destructive thyroiditis**, are (a) the sudden onset, (b) sometimes the presence of a small painful goiter, **(c) low or absent thyroidal radio-iodine uptake,** (d) frequently a self-limiting course and (d) high incidence of a subsequent subclinical hypothyroid stage. (102)

Note: I would add here Hashitoxicosis and Painless Thyroiditis also have similar pathophysiology to Type II Amiodarone thyroiditis, sharing the main features of destructive thyroiditis with the release of preformed thyroid hormone from ruptured follicles, with low radioiodine uptake.

Treatment of Amiodarone Associated Thyrotoxicosis

In 2018, Dr. Virginia Li Volsi discussed the treatment of amiodarone-induced thyrotoxicosis is different for each type. Type I is treated with thyroid-blocking drugs, such as methimazole. Type II is treated with glucocorticoids or thyroidectomy if severe. Dr. Virginia Li Volsi writes:

Amiodarone-induced thyrotoxicosis (AIT) is classified as type I and type II; the former occurs in patients with underlying thyroid disease such as nodular goiter, autonomous nodular goiter, or Graves' disease, whereas Type II is caused by iodine-led destruction of the thyroid follicular epithelium in a normal thyroid gland. Because amiodarone is vital to control cardiac problems, it is often not possible to wean the patient from the medication or to change to another drug. The first line of therapy in amiodarone-induced thyrotoxicosis is treatment with **thionamides [methimazole] in AIT I and glucocorticoids in AIT II**. Thyroid excision is undertaken in patients who do not respond to medical therapy in order to treat hyperthyroidism, which often worsens cardiac symptoms. (103-104)

Note both propranolol and glucocorticoids (corticosteroids, dexamethasone) reduce peripheral conversion of T4 to T3. (105-106)

Serum Thyroglobulin as Sensitive Marker of Thyroiditis

In various inflammatory conditions of the thyroid, the ruptured follicles release thyroglobulin (Tg) into the bloodstream, and measurement of thyroglobulin may indicate severity of thyroiditis. In 1978, Dr. Izumi writes:

Serum Tg (thyroglobulin) appears to be a sensitive indicator of acute thyroidal damage due to surgical, radiation, or inflammatory trauma. (107-109)

Conclusion

The autonomous nodule and toxic nodular goiter are the two most common causes of iodine-induced hyperthyroidism in the U.S. Unlike Graves' disease, in which potassium iodide may serve as a thyroid-blocking agent, iodide is contraindicated for the autonomous nodule and toxic nodular goiter patient. In these cases, iodide causes thyrotoxicosis, which may represent a life-threatening medical emergency. Another important cause of thyrotoxicosis is the cardiology drug amiodarone which causes destructive thyroiditis strikingly similar to Painless Thyroiditis and Hashitoxicosis, all three characterized by low radio-iodine uptake. (110-121)

◆ References for Chapter 19

1) Joseph, K., J. Mahlstedt, and U. Welcke. "Early Recognition of Autonomous Thyroid Tissue by a Combination of Quantitative Thyroid Pertechnetate Scintigraphy with the Free T4 Equivalent (Author's Transl)." Nuklearmedizin. Nuclear Medicine 19.2 (1980): 54-63.

2) Fricke, Eva, et al. "Scintigraphy for Risk Stratification of Iodine-Induced Thyrotoxicosis in Patients Receiving Contrast Agent for Coronary Angiography: A Prospective Study of Patients with Low Thyrotropin." The Journal of Clinical Endocrinology & Metabolism 89.12 (2004): 6092-6096.

3) Ratnos, Celso D., et al. "Thyroid Suppression Test with L-Thyroxine and [99mtc] Pertechnetate." Clinical Endocrinology 52.4 (2000): 471-477.

4) Meller, J., and W. Becker. "Scintigraphy with (99m) Tc-Pertechnetate in the Evaluation of Functional Thyroidal Autonomy." The Quarterly Journal of Nuclear Medicine and Molecular Imaging 43.3 (1999): 179.

5) Meller, J., and W. Becker. "The Continuing Importance of Thyroid Scintigraphy in the Era of High-Resolution Ultrasound." European Journal of Nuclear Medicine and Molecular Imaging 29.2 (2002): S425-S438.

6) Meller, J., and W. Becker. "Scintigraphic Evaluation of Functional Thyroidal Autonomy." Experimental and clinical endocrinology & diabetes 106.S 04 (1998): S45-S51.

7) Stanbury, John Burton, et al. "Iodine-Induced Hyperthyroidism: Occurrence and Epidemiology." Thyroid 8.1 (1998): 83-100.

8) Tonacchera, Massimo, et al. "Activating Thyrotropin Receptor Mutations Are Present in Nonadenomatous Hyperfunctioning Nodules of Toxic or Autonomous Multinodular Goiter." The Journal of Clinical Endocrinology & Metabolism 85.6 (2000): 2270-2274.

9) Bülow Pedersen, Inge, et al. "Large Differences in Incidences of Overt Hyper-and Hypothyroidism Associated with a Small Difference in Iodine Intake: A Prospective Comparative Register-Based Population Survey." The Journal of Clinical Endocrinology & Metabolism 87.10 (2002): 4462-4469.

10) Bülow Pedersen, Inge, et al. "Increase in Incidence of Hyperthyroidism Predominantly Occurs in Young People After Iodine Fortification of Salt in Denmark." The Journal of Clinical Endocrinology & Metabolism 91.10 (2006): 3830-3834.

11) Davies, Terry F., et al. "Thyrotropin Receptor–Associated Diseases: From Adenomata to Graves' Disease." The Journal of Clinical Investigation 115.8 (2005): 1972-1983.

12) Gozu, Hulya Ilıksu, et al. "Similar Prevalence of Somatic TSH Receptor and Gsα Mutations in Toxic Thyroid Nodules in Geographical Regions with Different Iodine Supply in Turkey." European Journal of Endocrinology 155.4 (2006): 535-545.

13) Krohn, Knut, and Ralf Paschke. "Progress in Understanding the Etiology of Thyroid Autonomy." The Journal of Clinical Endocrinology & Metabolism 86.7 (2001): 3336-3345.

14) Krohn, Knut, et al. "Mechanisms of Disease: Hydrogen Peroxide, DNA Damage and Mutagenesis in The Development of Thyroid Tumors." Nature Clinical Practice Endocrinology & Metabolism 3.10 (2007): 713-720.

15) Maier, J. et al. "Iodine Deficiency Activates Anti-Oxidant Genes and Causes DNA Damage in The Thyroid Gland of Rats and Mice." Biochimica et Biophysica Acta (BBA)-Molecular Cell Research 1773.6 (2007): 990-999.

16) Song, Yue, et al. "Roles of Hydrogen Peroxide in Thyroid Physiology and Disease." The Journal of Clinical Endocrinology & Metabolism 92.10 (2007): 3764-3773.

17) Zimmermann, Michael B. "Iodine and the Iodine Deficiency Disorders." Present Knowledge in Nutrition. Academic Press, 2020. 429-441.

18) Zimmermann, Michael B., and Kristien Boelaert. "Iodine Deficiency and Thyroid Disorders." The Lancet Diabetes & Endocrinology 3.4 (2015): 286-295.

19) Leung, Angela M., et al. "History of U.S. Iodine Fortification and Supplementation." Nutrients 4.11 (2012): 1740-1746.

20) Carpenter, Kenneth J. "David Marine and the Problem of Goiter." The Journal of Nutrition 135.4 (2005): 675-680.

21) Azizi, F. "Iodized Oil: Its Role in the Management of Iodine Deficiency Disorders." International Journal of Endocrinology and Metabolism 5.2 (2007): 91-98.

22) Kohn, Lawrence A. "The Midwestern American "Epidemic" of Iodine-Induced Hyperthyroidism in the 1920s." Bulletin of the New York Academy of Medicine 52.7 (1976): 770.

23) Connolly, R. J., et al. "Increase in Thyrotoxicosis in Endemic Goiter Area After Iodation of Bread." The Lancet 295.7645 (1970): 500-502.

24) Vidor, G. I., et al. "Pathogenesis of Iodine-Induced Thyrotoxicosis: Studies in Northern Tasmania." The Journal of Clinical Endocrinology & Metabolism 37.6 (1973): 901-909.

25) Todd, C. H., et al. "Increase in Thyrotoxicosis Associated with Iodine Supplements in Zimbabwe." The Lancet 346.8989 (1995): 1563-1564.

26) Bourdoux, Pierre, et al. "Iodine-Induced Thyrotoxicosis in Kivu, Zaire." Lancet 347.9000 (1996): 552-553.

27) Delange François M., et al. "Risks of Iodine-Induced Hyperthyroidism After Correction of Iodine Deficiency by Iodized Salt." Thyroid 9.6 (1999): 545-556.

28) Livadas, D. P., et al. "The Toxic Effects of Small Iodine Supplements in Patients with Autonomous Thyroid Nodules." Clinical Endocrinology 7.2 (1977): 121-127.

29) Kohn, Lawrence A. "The Midwestern American "Epidemic" of Iodine-Induced Hyperthyroidism in the 1920s." Bulletin of the New York Academy of Medicine 52.7 (1976): 770.

30) Baltisberger, Benedikt L., et al. "Decrease of Incidence of Toxic Nodular Goitre in a Region of Switzerland After Full Correction of Mild Iodine Deficiency." European Journal of Endocrinology 132.5 (1995): 546-549.

31) Mostbeck, Adolf, et al. "The Incidence of Hyperthyroidism in Austria from 1987 to 1995 Before and After an Increase in Salt Iodization in 1990." European Journal of Nuclear Medicine 25 (1998): 367-374.

32) Vidor, G. I., et al. "Pathogenesis of Iodine-Induced Thyrotoxicosis: Studies in Northern Tasmania." The Journal of Clinical Endocrinology & Metabolism 37.6 (1973): 901-909.

33) Gołkowski, Filip, et al. "Increased Prevalence of Hyperthyroidism as an Early and Transient Side-Effect of Implementing Iodine Prophylaxis." Public Health Nutrition 10.8 (2007): 799-802.

34) Stanbury, John Burton, et al. "Iodine-Induced Hyperthyroidism: Occurrence and Epidemiology." Thyroid 8.1 (1998): 83-100.

35) Corvilain, Bernard, et al. "Autonomy in Endemic Goiter." Thyroid 8.1 (1998): 107-113.

36) Schwarzfischer, P., et al. "Iodine-Induced Hyperthyroidism in The Aged. 2. Pathomechanism, Differential Diagnosis, and Therapy Problems." Fortschritte der Medizin 100.5 (1982): 153-158.

37) Daniels, Gilbert H. "Amiodarone-Induced Thyrotoxicosis." The Journal of Clinical Endocrinology & Metabolism 86.1 (2001): 3-8.

38) Dunne, Paul, et al. "Iodinated Contrast–Induced Thyrotoxicosis." CMAJ 185.2 (2013): 144-147.

39) Savoie, J. C., et al. "Iodine-Induced Thyrotoxicosis in Apparently Normal Thyroid Glands." The Journal of Clinical Endocrinology & Metabolism 41.4 (1975): 685-691.

40) Shilo, Shmuel, and Harry J. Hirsch. "Iodine-Induced Hyperthyroidism in a Patient with a Normal Thyroid Gland." Postgraduate Medical Journal 62.729 (1986): 661-662.

41) Yoshihara, Ai, et al. "Substituting Potassium Iodide for Methimazole as the Treatment for Graves' Disease During the First Trimester May Reduce the Incidence of Congenital Anomalies: A Retrospective Study at a Single Medical Institution in Japan." Thyroid 25.10 (2015): 1155-1161.

42) Nishikawa, Mitsushige, et al. "Coexistence of an Autonomously Functioning Thyroid Nodule in a Patient with Graves' Disease an Unusual Presentation of Marine-Lenhart Syndrome." Endocrine Journal 44.4 (1997): 571-574.

43) Charkes, N. David. "Graves' Disease with Functioning Nodules (Marine-Lenhart Syndrome)." Journal of Nuclear Medicine 13.12 (1972): 885-892.

44) Danno, Hirosuke, et al. "Prevalence and Treatment Outcomes of Marine-Lenhart Syndrome in Japan." European Thyroid Journal 10.6 (2021): 461-467.

45) Miyazaki, Megumi, et al. "A Case of Marine-Lenhart Syndrome with Predominance of Plummer Disease." Journal of UOEH 41.2 (2019): 165-170. Note: UOEH is the University of Occupational and Environmental Health.

46 Lima, N., and G. Medeiros-Neto. "Transient Thyrotoxicosis in Endemic Goiter Patients Following Exposure to a Normal Iodine Intake." Clinical Endocrinology 21.6 (1984): 631-637.

47) Taylor, Jayme E., et al. "A Case of Hyperthyroidism in a Patient Using the Nutritional Supplement "Survival Shield"." AACE Clinical Case Reports 4.5 (2018): e398-e401.

48) Patel, Richa, et al. "SUN-574 Exogenous Iodine Supplementation-Induced Thyroid Storm in a Patient with Multinodular Goiter." Journal of the Endocrine Society 3. Suppl 1 (2019).

49) Brotfain, E., et al. "Iodine-Induced Hyperthyroidism—An Old Clinical Entity That Is Still Relevant to Daily ICU Practice: A Case Report." Case Reports in Endocrinology 2013 (2013).

50) Abraham, Guy E. "The Safe and Effective Implementation of Orthoiodosupplementation in Medical Practice." The Original Internist 11.1 (2004): 17-36.

51) Azizi, Fereidoun. "Long-Term Treatment of Hyperthyroidism with Antithyroid Drugs: 35 Years of Personal Clinical Experience." Thyroid 30.10 (2020): 1451-1457.

52) Ross, Douglas S. "Treatment of Toxic Adenoma and Toxic Multinodular Goiter." UpToDate. 12th ed. Waltham, MA: Wolters Kluwer (2019).

53) Płazińska, Maria Teresa, et al. "Lithium Carbonate Pre-Treatment in 131-I Therapy of Hyperthyroidism." Nuclear Medicine Review 14.1 (2011): 3-8.

54) Wiersinga, W. M. "Propranolol and Thyroid Hormone Metabolism." Thyroid 1.3 (1991): 273-277.

55) Heyma, P., R. G. Larkins, and D. G. Campbell. "Inhibition by Propranolol of 3, 5, 3'-Triiodothyronine Formation from Thyroxine in Isolated Rat Renal Tubules: An Effect Independent of Beta-Adrenergic Blockade." Endocrinology 106.5 (1980): 1437-1441.

56) Azizi, Fereidoun, et al. "Treatment of Toxic Multinodular Goiter: Comparison of Radio-Iodine and Long-Term Methimazole Treatment." Thyroid 29.5 (2019): 625-630.

57) Bawand, Rashed, et al. "Comparison of Clinical Efficacy of Antithyroid Drugs, Radioactive Iodine, and Thyroidectomy for Treatment of Patients with Graves' Disease, Toxic Thyroid Adenoma, and Toxic Multinodular Goiter." Biomedical and Biotechnology Research Journal (BBRJ) 6.4 (2022): 569.

58) Roque, Catarina, et al. "Long-Term Effects of Radio-Iodine in Toxic Multinodular Goiter: Thyroid Volume, Function, and Autoimmunity." The Journal of Clinical Endocrinology & Metabolism 105.7 (2020): e2464-e2470.

59) Racaru, L. Vija, et al. "Management of Adenomas and Toxic Multinodular Goiters with Iodine 131." Médecine Nucléaire 44.4 (2020): 272-276.

60) Ross, Douglas S., et al. "Successful Treatment of Solitary Toxic Thyroid Nodules with Relatively Low-Dose Iodine-131, With Low Prevalence of Hypothyroidism." Annals of Internal Medicine 101.4 (1984): 488-490.

61) Huysmans, Dyde A., et al. "Long-term Follow-Up in Toxic Solitary Autonomous Thyroid Nodules Treated with Radioactive Iodine." Journal of Nuclear Medicine 32.1 (1991): 27-30.

62) Kırdak, Türkay. "Surgery in Hyperthyroidism: Toxic Adenoma and/or Multinodular Goiter." Thyroid and Parathyroid Diseases. Springer, Cham, 2019. 45-49.

63) Hisham, A. N., et al. "Total thyroidectomy: The Procedure of Choice for Multinodular Goitre." European Journal of Surgery 167.6 (2001): 403-405.

64) Kapre, Madan Laxman, et al. "Surgery for Multinodular Goiter." Thyroid Surgery. CRC Press, 2020. 75-77.

65) Monzani, Fabio, et al. "Five-Year Follow-Up of Percutaneous Ethanol Injection for the Treatment of Hyperfunctioning Thyroid Nodules: A Study Of 117 Patients." Clinical Endocrinology 46.1 (1997): 9-15.

66) Tarantino, Luciano, et al. "Percutaneous Ethanol Injection of Hyperfunctioning Thyroid Nodules: Long-Term Follow-Up In 125 Patients." American Journal of Roentgenology 190.3 (2008): 800.

67) Lippi, Francesco, et al. "Treatment of Solitary Autonomous Thyroid Nodules by Percutaneous Ethanol Injection: Results of An Italian Multicenter Study. The Multicenter Study Group." The Journal of Clinical Endocrinology & Metabolism 81.9 (1996): 3261-3264.

68) Kelly, Francis C. "Iodine in Medicine and Pharmacy Since its Discovery—1811-1961." Proceedings of the Royal Society of Medicine 54.10 (1961): 831.

69) Abraham, Guy E. "The History of Iodine in Medicine Part I: From Discovery To Essentiality." The Original Internist 13.1 (2006): 29-36.

70) Fuse, Yozen, et al. "Smaller Thyroid Gland Volume with High Urinary Iodine Excretion in Japanese Schoolchildren: Normative Reference Values in an Iodine-Sufficient Area and Comparison with the WHO/ICCIDD Reference." Thyroid 17.2 (2007): 145-155.

71) Nagataki, Shigenobu. "The Average of Dietary Iodine Intake Due to the Ingestion of Seaweeds Is 1.2 Mg/Day in Japan." Thyroid 18.6 (2008): 667-668.

72) Zava, Theodore T., and David T. Zava. "Assessment of Japanese Iodine Intake Based on Seaweed Consumption in Japan: A Literature-Based Analysis." Thyroid research 4.1 (2011): 14.

73) Patrick, Lyn. "Iodine: Deficiency and Therapeutic Considerations." Alternative Medicine Review 13.2 (2008).

74) Roti, Elio, and Ettore Degli Uberti. "Iodine Excess and Hyperthyroidism." Thyroid 11.5 (2001): 493-500.

75) Roti, E., et al. "Iodine-Induced Hypothyroidism in Euthyroid Subjects with a Previous Episode of Subacute Thyroiditis." The Journal of Clinical Endocrinology and Metabolism 70.6 (1990): 1581-1585.

76) Basaria, Shehzad, and David S. Cooper. "Amiodarone and the Thyroid." The American Journal of Medicine 118.7 (2005): 706-714.

77) Bervini, Sandrina, et al. "Prevalence of Iodine-Induced Hyperthyroidism After Administration of Iodinated Contrast During Radiographic Procedures: A Systematic Review and Meta-Analysis of the Literature." Thyroid 31.7 (2021): 1020-1029.

78) Leung, Angela M., et al. "American Thyroid Association Scientific Statement on the Use of Potassium Iodide Ingestion in a Nuclear Emergency." Thyroid 27.7 (2017): 865-877.

79) Aaseth, Jan, et al. "Medical Therapy of Patients Contaminated with Radioactive Cesium or Iodine." Biomolecules 9.12 (2019): 856.

80) Bishop, Kristen A., and Catherine E. Shuster. "Update to Current Policies for Use of Radiation Therapy Drugs." (2020).

81) Acosta, Robert, and Steven J. Warrington. "Radiation Syndrome." StatPearls [Internet]. StatPearls Publishing, 2022.

82) Okamura, Ken, et al. "Painless Thyroiditis Mimicking Relapse of Hyperthyroidism During or After Potassium Iodide or Thionamide Therapy for Graves' Disease Resulting in Remission." Endocrine Journal (2022): EJ22-0207.

83) Ishii, Hiroaki, et al. "A Case of Severe and Recurrent Painless Thyroiditis Requiring Thyroidectomy." Medical Principles and Practice 22.4 (2013): 408-410.

84) Stanbury, J. B., et al. "Iodine-Induced Hyperthyroidism: Occurrence and Epidemiology." Thyroid: Official Journal of the American Thyroid Association 8.1 (1998): 83-100.

85) Bray, George A. "Increased Sensitivity of the Thyroid in Iodine-Depleted Rats to the Goitrogenic Effects of Thyrotropin." The Journal of Clinical Investigation 47.7 (1968): 1640-1647.

86) Barakat, Russell M., and Sidney H. Ingbar. "The Effect of Acute Iodide Depletion on Thyroid Function in Man." The Journal of Clinical Investigation 44.7 (1965): 1117-1124.

87) Bonnema, Steen Joop, and Laszlo Hegedüs. "Radio-Iodine Therapy in Benign Thyroid Diseases: Effects, Side Effects, and Factors Affecting Therapeutic Outcome." Endocrine Reviews 33.6 (2012): 920-980.

88) Sawka, Anna M., et al. "Dietary Iodine Restriction in Preparation for Radioactive Iodine Treatment or Scanning in Well-Differentiated Thyroid Cancer: A Systematic Review." Thyroid 20.10 (2010): 1129-1138.

89) Corvilain, Bernard, et al. "Stimulation by Iodide of H2O2 Generation in Thyroid Slices from Several Species." American Journal of Physiology-Endocrinology and Metabolism 278.4 (2000): E692-E699.

92) Goyal, Itivrita, et al. "Hypothyroidism and Goiter in a Young Male with Suspected Dietary Iodine Deficiency Followed by Thyrotoxicosis After Iodine Supplementation." AACE Clinical Case Reports 6.1 (2020): e19-e22.

93) Heyma, Paul, et al. "D-Propranolol and DL-Propranolol Both Decrease Conversion of L-Thyroxine to L-Triiodothyronine." Br Med J 281.6232 (1980): 24-25.

94) Mittra, Erik S., et al. "Uncommon Causes of Thyrotoxicosis." Journal of Nuclear Medicine 49.2 (2008): 265-278.

95) Trohman, Richard G., et al. "Amiodarone and Thyroid Physiology, Pathophysiology, Diagnosis and Management." Trends in Cardiovascular Medicine 29.5 (2019): 285-295.

96) Mahmoud, Insaf, et al. "Direct Toxic Effect of Iodide in Excess on Iodine-Deficient Thyroid Glands: Epithelial Necrosis and Inflammation Associated with Lipofuscin Accumulation." Experimental and Molecular Pathology 44.3 (1986): 259-271.

97) Belshaw, Bruce E., and David V. Becker. "Necrosis of Follicular Cells and Discharge of Thyroidal Iodine-Induced by Administering Iodide to Iodine-Deficient Dogs." The Journal of Clinical Endocrinology & Metabolism 36.3 (1973): 466-474.

98) Newman, C. M., et al. "Amiodarone and the Thyroid: A Practical Guide to The Management of Thyroid Dysfunction Induced by Amiodarone Therapy." Heart 79.2 (1998): 121-127.

99) Pitsiavas, Vicki, et al. "Amiodarone Compared with Iodine Exhibits a Potent and Persistent Inhibitory Effect on TSH-Stimulated cAMP Production in Vitro: A Possible Mechanism to Explain Amiodarone-Induced Hypothyroidism." European Journal of Endocrinology 140.3 (1999): 241-249.

100) Yamazaki, Kazuko, et al. "Amiodarone Reversibly Decreases Sodium-Iodide Symporter mRNA Expression at Therapeutic Concentrations and Induces Anti-Oxidant Responses at Supraphysiological Concentrations in Cultured Human Thyroid Follicles." Thyroid 17.12 (2007): 1189-1200.

101) Vanderpas, Jean B., et al. "Iodine and Selenium Deficiency Associated with Cretinism in Northern Zaire." The American Journal of Clinical Nutrition 52.6 (1990): 1087-1093.

102) Eskes, Silvia A., and Wilmar M. Wiersinga. "Amiodarone and Thyroid." Best Practice & Research Clinical Endocrinology & Metabolism 23.6 (2009): 735-751.

103) LiVolsi, Virginia A., and Zubair W. Baloch. "The Pathology of Hyperthyroidism." Frontiers in Endocrinology 9 (2018): 737.

104) Sato, Kanji, et al. "Differential Diagnosis and Appropriate Treatment of Four Thyrotoxic Patients with Graves' Disease Required to Take Amiodarone Due to Life-Threatening Arrhythmia." Internal Medicine 47.8 (2008): 757-762.

105) Baharudin, M. S., et al. "Refractory Thyrotoxicosis: Report of Two Cases and Literature Review." Asian Journal of Case Reports in Surgery 15.3 (2022).

106) Heyma, P., and R. G. Larkins. "Glucocorticoids Decrease Conversion of Thyroxine Into 3, 5, 3'-Tri-Iodothyronine by Isolated Rat Renal Tubules." Clinical Science (London, England: 1979) 62.2 (1982): 215-220.

107) Izumi, M., and P. R. Larsen. "Correlation of Sequential Changes in Serum Thyroglobulin, Triiodothyronine, and Thyroxine in Patients with Graves' Disease and Subacute Thyroiditis." Metabolism 27.4 (1978): 449-460.

108) Yamamoto, M., et al. "Effect of Prednisolone and Salicylate on Serum Thyroglobulin Level in Patients with Subacute Thyroiditis." Clinical Endocrinology 27.3 (1987): 339-344.

109) Madeddu, Giuseppe, et al. "Serum Thyroglobulin Levels in the Diagnosis and Follow-Up of Subacute 'Painful' Thyroiditis: A Sequential Study." Archives Of Internal Medicine 145.2 (1985): 243-247.

110) Beck-Peccoz, Paolo. "Antithyroid Drugs Are 65 Years Old: Time for Retirement?" Endocrinology 149.12 (2008): 5943-5944.

111) Leung, Angela M., and Lewis E. Braverman. "Iodine-Induced Thyroid Dysfunction." Current Opinion in Endocrinology, Diabetes, And Obesity 19.5 (2012): 414.

112) Hehrmann, R., et al. "Risk of Hyperthyroidism in Examinations with Contrast Media." Aktuelle Radiologie 6.5 (1996): 243-248.

113) Iagaru, Andrei, and I. Ross McDougall. "Treatment of Thyrotoxicosis." Journal Of Nuclear Medicine 48.3 (2007): 379-389.

114) Rose, Noel R., et al. "Linking Iodine with Autoimmune Thyroiditis." Environmental Health Perspectives 107.suppl 5 (1999): 749-752.

115) Xue, Haibo, et al. "Selenium Upregulates CD4+ CD25+ Regulatory T Cells in Iodine-Induced Autoimmune Thyroiditis Model of NOD. H-2h4 Mice." Endocrine Journal 57.7 (2010): 595-601.

116) Ratcliffe, Guy E., et al. "Radio-Iodine Treatment of Solitary Functioning Thyroid Nodules." The British Journal of Radiology 59.700 (1986): 385-387.

117) Nygaard, Birte, et al. "Long-Term Effect of Radioactive Iodine on Thyroid Function and Size in Patients with Solitary Autonomously Functioning Toxic Thyroid Nodules." Clinical Endocrinology 50.2 (1999): 197-202.

118) Ross, Douglas S. "Syndromes of Thyrotoxicosis with Low Radioactive Iodine Uptake." Endocrinology and Metabolism Clinics of North America 27.1 (1998): 169-185.

119) Gluck, Franklin B., et al. "Chronic Lymphocytic Thyroiditis, Thyrotoxicosis, and Low Radioactive Iodine Uptake: Report of Four Cases." New England Journal of Medicine 293.13 (1975): 624-628.

120) Skare, Ståle, and Harald MM Frey. "Iodine-Induced Thyrotoxicosis in Apparently Normal Thyroid Glands." European Journal of Endocrinology 94.3 (1980): 332-336.

121) Edmunds, H. Tudor. "Acute Thyroiditis from Potassium Iodide." British Medical Journal 1.4909 (1955): 354.

122) de Boer, H., et al. "Hyperactive Thyroid Nodules Treated by Radiofrequency Ablation: A Dutch Single-Centre Experience." Neth J Med 78.2 (2020): 64-70.

123) Hussain, Iram, et al. "Safety and Efficacy of Radiofrequency Ablation of Thyroid Nodules—Expanding Treatment Options in the United States." Journal of the Endocrine Society 5.8 (2021): bvab110.

124) Spiezia, Stefano, et al. "Ultrasound-Guided Laser Thermal Ablation in the Treatment of Autonomous Hyperfunctioning Thyroid Nodules and Compressive Nontoxic Nodular Goiter." Thyroid 13.10 (2003): 941-947.

125) Døssing, Helle, et al. "Randomized Prospective Study Comparing a Single Radioiodine Dose and a Single Laser Therapy Session in Autonomously Functioning Thyroid Nodules." European Journal of Endocrinology 157.1 (2007): 95-100.

Chapter 20

Hashimoto's, Iodine and Selenium Part One

Iodine Supplementation in Hashimoto's Thyroiditis

IODINE SUPPLEMENTATION IN HASHIMOTO'S PATIENTS is a special case. As discussed in previous chapters, patients with autoimmune thyroid disease are unable to escape from the inhibitory actions of iodine supplements, meaning iodine will make them hypothyroid with high TSH. However, another less common outcome of excess iodine supplementation in Hashimoto's patients is Hashitoxicosis. This is a form of acute thyroiditis caused by oxidative damage from excess H2O2 generation, with rupture of follicles and release of preformed thyroid hormone. In Hashitoxicosis, as in other forms of thyroiditis, five-hour radio-iodine uptake will be very low, less than 5 percent.

What Are the Conditions for Iodine-Induced Hashitoxicosis?

As discussed in previous chapters, iodine decreases H2O2 production and inhibits its own organification, the Wolff-Chaikoff Effect. However, under conditions of iodine deficiency, the opposite occurs, and iodine intake will increase H2O2 generation, thus creating the conditions for excess oxidative damage, especially when selenium deficiency renders the anti-oxidant system dysfunctional. High TSH stimulates H2O2 generation, and this may also play a role in oxidative damage. Thus, we have created the conditions for Hashitoxicosis. (1-5)

Selenium is Protective

Selenium is a key component of the selenoprotein antioxidant system in the thyrocytes which quenches reactive oxygen species (ROS) and free radicles associated with hydrogen peroxide generation, a critical step in production of thyroid hormone. Hydrogen peroxide is a damaging oxidizing agent. Since selenium deficiency is a prerequisite for iodine induced thyroid damage, providing the patient with selenium supplements (200-400 mcg/day) is beneficial in preventing thyroiditis.

TSH Suppression is Protective

Perhaps the most effective intervention for turning off hydrogen peroxide generation in the thyroid gland is to suppress TSH, the master controller of all steps in the production of thyroid hormone, including the generation of hydrogen peroxide. This is done in Hashimoto's patients with the use of thyroid hormone medication, NDT, or levothyroxine. Similarly, in Graves' disease patients, TSH may be quite elevated during treatment with Anti-Thyroid Drug (ATD) treatment which blocks thyroid function. Elevated TSH will generate damaging excess hydrogen peroxide. Block and Replace technique using levothyroxine or NDT will suppress the TSH to a lower level, inhibiting hydrogen peroxide generation. As mentioned in Chapter 15. Graves' Hyperthyroidism Remission with Iodine, Part One, Dr. Ken Okamura found Block and Replace superior to tapering ATD dosage in preventing relapse of hyperthyroidism. In Chapter 16, we learned that most of these relapses were Painless Thyroiditis, PT, a form of inflammatory thyroiditis related to excess hydrogen peroxide generation. Block and Replace works because it suppresses TSH and turns off hydrogen peroxide generation. (6-8)

Supportive Animal Studies

In 2011, Dr. Xu performed supportive animal studies. In these studies, mice were given varying amounts of iodine as well as varying amounts of selenium, finding iodine excess causes autoimmune thyroiditis only if selenium is deficient or in excess. Dr Xu writes in his 2011 report:

> **Excess iodine intake can cause an autoimmune thyroiditis that bears all the characteristics of Hashimoto's.** However, in animal studies this occurs **only if selenium is deficient** or in excess. **Similarly, in animal studies very high iodine intake can exacerbate a pre- existing autoimmune thyroiditis, but only if selenium is deficient** or in excess. With optimal selenium status, thyroid follicles are healthy, goiter is eliminated, and autoimmune markers like Th1/Th2 ratio and CD4+/CD8+ ratio are normalized over a wide range of iodine intake... It seems that **optimizing selenium intake provides powerful protection against autoimmune thyroid disease, and provides tolerance of a wide range of iodine intakes.** Emphasis Mine. (9-11)

Iodine Excess Causes Selenium Deficiency

In 2006, Dr. Yang studied selenium supplementation in mice given excessive doses of iodine and finds that excess iodine contributes to selenium deficiency in the experimental mice. The selenium stores are exhausted in these mice while neutralizing excess hydrogen peroxide generated to process the iodine. Dr. Yang writes:

> Relative selenium deficiency caused by excessive iodine plays an essential role in the mechanism of iodine-induced abnormalities. An appropriate dose of selenium supplementation exercises a beneficial intervention. (11)

Iodine Excess- Mechanism for Thyroid Failure

in 2006, Dr. Na Man studied mice with varying doses of iodine intake. In these mice, Dr. Man studied TPO (thyroid peroxidase enzyme) activity and NIS (sodium-iodide symporter) protein levels, finding both are reduced by the iodine intake. As we have discussed elsewhere in this book, iodine excess inhibits thyroid function, the Wolff-Chaikoff effect. Dr. Na Ma writes:

> The iodine content of thyroid tissue was negatively correlated with TPO activity, iodine intake rate, NIS protein positive rate, and expression intensity...Moderate iodine excess continuously suppresses the thyroid iodine uptake and organification, which presents a mechanism for iodine-induced thyroid failure. Note: NIS (sodium-iodide symporter) is the active transport mechanism for iodine into the thyroid cells. (12)

Role of Selenium in Hashimoto's

In 2007, Dr. Elias E. Mazokopakis from Greece studied the benefits of selenium supplementation in autoimmune thyroid disease. These benefits are related to the incorporation of selenium into various selenoproteins involved in the anti-oxidant system of the thyroid gland which protects thyroid cells from the damaging effects of excess hydrogen peroxide, a substance playing a key role in the production of thyroid hormones. Indeed, hydrogen peroxide is necessary for the organification of iodine, the attachment of iodine to the thyroglobulin molecule by the TPO enzyme. The antioxidant selenoproteins are glutathione peroxidase (GPX) and thioredoxin reductase (TR). Dr Elias E. Mazokopakis writes:

> Selenium (Se) supplementation in patients with AITD [autoimmune thyroid disease], including HT [Hashimoto's Thyroiditis], seems to modify the inflammatory and immune responses, probably by enhancing plasma glutathione peroxidase (GPX) and thioredoxin reductase (TR) activity and by **decreasing toxic concentrations of hydrogen peroxide ($H2O2$)** and lipid hydroperoxides, resulting from thyroid hormone synthesis. (13)

Benefits of Iodine, Is Iodine the Next Vitamin D3?

Iodine is an essential nutrient, and globally, iodine deficiency is a massive health problem. Some researchers believe that iodine supplementation will become the "next Vitamin D," an example of a vitamin initially thought to be toxic, and now accepted in much higher doses as beneficial for health. Not only is iodine deficiency a leading cause of mental retardation in developing children, and miscarriage in mothers, but it is also implicated in the etiology of thyroid cancer, breast cancer, and gastric cancer in adults. Screening programs to detect iodine deficiency, and provide iodine supplements have an enormous benefit for public health. In 2011, Dr Zimmerman studied the benefits of iodine supplementation and concludes:

> Iodine prophylaxis of deficient populations with periodic monitoring is an extremely cost-effective approach to reduce the substantial adverse effects of iodine deficiency throughout the life cycle. (14-17)

World Health Organization Definition of Iodine Deficiency

Guidelines for Spot Urinary Iodine Levels (14)

50-99 mcg/L – mild iodine deficiency,

20-49 mcg/L – moderate iodine deficiency,

< 20 mcg/L – severe iodine deficiency.

As mentioned in Chapter 5, Quest, LabCorp and most other commercial laboratories will do a test called the spot urinary iodine. This is a single urine sample obtained at the same session as the blood draw. This is quick and easy way to get a measurement of the patient's iodine level. The spot urine is more convenient for the patient. No need to do a 24-hour sample which requires the patient to carry around a collection bucket all day.

Always Give Selenium Before Iodine Supplements

Selenium testing and supplementation when low is a prerequisite in all patients with elevated anti-thyroid antibody levels and Hashimoto's thyroiditis. Iodine deficiency is a health risk and iodine supplementation is beneficial. However, selenium supplementation is required before giving iodine to Hashimoto's patients. Selenium is inexpensive and readily available as a supplement in tablet or capsule form. The usual dosage is 200-400 mcg/day of seleno-methionine. Selenium can be toxic at excessive dosage, so it is best to measure selenium blood levels and work closely with a knowledgeable physician.

Iodine Supplementation for the Hashimoto's Patient

For iodine supplementation in autoimmune thyroiditis (Hashimoto's) patients, we follow a protocol described here. Both serum selenium and urinary spot iodine levels are determined on the initial laboratory panel. For selenium levels below 135 ng/mL, we give selenium supplementation (200-400 mcg/d) based on the 2008 study by Dr. Joachim Bleys. (18)

For spot urinary iodine levels below 100 mcg/L, we start low-dose iodine 225 mcg/day based on work by Dr. Reinhardt of Germany. (5)

Healthy Patients May Use Iodoral

For patients who do not have autoimmune thyroid disease, with normal anti-thyroid antibody levels, we use a higher dose iodine supplement called Iodoral, 12.5 mg tablets from Optimox, widely available over-the-counter without a prescription. Follow-up spot urine tests in patients on Iodoral will show levels far in excess of the laboratory reference range. This is to be expected and indicates the patient is taking a high-dose iodine supplement. For certain types of testing, we do not use the reference range. This is one of those. Again, it is best to work with a knowledgeable physician who can monitor laboratory testing.

Conclusion

One of the errors of modern endocrinology is ignoring the use of selenium for auto-immune thyroid patients. Selenium supplementation alleviates the adverse effects of excess iodine intake. (19-21)

♦ **References for Chapter 20:**

1) Wolff J, Chaikoff IL. Plasma Inorganic Iodide as a Homeostatic Regulator of Thyroid Function. J Biol Chem 1948; 174:555-564.

2) Rose, Noel R., Raphael Bonita, and C. Lynne Burek. "Iodine: An Environmental Trigger of Thyroiditis." Autoimmunity Reviews 1.1-2 (2002): 97-103.

3) Yoon, Soo Jee, et al. "The Effect of Iodine Restriction on Thyroid Function in Patients with Hypothyroidism Due to Hashimoto's Thyroiditis." Yonsei Medical Journal 44.2 (2003): 227-235.

4) Fountoulakis, Stelios, et al. "The Role of Iodine in the Evolution of Thyroid Disease in Greece: From Endemic Goiter to Thyroid Autoimmunity." Hormones-Athens- 6.1 (2007): 25.

5) Reinhardt, W., et al. "Effect of Small Doses of Iodine on Thyroid Function in Patients with Hashimoto's Thyroiditis Residing in an Area of Mild Iodine Deficiency." European Journal of Endocrinology 139.1 (1998): 23-28.

6) Okamura, Ken, et al. "Iodide-Sensitive Graves' Hyperthyroidism and the Strategy for Resistant or Escaped Patients During Potassium Iodide Treatment." Endocrine Journal (2022): EJ21-0436.

7) Vigone, M. C., et al. "Block-and-Replace" Treatment in Graves' Disease: Experience in a Cohort of Pediatric Patients." Journal Of Endocrinological Investigation 43 (2020): 595-600.

8) Dinauer, Catherine A. "The Block-and-Replace Method May Have a Role in the Management of Pediatric Graves' Disease." Clinical Thyroidology 32.1 (2020): 17-19.

9) Xu, Jian, et al. "Supplemental Selenium Alleviates the Toxic Effects of Excessive Iodine on Thyroid." Biological Trace Element Research 141.1 (2011): 110-118.

10) Xu, Jian, et al. "Selenium Supplement Alleviated the Toxic Effects of Excessive Iodine in Mice." Biological Trace Element Research 111.1 (2006): 229-238.

11) Yang, Xue-feng, et al. "Effect of Selenium Supplementation on Activity and mRNA Expression of Type 1 Deiodinase in Mice with Excessive Iodine Intake." Biomedical and Environmental Sciences 19.4 (2006): 302.

12) Man, Na, et al. "Long-Term Effects of High Iodine Intake: Inhibition of Thyroid Iodine Uptake and Organification in Wistar rats." Zhonghua Yi Xue Za Zhi 86.48 (2006): 3420-3424.

13) Mazokopakis, Elias E., and Vasiliki Chatzipavlidou. "Hashimoto's Thyroiditis and the Role of Selenium. Current Concepts." Hell J Nucl Med 10.1 (2007): 6-8.

14) Pizzorno, Lara and Meletis, Chris. "Iodine: The Next Vitamin D? Part II." https://biolargo.blogspot.com/2009_05_01_archive.html

15) Zimmermann, Michael B. "The Role of Iodine in Human Growth and Development." Seminars In Cell & Developmental Biology. Vol. 22. No. 6. Academic Press, 2011.

16) Zimmermann, Michael B. "Iodine Deficiency in Pregnancy and the Effects of Maternal Iodine Supplementation on the Offspring: A Review." The American Journal of Clinical Nutrition 89.2 (2009): 668S-672S.

17) Zimmermann, Michael B. "Efficacy and Safety of Iodine Fortification." Food Fortification in a Globalized World. Academic Press, 2018. 221-230.

18) Bleys, Joachim, et al. "Serum Selenium Levels and All-Cause, Cancer, and Cardiovascular Mortality Among US Adults." Archives of Internal Medicine 168.4 (2008): 404-410.

19) Mseddi, Malek, et al. "Lipid Peroxidation, Proteins Modifications, Anti-Oxidant Enzymes Activities and Selenium Deficiency in the Plasma of Hashitoxicosis Patients." Therapeutic Advances in Endocrinology and Metabolism 6.5 (2015): 181-188.

20) Zimmermann, Michael B., and Josef Köhrle. "The Impact of Iron and Selenium Deficiencies on Iodine and Thyroid Metabolism: Biochemistry and Relevance to Public Health." Thyroid 12.10 (2002): 867-878.

21) Triggiani, Vincenzo, et al. "Role of Iodine, Selenium and Other Micronutrients in Thyroid Function and Disorders." Endocrine, Metabolic & Immune Disorders-Drug Targets 9.3 (2009): 277-294.

Chapter 21

Hashimoto's Iodine and Selenium Part Two

Susan has Hashimoto's thyroiditis, an autoimmune thyroid disorder causing fatigue, puffy face, and muscle weakness. For the past year, she had been under the care of an endocrinologist who started thyroid medication called levothyroxine, generic Synthroid, and did follow-up testing for thyroid antibody levels. Susan found it disturbing that her anti-thyroid antibody levels kept climbing higher on each subsequent lab test. The doctors had no explanation, so she asked me if there was something else that could be done. Yes, there is a very good treatment called selenium, an essential trace mineral, available at the health food store as 200 mcg tablets.

Selenium Studies Showing Selenium Beneficial

By 2021, twenty clinical trials had been performed investigating the use of selenium in Hashimoto's thyroiditis. Here are a few of them:

In 2007, Dr. Mazokopakis from Crete reported in Thyroid a 21 percent reduction in the TPO antibodies after one year of selenomethionine, 200 mcg per day. (1)

In 2002, Dr. Roland Gärtner from Germany in the Journal of Clinical Endocrinology and Metabolism showed a 40 percent reduction in anti-thyroid antibody levels after selenium supplementation. Nine of thirty-six patients, twenty-five percent, completely normalized their antibody levels. (2)

In 2006, Dr. Omer Turker from Turkey in the Journal of Endocrinology showed a thirty percent decrease in anti-thyroid antibodies after three months of L-selenomethionine supplementation at 200 mcg per day in women with Hashimoto's thyroiditis. The starting average TPO antibodies was 803 IU/mL and after three months the average was 572 IU/mL. (3)

Combined Use of Levothyroxine and Selenium More Effective

In 2003, Dr. Duntas from Athens, Greece studied selenomethionine supplementation in 65 patients with Hashimoto's thyroiditis. Thirty-four patients in Group One were given selenomethionine 200 mcg, plus levothyroxine (to maintain TSH between 0.3-2.0 mU/l). Group Two patients received levothyroxine alone. In Group One receiving the selenium plus levothyroxine, anti-TPO levels decreased forty-six percent at three months (from roughly 1900 to 1000 IU/ml) and decreased fifty-five percent at six months. In group 2 with levothyroxine alone, TPO antibody declines were only twenty-one percent at three months and twenty-seven percent at six months. The combined use of selenium with levothyroxine was more effective than levothyroxine alone for a reduction in antibody levels. (4)

In 2021, Dr Hu conducted a prospective randomized trial in 43 Hashimoto's patients who received 200 µg/day selenized yeast tablets for six months, and 47 control patients who received no treatment. None were treated with levothyroxine. Patients were instructed to adjust dietary iodine intake to correspond with a urine output of 100–199 µg/L. After 6 months, for the selenium-treated group, serum selenium more than doubled from 74 to 187.2 µg/L. Glutathione peroxidase (GPx3) and selenoprotein P1 (SePP1) increased in the selenium-treated group. Both TPO and Thyroglobulin antibodies decreased significantly in the selenium-treated group compared to controls. Activated Tregs (aTreg) cells in the selenium group were significantly higher than the control group at 6 months. TSH was decreased in the selenium group, while increased in the control group. Note: Treg cells are immune cells involved in immune tolerance, protecting against auto-immune disease. Dr Hu writes:

> The thyroid gland contains the highest concentration of Se [selenium], which is incorporated into selenoproteins, such as glutathione peroxidase (GPx), selenoprotein P (SePP), thioredoxin reductase, and iodothyronine deiodinases... iodine as the primary factor to thyroid hormone synthesis is closely related to pathogenesis of autoimmune thyroiditis. The status of iodine deficiency or excessive iodine intake results in an increase in the prevalence of HT [Hashimoto's thyroiditis]... This study suggested that Se has the potential to reduce thyroid antibodies and TSH levels in the development of HT [Hashimoto's Thyroiditis], and ... low Se status is associated with increased risk of thyroid disease... GPx3 showed statistical difference between groups, implying the **reduced antioxidation ability in patients with HT...**In conclusion, **Se supplementation is associated with reductions in TPOAb [thyroperoxidase antibody], TGAb [thyroglobulin antibody], and TSH [thyroid stimulating hormone] levels, as well as increases in Se [selenium], GPx3, and SePP1 concentrations in patients with HT without levothyroxine replacement... HT patients whose selenium levels less than 120 µg/L may** be susceptible to the beneficial effect of Se supplementation... Se may have the potential to enhance antioxidant ability and upregulated activated Treg cells in vivo of patients with HT. (5-7)

Note: Dr. Hu is suggesting selenium supplementation if the blood level is less than 120 mcg/L. We use a selenium level of 135 mcg/L as our cut-off based on a 2008 study by Dr. Joachim Bleys. (8)

Why is Selenium So Important for Thyroid Function?

Recent research in thyroid cell physiology shows that selenium is very important for thyroid function. There are at least 30 selenium-de-pendent proteins, including the glutathione peroxidase enzyme, and the D1 and D2 iodo-thyronine deiodinases enzymes, which convert T4 (thyroxine) to the more bioactive T3. These enzymes all need selenium as a co-factor. The selenoprotein, glutathione peroxidase, protects thyroid cells from damage by hydrogen peroxide ($H2O2$) produced by the thyroid cell. $H2O2$ is needed as a normal step in thyroid hormone production, However, too much $H2O2$ can damage the thyroid cell. In the event of selenium deficiency, the glutathione peroxidase enzyme cannot do its job protecting the thyroid cell, and the thyroid cells are damaged by excess $H2O2$. The current theory is that these damaged proteins, thyroglobulin, and TPO enzyme, are then recognized by the immune system as foreign, leading to Hashimoto's autoimmune disease. In addition, excess hydrogen peroxide is mutagenic, leading to thyroid nodules, autonomous nodules, and thyroid malignancy. (9-12)

Link to Wheat Consumption, Leaky Gut and Molecular Mimicry

Although selenium deficiency is a predisposing factor, wheat gluten consumption is the other major culprit. As discussed in Chapter 18, Addressing the Auto-Immune Component of Thyroid Disease, wheat gluten consumption in genetically predisposed individuals causes Leaky Gut, with leakage of bacterial antigens into the bloodstream. Via a mechanism called molecular mimicry, the immune system then attacks the thyroid gland, explaining the underlying causation of Hashimoto's, and Graves' disease. Yersinia and H. Pylori are two such bacterial organisms that have been implicated. In addition, there is a high correlation between Hashimoto's thyroiditis and Celiac Disease, an autoimmune disease caused by wheat gluten consumption. Obviously, the elimination of wheat gluten from the diet is beneficial and highly recommended for the autoimmune thyroid patient.

Back to the Patient

Susan was started on selenium, 200 mcg per day. In addition, Susan's thyroid medication was switched from Synthroid to NDT, natural desiccated thyroid. In my opinion, NDT is a more robust and clinically superior thyroid preparation. Three months later, Susan returned for follow-up labs which showed a significant decline in antibody levels.

Thyroid Testing and Treatment

A good thyroid testing protocol includes the following lab values, TSH, Free T3, Free T4, TPO Abs, Thyroglobulin Abs, reverse T3, serum selenium level, and spot urinary iodine level. The thyroid panel is usually part of a larger evaluation with additional lab tests tailored to the clinical history and examination. We also check Vitamin D3, RBC magnesium, Iron, Ferritin, and H. Pylori breath test. A good thyroid treatment protocol uses NDT, a natural desiccated thyroid medication. Dosage for natural desiccated thyroid medication varies, based on body weight, thyroid lab values, and thyroid function.

Selenium Safety or Toxicity Depends on Dosage

Although selenium is an inexpensive supplement available without a prescription at the health food store, I would recommend working closely with your physician if you are considering selenium supplementation. Selenium is generally considered safe at standard doses of 200-400 mcg per day. However, very high dosages can cause selenium toxicity. By the way, a good dietary source of selenium is the Brazil nut, high in selenium. (13-16)

Testing and Treatment in Hashimoto's Thyroiditis

Thyroid function in Hashimoto's thyroiditis can have a variable course, with thyroid function varying over time. Thyroid function may emulate a "Roller Coaster Effect", caused by intermittent episodes of thyroiditis (also called Hashitoxicosis), thyrotoxicosis caused by the inflammatory release of preformed thyroid hormone from ruptured follicles. These hyperthyroid episodes alternate with longer periods of hypothyroidism requiring thyroid hormone replacement. The need for thyroid medication varies depending upon thyroid function which can change over time. Lab studies at any one time may show low, normal, or high thyroid function in patients with elevated antibody levels and Hashimoto's thyroid disease.

Conclusion

Ignoring the role of selenium is another error in modern thyroid endocrinology. The benefits of selenium supplementation for Hashimoto's patients are well-established in the medical literature. (17-19)

♦ **References for Chapter 21**

1) Mazokopakis, Elias E., et al. "Effects of 12 Months Treatment with L-Selenomethionine on Serum Anti-TPO Levels in Patients with Hashimoto's Thyroiditis." Thyroid 17.7 (2007): 609-612.

2) Gärtner, Roland, et al. "Selenium Supplementation in Patients with Autoimmune Thyroiditis Decreases Thyroid Peroxidase Antibodies Concentrations." The Journal of Clinical Endocrinology & Metabolism 87.4 (2002): 1687-1691.

3) Turker, Omer, et al. "Selenium Treatment in Autoimmune Thyroiditis: 9-Month Follow-Up with Variable Doses." Journal of Endocrinology 190.1 (2006): 151-156

4) Duntas, Leonidas H., et al. "Effects of a Six-Month Treatment with Selenomethionine in Patients with Autoimmune Thyroiditis." European Journal of Endocrinology 148.4 (2003): 389-393.

5) Hu, Y., et al. "Effect of Selenium on Thyroid Autoimmunity and Regulatory T Cells in Patients with Hashimoto's Thyroiditis: A Prospective Randomized-Controlled Trial." Clinical and Translational Science 14.4 (2021): 1390-1402.

6) Li, Qian, et al. "The Pathogenesis of Thyroid Autoimmune Diseases: New T Lymphocytes–Cytokines Circuits Beyond the Th1– Th2 Paradigm." Journal of Cellular Physiology 234.3 (2019): 2204-2216.

---

7) Duntas, L. H. "The Role of Iodine and Selenium in Autoimmune Thyroiditis." Hormone And Metabolic Research 47.10 (2015): 721-726.

8) Bleys, Joachim, et al. "Serum Selenium Levels and All-Cause, Cancer, and Cardiovascular Mortality Among US Adults." Archives of Internal Medicine 168.4 (2008): 404-410.

9) Song, Yue, et al. "Roles of Hydrogen Peroxide in Thyroid Physiology and Disease." The Journal of Clinical Endocrinology & Metabolism 92.10 (2007): 3764-3773.

10) Driessens, Natacha, et al. "Hydrogen Peroxide Induces DNA Single-and Double-Strand Breaks in Thyroid Cells and is Therefore a Potential Mutagen for this Organ." Endocrine-related cancer 16.3 (2009): 845.

11) Mseddi, Malek, et al. "Proteins Oxidation and Autoantibodies' Reactivity Against Hydrogen Peroxide and Malondialdehyde-Oxidized Thyroid Antigens in Patients' Plasmas with Graves' Disease and Hashimoto Thyroiditis." Chemico-Biological Interactions 272 (2017): 145-152.

12) Da Silva, Maurício Martins, et al. "Bisphenol A Increases Hydrogen Peroxide Generation by Thyrocytes Both in Vivo and in Vitro." Endocrine Connections 7.11 (2018): 1196.

13) Thomson, Christine D., et al. "Brazil Nuts: An Effective Way to Improve Selenium Status." The American Journal of Clinical Nutrition 87.2 (2008): 379-384.

14) Cheng, Wen-Hsing. "Revisiting Selenium Toxicity." The Journal of Nutrition 151.4 (chapter021): 747-748.

15) Aldosary, Barrak M., et al. "Case Series of Selenium Toxicity from a Nutritional Supplement." Clinical Toxicology 50.1 (2012): 57-64.

16) Hadrup, Niels, and Gitte Ravn-Haren. "Acute Human Toxicity and Mortality After Selenium Ingestion: A Review." Journal of Trace Elements in Medicine and Biology 58 (2020): 126435.

17) Zimmermann, Michael B., and Josef Köhrle. "The Impact of Iron and Selenium Deficiencies on Iodine and Thyroid Metabolism: Biochemistry and Relevance to Public Health." Thyroid 12.10 (2002): 867-878.

18) Mazokopakis, Elias E., and Vassiliki Chatzipavlidou. "Hashimoto's Thyroiditis and the Role of Selenium. Current Concepts." Hell J Nucl Med 10.1 (2007): 6-8.

19) Kohrle, J., et al. "Selenium, the Thyroid, and the Endocrine System." Endocrine Reviews 26.7 (2005): 944-984.

Chapter 22

Selenium and the Thyroid, More Good News Part Three

IN 2013 CLINICAL ENDOCRINOLOGY, DR. Anne Drutel wrote "More Good News!" on selenium supplementation decreasing antibody levels in Hashimoto's autoimmune thyroiditis:

> The thyroid is the organ with the highest selenium content per gram of tissue because it expresses specific selenoproteins...In patients with Hashimoto's disease and in pregnant women with anti-TPO antibodies, selenium supplementation decreases anti-thyroid antibody levels and improves the ultrasound structure of the thyroid gland. (1)

In my office, we routinely test for selenium levels and give 200 mcg/day selenomethionine when found below 130 mcg/L based on the 2008 study by Dr. Joachim Bleys. We follow serum selenium levels on serial laboratory studies in all patients routinely. (2)

The Rarity of Selenium Toxicity

Selenium overdose with selenium toxicity is a theoretical possibility, however, this is extremely rare. Over the time span of my medical career from 1976 to the present, working in multiple hospitals over several states as a diagnostic radiologist, I have never seen a patient admitted to the hospital with a diagnosis of selenium toxicity. If one does a medical literature search, there have been a few reports of selenium toxicity from manufacturing errors and misbranding made by fringe supplement companies. These have been promptly shut down by the FDA. In 2010, Dr. Jennifer MacFarquhar reported an "outbreak" of 201 patients with selenium toxicity from a liquid mineral supplement that contained 200 times the labeled concentration of selenium, providing a massive overdose of 41,749 mcg per day. The usual daily dosage for selenium is 200-400 mcg/day. In 8 of the patients of the 201 with selenium toxicity, the mean serum selenium was 751 mcg/L. The lab range for selenium is 63-160 mcg/L (Quest lab). Dr. Jennifer MacFarquhar writes:

> The source of the outbreak was identified as a liquid dietary supplement that contained 200 times the labeled concentration of selenium. Of 201 cases identified in 10 states, 1 person was hospitalized. The median estimated dose of selenium consumed was 41,749 mcg/d (recommended dietary allowance is 55 mcg/d). Frequently reported symptoms included diarrhea (78%), fatigue (75%), hair loss (72%), joint pain (70%), nail discoloration or brittleness (61%), and nausea (58%). Symptoms persisting 90 days or longer included fingernail discoloration and loss (52%), fatigue (35%), and hair loss (29%). The mean initial serum selenium concentration of 8 patients was 751 mcg/L (reference range, ≤125 mcg/L). The mean initial urine selenium concentration of 7 patients was 166 mcg/24 h (reference range, ≤55 mcg/24 h). (37-39)

The take-home message is to stick with reputable supplement companies, avoid fringe supplement manufacturers, and work with a knowledgeable physician who can monitor selenium levels.

The Iodine in Hashimoto's Controversy

Iodine supplementation in Hashimoto's autoimmune thyroiditis patients is controversial, and many patients read on the internet that iodine should never be given to Hashimoto's patients. However, iodine is an essential mineral, and iodine deficiency is associated with adverse health outcomes. Maternal iodine deficiency can lead to fetal neurodevelopment delay or even cretinism. As you will read in Chapters 31 and 32, iodine is useful in the treatment of fibrocystic breast disease and the prevention of breast cancer. (3) (55-60)

Starting Selenium First Before Iodine Supplementation!

Many Hashimoto's patients have normal iodine levels on testing. However, for the iodine-deficient patient, we would like to devise a protocol to provide iodine supplementation safely without aggravating inflammatory thyroid disease. This can be done by first supplementing with selenium before the iodine. Selenium supplementation protects the thyroid cells from oxidative damage arising from hydrogen peroxide production, an essential substrate in the production of thyroid hormone.

The Selenoproteins

In 2018, Dr. Agathocles Tsatsoulis studied the role of selenium and iodine in autoimmune thyroid disease, finding excess iodine intake triggers autoimmune thyroiditis, mainly by increasing the generation of H2O2, hydrogen peroxide. However, selenium supplementation is protective. Dr. Agathocles Tsatsoulis writes:

> Iodine is a trace element that is essential for the synthesis of thyroid hormones in the thyroid gland. Evidence suggests that **excess iodine intake exerts a triggering effect on the development of autoimmune thyroiditis** (AT), with many studies reporting a rising incidence in iodine-sufficient countries. **Processing excess iodine in thyroid follicular cells during thyroid hormone synthesis may result in increased amounts of reactive oxygen species [hydrogen peroxide], leading to thyroid cell damage and the triggering of thyroid autoimmunity.** Another trace element, selenium, found in high amounts in the thyroid, is very important for thyroid physiology. Selenium is incorporated into **selenoproteins that are involved in the protection of thyroid cells from oxidative damage incurred by exposure to hydrogen peroxide** (H2O2) originating during thyroid hormone synthesis. **Population studies suggest an increased prevalence of thyroid autoimmunity in areas following iodine fortification and a possible protective effect with selenium adequacy. In animal models, selenium has been shown to reverse the induction of autoimmune thyroiditis caused by excess iodine intake.** It appears therefore, that an optimal balance between iodine and selenium is important for maintaining normal thyroid function, and that the loss of such balance in favor of iodine, may play a role for the rising trend of autoimmune thyroiditis, currently seen in iodine sufficient countries. (4)

For Hashimoto's patients who test low for iodine, our office protocol starts with selenium supplementation of 200-400 mcg per day for two to four weeks, after which low dose iodine (225 mcg per day) is started. Several studies have shown that this dosage of iodine is safe and causes no harm in autoimmune thyroiditis patients. (5-8)

How to Reduce Antibody Levels in Hashimoto's

The most useful interventions for reducing antibody levels in Hashimoto's thyroiditis patients are:

1) TSH suppression with thyroid medication. Conventional endocrinologists use levothyroxine (generic Synthroid) with a treatment goal of TSH in the lower half of the normal range. In our treatment protocol, we use natural desiccated thyroid (NDT), and our goal is to suppress the TSH below the normal range. Studies show suppressive doses of thyroid medication beneficial for reducing antibody levels. We have found this true in clinical practice as well. See Chapter 7 on TSH Suppression Benefits and Adverse Effects. (4-5) (9-12)

2) Selenium supplementation, as discussed above. (13-42) (63-65)

3) Gluten-Free Diet. (43-45)

4) Myo-Inositol Supplements. See Chapter 28 on Myo-inositol for Hashimoto's Thyroiditis.

5) Vitamin D supplementation. (46-51)

6) LDN Low Dose Naltrexone: Some patients report LDN has benefits, but there are no medical studies to support this yet. The absence of adverse effects has liberalized use. (62)

TSH Suppression for the Hashimoto's Patient

In 1999, Dr. Rink studied 375 Euthyroid Hashimoto's patients given 200 mcg of iodide over 28 months. Despite the iodide intake, there was no increase in antibody levels over 28 months. However, for the high iodide group, a 1.5 mg dose of iodide given once a week had a "distinct increase in TPO and Thyroglobulin Antibodies." A second group of 377 Hashimoto's patients received levothyroxine, with or without the iodine. In the second group receiving levothyroxine, both anti-thyroglobulin antibodies and anti-TPO declined significantly, with the most significant decline in TPO in the TSH-suppressed group. Dr. Rink writes:

> The patients of the second collective [group] revealed a significant decrease of the TgAb in the subgroups treated with up to 200 micrograms iodide daily while the **reduction of the TPOAb depended on the thyrotropin level [TSH level] and was most significant in the suppressed group** (p < 0.0001). (5)

In 2007, Dr. Elias Mazokopakis discussed TSH suppression in Hashimoto's thyroiditis, writing suppressive doses of levothyroxine may be given to patients with enlarged thyroid and normal or elevated TSH levels:

> In HT [Hashimoto's Thyroiditis] patients with a large goiter and normal or elevated serum thyroid-stimulating hormone (TSH), L-T(4) [levothyroxine] may be given in doses sufficient to suppress serum TSH. (10)

In 2008, Dr. Matthias Schmidt did a retrospective observational study over 50 months of 38 patients (36 women and 2 men) on levothyroxine for Hashimoto's thyroiditis with elevated TPO antibody levels. Over the 50 months of the study, 92 percent of patients showed a decrease in TPO antibodies. After one year, the mean decrease was 45 percent, and after 5 years, the mean decrease was 70 percent. Dr. Schmidt writes:

> In the 35 patients with decreasing TPO-Ab values, the mean initial value was 4779 IU/mL ...The mean decrease after 3 months was 8%, and after 1 year it was 45%. Five years after the first value, TPO-Ab levels...decrease by 70%. (52)

In my opinion, the benefit of TSH suppression arises from the TSH control of H2O2 generation. As we read in Chapter 14, Production of Thyroid Hormones, TSH stimulates the generation of hydrogen peroxide. Suppressing TSH essentially turns off H2O2 hydrogen peroxide generation, thus eliminating the key element of thyroid damage and inflammation in autoimmune thyroid disease. In my opinion, this holds true for both Hashimoto's and Graves' disease. In Graves' Disease, this is called "Block and Replace," the practice of giving levothyroxine to suppress an elevated TSH in Graves' Disease patients. The elevated TSH results from over-treatment with thyroid-blocking drugs, a common occurrence. (53-54)

My Own Clinical Experience

In my experience, I have found TSH suppression, selenium, and vitamin D3 supplementation, and a gluten-free diet prevents anti-thyroid antibodies from increasing and prevents flare-ups of Hashitoxicosis. Thus, in my experience, we have seen no episodes of Hashitoxicosis in patients with TSH suppression. This is also true for Hashimoto's patients with suppressed TSH who commonly take 12.5 mg of iodine a day for treatment of fibrocystic breast disease. With a suppressed TSH, we have seen no episodes of Hashitoxicosis in this group despite the high dose of iodine for the treatment of fibrocystic breast disease. As mentioned in previous chapters, excess iodine has a strong inhibitory effect on thyroid function in

Hashimoto's patients, a mechanism for thyroid failure. This is called the Wolff-Chaikoff Effect. Negative feedback at the pituitary level will trigger a high TSH level, which then stimulates H202 generation, a damaging substance. If not neutralized by the selenium-based anti-oxidant system, excess H202 leads to an inflammatory attack, also known as Hashitoxicosis. TSH suppression prevents this from happening. (55-60)

Gluten Sensitivity and Gluten-Free Diet

In 2007, Dr. Muhammed Hadithi conducted a Dutch study of 104 patients with Hashimoto's thyroiditis; sixteen (15%) were positive for anti-gliadin antibodies and gluten sensitivity. The authors recommended routine testing of all Hashimoto's thyroiditis patients for gluten reactivity. We have done this, and our clinical experience agrees. (43)

Another study in 2003 by Dr. Akçay of four hundred patients with autoimmune thyroid disease (280 Graves' disease and 120 Hashimoto's thyroiditis) yielded a 5.5% positive test rate when tested for anti-gliadin antibodies. (44)

Note: Gliadin is a wheat protein. In some cases, serum anti-gliadin antibody testing may yield false negative results. I would surmise the actual positive test rate could be much higher when more sophisticated testing methods are used, such as the stool anti-gliadin antibody test, available at Enterolabs (223 W. 2nd St. Suite 104 Muenster, TX-76252. Phone: 972-686-6869). Since many patients report improvement on a gluten-free diet, it may be prudent for all autoimmune thyroid patients to avoid wheat gluten. For most patients following our entire protocol, we typically observe antibody levels decreasing on serial laboratory studies at 24-week intervals.

Conclusion

Ignoring the role of selenium in the prevention and treatment of autoimmune thyroid disease is another error of modern endocrinology. Testing for vitamin D3 and selenium levels is routine in our office practice. Our protocol for

Hashimoto's Thyroiditis also includes TSH suppression with thyroid medication, selenium, vitamin D3, and a gluten-free diet.

Financial Disclosure: I have no financial interest in Enterolabs, Quest Lab or LabCorp.

◆ References Chapter 22

1) Drutel, Anne, et al. "Selenium and the Thyroid Gland: More Good News for Clinicians." Clinical Endocrinology 78.2 (2013): 155-164.

2) Bleys, Joachim, et al. "Serum Selenium Levels and All-Cause, Cancer, and Cardiovascular Mortality Among US Adults." Arch Intern Med 168.4 (2008): 404-410.

3) Zimmermann, Michael B. "Iodine and the Iodine Deficiency Disorders." Present Knowledge in Nutrition. Academic Press, 2020. 429-441.

4) Tsatsoulis, Agathocles. "The Role of Iodine Vs Selenium on the Rising Trend of Autoimmune Thyroiditis in Iodine Sufficient Countries-An Opinion Article." Open Access J Thy Res 2.1 (2018): 12-14.

5) Rink, T., et al. "Effect of Iodine and Thyroid Hormones in the Induction and Therapy of Hashimoto's Thyroiditis." Nuklearmedizin. Nuclear Medicine 38.5 (1999): 144-149.

6) Reinhardt, W., et al. "Effect of Small Doses of Iodine on Thyroid Function in Patients with Hashimoto's Thyroiditis Residing in an Area of Mild Iodine Deficiency." European Journal of Endocrinology 139.1 (1998): 23-28.

7) Feldkamp, J., et al. "Therapy of Endemic Goiter with Iodide or L-Thyroxine in Older Patients." Deutsche Medizinische Wochenschrift (1946) 121.51-52 (1996): 1587-1591

8) Meng, Wieland, et al. "Iodine Therapy for Iodine Deficiency Goiter and Autoimmune Thyroiditis. A Prospective Study." Medizinische Klinik (Munich, Germany: 1983) 94.11 (1999): 597-602.

9) Krysiak, Robert, and Boguslaw Okopien. "The Effect of Levothyroxine and Selenomethionine on Lymphocyte and Monocyte Cytokine Release in Women with Hashimoto's Thyroiditis." The Journal of Clinical Endocrinology & Metabolism 96.7 (2011): 2206-2215.

10) Mazokopakis, Elias E., and Vassiliki Chatzipavlidou. "Hashimoto's Thyroiditis and the Role of Selenium. Current Concepts." Hell J Nucl Med 10.1 (2007): 6-8.

11) Romaldini, J. H., et al. "Effect of L-Thyroxine Administration on Antithyroid Antibody Levels, Lipid Profile, and Thyroid Volume in Patients with Hashimoto's Thyroiditis." Thyroid: Official Journal of the American Thyroid Association 6.3 (1996): 183-188.

12) Padberg S, Heller K, Usadel KH, Schumm Draeger PM. One-year Prophylactic Treatment of Euthyroid Hashimoto's Thyroiditis Patients with Levothyroxine: Is There a Benefit? Thyroid 2001; 11: 249-255.

13) Zheng, G., et al. "The Association Between Dietary Selenium Intake and Hashimoto's Thyroiditis Among US Adults: National Health and Nutrition Examination Survey (NHANES), 2007–2012." Journal of Endocrinological Investigation (2022): 1-11.

14) Schomburg, Lutz. "Selenium Deficiency Due to Diet, Pregnancy, Severe Illness, or COVID-19—A Preventable Trigger for Autoimmune Disease." International Journal of Molecular Sciences 22.16 (2021): 8532.

15) Zheng, Huijuan, et al. "Effects of Selenium Supplementation on Graves' Disease: A Systematic Review and Meta-Analysis." Evidence-Based Complementary and Alternative Medicine 2018 (2018).

16) Wichman, Johanna, et al. "Selenium Supplementation Significantly Reduces Thyroid Autoantibody Levels in Patients with Chronic Autoimmune Thyroiditis: A Systematic Review and Meta-Analysis." Thyroid 26.12 (2016): 1681-1692.

17) Vasiliu, Ioana, et al. "Protective Role of Selenium on Thyroid Morphology in Iodine-Induced Autoimmune Thyroiditis in Wistar Rats." Experimental and therapeutic medicine 20.4 (2020): 3425-3437.

18) Wang, Weiwei, et al. "Effects of Selenium Supplementation on Spontaneous Autoimmune Thyroiditis in NOD. H-2h4 Mice." Thyroid 25.10 (2015): 1137-1144.

19) Tsatsoulis, Agathocles. "The Role of Iodine Vs Selenium on the Rising Trend of Autoimmune Thyroiditis in Iodine Sufficient Countries-An Opinion Article." Open Access J Thy Res 2.1 (2018): 12-14.

20) Giammanco, Marco, and Manfredi M. Giammanco. "Selenium: A Cure for Autoimmune Thyroiditis." Endocrine, Metabolic & Immune Disorders-Drug Targets 21.8 (2021): 1377-1378.

21) Fountoulakis, Stelios, et al. "The Role of Iodine in the Evolution of Thyroid Disease in Greece: From Endemic Goiter to Thyroid Autoimmunity." Hormones-Athens- 6.1 (2007): 25.

22) Nielsen, Elsa, et al. "Iodine, Inorganic and Soluble Salts." The Danish Environmental Protection Agency, Copenhagen 290 (2014).

23) Li, Yang, et al. "Effects of Selenium Supplement on B Lymphocyte Activity in Experimental Autoimmune Thyroiditis Rats." International Journal of Endocrinology 2021 (2021).

24) Ruz, Manuel, et al. "Single and Multiple Selenium-Zinc-Iodine Deficiencies Affect Rat Thyroid Metabolism and Ultrastructure." The Journal of Nutrition 129.1 (1999): 174-180.

25) Liontiris, Michael I., and Elias E. Mazokopakis. "A Concise Review of Hashimoto Thyroiditis (HT) and the Importance of Iodine, Selenium, Vitamin D and Gluten on the Autoimmunity and Dietary Management of HT Patients. Points That Need More Investigation." Hell J Nucl Med 20.1 (2017): 51-56.

26) Mazokopakis, Elias E., et al. "Effects Of 12 Months Treatment with L-Selenomethionine on Serum Anti-TPO Levels in Patients with Hashimoto's Thyroiditis." Thyroid 17.7 (2007): 609-612.

27) Toulis, Konstantinos A., et al. "Selenium Supplementation in the Treatment of Hashimoto's Thyroiditis: A Systematic Review and a Meta-Analysis." Thyroid 20.10 (2010): 1163-1173.

28) Ferrari, Silvia Martina, et al. "Precision Medicine in Autoimmune Thyroiditis and Hypothyroidism." Frontiers in Pharmacology 12 (2021).

29) Ventura, Mara, et al. "Selenium and Thyroid Disease: From Pathophysiology to Treatment." International Journal of Endocrinology 2017 (2017).

30) Gärtner, Roland, et al. "Selenium Supplementation in Patients with Autoimmune Thyroiditis Decreases Thyroid Peroxidase Antibodies Concentrations." The Journal of Clinical Endocrinology & Metabolism 87.4 (2002): 1687-1691.

31) Gärtner, Roland, and Barbara CH Gasnier. "Selenium in the Treatment of Autoimmune Thyroiditis." Biofactors 19.3-4 (2003): 165-170.

32) Nacamulli, Davide, et al. "Influence of Physiological Dietary Selenium Supplementation on the Natural Course of Autoimmune Thyroiditis." Clinical Endocrinology 73.4 (2010): 535-539.

33) Mao, Jinyuan, et al. "Effect of Low-Dose Selenium on Thyroid Autoimmunity and Thyroid Function in UK Pregnant Women with Mild-To-Moderate Iodine Deficiency." European Journal of Nutrition 55.1 (2016): 55-61.

34) Negro, Roberto, et al. "The Influence of Selenium Supplementation on Postpartum Thyroid Status in Pregnant Women with Thyroid Peroxidase Autoantibodies." The Journal of Clinical Endocrinology & Metabolism 92.4 (2007): 1263-1268.

35) Karimi, F., and G. R. Omrani. "Effects of Selenium and Vitamin C on the Serum Level of Anti-Thyroid Peroxidase Antibody in Patients with Autoimmune Thyroiditis." Journal of Endocrinological Investigation 42.4 (2019): 481-487.

36) Tian, Xun, et al. "Selenium Supplementation May Decrease Thyroid Peroxidase Antibody Titer Via Reducing Oxidative Stress in Euthyroid Patients with Autoimmune Thyroiditis." International Journal of Endocrinology 2020 (2020).

37) MacFarquhar, Jennifer K., et al. "Acute Selenium Toxicity Associated with a Dietary Supplement." Archives of Internal Medicine 170.3 (2010): 256-261.

38) Aldosary, Barrak M., et al. "Case Series of Selenium Toxicity from a Nutritional Supplement." Clinical Toxicology 50.1 (2012): 57-64.

39) Morris, John Steven, and Stacy B. Crane. "Selenium Toxicity from a Misformulated Dietary Supplement, Adverse Health Effects, and the Temporal Response in the Nail Biologic Monitor." Nutrients 5.4 (2013): 1024-1057.

40) Goyens, Philippe, et al. "Selenium Deficiency as a Possible Factor in the Pathogenesis of Myxoedematous Endemic Cretinism." European Journal of Endocrinology 114.4 (1987): 497-502.

41) Hu, Y., et al. "Effect of Selenium on Thyroid Autoimmunity and Regulatory T Cells in Patients with Hashimoto's Thyroiditis: A Prospective Randomized Controlled Trial." Clinical and Translational Science 14.4 (2021): 1390-1402.

42) Duntas, Leonidas H., et al. "Effects of a Six-Month Treatment with Selenomethionine in Patients with Autoimmune Thyroiditis." European Journal of Endocrinology 148.4 (2003): 389-393.

43) Hadithi, Muhammed, et al. "Coeliac Disease in Dutch Patients with Hashimoto's Thyroiditis and Vice Versa." World Journal of Gastroenterology: WJG 13.11 (2007): 1715.

44) Akcay, Mufide Nuran, and Gungor Akcay. "The Presence of the Antigliadin Antibodies in Autoimmune Thyroid Diseases." Hepato-Gastroenterology 50 (2003): cclxxix-cclxxx.

45) Krysiak, Robert, et al. "The Effect of Gluten-Free Diet on Thyroid Autoimmunity in Drug-Naïve Women with Hashimoto's Thyroiditis: A Pilot Study." Experimental and Clinical Endocrinology & Diabetes 127.07 (2019): 417-422.

46) Mazokopakis, Elias E., and Vassiliki Chatzipavlidou. "Hashimoto's Thyroiditis and the Role of Selenium. Current Concepts." Hell J Nucl Med 10.1 (2007): 6-8.

47) Tamer, Gonca, et al. "Relative Vitamin D Insufficiency in Hashimoto's Thyroiditis." Thyroid 21.8 (2011): 891-896.

48) Bozkurt, Nujen Colak, et al. "The Association Between Severity of Vitamin D Deficiency and Hashimoto's Thyroiditis." Endocrine Practice 19.3 (2013): 479-484.

49) Botelho, Ilka Mara Borges, et al. "Vitamin D in Hashimoto's Thyroiditis and its Relationship with Thyroid Function and Inflammatory Status." Endocrine Journal 65.10 (2018): 1029-1037.

50) Zhao, Rui, et al. "Immunomodulatory Function of Vitamin D and its Role in Autoimmune Thyroid Disease." Frontiers in Immunology 12 (2021): 574967.

51) Krysiak, Robert, et al. "Selenomethionine Potentiates the Impact of Vitamin D on Thyroid Autoimmunity in Euthyroid Women with Hashimoto's Thyroiditis and Low Vitamin D Status." Pharmacological Reports 71 (2019): 367-373.

52) Schmidt, Matthias, et al. "Long-Term Follow-Up of Anti-Thyroid Peroxidase Antibodies in Patients with Chronic Autoimmune Thyroiditis (Hashimoto's Thyroiditis) Treated with Levothyroxine." Thyroid 18.7 (2008): 755-760.

53) Song, Yue, et al. "Roles of Hydrogen Peroxide in Thyroid Physiology and Disease." The Journal of Clinical Endocrinology & Metabolism 92.10 (2007): 3764-3773.

54) Ohye, Hidemi, and Masahiro Sugawara. "Dual Oxidase, Hydrogen Peroxide and Thyroid Diseases." Experimental Biology and Medicine 235.4 (2010): 424-433

55) Ghent, W. R., et al. "Iodine Replacement in Fibrocystic Disease of The Breast." Canadian Journal of Surgery. 36.5 (1993): 453-460.

56) Miller, D. W. "Extrathyroidal Benefits of Iodine." Journal of American Physicians and Surgeons 11.4 (2006): 106.

57) Venturi, Sebastiano. "Is There a Role for Iodine in Breast Diseases?" The Breast 10.5 (2001): 379-382.

58) Mansel, Robert E., et al. "A Randomized Controlled Multicenter Trial of an Investigational Liquid Nutritional Formula in Women with Cyclic Breast Pain Associated with Fibrocystic Breast Changes." Journal of Women's Health 27.3 (2018): 333-340.

59) Gantzer, Jen. "Bilateral Fibrocystic Breasts, Dysmenorrhea, and Anemia: A Case Report of Lugol's Iodine & GLA Borage Oil." Nutritional Perspectives: Journal of the Council on Nutrition 45.2 (2022).

60) Brownstein, David. "Clinical Experience with Inorganic, Non-Radioactive Iodine/Iodide." The Original Internist 12.3 (2005): 105-108.

62) McDermott, Michael T. "Low-dose Naltrexone Treatment of Hashimoto's Thyroiditis." Management of Patients with Pseudo-Endocrine Disorders: A Case-Based Pocket Guide (2019): 317-326.

63) Turker, Omer, et al. "Selenium Treatment in Autoimmune Thyroiditis: 9-Month Follow-Up with Variable Doses." Journal of Endocrinology 190.1 (2006): 151-156.12

64) Nacamulli, Davide, et al. "Influence of Physiological Dietary Selenium Supplementation on the Natural Course of Autoimmune Thyroiditis." Clinical Endocrinology 73.4 (2010): 535-539.

65) Zhu, Lin, et al. "Effects of Selenium Supplementation on Antibodies of Autoimmune Thyroiditis." Zhonghua Yi Xue Za Zhi 92.32 (2012): 2256-2260.

Chapter 23

Does Iodine Consumption Cause Hashimoto's Thyroiditis?

IN PREVIOUS CHAPTERS, WE DISCUSSED how generation of excess hydrogen peroxide and lack of degradation as the etiology of autoimmune thyroid disorders, goiter, nodules, and thyroid cancer. Iodine deficiency is the leading cause of excess hydrogen peroxide generation, primarily via increased TSH, which stimulates thyroid growth and goiter formation. If the patient is selenium deficient, with inadequate selenoprotein anti-oxidant system, then hydrogen peroxide will not be degraded. Excess H202 leads to oxidative damage, inflammation, and antigenicity of the nearby thyroglobulin and TPO. If this mechanism is accepted, combined iodine and selenium deficiency is the etiology of autoimmune thyroid disease.

However, it is also true that iodine excess will inhibit thyroid function and cause elevated TSH. This is the Wolff-Chaikoff Effect. In normal healthy people, there is an escape from the Wolff-Chaikoff Effect in a few days, thought to be related to down-regulation of the NIS, sodium iodide symporter, which reduces the entry of excess iodine into the thyrocyte. With restricted iodine entry into the thyrocyte, thyroid hormone levels, and TSH all return to normal. This is the escape from the Wolff-Chaikoff Effect. In 2010, Dr. Jerome Hershman wrote:

> Excess iodine intake, resulting in high intrathyroidal iodide, may cause a transient blockade of thyroid hormone synthesis (Wolff-Chaikoff effect). Normal subjects escape this blockade by down-regulation of iodide transport, probably by inhibition of gene expression of NIS (escape from the Wolff–Chaikoff effect), an autoregulatory process. (1)

However, a subset of patients has lost autoregulation and failed to escape. Their thyroid tissue cannot down-regulate the NIS, sodium iodide symporter, and cannot block entry of excess iodide into the thyrocytes. In 2010, Dr. Jerome Hershman wrote:

> Iodine-induced hypothyroidism can occur in patients who ingest large quantities of inorganic iodide (typically greater than 1–2 mg/day) and fail to escape from the acute Wolff–Chaikoff effect. These patients usually have underlying thyroid diseases, such as a history of autoimmune, subacute, or post-partum thyroiditis or Graves' disease that has been treated with partial thyroidectomy or radioactive iodine ablation. (1)

Loss of Autoregulation in Autoimmune Thyroid Disease

Patients with underlying autoimmune thyroid disease have lost autoregulation and cannot escape from the Wolff-Chaikoff Effect. In these patients, iodine excess continues to inhibit thyroid function, with elevation of TSH, stimulating the generation of H202 (hydrogen peroxide), which may then trigger a vicious cycle of further inflammation and antigenicity.

Severe iodine deficiency may also cause elevated TSH. If the thyroid lacks the iodine to make thyroid hormone, this causes hypothyroidism with high TSH. So, as we can see, both extremes of iodine intake, deficiency, and excess may cause elevated TSH.

As mentioned above, iodine excess will cause thyroid failure and elevated TSH only in a subset of patients with underlying autoimmune thyroid disease and a few other thyroid disorders. The vast majority of the population consuming excess iodine escape from its inhibitory effect, TSH levels normalize, and these patients return to normal and are perfectly fine.

Excess Iodine Dietary Intake

In 2019, Dr. Jessica Farebrother discussed the effect of excess iodine on thyroid function, reiterating the above-mentioned points. Notice Dr. Farebrother states that most healthy individuals tolerate high iodine intake. This is because of normal autoregulation and normal escape from the Wolff-Chaikoff effect. Autoregulation has been lost in people with pre-existing thyroid disease, and excess iodine will precipitate hyperthyroidism, hypothyroidism, goiter, or thyroid autoimmunity. For our discussion, we are concerned with autoimmune thyroid disease caused initially by iodine deficiency, as the pre-existing thyroid disease mentioned by Dr. Farebrother.

Two Mechanisms at Play

There are two mechanisms at play. For autoimmune thyroid patients with loss of autoregulation, unable to escape from the Wolff-Chaikoff effect, excess iodine intake inhibits thyroid function, causing thyroid failure with low serum hormone levels and elevation of TSH. The elevated TSH turns on hydrogen peroxide generation, aggravating thyroid inflammation and auto-immunity. Notice the mechanism of high TSH is the same common denominator for both iodine deficiency (in the general population) and iodine excess in a subset of patients who have lost the ability to escape from the Wolf Chaikoff effect. Both groups will have high TSH, stimulating thyroid enlargement (goiter) and excess hydrogen peroxide generation with inflammatory, antigenic, and mutagenic effects.

The second mechanism is for patients with autonomous nodules from mutations in the TSH receptor. These mutations were caused by iodine deficiency, high TSH, and the mutagenic effects of excess hydrogen peroxide, resulting in TSH receptor mutation. Even modest iodine intake in autonomous nodule patients will precipitate an episode of hyperthyroidism, which can result in a visit to the emergency room. Dr. Jessica Farebrother writes:

> Iodine is essential for thyroid hormone

synthesis. **High iodine intakes are well tolerated by most healthy individuals, but in some people**, excess iodine intakes may precipitate hyperthyroidism, hypothyroidism, goiter, and/or thyroid autoimmunity. Individuals with pre-existing thyroid disease or those previously exposed to iodine deficiency may be more susceptible to thyroid disorders due to an increase in iodine intake, in some cases at intakes only slightly above physiological needs. Thyroid dysfunction due to excess iodine intake is usually mild and transient, but iodine-induced hyperthyroidism can be life-threatening in some individuals. (2)

In agreement with the above is Dr. Karbownik-Lewińska, who wrote in 2022:

> It should be stressed that compared to iodine deficiency, **iodine in excess…is much less harmful** in such a sense that **it affects only a small percentage of sensitive individuals** [pre-existing autoimmune disease, etc.], whereas the former affects whole populations; therefore, it causes endemic consequences. (3)

Also in agreement is Dr. Dijck-Brouwer, who feels that guidelines for optimal iodine intake should be based on healthy adults, not adults with underlying autoimmunity or thyroid autonomy. Dr Dijck-Brouwer writes in 2022:

> Some adults fail to escape from the usually transient Wolff–Chaikoff effect and remain hypothyroidic (iodide myxedema) or progress to hyperthyroidism (Jod–Basedow effect). They obviously lack appropriate thyroid autoregulation and **likely have thyroid autoimmunity**, often unrecognized or subclinical, or another underlying thyroid disease. Basing optimal intakes [for iodine] on them closes a perfect vicious circle because many of those may have contracted this condition because of an iodine/selenium disbalance in the past. Moreover, dietary reference intakes are made for the healthy population, and it is questionable whether those who fail to escape from the Wolff–Chaikoff effect are healthy… (4)

Does Iodine Excess Cause Hyperthyroid Auto-Immunity?

In 2007, Dr. Fan Yang conducted a 5-year population study of 3700 people in three rural communities of China thyroid function tests, and urinary iodine excretion tests were obtained. Median urinary iodine excretion was 88 (low), 214 (medium), and 634 (high) mg/L. Cumulative incidence of hyperthyroidism was not increased for the higher iodine excretion cohort, which was 1.4, 0.9 and 0.8 per cent in three respective areas. This study shows chronic iodine excess does not increase autoimmune hyperthyroidism. Dr. Fan Yang concludes:

> Conclusion: Iodine supplementation may not induce an increase in hyperthyroidism in a previously mildly iodine-deficient population. Chronic iodine excess does not apparently increase the risk of autoimmune hyperthyroidism, suggesting that excessive iodine intake may not be an environmental factor involved in the occurrence of autoimmune hyperthyroidism. (5)

Note: In Chapter 19, Iodine Induced Hyperthyroidism - the Autonomous Thyroid Nodule, the introduction of iodine-fortified salt in the US and other countries triggered a sudden increase in mortality from thyrotoxicosis. This was traced back to patients harboring autonomous nodules and multinodular goiters. Dr. Fan Yang accepted this as a given and was not studying this. He was concerned with the new appearance of Graves' disease (auto-immune hyperthyroidism) with low, medium, and high iodine intake of iodized salt, and Dr. Fan Yang found there was no correlation.

Dr. Zimmermans' Study

In 2003, Dr. Michael Zimmerman conducted a one-year prospective study on 323 iodine-deficient Moroccan schoolchildren. Dr. Zimmerman's plan was to determine if the introduction of iodized salt induces thyroid autoimmunity in goitrous iodine deficient children. Although there was a transient rise in TPO antibodies in 1% of children after the introduction of iodized salt, this returned to normal after one year. I assume this population of children had adequate selenium levels. However, this was not studied. It would be prudent to measure serum selenium levels in all such future studies. Dr. Michael Zimmerman concludes the introduction of iodized salt to iodine-deficient children does not provoke significant thyroid auto-immunity, and he writes:

> At baseline, median UI [urinary iodine] was 17 microg/L and the prevalence of goiter and hypothyroidism was 72% and 18%, respectively. Provision of iodized salt maintained median UI at 150-200 microg/L for the year. There was a significant increase in mean total thyroxine (T(4)) and a significant reduction in the prevalence of hypothyroidism. There was a transient increase in the prevalence of detectable antibodies after introduction of iodized salt with levels returning to baseline at 1 year. Only congruent with 1% of children had elevated TPO-Ab and none had elevated Tg-Ab over the course of the study, and no child with elevated TPO-Ab had abnormal thyrotropin (TSH) or T(4) concentrations. None developed clinical or ultrasonographic evidence of thyroid autoimmune disease and/or iodine-induced hypothyroidism or hyperthyroidism. Rapid introduction of iodized salt does not provoke significant thyroid autoimmunity in severely iodine-deficient children followed for 1 year. (6-7)

Evidence for Iodine Deficiency as Etiology of Autoimmune Thyroid Disease

In 2015, Dr. Zimmerman reviewed iodine deficiency disorders finding some studies show increased thyroid autoimmunity in iodine-deficient human populations after iodized salt introduction, and some studies do not. Dr. Zimmerman writes increases in thyroid auto-immunity (albeit low titer) in the wake of salt iodization is modest and may be transient:

> In summary, the link between iodine intake and thyroid autoimmunity is complex. Some

studies have noted raised concentrations of thyroid antibodies in areas of excessive iodine intake, but others have not. However, large oral doses of iodine in iodine-deficient individuals might precipitate the development of thyroid antibodies, and individuals with autoimmune thyroiditis are at increased risk of hypothyroidism when exposed to excess iodine [Wolff-Chaikoff Effect]. Most surveys have reported modest increases in the occurrence of thyroid autoimmunity (albeit antibodies are at a low titre) in the wake of iodisation; whether these increases are transient is unclear. (7)

Iodine Deficiency in Animal Studies as Etiology of Autoimmune Thyroid Disease

In 1993, Dr. Mooij studied normal mice (nonautoimmune normal euthyroid female Wistar rats) kept on four iodine regimens, an iodine-enriched diet (EID), a normal conventional diet (COD), a low iodine diet (LID), and an Extremely Low iodine diet (LID+), for periods of up to 18 weeks. As expected, the mice fed a low-iodine diet developed thyroid enlargement (goiter). As expected, the TSH was markedly elevated in the Extremely Low iodine diet, and thyroid hormone levels (Free T3 and Free T4) were markedly reduced. The Low and Extremely Low iodine diets showed thyroid autoimmunity with elevated thyroglobulin antibodies. Dr. Mooij concludes iodine deficiency precipitates thyroid auto-immunity in his animal model and in humans, writing:

> The Wistar rats **supplemented with iodine showed a very low** local thyroid immune response (few intrathyroidal DC and T-cells) [immune cells] and a **very low** production of anticolloid [thyroglobulin] antibodies. The higher incidence of anticolloid antibodies in the iodine-deficient goitrous Wistar rats is in accordance with the higher prevalences of anti-Tg antibodies reported in endemic goiter patients with iodine deficiency.... The observed increases in the number of intrathyroidal DC [Dendritic Cells] and homotypic clusters of these cells in the rat goiters find their human parallel in

the reported increases in DC infiltration and clustering of these cells in thyroids of iodine deficient endemic goiter patients... In conclusion, the data reported here show that an **insufficient dietary iodine intake is capable of precipitating a thyroid autoimmune response in normal nonautoimmune Wistar rats, as in normal human populations. Evidence is also accumulating that iodine deficiency is able to precipitate thyroid autoimmune reactivity in humans.** (8)

Selenium Deficiency Increases Risk for Hashimoto's Thyroiditis

In 2022, Dr. Zheng studied the association of selenium deficiency with Hashimoto's disease. He concludes there is indeed a correlation of selenium deficiency with thyroid auto-immunity, and dietary selenium intake is a safe and low-cost prevention and treatment for Hashimoto's thyroiditis, writing:

> Dietary selenium intake is independently and inversely associated with HT [Hashimoto's Thyroiditis] risk. Moreover, dietary selenium intake is negatively correlated with TPOAb [Thyro-Per-Oxidase antibody] levels and non-linearly correlated with TGAb [Thyroglobulin antibody] levels. Therefore, dietary selenium intake may be a safe and low-cost alternative for the prevention and treatment of HT. (9-12)

Iodine Deficiency with Loss of Autoregulation, Followed by Iodine Repletion, Causes Autoimmune Thyroid Disease

In 2016, Dr. Robyn Murphy explained excess dietary iodine intake is not the cause of thyroid autoimmunity. Loss of autoregulation caused by pre-existing iodine deficiency, followed by iodine repletion, is the cause of autoimmune thyroid disease, writing:

> Universal salt iodization programs were successfully implemented to reduce the incidence of iodine deficiency disorders; however, **unexpected increases in the**

prevalence of thyroid autoimmunity occurred, and iodine excess was implicated as the causative factor. A review of observational and in vitro studies revealed that iodine alone is not responsible for thyroid autoimmunity. Experimental models used to explain iodine excess as the culprit in thyroid autoimmunity fail to induce thyroid autoantibodies unless iodine is in the presence of excess inflammatory cytokines (interferon [IFN]-γ) and hydrogen peroxide (H2O2) [high TSH, and selenium deficiency]. Within iodine-deficient populations, regulatory mechanisms to limit oxidative stress and excess iodine are lost. Thyroid-stimulating hormone [TSH] persistently activates the sodium-iodide symporter. At the same time, iodine concentrations fail to achieve levels high enough to produce iodolactones, which are responsible for modulating NADPH oxidase and H2O2 production. Subsequently, the thyroid becomes susceptible to oxidative stress as iodine is reintroduced. Oxidation of thyroid peroxidase and thyroglobulin [by H2O2] initiate the release of inflammatory cytokines (IFN-γ) and lymphocytic infiltration, which induce autoantibody production and thyroid autoimmunity. Population studies revealed that iodine administration, even below the recommended dietary allowance, alters thyroid autoimmunity. Despite increases in thyroid antibodies, these changes are found to be transient. Interestingly, reports of iodine in combination with other nutrients and standardized botanical extracts have been used successfully to restore thyroid function. On the basis of our review of the literature, it is apparent that a loss of regulatory mechanisms due to pre-existing iodine deficiency followed by iodine repletion, as opposed to iodine excess, is a causal factor in the development of thyroid autoimmunity. (13-14)

Conclusion

A combination of iodine and selenium deficiency causes thyroid oxidative damage from excess hydrogen peroxide. This leads to loss of autoregulation, which upon iodine repletion, leads to thyroid autoimmunity. (15-23)

♦ References for Chapter 23

1) Hershman, Jerome M. "Regulation of Thyroid Hormone Production and Measurement of Thyrotropin." Thyroid Function Testing. Springer, Boston, MA, 2010. 71-84.

2) Farebrother, Jessica, et al. "Excess Iodine Intake: Sources, Assessment, and Effects on Thyroid Function." Annals of the New York Academy of Sciences 1446.1 (2019): 44-65.

3) Karbownik-Lewińska, Małgorzata, et al. "Iodine as a Potential Endocrine Disruptor—A Role of Oxidative Stress." Endocrine (2022): 1-22.

4) Dijck-Brouwer, DA Janneke, et al. "Thyroidal and Extrathyroidal Requirements for Iodine and Selenium: A Combined Evolutionary and (Patho) Physiological Approach." Nutrients 14.19 (2022): 3886.

5) Yang, Fan, et al. "Chronic Iodine Excess Does Not Increase the Incidence of Hyperthyroidism: A Prospective Community-Based Epidemiological Survey in China." European Journal of Endocrinology 156.4 (2007): 403-408.

6) Zimmermann, Michael B., et al. "Introduction of Iodized Salt to Severely Iodine-Deficient Children Does Not Provoke Thyroid Autoimmunity: A One-Year Prospective Trial in Northern Morocco." Thyroid 13.2 (2003): 199-203.

7) Zimmermann, Michael B., and Kristien Boelaert. "Iodine Deficiency and Thyroid Disorders." The Lancet Diabetes & Endocrinology 3.4 (2015): 286-295.

8) Mooij, P., et al. "Iodine Deficiency Induces Thyroid Autoimmune Reactivity in Wistar Rats." Endocrinology 133.3 (1993): 1197-1204.

9) Zheng, G., et al. "The Association Between Dietary Selenium Intake and Hashimoto's Thyroiditis Among US Adults: National Health and Nutrition Examination Survey (NHANES), 2007–2012." Journal of Endocrinological Investigation (2022): 1-11.

10) Ruggeri, Rosaria M., et al. "Selenium Exerts Protective Effects Against Oxidative Stress and Cell Damage in Human Thyrocytes and Fibroblasts." Endocrine 68.1 (2020): 151-162.

11) Wu, Qian, et al. "Increased Incidence of Hashimoto Thyroiditis in Selenium Deficiency: A Prospective 6-Year Cohort Study." The Journal of Clinical Endocrinology & Metabolism 107.9 (2022): e3603-e3611.

12) Mayunga, K. Clara, et al. "Pregnant Dutch Women Have Inadequate Iodine Status and Selenium Intake." Nutrients 14.19 (2022): 3936.

13) Murphy, Robyn, et al. "The Role of Iodine Deficiency and Subsequent Repletion in Autoimmune Thyroid Disease and Thyroid Cancer." Journal of Restorative Medicine 5.1 (2016): 32.

14) Flechas, Jorge. "Autoimmune Thyroiditis and Iodine Therapy." Journal of Restorative Medicine 2.1 (2013): 54-59.

15) Song, Yue, et al. "Roles of Hydrogen Peroxide in Thyroid Physiology and Disease." The Journal of Clinical Endocrinology & Metabolism 92.10 (2007): 3764-3773.

16) Ruwhof, C., and H. A. Drexhage. "Iodine and Thyroid Autoimmune Disease in Animal Models." Thyroid 11.5 (2001): 427-436.

17) Teti, Claudia, et al. "Iodoprophylaxis and Thyroid Autoimmunity: An Update." Immunologic Research 69.2 (2021): 129-138.

18) Liu, Jiameng, et al. "Excessive Iodine Promotes Pyroptosis of Thyroid Follicular Epithelial Cells in Hashimoto's Thyroiditis Through the ROS-NF-Kb-NLRP3 Pathway." Frontiers in Endocrinology 10 (2019): 778.

19) Teng, Xiaochun, et al. "More Than Adequate Iodine Intake May Increase Subclinical Hypothyroidism and Autoimmune Thyroiditis: A Cross-Sectional Study Based on Two Chinese Communities with Different Iodine Intake Levels." European Journal of Endocrinology 164.6 (2011): 943-950.

20) Doğan, Murat, et al. "The Frequency of Hashimoto Thyroiditis in Children and the Relationship Between Urinary Iodine Level and Hashimoto Thyroiditis." (2011): 75-80.

21) Wang, Bin, et al. "U-Shaped Relationship Between Iodine Status and Thyroid Autoimmunity Risk in Adults." European Journal of Endocrinology 181.3 (2019): 255-266.

22) Mikulska, Aniceta A., et al. "Metabolic Characteristics of Hashimoto's Thyroiditis Patients and the Role of Microelements and Diet in the Disease Management—An Overview." International Journal of Molecular Sciences 23.12 (2022): 6580.

23) Zhao, Hengqiang, et al. "Correlation Between Iodine Intake and Thyroid Disorders: A Cross-Sectional Study from The South of China." Biological Trace Element Research 162 (2014): 87-94.

Chapter 24

Origin and Features of Hashimoto's Autoimmune Thyroid Disease

Hashimoto's thyroiditis was originally described in 1912 by a Japanese surgeon, Hakaru Hashimoto, for whom the disease is named. Hashimoto's thyroiditis is an autoimmune disease in which our immune system attacks the thyroid gland causing inflammation and eventual destruction. Initially, thyroid function may be normal. In later stages, there is a loss of thyroid function and hypothyroidism severe enough to require thyroid hormone replacement. Medical science claims the cause of autoimmune thyroid disease is not completely known, citing a combination of genetic and environmental factors. As mentioned in Chapter 23, iodine deficiency, selenium deficiency, and molecular mimicry are the most compelling theories for the etiology of autoimmune thyroid disease. (1-2)

"Molecular Mimicry"

"Molecular Mimicry" is the theory that explains how our immune system can be "tricked "into attacking the thyroid cells. A bacterial organism called Yersinia, residing in our intestinal tract, has been found to share identical amino acid sequences compared to the TSH receptor, thyroglobulin, thyroid peroxidase [TPO], and the sodium iodide symporter [NIS]. Also, a spirochete called Borrelia burgdorferi has been implicated, thus explaining increased thyroglobulin and thyroperoxidase (TPO) antibodies in Hashimoto's patients. (1-7)

H2O2 Excess Damages TPO and Thyroglobulin

What is the cause of autoimmune thyroid disease? Iodine deficiency and the resulting damaging effect of high TSH and excess H2O2 production, or lack of neutralization from a dysfunctional anti-oxidant system from sele-

nium and magnesium deficiency, cause autoimmune thyroid disease, as discussed in previous chapters.

TSH Receptor Antibodies, TPO Antibodies

The anti-thyroid antibodies come in two varieties. In the first type, the TSH Receptor is stimulated by TSI and TRAb, giving rise to Graves' Disease and hyperthyroidism. In the second variety, TPO and Thyroglobulin antibodies give rise to Hashimoto's disease, which causes thyroid destruction, and, ultimately, hypothyroidism. Although Graves' and Hashimoto's may have a common origin, namely iodine, selenium, and Vitamin D deficiency, gluten sensitivity with leaky gut, and molecular mimicry, they differ in thyroid function. Graves' disease causes a hyperthyroid state, and Hashimoto's disease causes a hypothyroid state. Both have very different outcomes. Note: in rare exceptions, a transient hyperthyroid state can be seen in Hashimoto's thyroiditis, termed Hashitoxicosis, a form of thyroiditis with reduced radioactive iodine uptake. Hashitoxicosis can be prevented by TSH suppression with thyroid hormone replacement. TSH suppression prevents excessive hydrogen peroxide formation, thus preventing oxidative damage to thyrocytes which can cause thyroiditis.

Antibodies to the NIS in the Basolateral Membrane

In 2020, Dr. Anna-Maria Eleftheriadou studied antibodies to the NIS, sodium iodide symporter (NIS-aAb), finding NIS-aAb were more prevalent in Hashimoto's 7.7% and Graves' 12.3% compared to controls 1.8%. Unfortunately, routine clinical testing is not yet available. One might speculate the presence of anti-NIS antibodies in Graves' disease might create NIS dysfunction, and interfere with the uptake of iodine, rendering the Graves' disease patient resistant to treatment with iodine. (8)

Graves' and Hashimoto's antibodies can coexist in the same patient, and one can transform into another. Some authors consider the two to be different manifestations of the same disease. (9)

Hashitoxicosis

In early Hashimoto's disease, inflammatory episodes may cause a transient release of thyroid hormone into the circulation, causing hyperthyroidism and thyrotoxicosis. This is a form of thyroiditis called Hashitoxicosis, in which inflammation causes the rupture of follicles with the release of preformed thyroid hormone. Differentiation from Graves' thyrotoxicosis can be made with a radio-iodine uptake scan. In Hashitoxicosis, the radio-iodine uptake of the thyroid gland is very low, while markedly increased in Graves's thyrotoxicosis. (10-13)

Gluten and Leaky Gut

How do micro-organisms get into the bloodstream to incite an immune response? The answer is they can "leak in" from the bowel lumen into the bloodstream in patients with leaky gut. What causes a leaky gut? The most common cause is gluten consumption in genetically predisposed individuals. This explains the connection between Hashimoto's, Graves', and gluten sensitivity. A gluten-free diet is advised for all patients with Hashimoto's and Graves' disease.

Gluten sensitivity in predisposed individuals may lead to a leaky gut, a condition in which the tight junctions remain open with leakage of lumen contents such as gut bacteria and undigested food particles into the bloodstream. This triggers an immune response with considerable inflammation in the wall of the gut, causing loss of micro-villi and malabsorption of key vitamins and minerals such as B12, calcium, and iron. This immune response may attack distant host tissues giving rise to various autoimmune diseases, including autoimmune thyroid disease. This is called molecular mimicry, the ability of various micro-organisms to cause autoimmune thyroid disease because they contain amino acid sequences identical to those in our thyroid gland. Molecular mimicry means a micro-organism leaks into the bloodstream, mimicking our own tissues' molecular pattern. These include micro-organisms such as Borrelia, Yersinia, Clostridium botulinum, Rickettsia prowazekii, and Helicobacter pylori, as discussed by Dr. Benvenga in 2016. The most widely accepted mechanism for molecular mimicry is infection with the H. Pylori organism. (7) (14-16)

Selenium Deficiency and Autoimmune Thyroid Disease

Selenium is an important mineral incorporated into seleno-proteins which comprise the anti-oxidant system which protects the thyrocytes from the damaging effects of hydrogen peroxide, required to iodinate thyroglobulin and manufacture thyroid hormone. Selenium deficiency has been implicated in the origin of autoimmune thyroid disease. In animal studies, selenium alleviates the toxic effects of excess iodine and reverses microscopic changes in the thyroid gland induced by iodine. (17-19)

Conclusion

The etiology of Hashimoto's thyroiditis is not iodine excess. It is combined iodine and selenium deficiency followed by iodine repletion. Modern endocrinology is concerned solely with managing thyroid function while ignoring the autoimmune component of Hashimoto's and Graves' Disease. This is yet another error of modern endocrinology. (20-37)

♦ References Chapter 24

1) Eschler, Deirdre Cocks, et al. "Cutting Edge: The Etiology of Autoimmune Thyroid Diseases." Clinical Reviews in Allergy & Immunology 41.2 (2011): 190-197.

2) Hiromatsu, Yuji, et al. "Hashimoto's Thyroiditis: History and Future Outlook." Hormones (Athens) 12.1 (2013): 12-8.

3) Chatzipanagiotou, S., et al. "Prevalence of Yersinia Plasmid-Encoded Outer Protein (Yop) Class-Specific Antibodies in Patients with Hashimoto's Thyroiditis." Clinical Microbiology and Infection 7.3 (2001): 138-143.

4) Tozzoli, R., et al. "Infections and Autoimmune Thyroid Diseases: Parallel Detection of Antibodies Against Pathogens with Proteomic Technology." Autoimmunity Reviews 8.2 (2008): 112-115.

5) Benvenga, Salvatore, et al. "Human Thyroid Autoantigens and Proteins of Yersinia and Borrelia Share Amino Acid Sequence Homology that Includes Binding Motifs to HLA-DR Molecules and T-Cell Receptor." Thyroid 16.3 (2006): 225-236.

6) Benvenga, Salvatore, et al. "Homologies Between Proteins of Borrelia Burgdorferi and Thyroid Autoantigens." Thyroid 14.11 (2004): 964-966.

7) Cuan-Baltazar, Yunam, and Elena Soto-Vega. "Micro-Organisms Associated with Thyroid Autoimmunity." Autoimmunity Reviews 19.9 (2020): 102614.

8) Eleftheriadou, Anna-Maria, et al. "Re-visiting Autoimmunity to Sodium-Iodide Symporter and Pendrin in Thyroid Disease." European Journal of Endocrinology 183.6 (2020): 571-580.

9) Ohye, Hidemi, et al. "Four Cases of Graves' Disease Which Developed After Painful Hashimoto's Thyroiditis." Internal Medicine 45.6 (2006): 385-389.

10) Dos Reis, Juliana Delfino, et al. "Assessment of Clinical and Laboratory Limits between Hashitoxicosis and Graves' Disease." Global Journal of Health Science 14.12 (2022): 28.

11) Ross, Douglas S. "Syndromes of Thyrotoxicosis with Low Radioactive Iodine Uptake." Endocrinology and metabolism clinics of North America 27.1 (1998): 169-185.

12) Gluck, Franklin B., et al. "Chronic Lymphocytic Thyroiditis, Thyrotoxicosis, and Low Radioactive Iodine Uptake: Report of Four Cases." New England Journal of Medicine 293.13 (1975): 624-628.

13) Baral, Neelam, et al. "SUN-560 Thyrotoxic Hashimoto's Disease: Is it Graves' Thyrotoxicosis or Hashitoxicosis?" Journal of the Endocrine Society 3. Supplement_1 (2019): SUN-560.

14) Benvenga, Salvatore, and Fabrizio Guarneri. "Molecular Mimicry and Autoimmune Thyroid Disease." Reviews in Endocrine and Metabolic Disorders 17.4 (2016): 485-498.

15) Avni, Orly, and Omry Koren. "Molecular (Me), Mimicry?" Cell Host & Microbe 23.5 (2018): 576-578.

16) Ihnatowicz, Paulina, et al. "The Importance of Nutritional Factors and Dietary Management of Hashimoto's Thyroiditis." Annals of Agricultural and Environmental Medicine 27.2 (2020).

17) Vasiliu, Ioana, et al. "Protective Role of Selenium on Thyroid Morphology in Iodine-Induced Autoimmune Thyroiditis in Wistar Rats." Experimental And Therapeutic Medicine 20.4 (2020): 3425-3437.

18) Tsatsoulis, Agathocles. "The Role of Iodine Vs Selenium on the Rising Trend of Autoimmune Thyroiditis in Iodine Sufficient Countries-An Opinion Article." Open Access J Thy Res 2.1 (2018): 12-14.

19) Giammanco, Marco, and Manfredi M. Giammanco. "Selenium: A Cure for Autoimmune Thyroiditis." Endocrine, Metabolic & Immune Disorders-Drug Targets 21.8 (2021): 1377-1378.

20) Klubo-Gwiezdzinska, Joanna, and Leonard Wartofsky. "Hashimoto Thyroiditis: An Evidence-Based Guide to Etiology, Diagnosis, and Treatment." Polish Archives of Internal Medicine 132.3 (2022): 16222-16222.

21) Quintero, Beatriz Martinez, et al. "Thyroiditis: Evaluation and Treatment." American Family Physician 104.6 (2021): 609-617.

22) Shukla, Sanjeev Kumar, et al. "Infections, Genetic and Environmental Factors in the Pathogenesis of Autoimmune Thyroid Diseases." Microbial pathogenesis 116 (2018): 279-288.

23) Lahner, Edith, et al. "Thyro-Enter-Gastric Autoimmunity: Pathophysiology and Implications for Patient Management." Best Practice & Research Clinical Endocrinology & Metabolism 34.1 (2020): 101373.

24) Ralli, Massimo, et al. "Hashimoto's Thyroiditis: An Update on Pathogenic Mechanisms, Diagnostic Protocols, Therapeutic Strategies, and Potential Malignant Transformation." Autoimmunity Reviews 19.10 (2020): 102649.

25) Wang, Weiwei, et al. "Effects of Selenium Supplementation on Spontaneous Autoimmune Thyroiditis In NOD. H-2h4 Mice." Thyroid 25.10 (2015): 1137-1144.

26) Wu, Qian, et al. "Increased Incidence of Hashimoto Thyroiditis in Selenium Deficiency: A Prospective 6-Year Cohort Study." The Journal of Clinical Endocrinology & Metabolism 107.9 (2022): e3603-e3611.

27) Mikulska, Aniceta A., et al. "Metabolic Characteristics of Hashimoto's Thyroiditis Patients and the Role of Microelements and Diet in the Disease Management—An Overview." International Journal of Molecular Sciences 23.12 (2022): 6580.

28) Gorini, Francesca, et al. "Selenium: An Element of Life Essential for Thyroid Function." Molecules 26.23 (2021): 7084.

29) Giammanco, Marco, and Gaetano Leto. "Selenium and Autoimmune Thyroiditis." EC Nutr 14 (2019): 449-450.

30) Wessels, Inga, and Lothar Rink. "Micronutrients in Autoimmune Diseases: Possible Therapeutic Benefits of Zinc and Vitamin D." The Journal of Nutritional Biochemistry 77 (2020): 108240.

31) Fountoulakis, Stelios, et al. "The Role of Iodine in The Evolution of Thyroid Disease in Greece: From Endemic Goiter to Thyroid Autoimmunity." Hormones-Athens- 6.1 (2007): 25.

32) Nielsen, Elsa, et al. "Iodine, Inorganic and Soluble Salts." The Danish Environmental Protection Agency, Copenhagen 290 (2014).

33) Lossow, Kristina, et al. "The Nutritional Supply of Iodine and Selenium Affects Thyroid Hormone Axis Related Endpoints in Mice." Nutrients 13.11 (2021): 3773.

34) Li, Yang, et al. "Effects of Selenium Supplement on B Lymphocyte Activity in Experimental Autoimmune Thyroiditis Rats." International Journal of Endocrinology 2021 (2021).

35) Ruz, Manuel, et al. "Single and Multiple Selenium-Zinc-Iodine Deficiencies Affect Rat Thyroid Metabolism and Ultrastructure." The Journal of Nutrition 129.1 (1999): 174-180.

36) Rostami, Rahim, et al. "Serum Selenium Status and Its Interrelationship with Serum Biomarkers of Thyroid Function and Anti-Oxidant Defense in Hashimoto's Thyroiditis." Anti-oxidants 9.11 (2020): 1070.

37) Zuo, Ying, et al. "The Correlation Between Selenium Levels and Autoimmune Thyroid Disease: A Systematic Review and Meta-Analysis." Ann. Palliat. Med 10 (2021): 4398-4408.

Chapter 25

Low Thyroid, Hashimoto's, and Pregnancy

TODAY IS A HAPPY DAY for Susan. She just delivered a healthy baby girl and sent me a cute baby photo with a thank you note. Twelve months before, Susan was weeping in my office, recounting her story of repeated miscarriages and fertility problems. Her lab panel showed a borderline low thyroid status and elevated anti-thyroid antibodies indicating Hashimoto's autoimmune thyroiditis. After a complete evaluation, we started Susan on our usual program of natural desiccated thyroid (NDT) One and a Half Grains per day, selenium 200 mcg/day, iodine 450 mcg per day, and a good prenatal multivitamin. A few months later, Susan was expecting!

A Common Scenario

There are thousands of low-thyroid people like Susan, ignored by mainstream medicine and left to suffer through repeated miscarriages and other fertility problems, representing yet another tragic error by conventional endocrinology.

Dr. Peter Taylor Makes a Plea

Dr. Peter Taylor made precisely this point at a 2016 Endocrine Society Meeting, saying more pregnant women would benefit from thyroid hormone treatment to prevent miscarriages and stillborn babies. His pleas to screen all pregnant women were ignored, as they have been for many years. Further studies show that many women with anti-thyroid antibodies have better pregnancy outcomes when treated with thyroid hormones. (1-4)

The New York Times Gets the Story Right

A few years back, in 2009, Dr. Alex Stagnaro-Green gave the New York Times an accurate accounting of the role of thyroid hormone in pregnancy. (5-6)

These are Dr. Alex Stagnaro-Green's points:

1) Pregnancy is like a stress test for the thyroid, increasing thyroid hormone requirement by 50%.
2) Hypothyroidism during pregnancy is linked to miscarriage and preterm delivery. Compared to aged-matched controls, children of hypothyroid mothers have lower IQs by seven points on average when tested seven to nine years later. Nineteen percent of these children had IQs of 85 or less.
3) Even though thyroid hormone levels may be completely normal, Hashimoto's anti-thyroid antibodies are associated with a 200-300% increase in miscarriage. (5-9)

Ten to twenty percent of reproductive-age women have elevated thyroid antibodies. Dr. Roberto Negro from Italy published a study in 2006 of women who were thyroid antibody-positive. Treatment of these women with thyroid hormone resulted in a dramatic reduction in stillbirths and preterm deliveries. (8)

How to Make Smarter Babies

As mentioned above, children born to hypothyroid mothers have lower IQs when tested 7-9 years later. Giving thyroid hormones to the mother makes babies smarter. In addition, maternal iodine deficiency is associated with reduced educational outcomes in the offspring. This is precisely why we screen women for iodine levels and make sure they have adequate iodine supplementation. In Hashimoto's patients, we use low-dose iodine supplementation of 225-450 mcg per day, which is a safe level. (7) (10-11)

Unexplained Fertility, Higher TSH

In 2017, Dr. Tahereh found women with unexplained infertility had lower thyroid function than control patients. They had higher TSH values. In 2017, Dr Tahereh writes:

Women with Unexplained Infertility (UI) had significantly higher TSH levels than controls. Nearly twice as many women with UI (26.9%) had a TSH >2.5mIU/L compared to controls (13.5%; p<0.05). (12)

Hypothyroid MOM

Perhaps the one person most dedicated to getting this message out is Dana Trentini, who runs the HypoThyroidMom website. After suffering a miscarriage, she discovered the importance of thyroid hormone replacement in pregnancy and has been a tireless advocate ever since. Regretting her misplaced trust in doctors who failed to treat her low thyroid condition, Hypothyroid Mom now encourages all women to take charge of their thyroid health. (13)

Conclusion

Another of the errors and tragedies of modern endocrinology is ignoring the role of thyroid hormone in women of childbearing age, the hypothyroid mom, leading to unnecessary suffering. All pregnant women should be screened for anti-thyroid antibodies, and more pregnant women should be treated with thyroid hormones which will result in a reduction in miscarriages, a reduction in preterm infants, and an improvement in IQ and educational outcomes in the newborn. (14-25)

Infertility workup should include a prolactin level to exclude prolactin-secreting microadenoma. However, elevated prolactin is common in hypothyroidism with elevated TSH. The increased hypothalamic secretion of TRH (thyrotropin-releasing hormone) also stimulates prolactin secretion. In these cases, prolactin levels decline after treatment with thyroid hormones. (26-32)

♦ References for Chapter 25

1) Society for Endocrinology. "Giving More Pregnant Women Common Thyroid Medicine May Reduce Risk of Complications." ScienceDaily. ScienceDaily, November 9, 2016. www.sciencedaily.com/releases/2016/11/161109090353.htm

2) Taylor, Peter N., et al. "Should All Women Be Screened for Thyroid Dysfunction in Pregnancy?" Women's Health 11.3 (2015): 295-307.

3) Taylor, Peter, et al. "Controlled Antenatal Thyroid Screening Study; Obstetric Outcomes." Endocrine Abstracts. Vol. 44. Bioscientifica, 2016.

4) Thangaratinam, Shakila, et al. "Association Between Thyroid Autoantibodies and Miscarriage and Preterm Birth: Meta-Analysis Of Evidence." BMJ 342 (2011): d2616.

5) Pregnancy and the Thyroid by Ingfei Chen, New York Times, 3/13/2009.

6) Stagnaro-Green, Alex, et al. "Detection of At-Risk Pregnancy by Means of Highly Sensitive Assays for Thyroid Autoantibodies." JAMA 264.11 (1990): 1422-1425.

7) Haddow, James E., et al. "Maternal Thyroid Deficiency During Pregnancy and Subsequent Neuropsychological Development of The Child." New England Journal of Medicine 341.8 (1999): 549-555.

8) Negro, Roberto, et al. "Levothyroxine Treatment in Euthyroid Pregnant Women with Autoimmune Thyroid Disease: Effects on Obstetrical Complications." The Journal of Clinical Endocrinology & Metabolism 91.7 (2006): 2587-2591.

9) Liu, Haixia, et al. "Maternal Subclinical Hypothyroidism, Thyroid Autoimmunity, and the Risk of Miscarriage: A Prospective Cohort Study." Thyroid 24.11 (2014): 1642-1649.

10) Hynes, Kristen L., et al. "Mild Iodine Deficiency During Pregnancy Is Associated with Reduced Educational Outcomes in The Offspring: 9-Year Follow-Up of The Gestational Iodine Cohort." The Journal of Clinical Endocrinology & Metabolism 98.5 (2013): 1954-1962.

11) Abel, Marianne Hope, et al. "Insufficient Maternal Iodine Intake Is Associated with Subfecundity, Reduced Fetal Growth, and Adverse Pregnancy Outcomes in the Norwegian Mother, Father, and Child Cohort Study." BMC Medicine 18.1 (2020): 1-17.

12) Orouji Jokar, Tahereh, et al. "Higher TSH levels within the Normal Range Are Associated with Unexplained Infertility." The Journal of Clinical Endocrinology & Metabolism 103.2 (2018): 632-639.

13) What Every Pregnant Woman Needs To Know About Hypothyroidism by Dana Trentini October 8, 2012 https://hypothyroidmom.com/what-every-pregnant-woman-needs-to-know-about-hypothyroidism/

14) Bowan, R. A. "Thyroid hormones: Pregnancy and Fetal Development." Retrieved November 19 (1999): 2002. http://www.vivo.colostate.edu/hbooks/pathphys/endocrine/thyroid/thyroid_preg.html

15) Dal Lago, Alessandro, et al. "Positive Impact of Levothyroxine Treatment on Pregnancy Outcome in Euthyroid Women with Thyroid Autoimmunity Affected by Recurrent Miscarriage." Journal of Clinical Medicine 10.10 (2021): 2105.

16) Dhillon-Smith, Rima K., et al. "Subclinical Hypothyroidism and Anti-Thyroid Autoantibodies In Women With Subfertility Or Recurrent Pregnancy Loss: Scientific Impact Paper No. 70 June 2022." BJOG: An International Journal of Obstetrics & Gynaecology (2022).

17) Konishi, Shoko, and Yuki Mizuno. "Pre-Conceptional Anti-Thyroid Antibodies and Thyroid Function in Association with Natural Conception Rates." International Journal of Environmental Research and Public Health 19.20 (2022): 13177.

18) Mild Thyroid Dysfunction in Early Pregnancy Is Linked to Serious Complications. Newswise. Endocrine Society (2012, June 23). http://www.newswise.com/articles/mild-thyroid-dysfunction-in-early-pregnancy-linked-to-serious-complications

19) Allan, W. C., et al. "Maternal Thyroid Deficiency and Pregnancy Complications: Implications for Population Screening." Journal Of Medical Screening 7.3 (2000): 127-130.

20) Rao, V., A. Lakshmi, and M. D. Sadhnani. "Prevalence of Hypothyroidism in Recurrent Pregnancy Loss in The First Trimester." Indian Journal of Medical Sciences 62.9 (2008): 359-363.

21) Unuane, David, and Brigitte Velkeniers. "Impact of Thyroid Disease on Fertility And Assisted Conception." Best Practice & Research Clinical Endocrinology & Metabolism 34.4 (2020): 101378.

22) Cleary-Goldman, Jane, et al. "Maternal Thyroid Hypofunction and Pregnancy Outcome." Obstetrics and gynecology 112.1 (2008): 85.

23) Panwar, Mr. Ekagra, et al. "Thyroid Dysfunction & Pregnancy." Journal of Coastal Life Medicine 10 (2022): 57-67.

24) De Groot, Leslie, et al. "Management of Thyroid Dysfunction During Pregnancy and Postpartum: An Endocrine Society Clinical Practice Guideline." The Journal of Clinical Endocrinology & Metabolism 97.8 (2012): 2543-2565.

25) Eligar, Vinay, et al. "Thyroxine Replacement: A Clinical Endocrinologist's Viewpoint." Annals Of Clinical Biochemistry 53.4 (2016): 421-433.

26) Honbo, Ken S., Andre J. Van Herle, and Katherine A. Kellett. "Serum Prolactin Levels in Untreated Primary Hypothyroldism." The American Journal of Medicine 64.5 (1978): 782-787.

27) Sokhadze, Khatuna, et al. "Efficacy of Thyroxine Treatment in Women with Reproductive Disorders and Hyperprolactinemia Developed on the Background of Primary Hypothyroidism and Correlations Between Prolactin and Thyroid Hormones." Translational and Clinical Medicine-Georgian Medical Journal 5.2 (2020): 22-26.

28) Ansari, Mohd Saleem, and Mussa H. Almalki. "Primary Hypothyroidism with Markedly High Prolactin." Frontiers in Endocrinology 7 (2016): 35.

29) Shukla, Prateek, et al. "Pituitary Hyperplasia in Severe Primary Hypothyroidism: A Case Report and Review of the Literature." Case Reports in Endocrinology 2019 (2019).

30) Sheikhi, Vahid, and Zahra Heidari. "Increase in Thyrotropin Is Associated with an Increase in Serum Prolactin in Euthyroid Subjects and Patients with Subclinical Hypothyroidism." Medical Journal of the Islamic Republic of Iran 35 (2021).

31) Koner, Samarjit, et al. "A Study on Thyroid Profile and Prolactin Level in Hypothyroid Females of a Rural Population of a Developing Country." Medical Journal of Dr. DY Patil University 12.3 (2019): 217-224.

32) ILyas, Amber, et al. "Study of Serum FSH, LH and Prolactin in Female Albino Rats by Experimentally Creating Hypothyroidism." Annals of Abbasi Shaheed Hospital and Karachi Medical College 25.4 (2020): 225-230.

Chapter 26

Hashimoto's Thyroiditis with Normal TSH, When to Treat?

A 15-YEAR-OLD HIGH SCHOOL STUDENT, Kathy, arrived at my office with her mother. She carried the diagnosis of Hashimoto's autoimmune thyroid disease. Her laboratory studies showed a TSH within the normal range, with elevated thyroid antibodies. The thyroid antibodies were markedly elevated, anti-thyroglobulin 425 IU/mL and anti-thyro-peroxidase (TPO) 350 IU/mL. Her thyroid gland was moderately enlarged, indicating goiter. Additional laboratory testing showed low vitamin D3 and low vitamin B12 levels.

This young lady had previously seen multiple endocrinologists, all of whom declined to give thyroid medication, saying it was unnecessary. This decision, of course, was based on her normal TSH. All the doctors said they would wait and give thyroid medication at some future time when the TSH rises above the lab range, which will then serve as an indication of low thyroid function requiring treatment.

The Patient is Symptomatic

Despite the TSH in the normal range, this 15-year-old girl was symptomatic with menstrual irregularities, mood disorders, weight gain, and acne. By the way, she also consumed a steady diet of junk food and carbonated sodas with high fructose corn syrup.

Another Error in Endocrinology

My previous Chapter 5 on Errors in Modern Thyroid Endocrinology discussed several errors endocrinologists commonly make. This is another one of them, **NOT TREATING** the Euthyroid Hashimoto's patient, i.e., the Hashimoto's patient with a TSH in the normal range. This is an obvious error in the practice of modern endocrinology.

Treating the Euthyroid Hashimoto's Patient

In my office, we make a point of starting the Euthyroid Hashimoto's patients on thyroid medication right away. We do not wait. This is a practice supported by massive numbers of studies published in the endocrinology medical literature, the same medical literature your endocrinologist should be reading to keep up to date in his field. (1-7) (43-48)

The Endocrinology Medical Literature, What Does It Say?

In 2013, Dr. Katarzyna Korzeniowska found that thyroid medication (in this case, levothyroxine) stabilizes the autoimmune inflammatory process in euthyroid non-goitrous children with Hashimoto's thyroiditis and type 1 diabetes mellitus. Dr. Korzeniowska writes that treatment with L-thyroxine should be started right away. Dr. Korzeniowska writes:

> Treatment with L-T4 [levothyroxine] in euthyroid pediatric patients with T1DM [type one diabetes] and AIT [auto immune thyroid] stabilizes autoimmune inflammation in the thyroid gland and is to be recommended as soon as the diagnosis is established…. To sum up, our findings also indicate that the treatment of patients with autoimmune polyglandular syndrome type 3a who are euthyroid or sub-clinically hypothyroid is to be recommended. This treatment needs to be started as soon as Hashimoto's disease is diagnosed. (1)

Lymphocytic Infiltration of Thyroid Gland in Hashimoto's Thyroid Disease

In 2001, Dr. Padberg published a study in Thyroid, the official journal of the American Thyroid Association. Dr. Padberg studied 21 euthyroid Hashimoto's patients for one year. Half were treated with levothyroxine, and the other half were untreated. Healthy controls were used for comparison. (2). Dr. Padberg remarks that:

> Studies in animal models of spontaneous Hashimoto's autoimmune thyroiditis (HT) show that prophylactic treatment with levothyroxine (LT4) can reduce the incidence and degree of lymphocytic infiltration in HT. (2)

Dr. Padberg found considerable benefit after one year of treatment with levothyroxine (LT4). The TPO Antibody levels and B lymphocytes declined. Dr. Padberg writes:

> After one year of therapy with LT4, TPO-Abs and B lymphocytes decreased significantly only in the treated group of euthyroid patients with HT [Hashimoto's Thyroiditis] ... In contrast, TPO-Abs levels did not change or even increased in untreated euthyroid patients with HT... Prophylactic treatment of euthyroid patients with HT reduced both serological and cellular markers of autoimmune thyroiditis. Therefore, prophylactic LT4 treatment might be useful to stop the progression or even manifestation of the disease. (2)

In 2008, Dr. Matthias Schmidt published in Thyroid a retrospective study of 38 patients with Hashimoto's disease taking levothyroxine long term. 92% of the patients had a decrease in TPO antibody levels, with a mean reduction of 8% after three months and a 45% decrease after one year. Dr. Schmidt writes:

> In the 35 patients in whom there were decreasing TPO-Ab values, the mean of the first value was 4779 IU/mL... The mean decrease after 3 months was 8%, and after 1 year it was 45%. Five years after the first value, TPO-Ab levels were 1456 +/- 1219 IU/mL, a decrease of 70%. (3)

In 2005 Dr. Aksoy published a study in the Journal of Endocrinology of 33 patients with euthyroid Hashimoto's thyroiditis followed over 15 months. Half received prophylactic levothyroxine treatment, and the other half had no treatment. Dr. Aksoy found considerable benefit both in serological markers of thyroid function and auto-immunity, as well as thyroid volume only in the levothyroxine-treated group, and he recommended prophylactic (preventive) treatment for euthyroid Hashimoto's patients: Dr. Aksoy writes:

> After 15 months of levothyroxine treatment, there was a significant increase in free T4 and a significant decrease in TSH and anti-thyroglobulin antibody anti-thyroid peroxidase antibody levels. CD8+ cell counts increased in both groups, and CD4/CD8 levels decreased significantly because of the increase in CD8+ cell count levels. Though there was no change in cytological findings, ultrasonography showed a decrease in thyroid volume in levothyroxine-receiving patients, whereas an increase was detected in patients who were followed without treatment. In conclusion, prophylactic thyroid hormone therapy can be used in patients with Hashimoto's thyroiditis, even if they are euthyroid. (4)

Combining Levothyroxine with Selenium

In 2011, Dr. Robert Krysiak published his study in the Journal of Clinical Endocrinology & Metabolism on the beneficial effect of combining levothyroxine and selenomethionine (selenium) for reducing the severity of autoimmune disease in women with Hashimoto's thyroiditis. This was a randomized clinical trial of 170 previously untreated euthyroid Hashimoto's women and 41 matched healthy subjects. Half the participants received a 6-month treatment with levothyroxine plus selenomethionine and half a placebo. They found a considerable reduction in inflammatory markers such as cytokines and CRP, with both agents, levothyroxine plus selenomethionine, working synergistically for even greater benefit. Dr. Robert Krysiak writes:

The decrease in cytokine release and in plasma CRP levels was strongest when both drugs were given together...levothyroxine and selenomethionine exhibit a similar systemic anti-inflammatory effect in euthyroid females with Hashimoto's thyroiditis. This action, which correlates with a reduction in thyroid peroxidase antibody titers, may be associated with clinical benefits in the prevention and management of Hashimoto's thyroiditis, particularly in subjects receiving both agents. (5)

IVF for Euthyroid Hashimoto's Patients

In 2009, Dr. Alberto Revelli, a reproductive endocrinologist, published his study in Reproductive Biology and Endocrinology, finding better IVF (in vitro fertilization) outcomes in euthyroid Hashimoto's patients when treated with a combination of levothyroxine plus anti-inflammatory drugs, aspirin, and prednisone. Dr. Revelli found that euthyroid Hashimoto's patients had reduced IVF outcomes. However, when treated with levothyroxine, the IVF outcomes improved to equal that of normal females (without ATA – anti-thyroid antibodies). He writes:

Anti-thyroid antibodies (ATA), even if not associated with thyroid dysfunction, are suspected to cause poorer outcome of in vitro fertilization (IVF)...The prevalence of ATA in euthyroid, infertile patients was 10.5%, similar to the one reported in euthyroid women between 18 and 45 years. ATA+ patients [with thyroid auto antibodies] who did not receive any adjuvant treatment showed significantly poorer ovarian responsiveness to stimulation and IVF results than controls. ATA+ patients receiving LT [levothyroxine] responded better to ovarian stimulation but had IVF results as poor as untreated ATA+ women...Patients receiving LT+ASA+P had significantly higher pregnancy and implantation rates than untreated ATA+ patients...and overall IVF results comparable to patients without ATA. (6-7)

Back to the Patient's Low B12 Level- Gastric Achlorhydria

This patient had a low B12 level, raising the question of pernicious anemia. Thyroid disease has been linked to pernicious anemia going back to 1881, and in 1960 this connection was renamed the hypogastric syndrome, autoimmune destruction of parietal cells of the gastric mucosa leads to gastric achlorhydria, loss of intrinsic factor, and inability to absorb B12. Iron deficiency and other malabsorption-related micronutrient deficiencies may be present. Treatment with iron supplements and B12 sublingual tablets or injections is straightforward. The hypogastric syndrome is sometimes reversible if underlying H. Pylori infection is found and eradicated with triple therapy. (8-10)

Observations in Our Office

Over the years of treating Hashimoto's patients, we have seen anti-thyroid antibody levels decline in most patients under treatment with selenium and TSH suppressive doses of thyroid hormone. In my opinion, NDT, natural desiccated thyroid, is preferred over levothyroxine. Clinical results are better with the use of NDT containing both T3 and T4 rather than the T4-only levothyroxine. Evaluation for gluten sensitivity, deficiencies in B12 and iron, and H. Pylori infection are routine for all patients with autoimmune thyroid disease.

Our treatment protocol for Hashimoto's thyroid patients also includes the following:

- TSH Suppression with NDT (Natural Desiccated Thyroid) (1-7) (43-48)
- Gluten-Free Diet with the elimination of junk food and sodas. (11-16)
- Optimize Vitamin D3 to the upper end of the laboratory reference range. (17-26)
- Selenium Supplementation when found low on blood testing. (27-31)

- B12 Testing and Supplementation when deficient. (26) (32-37)
- Low Dose Iodine Supplementation (225 mcg per day) (38-39)
- LDN (low-dose naltrexone) in selected cases. (40-42)

Conclusion

Another Error in Modern Endocrinology is the common practice of NOT TREATING euthyroid Hashimoto's patients with thyroid medication (NDT or Levothyroxine). Such treatment is supported by massive evidence in the medical literature and is even more beneficial when combined with selenium, D3, B12, and a Gluten-Free Diet. (43-45)

♦ References for Chapter 26

1) Korzeniowska, Katarzyna, et al. "L-Thyroxine Stabilizes Autoimmune Inflammatory Process in Euthyroid Non Goitrous Children with Hashimoto's Thyroiditis and Type 1 Diabetes Mellitus." Journal of Clinical Research in Pediatric Endocrinology 5.4 (2013): 240.

2) Padberg, S., et al. "One-Year Prophylactic Treatment of Euthyroid Hashimoto's Thyroiditis Patients with Levothyroxine: Is There a Benefit?" Thyroid: Official Journal of the American Thyroid Association 11.3 (2001): 249-255.

3) Schmidt, Matthias, et al. "Long-Term Follow-Up of Anti-Thyroid Peroxidase Antibodies in Patients with Chronic Autoimmune Thyroiditis (Hashimoto's Thyroiditis) Treated with Levothyroxine." Thyroid: Official Journal of the American Thyroid Association 18.7 (2008): 755-760.

4) Aksoy, Duygu Yazgan, et al. "Effects of Prophylactic Thyroid Hormone Replacement in Euthyroid Hashimoto's Thyroiditis." Endocrine Journal 52.3 (2005): 337-343.

5) Krysiak, Robert, and Boguslaw Okopien. "The Effect of Levothyroxine and Selenomethionine on Lymphocyte and Monocyte Cytokine Release in Women with Hashimoto's Thyroiditis." The Journal of Clinical Endocrinology & Metabolism 96.7 (2011): 2206-2215.

6) Revelli, Alberto, et al. "A Retrospective Study on IVF Outcome in Euthyroid Patients with Anti-Thyroid Antibodies: Effects of Levothyroxine, Acetylsalicylic Acid, and Prednisolone Adjuvant Treatments." Reproductive Biology and Endocrinology 7.1 (2009): 1-6.

7) Dörr, Helmuth G., et al. "Levothyroxine Treatment of Euthyroid Children with Autoimmune Hashimoto Thyroiditis: Results of a Multicenter, Randomized, Controlled Trial." Hormone Research in Pediatrics 84.4 (2015): 266-274.

8) Lahner, Edith, et al. "Thyro-Enter-Gastric Autoimmunity: Pathophysiology and Implications for Patient Management." Best Practice & Research Clinical Endocrinology & Metabolism 34.1 (2020): 101373.

9) Valdes-Socin, H., et al. "Chronic Autoimmune Gastritis: A Multidisciplinary Management." Revue Medicale de Liege 74.11 (2019): 598-605.

10) Henao, Sandra Consuelo, et al. "Thyrogastric Syndrome: Case Series." Revista Colombiana de Gastroenterología 34.4 (2019): 350-355.

11) Pobłocki, Jakub, et al. "Whether a Gluten-Free Diet Should Be Recommended in Chronic Autoimmune Thyroiditis or Not? —A 12-Month Follow-Up." Journal of Clinical Medicine 10.15 (2021): 3240.

12) Krysiak, Robert, et al. "The Effect of Gluten-Free Diet on Thyroid Autoimmunity in Drug-Naïve Women with Hashimoto's Thyroiditis: A Pilot Study." Experimental and Clinical Endocrinology & Diabetes 127.07 (2019): 417-422.

13) Wojtas, Natalia, et al. "Evaluation of Qualitative Dietary Protocol (Diet4hashi) Application in Dietary Counseling in Hashimoto Thyroiditis: Study Protocol of a Randomized Controlled Trial." International Journal of Environmental Research and Public Health 16.23 (2019): 4841.

14) Agardh, Daniel, et al. "Reduction of Tissue Transglutaminase Autoantibody Levels by Gluten-Free Diet Is Associated with Changes in Subsets of Peripheral Blood Lymphocytes in Children with Newly Diagnosed Coeliac Disease." Clinical & Experimental Immunology 144.1 (2006): 67-75.

15) Liontiris, Michael I., and Elias E. Mazokopakis. "A Concise Review of Hashimoto Thyroiditis (HT) and the Importance of Iodine, Selenium, Vitamin D and Gluten on the Autoimmunity and Dietary Management of HT Patients. Points That Need More Investigation." Hell J Nucl Med 20.1 (2017): 51-56.

16) Ihnatowicz, Paulina, et al. "The Importance of Nutritional Factors and Dietary Management of Hashimoto's Thyroiditis." Annals of Agricultural and Environmental Medicine 27.2 (2020): 184-193.

17) Piekarska, Małgorzata, et al. "The Correlation Between Vitamin D and Autoimmune Thyroid Function–Short Review." Journal of Education, Health and Sport 11.9 (2021): 401-408.

18) Vieira, Inês Henriques, et al. "Vitamin D and Autoimmune Thyroid Disease—Cause, Consequence, or a Vicious Cycle?" Nutrients 12.9 (2020): 2791.

19) Koehler, Viktoria F., et al. "Vitamin D Status and Thyroid Autoantibodies in Autoimmune Thyroiditis." Hormone and Metabolic Research 51.12 (2019): 792-797.

20) Mazokopakis, Elias E., et al. "Is Vitamin D Related to Pathogenesis and Treatment of Hashimoto's Thyroiditis." Hell J Nucl Med 18.3 (2015): 222-7.

21) Chahardoli, Reza, et al. "Can Supplementation with Vitamin D Modify Thyroid Autoantibodies (Anti-TPO Ab, Anti-Tg Ab) and Thyroid Profile (T3, T4, TSH) in Hashimoto's Thyroiditis? A Double-Blind, Randomized Clinical Trial." Hormone and Metabolic Research 51.05 (2019): 296-301.

22) Krysiak, Robert, et al. "The Effect of Vitamin D on Thyroid Autoimmunity in Levothyroxine-Treated Women with Hashimoto's Thyroiditis and Normal Vitamin D Status." Experimental and Clinical Endocrinology & Diabetes 125.04 (2017): 229-233.

23) Koehler, Viktoria F., et al. "Vitamin D Status and Thyroid Autoantibodies in Autoimmune Thyroiditis." Hormone and Metabolic Research 51.12 (2019): 792-797.

24) Fang, Fang, et al. "Vitamin D Deficiency Is Associated with Thyroid Autoimmunity: Results from An Epidemiological Survey in Tianjin, China." Endocrine 73.2 (2021): 447-454.

25) Mazokopakis, Elias E., et al. "Is Vitamin D Related to Pathogenesis and Treatment of Hashimoto's Thyroiditis." Hell J Nucl Med 18.3 (2015): 222-7.

26) Aktas, Hanife Serife. "Vitamin B12 and Vitamin D Levels in Patients with Autoimmune Hypothyroidism and Their Correlation with Anti-Thyroid Peroxidase Antibodies." Medical Principles and Practice 29.4 (2020): 364-370.

27) Wichman, Johanna, et al. "Selenium Supplementation Significantly Reduces Thyroid Autoantibody Levels in Patients with Chronic Autoimmune Thyroiditis: A Systematic Review and Meta-Analysis." Thyroid 26.12 (2016): 1681-1692.

28) Onal, Hasan, et al. "Effects of Selenium Supplementation in the Early Stage of Autoimmune Thyroiditis in Childhood: An Open-Label Pilot Study." Journal of Pediatric Endocrinology and Metabolism 25.7-8 (2012): 639-644.

29) Yu, L., et al. "Levothyroxine Monotherapy Versus Levothyroxine and Selenium Combination Therapy in Chronic Lymphocytic Thyroiditis." Journal of Endocrinological Investigation 40.11 (2017): 1243-1250.

30) Pirola, Ilenia, et al. "Selenium Supplementation Could Restore Euthyroidism in Subclinical Hypothyroid Patients with Autoimmune Thyroiditis." Endokrynologia Polska 67.6 (2016): 567-571.

31) Fan, Yaofu, et al. "Selenium Supplementation for Autoimmune Thyroiditis: A Systematic Review and Meta-Analysis." International Journal of Endocrinology 2014 (2014).

32) Kacharava, Tinatin, et al. "Correlation between Vitamin B12 Deficiency and Autoimmune Thyroid Diseases." Endocrine, Metabolic & Immune Disorders-Drug Targets 23.1 (2023): 86-94.

33) Benites-Zapata, Vicente A., et al. "Vitamin B12 levels in Thyroid Disorders: A Systematic Review and Meta-Analysis." Frontiers in Endocrinology 14 (2023).

34) Collins, Aryn B., and Roman Pawlak. "Prevalence of Vitamin B-12 Deficiency Among Patients with Thyroid Dysfunction." Asia Pacific Journal of Clinical Nutrition 25.2 (2016): 221-226.

35) Ness-Abramof, Rosane, et al. "Prevalence and Evaluation of B12 Deficiency in Patients with Autoimmune Thyroid Disease." The American Journal of the Medical Sciences 332.3 (2006): 119-122.

36) Jabbar, Abdul, et al. "Vitamin B12 Deficiency Common in Primary Hypothyroidism." Journal of the Pakistan Medical Association 58.5 (2008): 258.

37) Wang, Yi-Ping, et al. "Hemoglobin, Iron, and Vitamin B12 Deficiencies and High Blood Homocysteine Levels in Patients with Anti-Thyroid Autoantibodies." Journal of the Formosan Medical Association 113.3 (2014): 155-160.

38) Reinhardt, W., et al. "Effect of Small Doses of Iodine on Thyroid Function in Patients with Hashimoto's Thyroiditis Residing in an Area of Mild Iodine Deficiency." European Journal of Endocrinology 139.1 (1998): 23-28.

39) Braverman, Lewis E. "Adequate Iodine Intake-The Good Far Outweighs the Bad." European Journal of Endocrinology 139.1 (1998): 14-15.

40) Toljan, Karlo, and Bruce Vrooman. "Low-Dose Naltrexone (LDN)—Review of Therapeutic Utilization." Medical Sciences 6.4 (2018): 82.

41) McDermott, Michael T. "Low-Dose Naltrexone Treatment of Hashimoto's Thyroiditis." Management of Patients with Pseudo-Endocrine Disorders. Springer, Cham, 2019. 317-326.

42) Neuman, Daniel L., and Andrea L. Chadwick. "Utilization of Low-Dose Naltrexone for Burning Mouth Syndrome: A Case Report." A&A Practice 15.5 (2021): e01475.

43) Ozen, Samim, et al. "Clinical Course of Hashimoto's Thyroiditis and Effects of Levothyroxine Therapy on the Clinical Course of the Disease in Children and Adolescents." Journal of Clinical Research in Pediatric Endocrinology 3.4 (2011): 192.

44) Yamauchi, Keishi, et al. "Elevation of Serum Immunoglobulin G In Hashimoto's Thyroiditis and Decrease After Treatment With L-Thyroxine in Hypothyroid Patients." Internal Medicine 49.4 (2010): 267-271.

45) Romaldini, Joao H., et al. "Effect of L-Thyroxine Administration on Anti-Thyroid Antibody Levels, Lipid Profile, and Thyroid Volume in Patients with Hashimoto's Thyroiditis." Thyroid 6.3 (1996): 183-188.

46) Rink, T., et al. "Effect of Iodine and Thyroid Hormones in the Induction and Therapy of Hashimoto's Thyroiditis." Nuklearmedizin. Nuclear Medicine 38.5 (1999): 144-149.

47) Hegedüs, Laszlo, et al. "Influence of Thyroxine Treatment on Thyroid Size and Anti-Thyroid Peroxidase Antibodies in Hashimoto's Thyroiditis." Clinical Endocrinology 35.3 (1991): 235-238.

48) Schumm-Draeger, P-M., S. Padberg, and K. Heller. "Prophylactic Levothyroxine Therapy in Patients with Hashimoto's Thyroiditis." Experimental and Clinical Endocrinology & Diabetes 107.S 03 (1999): S84-S87.

Chapter 27

Hashimoto's Thyroiditis, Manic Depression, and Psychosis

Pathophysiology of Hashimoto's

HASHIMOTO'S THYROIDITIS IS AN AUTOIMMUNE disease in which the thyroid gland is infiltrated by lymphocytes that attack and destroy the functioning thyroid cells, called thyrocytes forming a single circumferential layer lining the colloid follicles. See the photomicrograph on the cover of this book showing the architectural pattern of thyroid follicles, the storage area for thyroglobulin, also called colloid, the protein backbone for thyroid hormone production. The thyrocytes concentrate iodide from the bloodstream, activate the iodide to iodine, and then combine it with thyroglobulin to form thyroid hormone (T4 and T3), which is then secreted into the bloodstream.

Microscopy of the thyroid gland in a typical case of Hashimoto's thyroiditis reveals lymphoid infiltration. Blood testing may reveal anti-thyroid peroxidase and anti-thyroglobulin antibodies. Although the cellular infiltrate in the thyroid gland is the hallmark of the disease, the diagnosis of Hashimoto's Thyroiditis is usually made by the detection of anti-thyroid antibodies in the blood, the TPO (thyroid peroxidase) and thyroglobulin antibodies.

In Graves' disease, antibodies to the TSH Receptor consist of two types. The TRAb (TSH Receptor Antibodies) may be blocking or stimulatory, while TSH Stimulating Antibodies (TSI) are stimulatory. As discussed in previous chapters, TSH Receptor stimulation causes hyperthyroidism. Other antibodies have also been detected against the NIS (sodium iodide symporter) and against Pendrin. Future investigation may yet reveal additional antibodies currently unknown. (1)

Clinical Course of Hashimoto's Thyroiditis

The clinical course of Hasshimoto's thyroiditis can be variable depending on the severity of the inflammatory attack and the amount of damaged thyroid tissue. Early on, Hashimoto's has a 20-27%% chance of spontaneous recovery. The late-stage disease is associated with a destroyed and fibrotic thyroid gland which functions poorly, rendering the patient hypothyroid, requiring thyroid hormone replacement. (2-9)

Thyroid Function May Vary – Hashitoxicosis

In Hashimoto's, thyroid function can be variable. The early-stage disease may have normal thyroid function, or episodic periods of transient hyperthyroidism, also called thyrotoxicosis or thyroid storm, which if severe, may represent a medical emergency requiring hospitalization. The hyperthyroidism of Hashimoto's disease has been named "Hashitoxicosis," an inflammatory process with rupture of follicles and release of preformed hormone associated with low 5-hour and 24-hour radio-iodine uptake. Treatment is with observation and Beta Blockers such as propranolol. Thyroid blocking drugs such as methimazole are not effective, since this is an inflammatory condition with rupture of follicles and release of preformed thyroid hormone. (10-14)

Indeed, in Hashimoto's, thyroid function may fluctuate up and down. The patient may cycle back and forth from low to high thyroid function, which can mimic various psychiatric syndromes such as Bi-Polar Syndrome and Manic-Depressive Psychosis. (15-16)

In 2013, Dr. Brian Morris described Hashitoxicosis as follows:

Thus, Hashimoto's can present either as overt hypothyroidism, subclinical hypothyroidism, or rarely during the hyperthyroid phase. This period of hyperthyroidism is called hashitoxicosis and is believed to result from uncontrolled release of thyroid hormone during the active inflammatory phase of the disease. Enlargement of the thyroid is common during the Hashitoxicosis phase and results from lymphocytic infiltration of the gland, which typically leads to eventual fibrosis. (17)

Radio-Iodine Scan

Useful for differentiating Hashitoxicosis from Graves' thyrotoxicosis is the radio-iodine uptake scan. Radio-iodine uptake in Hashitoxicosis is low, while in Graves' Disease significantly increased. In 2013, Dr. Brian Morris says that radio-iodine uptake is helpful to differentiate Hashitoxicosis from Graves' thyrotoxicosis. Dr. Brian Morris writes:

The differential diagnosis [of a patient with Hashitoxicosis] typically includes Graves' disease, toxic adenoma, multinodular goiter, other forms of thyroiditis, and exogenous ingestion of thyroid hormone. Because many of the symptoms are nonspecific, many patients are misdiagnosed so the diagnosis may be delayed for months or years. **Occasionally an I-131 uptake scan is necessary to clarify the diagnosis with low to normal uptake suggestive of Hashimoto's and high uptake favoring Graves' disease or toxic adenoma.** (17)

The T3/T4 Ratio

Another helpful feature to differentiate Graves' thyrotoxicosis from Hashitoxicosis is the T3/T4 ratio, usually increased in Graves' thyrotoxicosis and decreased in Hashitoxicosis. This is due to the upregulated intra-thyroidal D1 deiodinase in Graves' disease, which converts T4 to T3, thus increasing the amount of T3 secreted by the thyroid. (18-21)

Alternating Hyper and Hypothyroidism

Two explanations for Hashitoxicosis have been proposed. One is that cell death of thyrocytes (thyroid cells) releases preformed thyroid hormone into circulation, producing a transient thyroid storm. This is usually self-limiting once the inflammatory attack and cell death of thyrocytes cease. The second explanation is that there may be alternating dominance of TSH Receptor blocking antibodies (TRAb) with TSH Receptor stimulatory antibodies. The TSH Receptor blocking antibodies may cause hypothyroidism and the opposite for TSH stimulating antibodies which cause hyperthyroidism and thyrotoxicosis. Some Hashimoto's patients will develop high TSH Receptor antibody (TSI thyroid stimulatory immunoglobulins or TRAb) levels and transform into Graves' disease, a form of hyperthyroidism. About 70% of Graves' patients also have Hashimoto's antibodies. These two diseases may co-exist in the same patient and cause alternating episodes of hyper and hypothyroidism. (22-25)

Painless Thyroiditis and Wheat Gluten Exposure

Painless Thyroiditis (PT) bears a striking similarity to Hashitoxicosis. This was discussed in Chapter 21. Hashimoto's, Iodine and Selenium, Part Two with reference to Dr. Ken Okamura's 2023 study. When thyroid blocking drug dosage is decreased during treatment for thyrotoxicosis, this allows TSH elevation, and may be followed by an episode of PT (painless thyroiditis) with relapse of thyrotoxicosis. The possibility of selenium and magnesium deficiency as an aggravating factor was discussed. (26)

Another speculative explanation for acute flare-ups of thyroiditis is sudden exposure to an environmental antigen such as wheat gluten, viral, bacterial, or parasitic antigen which stimulates the immune system. The resulting inflammation in the thyroid gland leads to the release of pre-stored thyroid hormone into circulation. This effect is usually self-limited and subsides after a few weeks or so. (27-28)

Combined Selenium and Iodine Deficiency

Another possible explanation of Hashitoxicosis is related to combined selenium and iodine deficiency in a mechanism similar to myxoedematous cretinism in Zaire, Africa. In this syndrome, African children were found selenium deficient with only half the level of glutathione peroxidase as normal controls. The selenoprotein, glutathione peroxidase, is the primary antioxidant in the thyrocyte protecting the cells from the damaging effects of hydrogen peroxide used in the organification of iodide. The proposed mechanism of thyroid gland destruction is the following: iodine deficiency causes hypothyroidism, which causes elevated TSH, which stimulates the thyroid to make more thyroglobulin and hydrogen peroxide. Since the seleno-protein antioxidant system is dysfunctional, this results in massive oxidative damage to the thyroid gland leading to destruction and fibrosis. One might suggest a less severe yet similar mechanism in Hashimoto's thyroiditis, in which the damaging effects of hydrogen peroxide, not completely neutralized, could cause enough inflammation to worsen the autoimmune disease and release pre-stored thyroid hormone from the follicles into the bloodstream. (29-34)

Protocol for Prevention of Hashitoxicosis

Based on the above considerations, we have devised a protocol to prevent episodes of Hashitoxicosis, which uses TSH suppression to turn off hydrogen peroxide generation. We observe no episodes of Hashitoxicosis when this protocol is followed:

1) Selenium supplementation 200 mcg/day.

2) Iodine 225 mcg/day.

3) TSH suppression using thyroid hormone treatment. We prefer NDT, although levothyroxine may also be used.

4) Vitamin D3 supplementation. (90-92)

5) Gluten Free Diet

Hashimoto's Thyroiditis, Manic Depression, Psychosis, and Psychiatric Manifestations

Various psychiatric syndromes have been associated with Hashimoto's thyroiditis, including depression, anxiety, manic-depression, bipolar, acute psychosis, dementia, loss of cognitive function, etc. Most of these cases recover after treatment of Hashimoto's thyroiditis with thyroid medication and other measures. (35-59)

Steroid-Responsive Hashimoto's Encephalopathy

A more severe form of neuro-psychiatric disturbance has been recently described called Hashimoto's Encephalopathy. This diagnosis is crucial as it responds promptly to steroid therapy. This condition may mimic the usual psychiatric disturbances or present as a more severe neurologic disorder with dementia, ataxia, seizures, epilepsy, and cerebral vasculitis. Brain Perfusion Imaging and EEG studies may show abnormalities. (35-59)

Anti-NAE autoantibodies may be present in about half the cases. Recognition of Hashimoto's Encephalopathy is essential because the disorder is very responsive to corticosteroid treatment with prompt remission in most cases. Note: Anti-NAE autoantibodies are against the NH2-terminal of α-enolase. (48-49)

In 2011, Dr. Giulia Monti reviewed Hashimoto's encephalopathy writing that non-convulsive seizures, also called non-convulsive status epilepticus (NCSE), maybe the first manifestation:

Hashimoto's encephalopathy is an often misdiagnosed, life-threatening condition which improves promptly with steroid therapy. Since clinical manifestations are heterogeneous and nonspecific, the diagnosis is often difficult...We report two patients presenting with repetitive and prolonged seizures characterized by progressive reduction in contact and reactivity associated with frontal/diffuse polyspike-and-wave activities. This condition, which can be interpreted as a form of non-convulsive status epilepticus (NCSE) of frontal origin, **was refractory to antiepileptic drugs but responded promptly to high doses of intravenous steroid treatment.** In cases of unexplained encephalopathy with EEG documentation of NCSE, the early recognition and treatment of Hashimoto's encephalopathy may lead to a favorable prognosis. (54)

In 2008, Dr. Wilcox reviewed Hashimoto's encephalopathy masquerading as acute psychosis, writing:

Hashimoto's encephalopathy (HE) is a relapsing but exquisitely corticosteroid-responsive encephalopathy associated with autoimmune thyroiditis. Although a rare disease, with just over 100 cases reported, it may be under-recognized. Its presentation can be protean with prominent neuropsychiatric features, stroke-like episodes, seizures, and myoclonic jerks. Prompt corticosteroid treatment usually leads to rapid recovery. (55)

Antigens in Hashimoto's Cross-React with CNS Antigens

In 2020, Dr. Salvatore Benvenga found homology between the TSH Receptor, Thyroglobulin, and Thyroperoxidase (TPO) with auto-antigens in the CNS (Central Nervous System), suggesting cross-reactivity as an explanation for Hashimoto's Encephalopathy, writing:

These data suggest that cross-reactivity between CNS autoantigens and thyroid autoantigens might contribute to the HE [Hashimoto's Encephalopathy] pathogenesis. (60-61)

Gluten Encephalopathy

In genetically predisposed individuals, gluten consumption may cause neuropsychiatric disorders, ataxia, encephalopathies, sensory neuropathies, cranial neuropathies, cerebral vasculitis, etc. These may overlap with the clinical presentation of Hashimoto's related neuropsychiatric disorders. Note that ataxia, loss of balance due to cerebellar dysfunction, is a manifestation of both Gluten encephalopathy and Hashimoto's encephalopathy as noted in 2007 by Dr. Nakagawa and in 2001 by Dr. Burk. (47)(62)

Celiac disease and other forms of gluten sensitivity have a high correlation with Hashimoto's autoimmune thyroiditis. Indeed, testing for gluten sensitivity would be prudent for Hashimoto's patients. Even without testing, some practitioners advise a gluten-free diet for all Hashimoto's patients. Ingestion of wheat gluten in the gluten-sensitive individual is associated with prolonged Zonulin release, which opens the tight junctions between cells in the gut epithelial lining, thus producing a "leaky gut," allowing passage of gram-negative bacterial cell walls called LPS (short for lipopolysaccharide) into the bloodstream. In 2007, Dr. Qin showed that LPS released by the gut eventually crosses the blood-brain barrier and enters the brain, where it causes microglial activation, a hallmark of neuroinflammation. This inflammation in the brain causes depression, chronic fatigue, and neuropsychiatric disorders. (63-69)

Eating Disorders - Treatment with Thyroid Hormone?

Anorexia is an eating disorder and is considered a psychiatric disease. Patients with anorexia may appear cachectic from starvation, and as such, can represent a life-threatening medical emergency requiring hospitalization and hyper-alimentation. (70-72)

In 2011, Dr. Michelle Warren reviewed the endocrine manifestations of eating disorders, finding a similarity with the euthyroid sick syndrome, with low Free T3 and high reverse T3, a pattern suggesting central hypothyroidism, writing:

Also typical in anorexia are changes seen with the euthyroid sick syndrome. T3 levels are low, whereas rT3 [reverse T3] is elevated. In some patients, T4 is also decreased. TSH levels are normal or occasionally slightly reduced, suggesting a hypothalamic origin of the suppressed thyroid function...Treatment with thyroid hormone is inappropriate and leads to undesirable weight loss and loss of muscle mass. (73)

On the other hand, Dr. Richard Shames disagrees with Dr. Warren regarding thyroid hormone treatment for eating disorders. In 2022, Dr. Richard Shames found eating disorder patients have the low-T3 syndrome and should be treated with T3-containing thyroid medication with good results. He says T3 "acts directly on the hypothalamus to stimulate feeding." Dr. Richard Shames writes:

Calorie restriction reduces circulating triiodothyronine (T3) – the most active thyroid hormone – inducing hypothyroidism, constipation, and reduced appetite that inhibit eating, acting to sustain and sometimes precipitate eating disorders. **Thyroid-hormone treatment can be effective but is rarely employed**... Circulating T3 levels decrease in eating disorders (EDs) and in most severe and chronic illnesses in the eponymous medical condition low-T3 syndrome (LT3S)... LT3S occurs broadly in severe and chronic illnesses including trauma, sepsis, heart failure, COVID-19, and during calorie restriction aside from EDs... LT3S has major role in sustaining eating disorders by causing chronic constipation that inhibits eating and weight gain. **T3 also acts directly on the hypothalamus to stimulate feeding** (independent of energy expenditure). Reduced circulating T3 in LT3S is likely a factor in appetite suppression... **Though thyroid-hormone dysfunction is central to EDs, thyroid-hormone treatment is rarely considered by doctors or presented as an option to patients. Emphasis Mine** (Reference Shames 2022) Note: Euthyroid sick syndrome is synonymous with low-T3 syndrome. (74)

Conclusion

Ignoring the neuropsychiatric manifestations of Hashimoto's thyroiditis is another error of modern endocrinology. Gluten sensitivity and Hashimoto's are associated with neuropsychiatric disorders with considerable overlap. A gluten-free diet is beneficial. A frequently missed diagnosis is Hashimoto's Encephalopathy exquisitely sensitive to and reversible with corticosteroids. Anorexia eating disorders may be sensitive to T3-containing thyroid medication. However, this is controversial and applies only to those less severe patients with good muscle mass and body weight, ie. those whose condition is not life-threatening. For the anorectic patient with life-threatening cachexia, hyperalimentation should be the first priority. Obviously, we need more studies of T3 medication for eating disorders before this can be recommended. (75-92)

♦ References for Chapter 27

1) Akamizu, Takashi, and Nobuyuki Amino. "Hashimoto's Thyroiditis." Endotext [Internet] (2017).

2) Kaplowitz, Paul B. "Case Report: Rapid Spontaneous Recovery from Severe Hypothyroidism In 2 Teenage Girls." International Journal of Pediatric Endocrinology 2012.1 (2012): 1-3.

3) Takasu, Nobuyuki, et al. "Disappearance of Thyrotropin-Blocking Antibodies and Spontaneous Recovery from Hypothyroidism in Autoimmune Thyroiditis." New England Journal of Medicine 326.8 (1992): 513-518.

4) Takasu, Nobuyuki, and Mina Matsushita. "Changes of TSH-Stimulation Blocking Antibody (Tsbab) and Thyroid Stimulating Antibody (Tsab) Over 10 Years in 34 Tsbab-Positive Patients with Hypothyroidism and in 98 Tsab-Positive Graves' Patients with Hyperthyroidism: Reevaluation of Tsbab and Tsab In TSH-Receptor-Antibody (Trab)-Positive Patients." Journal of Thyroid Research 2012 (2012).

5) Alzahrani, Ali S., et al. "Autoimmune Thyroid Disease with Fluctuating Thyroid Function." PLoS medicine 2.5 (2005): e89.

6) Rallison, Marvin L., et al. "Natural History of Thyroid Abnormalities: Prevalence, Incidence, and Regression of Thyroid Diseases in Adolescents and Young Adults." The American Journal of Medicine 91.4 (1991): 363-370.

7) Yamamoto, Makiko, et al. "Recovery of Thyroid Function with a Decreased Titer of Anti Microsomal Antibody in a Hypothyroid Man with Hashimoto's Thyroiditis." European Journal of Endocrinology 102.4 (1983): 531-534.

8) Takasu, Nobuyuki, et al. "Disappearance of Thyrotropin-Blocking Antibodies and Spontaneous Recovery from Hypothyroidism in Autoimmune Thyroiditis." New England Journal of Medicine 326.8 (1992): 513-518.

9) Kaplowitz, Paul B. "Case Report: Rapid Spontaneous Recovery from Severe Hypothyroidism In 2 Teenage Girls." International Journal of Pediatric Endocrinology 2012.1 (2012): 1-3.

10) Unnikrishnan, A. G. "Hashitoxicosis: A Clinical Perspective." Thyroid Research and Practice 10.4 (2013): 5.

11) Harsch, Igor Alexander, et al. "Hashitoxicosis— Three Cases and A Review of The Literature." Eur Endocrinol 4.1 (2008): 70-2.

12) Wasniewska, Malgorzata, et al. "Outcomes of Children with Hashitoxicosis." Hormone research in pediatrics 77.1 (2012): 36-40.

13) Klubo-Gwiezdzinska, Joanna, and Leonard Wartofsky. "Hashimoto Thyroiditis: An Evidence-Based Guide to Etiology, Diagnosis, and Treatment." Pol. Arch. Intern. Med 132 (2022): 16222.

14) Dzagania, Ketevan, and Natia Vashakmadze. "A Rare Case of Autoimmune Thyroiditis with Frequent Episodes of Hashitoxicosis Requiring Thyroid Surgery." Endocrine Abstracts. Vol. 90. Bioscientifica, 2023.

15) Hall, Richard CW, et al. "Psychiatric Manifestations of Hashimoto's Thyroiditis." Psychosomatics 23.4 (1982): 337-342.

16) Barbuti, Margherita, et al. "Thyroid Autoimmunity in Bipolar Disorder: A Systematic Review." Journal of affective disorders 221 (2017): 97-106.

17) Morris, Brian S. "Hashitoxicosis: An Uncommon Presentation of Autoimmune Thyroid." Proceedings of UCLA Healthcare 17 (2013).

18) Ibrahim, Nesma A., and Ahmed M. Hamam. "Diagnostic Value of Estimating the Ratio of Serum Free Triiodothyronine to Free Thyroxine in Differentiating Graves' Disease from Thyroiditis." Suez Canal University Medical Journal 23.2 (2020): 135-142.

19) Sümbül, Hilmi Erdem, and Fettah ACIBUCU. "Graves' Disease and Thyroiditis Can Be Differentiated Using Only Free Thyroid Hormone Levels." The European Research Journal 6.4 (2020): 314-318.

20) Baral, Suman, Pradeep Krishna Shrestha, and Vivek Pant. "Serum free T3 to free T4 ratio as a Useful Indicator for Differentiating Destruction Induced Thyrotoxicosis from Graves' Disease." Journal of Clinical and Diagnostic Research: JCDR 11.7 (2017): OC12.

21) Sriphrapradang, Chutintorn, and Adikan Bhasipol. "Differentiating Graves' disease from Subacute Thyroiditis Using Ratio of Serum Free Triiodothyronine to Free Thyroxine." Annals of Medicine and Surgery 10 (2016): 69-72.

22) Wong, Mimi, and Warrick J. Inder. "Alternating Hyperthyroidism and Hypothyroidism in Graves' Disease." Clinical Case Reports 6.9 (2018): 1684.

23) Shrestha, Aakriti, et al. "Fluctuating Hyperthyroidism and Hypothyroidism in Graves' Disease: The Swinging Between Two Clinical Entities." Cureus 14.8 (2022).

24) Furqan, Saira, et al. "Conversion of Autoimmune Hypothyroidism to Hyperthyroidism." BMC Research Notes 7.1 (2014): 1-4.

25) Ahmad, Ehtasham, et al. "Hypothyroidism Conversion to Hyperthyroidism: It's Never Too Late." Endocrinology, Diabetes & Metabolism Case Reports 2018 (2018).

26) Okamura, Ken, et al. "Painless Thyroiditis Mimicking Relapse of Hyperthyroidism During or After Potassium Iodide or Thionamide Therapy for Graves' Disease Resulting in Remission." Endocrine Journal 70.2 (2023): 207-222.

27) Ihnatowicz, Paulina, et al. "The Importance of Gluten Exclusion in the Management of Hashimoto's Thyroiditis." Annals of Agricultural and Environmental Medicine 28.4 (2021): 558-568.

28) Liontiris, Michael I., and Elias E. Mazokopakis. "A Concise Review of Hashimoto Thyroiditis (HT) and the Importance of Iodine, Selenium, Vitamin D and Gluten on the Autoimmunity and Dietary Management of HT Patients. Points That Need More Investigation." Hell J Nucl Med 20.1 (2017): 51-56.

29) Vanderpas, Jean B., et al. "Iodine and Selenium Deficiency Associated with Cretinism in Northern Zaire." The American Journal of Clinical Nutrition 52.6 (1990): 1087-1093.

30) Boyages, Steven C., and Jean-Pierre Halpern. "Endemic Cretinism: Toward a Unifying Hypothesis." Thyroid 3.1 (1993): 59-69.

31) Contempre, Bernard, et al. "Effect of Selenium Supplementation in Hypothyroid Subjects of an Iodine and Selenium Deficient Area: The Possible Danger of Indiscriminate Supplementation of Iodine-Deficient Subjects with Selenium." The Journal of Clinical Endocrinology & Metabolism 73.1 (1991): 213-215.

32) Foster, HD. "The Iodine-Selenium Connection: Its Possible Roles in Intelligence, Cretinism, Sudden Infant Death Syndrome, Breast Cancer and Multiple Sclerosis." (1983).

33) Shahbaz, Amir, et al. "Prolonged Duration of Hashitoxicosis in a Patient with Hashimoto's Thyroiditis: A Case Report And Review Of Literature." Cureus 10.6 (2018).

34) Baral, Neelam, Leonard Wartofsky, and Meeta Sharma. "SUN-560 Thyrotoxic Hashimoto's Disease: Is It Graves' Thyrotoxicosis or" Hashitoxicosis"?" Journal of the Endocrine Society 3. Supplement_1 (2019): SUN-560.

35) Lee, Min-Joo, et al. "A Case of Hashimoto's Encephalopathy Presenting with Seizures and Psychosis." Korean Journal of Pediatrics 55.3 (2012): 111-113.

36) Lin, Shuai-Ting, et al. "Manic Symptoms Associated with Hashimoto's Encephalopathy: Response to Corticosteroid Treatment." The Journal of Neuropsychiatry and Clinical Neurosciences 23.1 (2011): E20-E21.

37) Bocchetta, Alberto, et al. "Affective Psychosis, Hashimoto's Thyroiditis, and Brain Perfusion Abnormalities: Case Report." Clinical Practice and Epidemiology in Mental Health 3.1 (2007): 1-5.

38) Tsai, Ching-Heng, et al. "Hashimoto's Encephalopathy Presenting as Catatonia in a Bipolar Patient." Asian Journal of Psychiatry 66 (2021): 102895.

39) Sporiš, Davor, et al. "Psychosis and EEG Abnormalities as Manifestations of Hashimoto Encephalopathy." Cognitive and Behavioral Neurology 20.2 (2007): 138-140.

40) Chong, Catherine Shiu-Yin, et al. "Presenile Dementia: A Case of Hashimoto's Encephalopathy." East Asian Archives of Psychiatry 21.1 (2011): 32-36.

41) Mocellin, Ramon, et al. "Reversible Dementia with Psychosis: Hashimoto's Encephalopathy." Psychiatry and Clinical Neurosciences 60.6 (2006): 761-763.

42) Montagna, Giacomo, et al. "Hashimoto's Encephalopathy: A Rare Proteiform Disorder." Autoimmunity Reviews 15.5 (2016): 466-476.

43) Degner, Detlef, et al. "Affective Disorders Associated with Autoimmune Thyroiditis." The Journal of Neuropsychiatry and Clinical Neurosciences 13.4 (2001): 532-533.

44) Teuber, Isabel, and Hans-Peter Volz. "Acute Schizophrenic Disorder in a Patient with Hashimoto's Thyroiditis." Psychiatrische Praxis 30.Suppl 2 (2003): 83-84.

45) Nayak, Hemanta Kumar, et al. "A Series Report of Autoimmune Hypothyroidism Associated with Hashimoto's Encephalopathy: An Underdiagnosed Clinical Entity with Good Prognosis." BMJ Case Reports 2010 (2010): bcr0120102630.

46) Yoneda, Makoto. "Hashimoto's Encephalopathy and Autoantibodies." Brain and Nerve= Shinkei Kenkyu No Shinpo 65.4 (2013): 365-376.

47) Nakagawa, H., et al. "Hashimoto's Encephalopathy Presenting with Progressive Cerebellar Ataxia." Journal of Neurology, Neurosurgery & Psychiatry 78.2 (2007): 196-197.

48) Matsunaga, Akiko, and Makoto Yoneda. "Anti-NAE Autoantibodies and Clinical Spectrum in Hashimoto's Encephalopathy." Rinsho byori. The Japanese Journal of Clinical Pathology 57.3 (2009): 271-278.

49) Matsunaga, Akiko, et al. "Hashimoto's Encephalopathy Associated with Anti-NAE Autoantibodies: Analysis of 101 Patients (S29. 002)." (2013): S29-002.

50) Ray, Munni, et al. "Hashimoto's Encephalopathy in an Adolescent Boy." The Indian Journal of Pediatrics 74.5 (2007): 492-494.

51) Erol, Ilknur, et al. "Hashimoto's Encephalopathy in Children and Adolescents." Pediatric Neurology 45.6 (2011): 420-422.

52) Chong, Catherine Shiu-Yin, et al. "Presenile Dementia: A Case of Hashimoto's Encephalopathy." East Asian Archives of Psychiatry 21.1 (2011): 32-36.

53) Kutlubaev, M. A., et al. "Hashimoto's Encephalopathy (A Brief Review of Literature and a Clinical Case)." Neurology, Neuropsychiatry, Psychosomatics 11.1 (2019): 79-83.

54) Monti, Giulia, et al. "Non-Convulsive Status Epilepticus of Frontal Origin as the First Manifestation of Hashimoto's Encephalopathy." Epileptic Disorders 13.3 (2011): 253-258.

55) Wilcox, R. A., et al. "Hashimoto's Encephalopathy Masquerading as Acute Psychosis." Journal of Clinical Neuroscience 15.11 (2008): 1301-1304.

56) Das, Soumitra, and Balaswamy Reddy. "Hashimoto's Encephalopathy Presented with Mutism: A Case Report." General Psychiatry 34.3 (2021).

57) Waliszewska-Prosół, Marta, and Maria Ejma. "Hashimoto Encephalopathy—Still More Questions than Answers." Cells 11.18 (2022): 2873.

58) DeBiase, Joseph M., and Deepti Avasthi. "Hashimoto's Encephalopathy: A Case Report and Literature Review of an Encephalopathy with Many Names." Cureus 12.8 (2020).

59) Churilov, Leonid P., et al. "Thyroid Gland and Brain: Enigma of Hashimoto's Encephalopathy." Best Practice & Research Clinical Endocrinology & Metabolism 33.6 (2019): 101364.

60) Benvenga, Salvatore, and Fabrizio Guarneri. "Homology between TSH-R/Tg/TPO and Hashimoto's Encephalopathy Autoantigens." Frontiers in Bioscience-Landmark 25.2 (2020): 229-241.

61) Blanchin, Stéphanie, et al. "Anti-Thyroperoxidase Antibodies from Patients with Hashimoto's Encephalopathy Bind to Cerebellar Astrocytes." Journal of Neuroimmunology 192.1-2 (2007): 13-20.

62) Bürk, K., et al. "Sporadic Cerebellar Ataxia Associated with Gluten Sensitivity." Brain 124.5 (2001): 1013-1019.

63) Qin, Liya, et al. "Systemic LPS Causes Chronic Neuroinflammation and Progressive Neurodegeneration." Glia 55.5 (2007): 453-462.

64) Chentouf, Amina, and Souad DAOUD. "Celiac Disease and Neuropsychiatric Disorders: A Systematic Review." Journal De La Faculté De Médecine d'Oran 3.2 (2019): 489-498.

65) Trovato, Chiara Maria, et al. "Neuropsychiatric Manifestations in Celiac Disease." Epilepsy & Behavior 99 (2019): 106393.

66) Dale, Hanna Fjeldheim, et al. "Non-Coeliac Gluten Sensitivity and the Spectrum of Gluten-Related Disorders: an Updated Overview." Nutrition Research Reviews 32.1 (2019): 28-37.

67) Sobolevskaia, Polina A., et al. "The Association of Neuropsychiatric Disorders and Endocrine Parameters in Hashimoto Thyroiditis." Pediatrician (St. Petersburg) 11.4 (2020): 55-68.

68) Lekurwale, Vedant, et al. "Neuropsychiatric Manifestations of Thyroid Diseases." Cureus 15.1 (2023).

69) Ihnatowicz, Paulina, et al. "The Importance of Gluten Exclusion in the Management of Hashimoto's Thyroiditis." Annals of Agricultural and Environmental Medicine 28.4 (2021): 558-568.

70) Tonoike, Takashi, et al. "Treatment with Intravenous Hyperalimentation for Severely Anorectic Patients and Its Outcome." Psychiatry and clinical neurosciences 58.3 (2004): 229-235.

71) Latzer, Yael, et al. "A Case Report: Treatment of Severe Anorexia Nervosa with Home Total Parenteral Hyperalimentation." International Journal of Eating Disorders 27.1 (2000): 115-118.

72) Maloney, Michael J., and Michael K. Farrell. "Treatment of Severe Weight Loss in Anorexia Nervosa with Hyperalimentation and Psychotherapy." The American Journal of Psychiatry (1980).

73) Warren, Michelle P. "Endocrine Manifestations of Eating Disorders." The Journal of Clinical Endocrinology & Metabolism 96.2 (2011): 333-343.

74) Shames, Richard, and Stuart Wenzel. "On the Fundamental Efficacy of Thyroid Hormone Therapy in Eating Disorders: Review of Mechanisms and Case Study." Journal of Restorative Medicine 12.1 (2022).

75) Rahhal, Samar N., and Erica A. Eugster. "Thyroid Stimulating Immunoglobulin Is Often Negative in Children with Graves' Disease." Journal of Pediatric Endocrinology and Metabolism 21.11 (2008): 1085-1088.

76) Nagasaki, Keisuke, et al. "Investigation of TSH Receptor Blocking Antibodies in Childhood-Onset Atrophic Autoimmune Thyroiditis." Clinical Pediatric Endocrinology 30.2 (2021): 79-84.

77) Giannone, Mariella, et al. "TSH-Receptor Autoantibodies in Patients with Chronic Thyroiditis and Hypothyroidism." Clinical Chemistry and Laboratory Medicine (CCLM) 60.7 (2022): 1020-1030.

78) Diana, Tanja, et al. "Thyrotropin Receptor Blocking Antibodies." Hormone and Metabolic Research 50.12 (2018): 853-862.

79) Hedstrand, Håkan, et al. "Identification of Tyrosine Hydroxylase as an Autoantigen in Autoimmune Polyendocrine Syndrome Type I." Biochemical and Biophysical Research Communications 267.1 (2000): 456-461.

80) Unnikrishnan, A. G. "Hashitoxicosis: A Clinical Perspective." Thyroid Research and Practice 10.4 (2013): 5.

81) Harsch, Igor A., et al. "Hashitoxicosis, Three Cases and a Review of the Literature." (2008): 70-2.

82) Menon, Vikas, et al. "Psychiatric Presentations Heralding Hashimoto's Encephalopathy: A Systematic Review and Analysis of Cases Reported in the Literature." Journal of Neurosciences in Rural Practice 8.02 (2017): 261-267.

83) Robles-Martínez, María, et al. "Psychosis, an Unusual Presentation of Hashimoto's Thyroiditis." Revista de Psiquiatria y Salud Mental 8.4 (2015): 243-244.

84) Correia, Inês, et al. "Encephalopathy Associated with Autoimmune Thyroid Disease: A Potentially Reversible Condition." Case Reports in Medicine 2016 (2016).

85) Jung, Kyong Yeun, et al. "Clinical Factors Predicting the Successful Discontinuation of Hormone Replacement Therapy in Patients Diagnosed with Primary Hypothyroidism." PLoS one 15.5 (2020): e0233596.

86) Gonzalez-Aguilera, Beatriz, et al. "Conversion to Graves' Disease from Hashimoto Thyroiditis: A Study Of 24 Patients." Archives of Endocrinology and Metabolism 62 (2018): 609-614.

87) Takasu, Nobuyuki, et al. "Thyroid-Stimulating Antibody and TSH-Binding Inhibitor Immunoglobulin in 277 Graves' Patients and in 686 Normal Subjects." Journal of Endocrinological Investigation 20.8 (1997): 452-461.

88) Lee, Michelle N., and Jeffrey A. Colburn. "A Grave Turn on Hashimoto's Thyroiditis-A Case Series on Four Patients with Autoimmune Hypothyroidism that Converted to Graves' Disease." Journal of the Endocrine Society 5.Supplement_1 (2021): A913-A914.

89) Trummer, Christian, et al. "Rapid Changes of Thyroid Function in a Young Woman with Autoimmune Thyroid Disease." Medical Principles and Practice 28.4 (2019): 397-400.

90) Mehdizadeh, Alireza, et al. "Comparing the Serum Level of Vitamin D in Patients with Autoimmune Hypothyroidism and Control Group Subjects." J Biochem Technol 2 (2019): 70-4.

91) Solhjoo, Mahdis, et al. "The Prevalence of Vitamin D Deficiency in Patients with Hashimoto's Hypothyroidism." Mathews Journal of Immunology & Allergy 2.1 (2018): 1-4.

92) Ke, Wencai, et al. "25-Hydroxyvitamin D Serum Level in Hashimoto's Thyroiditis, But Not Graves' Disease Is Relatively Deficient." Endocrine Journal 64.6 (2017): 581-587.

Chapter 28

Myo-inositol for Hashimoto's Thyroiditis

What is Myo-inositol?

MYO-INOSITOL IS A SUGAR-LIKE MOLECULE involved in cell signaling, making the TSH signal more effective in thyroid cells. This is useful in Hashimoto's thyroiditis, where myo-inositol is given with selenium and vitamin D3 to improve efficacy. Myo-inositol is present in our diet or as a nutritional supplement at the health food store. (1-12) (76-84)

Hashimoto's Thyroiditis Elevated Antibodies

Hashimoto's thyroiditis is an autoimmune disease affecting 10 percent of females and 2 percent of males. It is usually detected by finding characteristic anti-thyroid antibodies, the TPO (thyro-peroxidase), and thyroglobulin antibodies on routine blood tests. (1-12)

Hashimoto's Microscopic Histology of Thyroid Gland

Hashimoto's thyroiditis is characterized by diffuse lymphocyte and plasma cell infiltration, fibrous replacement, and eventual atrophy of the thyroid gland. Microscopic evaluation of the thyroid gland shows lymphocytic infiltration, plasma cell infiltration, fibrotic scarring, and over time, atrophic changes. In about 20 percent of patients with Hashimoto's autoimmune thyroiditis, there is lymphocytic infiltration alone without the tell-tale elevation of TPO or thyroglobulin antibodies. This is called seronegative Hashimoto's thyroiditis. The decreased echogenicity of the thyroid gland on ultrasound imaging is predictive of hypothyroidism in Hashimoto's with a high probability. In 2002, Dr. Wolfgang Raber writes:

Abnormal thyroid ultrasound [hypoechoic] patterns were highly indicative of

autoimmune thyroiditis and allowed the detection of thyroid dysfunction [hypothyroidism] with 96% probability. (13-16)

Inositol Involved in TSH Signaling Cascade

In 2023, Dr. Sabrina Rosaria Paparo reviewed the role of inositol in the signaling cascade for TSH- generation of hydrogen peroxide. TSH does not work directly. Instead TSH signal activates two separate signaling cascades. One signaling cascade uses inositol phosphate to generate H2O2, used by TPO to organify iodine to thyroglobulin, thus producing thyroid hormone. Note: myo-inositol will be discussed more fully below. The other TSH cascade uses cAMP to regulate cell growth and thyroid hormone secretion. Note: cAMP is Cyclic AMP. TSH activates both cascades, while TSH Receptor antibodies in Graves' disease activate only the cAMP cascade and not the H2O2-generating inositol phosphate cascade. Increasing TSH causes a greater accumulation of myo-inositol phosphate within thyrocytes. Patients with hypothyroidism require higher levels of myo-inositol than controls. Myo-inositol improves iodine availability for organification, which is of benefit in Hashimoto's patients who typically have an organification defect as demonstrated by the perchlorate discharge test. Dr. Sabrina Rosaria Paparo writes that myo-inositol is essential for thyroid physiology:

Thyroid hormone (TH) homeostasis is controlled through both the PLC-dependent **inositol phosphate** Ca2+/DAG and the cyclic AMP (cAMP) cascade, both activated by the TSH and its receptor (TSHR) binding. The cAMP cascade regulates thyrocyte development and differentiation and TH secretion, **while the PLC-dependent inositol** phosphate Ca2+/DAG pathway results in enhanced H2O2 production, which is needed for iodine incorporation and TH synthesis. Therefore, Myo [myo-inositol] and its derivates are essential in thyroid physiology, as demonstrated in vitro, by active accumulation of myo-inositol phosphate formation in thyrocytes under increased TSH level. Moreover, metabolomic studies indicate that hypothyroid patients require higher Myo levels than healthy subjects, suggesting that Myo may limit thyroid function impairment by increasing iodine availability for thyrocytes (3).

Inositol in Signaling Cascade for Many Other Hormones

As it turns out, inositol is a key player in many other signaling cascades transducing the cellular effects of pituitary hormones LH and FSH, which stimulate ovarian function, and pancreatic hormone, insulin involved in glucose uptake metabolism, thus playing a role in PCOS, Obesity, and Adult-Onset Diabetes Mellitus (AODM). In 2023, Dr. Sabrina Rosaria Paparo reviewed the role of inositol in signal transduction, opening calcium channels, writing:

> numerous hormones, such as thyroid stimulating hormone (TSH), luteinizing hormone (LH), follicle-stimulating hormone (FSH), and insulin, transmit their function through the PI [phospho-inositol] signal pathway where the phospholipase C (PLC) hydrolyzes phosphatidylinositol-4,5-biphosphate (PIP2) in two-second messengers: IP3, and diacylglycerol (DAG), which in turn, open Ca2+ channels of the smooth endoplasmic reticulum and mitochondria membranes and induce protein kinase C (PKC), with subsequent cellular responses. (3)

Myo-inositol and Selenium Reduce Antibodies and TSH in Hashimoto's

In 2013, Maurizio Nordio conducted a 6-month randomized, controlled trial (RCT) on the combined use of myo-inositol (600 mg/day) and selenomethionine (83mcg/day) in 46 women with Hashimoto's thyroiditis with high thyroglobulin antibodies (TgAb). After six months of combined use, TPO and thyroglobulin antibodies were reduced by about 40% from around 900 to 500 mIU/mL. Surprisingly, the elevated TSH normalized in the group taking both supplements, not achieved with selenium alone. Only in the combined use group, TSH levels decreased by about 31 percent from 4.4 to 3.1 mIU/mL. Dr. Maurizio Nordio writes:

> We demonstrated that the beneficial effects obtained by selenomethionine treatment on patients affected by subclinical hypothyroidism, likely due to the presence of autoantibody (TPOAb and TgAb), are further improved by cotreatment with myo-inositol. Conclusions. Indeed, due to its action as TSH's second messenger, myo-inositol treatment reduces TSH levels closer to physiological concentrations. (1) (76-84)

Myo-Inositol and TSH Suppression is Beneficial in Hashimoto's

As seen above, the post-treatment TSH in Dr. Maurizio Nordio's study was 3.1 mIU/mL. Although this TSH is within the reference range for normal, this is not a suppressed TSH, defined as TSH below the reference range. Our treatment plan for Hashimoto's patients includes TSH suppression below the reference range with a suitable dosage of thyroid hormone medicine, preferably NDT (natural desiccated thyroid). The lower the TSH, the less stimulation of the thyroid gland to produce hydrogen peroxide, a damaging oxidizing agent. A suppressed TSH turns off hydrogen peroxide generation. This was discussed in Chapter 26 on Hashimoto's Thyroiditis with Normal TSH When to Treat? (17-19) (76-84)

Myo-inositol and Selenium for Subclinical Hypothyroidism (SCH)

In 2017, Dr Maurizio Nordio conducted a more extensive study of 85 Hashimoto's patients with subclinical hypothyroidism, with

TSH between 3 and 6 mIU/L. The 85 patients had elevated anti-thyroid antibodies and normal Free T3 and Free T4 hormone levels. Again, the combined use of selenium and myo-inositol restored normal TSH levels and increased Free T3 and Free T4 levels. The one hyperthyroid patient showed improvement in TSH, which increased into the normal range. Dr. Nordio writes:

> Patients were assigned to receive Myo-Ins-Se (myoinositol and selenium). TSH, TPOAb, and TgAb levels were significantly decreased in patients treated with combined Myo-Ins-Se after 6 months of treatment. In addition, a significant fT3 and fT4 increase, along with an amelioration of their quality of life, was observed...**Remarkably, TSH values of the hyperthyroid patient increased from 0.14 µU/ml up to 1.02 µU/ml, showing a complete restoration of TSH values at a normal range.** In conclusion, the administration of Myo-Ins-Se is significantly effective in decreasing TSH, TPOAb, and TgAb levels, as well as enhancing thyroid hormones and personal well-being, therefore restoring euthyroidism in patients diagnosed with autoimmune thyroiditis. (2)

Note: this is the first and only reference I have seen reporting the benefits of myo-inositol in Graves' disease. This beneficial effect may be due to myo-inositol ability to reduce pro-inflammatory Chemokines CXCL10 found in Graves' disease (GD) and Hashimoto's thyroiditis (HT). Chemokines stimulate the movement of immune cells to a particular location, perpetuating the autoimmune process. In 2019, Dr. Silvia Martina Ferrari writes:

> In GD, recruited Th1 lymphocytes are responsible for enhanced IFN-γ [interferon gamma] and TNF-α [tumor necrosis factor alpha] production, which in turn stimulates Th1 chemokines release from thyrocytes, initiating and perpetuating the autoimmune process. Circulating levels of these chemokines are associated with the active phase of GD. (20)

In 2018, Dr. Silvia Martina Ferrari studied surgically removed tissue obtained after thyroidectomy from three Hashimoto's patients and three benign goiter patients. This in-vitro thyrocyte study used cytokines to stimulate chemokine CXCL10 secretion in the presence or absence of H2O2. Dr. Silvia Martina Ferrari found myo-inositol, but not selenium, decreased the secretion of CXCL10 chemokines, providing a protective effect, writing:

> The secretion of CXCL10 chemokine induced by IFN-γ+tumor necrosis factor alpha (TNF)-α has been decreased by Myo+Ins [myo-inositol], both in the presence or absence of H2O2. (5)

In 2020 and 2021, Dr. Salvatore Benvenga showed that myo-inositol combined with selenium had protective effects on cadmium-induced thyroid toxicity in mice, reducing C cell hyperplasia and hypertrophy. Note: C cells produce calcitonin, and C cell hyperplasia is considered a precursor to medullary carcinoma of the thyroid. Serum calcitonin is a screening test for medullary thyroid cancer, while serum thyroglobulin is the gold standard cancer marker for recurrent thyroid cancer post thyroidectomy.(21-22) (85-86)

Myo-Inositol for Benign Thyroid Nodules

Thyroid nodules are quite common in the general population, prevalent in up to two-thirds of healthy patients screened with thyroid ultrasound. Typically, these are benign and of no clinical significance. In 2018, Dr. Nordio did a retrospective study of thyroid nodules detected by ultrasound in 34 of 642 patients with suspected hypothyroidism. Half were treated with myo-inositol 600 mg plus Selenium 83 mcg over six months. The other half served as controls. Final data in 34 patients showed a significant reduction in size for 76% of thyroid nodules in the treated group, compared to only 38% in the untreated group. The treated group had a significant decrease in nodule diameter from 16.7 mm to 12.4 mm. However, in the control group nodule size reduction was not significant, from only 19.5 mm to 17.5 mm. In the treated group, TSH levels dropped from 4.2 to 2.1 mIU/L after six months. However, in the control group, TSH levels significantly increased from 3.95 to 4.30 mIU/L after six months. (7)

Management of Thyroid Nodules with Suppression of TSH

Results such as Dr. Nordio's 2018 study above can be improved by adding TSH suppression with thyroid hormone medication, as is commonly done by mainstream endocrinology using levothyroxine. In 2003, Dr. Mary Jo Welker writes in American Family Physician, TSH suppression for the thyroid nodule patient is controversial, yet remains optional:

> The use of TSH suppressive therapy with thyroxine to manage benign, solitary thyroid nodules remains controversial. The lack of universal efficacy makes such therapy optional in most patients. Some randomized, controlled studies suggest that short-term thyroxine therapy is not superior to placebo in patients with a solitary hypofunctioning colloid nodule. The efficacy of thyroxine is less certain for solitary nodules than for a diffuse or multinodular goiter. However, some patients may benefit, and suppressive therapy is considered an appropriate alternative if the patient is followed carefully at six-month intervals. (23-26)

The prudent physician will follow Dr. Mary Jo Welker's advice to carefully follow nodules with serial ultrasound for any increase in size, which raises suspicion of malignancy. Enlarging nodules are referred for biopsy or surgery. Referral for surgical removal is usually justified for large nodules that protrude from or cause bulging in the neck. In my experience over 20 years following thyroid nodules with serial ultrasound in patients under medical treatment, not a single one has required rebiopsy or surgical intervention. For further discussion of thyroid nodule management, see Chapter 33 on the Thyroid Nodule Epidemic.

Inhibition of Secretion of Chemokines

One might object to an intervention such as myo-inositol, which makes TSH signaling more effective and increases hydrogen peroxide generation in the thyroid. Yet paradoxically, such an intervention with myo-inositol protects thyrocytes by reducing chemokines. In 2019 and 2023, Dr. Daniele Barbaro suggested myo-inositol was useful in the treatment of autoimmune thyroiditis, prevention of thyroid tumors, and treatment of iodine deficiency, writing:

> As myo-inositol plays a crucial role in the regulation of iodine organification, supplementation may promote faster recovery from ID [iodine deficiency]. Indeed, H2O2 generated under the stimulus of myo-inositol is available for iodine incorporation inside the thyroid. Such activity makes myo-inositol very appealing as a novel molecule to increase iodine availability....myo-inositol, when administered with selenium in patients affected by autoimmune thyroiditis, contributes to restoring the euthyroid status, reducing the titer of the autoantibodies and preventing the progression of SCH [subclinical hypothyroidism] to overt hypothyroidism. This positive activity of myo-inositol is further demonstrated in cases of hypothyroidism during pregnancy. Moreover, preliminary evidence on the role of myo-inositol on thyroid cancer has also been investigated, and the data on thyroid nodules appear promising. Also, animal studies suggest a protective effect of myo-inositol against proliferation of cancer cells and indirectly by inhibition of secretion of chemokines... (27-28)

PCOS-Polycystic Ovary Syndrome

PCOS affects 6-18 percent of adolescent girls. The two main features of PCOS are:

1) Irregular, anovulatory menstrual cycles.

2) Hyperandrogenism (high testosterone and DHEA) causing Hirsutism and Acne.

In the thyroid gland, myo-inositol acts as a second messenger to TSH, a pituitary hormone.

Similarly, in the ovary, myo-inositol acts as a second messenger to FSH (follicle-stimulating hormone) and LH (luteinizing hormone), pituitary hormones which stimulate ovulation and estrogen production. Myo-inositol is very effective in PCOS (polycystic ovary syndrome), improving insulin sensitivity, reducing acne and hirsutism, and restoring ovulation, regular cycling, and fertility. (29-45)

In 2013, Dr. Paolo Giovanni Artini did a randomized study in 50 overweight PCOS patients using myo-inositol 2 grams/day plus folic acid 200 mg/ day. After 12 weeks, the LH (Luteinizing Hormone), Prolactin, and Insulin levels were reduced. Insulin sensitivity improved, and normal menstrual cycles were restored in all subjects. (31)

Alpha Lactalbumin Added to Myo-Inositol

Myo-inositol has been effective in restoring ovulation in women with PCOS. However, some women are resistant. In 2018, Dr. Mario Montanino Oliva used myoinositol to treat 37 anovulatory women with PCOS. Two-thirds of the women ovulated with myo-inositol treatment, while one-third were resistant and did not ovulate. However, by adding 50 milligrams of α-LA (alpha lactalbumin) to 2 g of myo-inositol twice a day, ovulation was restored in 86 percent of inositol-resistant women. (29)

Myo-inositol combined with D-chiro-inositol in a 40:1 ratio improved efficacy for restoring ovulation in PCOS patients. (40)

Panic Disorder, Depression, OCD

Myo-inositol is also effective for panic disorder. A small study published in 2001 showed it was more effective than SSRI antidepressants. Large doses, up to 16 grams per day, were used. It may also be effective for depression and OCD (obsessive-compulsive disorder), acting as a second messenger for dopamine, serotonin, or norepinephrine receptors in the brain. (41-54)

In 2002, Dr. Brian Harvey writes:

Despite a mode of action that remains elusive, MI [myo-inositol] has demonstrated therapeutic efficacy in obsessive-compulsive disorder (OCD), putative OCD-spectrum disorders, as well as panic and depression. (52)

In 2023, Dr. Carmen Concerto writes:

The interest in inositol as a possible antidepressant molecule began in 1978 when Barkai and colleagues showed a reduced concentration of inositol in the CSF of patients with mood disorders. Afterward, several studies measured levels of myo-inositol in different brain areas of patients with major depressive disorder (MDD) and bipolar disorder (BD), highlighting how low levels of inositol were associated with depressive symptoms, while high levels with (hypo) manic symptoms...It has been suggested that the therapeutic activity of inositol may be related to the modulation of serotonin and/or norepinephrine receptors and to an effect on the signal transduction pathway. Indeed, from the data available in the literature, inositol acts as a precursor of the inositol phosphate-phosphoinositide (IPP) cycle...The IPP cycle and its derived second messengers are involved in several receptor systems, including noradrenergic (α-1), serotonergic (5-HT2A and 5-HT2C), cholinergic (muscarinic), and dopaminergic (D1) receptors [96,97]...Overall, encouraging results seem to emerge for inositol in panic disorders, likely through its peculiar second messenger characteristics, which are different from the transmitter-receptor mechanism of SSRIs used for this disorder... findings have been demonstrated in animal models...to date, literature evidence on the efficacy of inositol in the treatment of psychiatric disorders is still controversial... partly due to the heterogeneity of supporting studies. ... systematic use of inositol in routine clinical practice cannot be recommended yet... (54)

Myo-Inositol for Type Two Diabetes and Obesity

Myo-inositol is a second messenger for insulin and has an insulin-sensitizing effect similar to metformin. Several studies have shown beneficial effects in Adult-Onset Diabetes Miletus (AODM, Type 2) with improvement in insulin sensitivity, with reduction in blood glucose and HgbA1C. Myo-inositol was found useful in the prevention of gestational diabetes. (55-63)

Myo-Inositol Broad Spectrum Anti-Cancer Effects

In 2016, Dr. Mariano Bizzarri reviewed inositol and inositol hexaphosphate (InsP6) as broad-spectrum anti-cancer agents, writing:

> Further investigation demonstrated that InsP6 [inositol-6-phophate] had unequivocal apoptotic effects on both solid and hematogenous tumors. Indeed, InsP6 has been shown to trigger programmed cell death both *in vitro* and *in vivo* in numerous cancer cell lines, including Kaposi's sarcoma and prostate, breast, cervical, pancreas, melanoma, and colon cancer. This apoptotic effect is frequently associated with growth inhibition...[Note: apoptosis is programmed cell death]. (64-69)

In Conclusion: In 2022, Dr. Paparo writes,

> Myo [myo-inositol] homeostasis impairment could potentially affect several physiological cellular mechanisms that may translate to a broad range of disorders, ranging from thyroid diseases, fertility impairment, polycystic ovary syndrome (PCOS), neurological diseases, and diabetes. (3)

Myo-inositol is an effective tool in treating Hashimoto's thyroiditis, normalizing TSH and anti-thyroid antibody levels. Efficacy is improved when combined with selenium, vitamin D3 and alpha-lactalbumin. By virtue as a signaling molecule in various cascades, myo-inositol plays a role in multiple areas of human health. (70-75)

◆ References for Chapter 28

1) Nordio, Maurizio, and Raffaella Pajalich. "Combined Treatment with Myo-Inositol and Selenium Ensures Euthyroidism in Subclinical Hypothyroidism Patients with Autoimmune Thyroiditis." Journal of Thyroid Research 2013 (2013).

2) Nordio, Maurizio, and Sabrina Basciani. "Treatment with Myo-Inositol and Selenium Ensures Euthyroidism in Patients with Autoimmune Thyroiditis." International Journal of Endocrinology 2017 (2017).

3) Paparo, Sabrina Rosaria, et al. "Myoinositol in Autoimmune Thyroiditis." Frontiers in Endocrinology 13 (2022).

4) Fallahi, Poupak, et al. "Myo-inositol in Autoimmune Thyroiditis, and Hypothyroidism." Reviews in Endocrine and Metabolic Disorders 19.4 (2018): 349-354.

5) Ferrari, Silvia Martina, et al. "The Protective Effect of Myoinositol on Human Thyrocytes." Reviews in Endocrine and Metabolic Disorders 19.4 (2018): 355-362.

6) Porcaro, G., and P. Angelozzi. "Myo-inositol and Selenium Prevent Subclinical Hypothyroidism During Pregnancy: An Observational Study." IJMDAT 1.2 (2018): e164.

7) Nordio, M., and S. Basciani. "Evaluation of Thyroid Nodule Characteristics in Subclinical Hypothyroid Patients Under a Myo-Inositol Plus Selenium Treatment." Eur Rev Med Pharmacol Sci 22.7 (2018): 2153-9.

8) Pace, Cinzia, et al. "Role of Selenium and Myo-Inositol Supplementation on Autoimmune Thyroiditis Progression." Endocrine Journal (2020): EJ20-0062.

9) Benvenga, Salvatore, et al. "The Role of Inositol in Thyroid Physiology and in Subclinical Hypothyroidism Management." Frontiers in Endocrinology (2021): 458.

10) Pankiv, Ivan, et al. "Efficacy of a Combined Administration of Myoinositol and Vitamin D In Patients with Autoimmune Thyroiditis." Endocrine Abstracts. Vol. 73. Bioscientifica, 2021.

11) Krysiak, Robert, et al. "The Impact of Vitamin D on Thyroid Autoimmunity and Hypothalamic–Pituitary–Thyroid Axis Activity in Myo-Inositol-Treated and Myo-Inositol-Naïve Women with Autoimmune Thyroiditis: A Pilot Study." Journal of Clinical Pharmacy and Therapeutics (2022).

12) Pasyechko, Nadiya, and Veronika Kulchinska. "Myo-Inositol Supplementation in Autoimmune Thyroiditis and Subclinical Hypothyroidism on the Background of Vitamin D Deficiency." Endocrine Abstracts. Vol. 81. Bioscientifica, 2022.

13) Lenti, Marco Vincenzo, et al. "Seronegative Autoimmune Diseases: A Challenging Diagnosis." Autoimmunity Reviews (2022): 103143.

14) Croce, L., et al. "Compared with Classic Hashimoto's Thyroiditis, Chronic Autoimmune Serum-Negative Thyroiditis Requires a Lower Substitution Dose Of L-Thyroxine to Correct Hypothyroidism." Journal of Endocrinological Investigation 43 (2020): 1631-1636.

15) Jeong, Sun Hye, et al. "The Association Between Thyroid Echogenicity and Thyroid Function in Pediatric and Adolescent Hashimoto's Thyroiditis." Medicine 98.14 (2019).

16) Raber, Wolfgang, et al. "Thyroid Ultrasound Versus Anti-Thyroid Peroxidase Antibody Determination: A Cohort Study of Four Hundred Fifty-One Subjects." Thyroid 12.8 (2002): 725-731.

17) Björkman, U., and R. Ekholm. "Hydrogen Peroxide Generation and its Regulation in FRTL-5 and Porcine Thyroid Cells." Endocrinology 130.1 (1992): 393-399.

18) Ohye, Hidemi, and Masahiro Sugawara. "Dual Oxidase, Hydrogen Peroxide and Thyroid Diseases." Experimental Biology and Medicine 235.4 (2010): 424-433.

19) Song, Yue, et al. "Roles of Hydrogen Peroxide in Thyroid Physiology and Disease." The Journal of Clinical Endocrinology & Metabolism 92.10 (2007): 3764-3773.

20) Ferrari, Silvia Martina, et al. "Chemokines in Hyperthyroidism." Journal Of Clinical & Translational Endocrinology 16 (2019): 100196.

21) Benvenga, Salvatore, et al. "Protective Effects of Myo-Inositol and Selenium on Cadmium-Induced Thyroid Toxicity in Mice." Nutrients 12.5 (2020): 1222.

22) Benvenga, Salvatore, et al. "The Association of Myo-Inositol and Selenium Contrasts Cadmium-Induced Thyroid C Cell Hyperplasia and Hypertrophy in Mice." Frontiers in Endocrinology 12 (2021): 608697.

23) Welker, Mary Jo, and Diane Orlov. "Thyroid Nodules." American Family Physician 67.3 (2003): 559-566.

24) Clark, Orlo H. "TSH Suppression in the Management of Thyroid Nodules and Thyroid Cancer." World Journal of Surgery 5.1 (1981): 39-46.

25) Wémeau, Jean-Louis, et al. "Effects of Thyroid-Stimulating Hormone Suppression with Levothyroxine in Reducing the Volume of Solitary Thyroid Nodules and Improving Extraocular Nonpalpable Changes: A Randomized, Double-Blind, Placebo-Controlled Trial by the French Thyroid Research Group." The Journal of Clinical Endocrinology & Metabolism 87.11 (2002): 4928-4934.

26) Castro, M. Regina, Pedro J. Caraballo, and John C. Morris. "Effectiveness of Thyroid Hormone Suppressive Therapy in Benign Solitary Thyroid Nodules: A Meta-Analysis." The Journal of Clinical Endocrinology & Metabolism 87.9 (2002): 4154-4159.

27) Barbaro, Daniele, et al. "Iodine and Myo-inositol: a Novel Promising Combination for Iodine Deficiency." Frontiers in Endocrinology 10 (2019): 457.

28) Barbaro, Daniele, et al. "Myo-Inositol for Subclinical Hypothyroidism and Potential Prevention of Thyroid Tumors." A Clinical Guide to Inositols. Academic Press, 2023. 213-231.

29) Montanino Oliva, Mario, et al. "Effects of Myo-Inositol Plus Alpha-Lactalbumin in Myo-Inositol-Resistant PCOS Women." Journal of Ovarian Research 11.1 (2018): 1-7.

30) Mendoza, Nicolas, et al. "Comparison of the Effect of Two Combinations of Myo-Inositol and D-Chiro-Inositol in Women with Polycystic Ovary Syndrome Undergoing ICSI: A Randomized Controlled Trial." Gynecological Endocrinology (2019).

31) Artini, Paolo Giovanni, et al. "Endocrine and Clinical Effects of Myo-Inositol Administration in Polycystic Ovary Syndrome. A Randomized Study." Gynecological Endocrinology 29.4 (2013): 375-379.

32) Unfer, V., et al. "Effects of Myo-Inositol in Women with PCOS: A Systematic Review of Randomized Controlled Trials." Gynecological Endocrinology 28.7 (2012): 509-515.

33) Genazzani, Alessandro D., et al. "Differential Insulin Response to Myo-Inositol Administration in Obese Polycystic Ovary Syndrome Patients." Gynecological Endocrinology 28.12 (2012): 969-973.

34) Zacchè, Martino M., et al. "Efficacy of Myo-Inositol in the Treatment of Cutaneous Disorders in Young Women with Polycystic Ovary Syndrome." Gynecological Endocrinology 25.8 (2009): 508-513.

35) Roxas, Mario. "Myo-inositol in Patients with Polycystic Ovary Syndrome: A Novel Method for Ovulation Induction." Alternative Medicine Review 12.4 (2007): 381-382.

36) Bizzarri, Mariano, et al. "An Innovative Approach to Polycystic Ovary Syndrome: Vittorio Unfer and His Pioneering Research on Inositols." Journal of Obstetrics and Gynaecology 42.4 (2022): 546-556.

37) Unfer, Vittorio. "D-Chiro-Inositol In PCOS: The Myths and What We Know About the Reality." International Journal of Food Sciences and Nutrition 73.7 (2022): 989-991.

38) Facchinetti, Fabio, et al. "Experts' Opinion on Inositols in Treating Polycystic Ovary Syndrome and Non-Insulin-Dependent Diabetes Mellitus: A Further Help for Human Reproduction and Beyond." Expert Opinion on Drug Metabolism & Toxicology 16.3 (2020): 255-274.

39) Merviel, Philippe, et al. "Impact of Myo-Inositol Treatment in Women with Polycystic Ovary Syndrome in Assisted Reproductive Technologies." Reproductive Health 18.1 (2021): 1-8.

40) Nordio, M., et al. "The 40: 1 Myo-Inositol/D-Chiro-Inositol Plasma Ratio Is Able to Restore Ovulation in PCOS Patients: Comparison with Other Ratios." Eur Rev Med Pharmacol Sci 23.12 (2019): 5512-5521.

41) Greff, Dorina, et al. "Inositol Is an Effective and Safe Treatment in Polycystic Ovary Syndrome: A Systematic Review and Meta-Analysis of Randomized Controlled Trials." Reproductive Biology and Endocrinology 21.1 (2023): 10.

42) Bevilacqua, Arturo, et al. "Treating PCOS With Inositols: Choosing the Most Appropriate Myo-To D-Chiro-Inositol Ratio." A Clinical Guide to Inositols. Academic Press, 2023. 53-64

43) Haghollahi, Fedyeh, et al. "Polycystic Ovary Syndrome in Adolescence: From the Cradle to the Grave." Fertility, Gynecology and Andrology 2.1 (2022).

44) Kamenov, Zdravko, and Mario Montanino Oliva. "Overcoming Inositol Resistance." A Clinical Guide to Inositols. Academic Press, 2023. 65-72.

45) Pkhaladze, Lali, et al. "Use of Myo-Inositol in The Treatment of PCOS Symptoms in Adolescents." A Clinical Guide to Inositols. Academic Press, 2023. 151-165.

46) Chhetri, Dhani Raj. "Myo-inositol and Its Derivatives: Their Emerging Role in the Treatment of Human Diseases." Frontiers in Pharmacology 10 (2019): 1172.

47) Palatnik, Alex, et al. "Double-blind, Controlled, Crossover Trial of Inositol Versus Fluvoxamine for the Treatment of Panic Disorder." Journal of Clinical Psychopharmacology 21.3 (2001): 335-339.

48) Benjamin, Jonathan, et al. "Double-Blind, Placebo-Controlled, Crossover Trial of Inositol Treatment for Panic Disorder." American Journal of Psychiatry 152.7 (1995): 1084-1086.

49) Fux, Mendel, et al. "Inositol Treatment of Obsessive-Compulsive Disorder." American Journal of Psychiatry 153.9 (1996): 1219-1221.

50) Levine, Joseph. "Controlled Trials of Inositol in Psychiatry." European neuropsychopharmacology 7.2 (1997): 147-155.

51) Levine, Joseph, et al. "Double-Blind, Controlled Trial of Inositol Treatment of Depression." American Journal of Psychiatry 152.5 (1995): 792-793.

52) Harvey, Brian H., et al. "Defining the Neuromuscular Action of Myoinositol: Application to Obsessive-Compulsive Disorder." Progress In Neuro-Psychopharmacology & Biological Psychiatry 26.1 (2002): 21-32.

53) Chiappelli, Joshua, et al. "Evaluation of Myo-Inositol as a Potential Biomarker for Depression in Schizophrenia." Neuropsychopharmacology 40.9 (2015): 2157-2164.

54) Concerto, Carmen, et al. "Neurobiology and Applications of Inositol in Psychiatry: A Narrative Review." Current Issues in Molecular Biology 45.2 (2023): 1762-1778.

55) D'Anna, R., et al. "Myo-Inositol May Prevent Gestational Diabetes in PCOS Women." Gynecological endocrinology 28.6 (2012): 440-442.

56) Motuhifonua, Soana K., et al. "Antenatal Dietary Supplementation with Myo-Inositol for Preventing Gestational Diabetes." Cochrane Database of Systematic Reviews 2 (2023).

57) Facchinetti, Fabio, et al. "Inositol Supplementation for Preventing Gestational Diabetes Mellitus." A Clinical Guide to Inositols. Academic Press, 2023. 123-150.

58) Pintaudi, Basilio, et al. "The Effectiveness of Myoinositol and D-Chiro Inositol Treatment in Type 2 Diabetes." International Journal of Endocrinology 2016 (2016).

59) Omoruyi, Felix O., et al. "New Frontiers for the Use of IP6 and Inositol Combination in Treating Diabetes Mellitus: A Review." Molecules 25.7 (2020): 1720.

60) Mashayekh-Amiri, Sepideh, et al. "Myo-Inositol Supplementation for Prevention of Gestational Diabetes Mellitus in Overweight and Obese Pregnant Women: A Systematic Review and Meta-Analysis." Diabetology & Metabolic Syndrome 14.1 (2022): 1-15.

61) Genazzani, Alessandro D., et al. "Modulatory Role of D-Chiro-Inositol (DCI) on LH and Insulin Secretion in Obese PCOS Patients." Gynecological Endocrinology 30.6 (2014): 438-443.

62) Chatree, Saimai, et al. "Role of Inositols and Inositol Phosphates in Energy Metabolism." Molecules 25.21 (2020): 5079.

63) Cabrera-Cruz, Heidy, et al. "The Insulin-Sensitizing Mechanism of Myo-Inositol Is Associated with AMPK Activation and GLUT-4 Expression in Human Endometrial Cells Exposed to a PCOS Environment." American Journal of Physiology-Endocrinology and Metabolism 318.2 (2020): E237-E248.

64) Bizzarri, Mariano, et al. "Broad Spectrum Anti-Cancer Activity of Myo-Inositol and Inositol Hexakisphosphate." International Journal of Endocrinology 2016 (2016).

65) Vucenik, Ivana, et al. "Inositol Hexaphosphate (IP6) and Colon Cancer: From Concepts and First Experiments to Clinical Application." Molecules 25.24 (2020): 5931.

66) Chen, Qian, Liangfang Shen, and Shan Li. "Emerging Role of Inositol Monophosphatase in Cancer." Biomedicine & Pharmacotherapy 161 (2023): 114442.

67) Vucenik, Ivana. "Anti-Cancer Properties of Inositol Hexaphosphate and Inositol: An Overview." Journal Of Nutritional Science and Vitaminology 65. Supplement (2019): S18-S22.

68) Vucenik, Ivana, and AbulKalam M. Shamsuddin. "Cancer Inhibition by Inositol Hexaphosphate (IP6) and Inositol: From Laboratory to Clinic." The Journal of Nutrition 133.11 (2003): 3778S-3784S.

69) Yuan, Guixin, et al. "Phosphatidyl Inositol 3-Kinase (PI3K)-mTOR Inhibitor PKI-402 Inhibits Breast Cancer-Induced Osteolysis." Cancer Letters 443 (2019): 135-144.

70) Gambioli, R., et al. "The Use of D-Chiro-Inositol in Clinical Practice." Eur. Rev. Med. Pharmacol. Sci 25.1 (2021): 438-446.

71) Tutunchi, Helda, et al. "Clinical Effectiveness of alpha-Lipoic Acid, Myo-Inositol and Propolis Supplementation on Metabolic Profiles and Liver Function in Obese Patients with NAFLD: A Randomized Controlled Clinical Trial." Clinical Nutrition ESPEN (2023).

72) Arefhosseini, Sara, et al. "Myo-inositol Supplementation Improves Cardiometabolic Factors, Anthropometric Measures, and Liver Function in Obese Patients with Non-Alcoholic Fatty Liver Disease." Frontiers in Nutrition 10 (2023).

73) Diamanti-Kandarakis, Evanthia, et al. "Effectiveness of Myo-and D-Chiro-Inositol in the Treatment of Metabolic Disorders." A Clinical Guide to Inositols. Academic Press, 2023. 31-51.

74) Cantelmi, Tonino, and Cherubino Di Lorenzo. "Myo-inositol Could Restore Peripheral Inositol Depletion Induced by Treatments for Psychiatric and Neurological Conditions." A Clinical Guide to Inositols. Academic Press, 2023. 73-85.

75) Korkmaz, Serol, et al. "The Potential Antiviral Activity of Inositol (Vitamin B8) as a Dietary Supplement in Human and Animal Nutrition." Journal of Health Sciences and Management 2.3 (2022): 68-72.

76) Fallahi, Poupak, et al. "Myo-inositol in Autoimmune Thyroiditis, and Hypothyroidism." Reviews in Endocrine and Metabolic Disorders 19.4 (2018): 349-354.

77) Pace, Cinzia, et al. "Role of Selenium and Myo-Inositol Supplementation on Autoimmune Thyroiditis Progression." Endocrine Journal 67.11 (2020): 1093-1098.

78) Pankiv, Ivan, et al. "Efficacy of a Combined Administration of Myoinositol and Vitamin D In Patients with Autoimmune Thyroiditis." Endocrine Abstracts. Vol. 73. Bioscientifica, 2021.

79) Ferrari, Silvia Martina, et al. "Precision Medicine in Autoimmune Thyroiditis and Hypothyroidism." Frontiers in Pharmacology (2021): 3123.

80) Martina, Ferrari Silvia, et al. "Autoimmune Thyroiditis and Hypothyroidism: A Personalized Medical Approach." Endocrine Abstracts. Vol. 81. Bioscientifica, 2022.

81) Krysiak, Robert, et al. "The Impact of Vitamin D on Thyroid Autoimmunity and Hypothalamic–Pituitary–Thyroid Axis Activity in Myo-Inositol-Treated and Myo-Inositol-Naïve Women with Autoimmune Thyroiditis: A Pilot Study." Journal of Clinical Pharmacy and Therapeutics 47.11 (2022): 1759-1767.

82) Payer, Juraj, et al. "Supplementation with Myo-Inositol and Selenium Improves the Clinical Conditions and Biochemical Features of Women with or at Risk for Subclinical Hypothyroidism." Frontiers in Endocrinology 13 (2022).

83) Barbaro, Daniele, et al. "Myo-Inositol for Subclinical Hypothyroidism and Potential Prevention of Thyroid Tumors." A Clinical Guide to Inositols. Academic Press, 2023. 213-231.

84) Barbaro, Daniele, et al. "Iodine and Myo-Inositol: A Novel Promising Combination for Iodine Deficiency." Frontiers in Endocrinology 10 (2019): 457.

85) Garo, Maria Luisa, et al. "Evolution of Thyroid Cancer Biomarkers: From Laboratory Test to Patients' Clinical Management." Clinical Chemistry and Laboratory Medicine (CCLM) 61.5 (2023): 935-945.

86) Giannetta, Elisa, et al. "Endocrine Tumours: Calcitonin in Thyroid and Extra-Thyroid Neuroendocrine Neoplasms: The Two-Faced Janus." European Journal of Endocrinology 183.6 (2020): R197-R215.

Chapter 29

Bromine Detoxification with Unrefined Sea Salt

CREDIT AND THANKS GO TO Dr. David Brownstein, who, over the years, has served as my mentor on the topics of iodine and thyroid. One of the things I learned from Dr. Brownstein is the use of unrefined sea salt for bromine detoxification prior to and during high-dose iodine supplementation with Iodoral or Lugol's Solution. Iodoral is a commercially available iodine supplement. Each 12.5 mg tablet contains 7.5 mg of potassium iodide and 5 mg of molecular iodine, in the same ratio as Lugol's. In other words, Iodoral is Lugol's Solution in tablet form. The patient typically starts the unrefined sea salt, half teaspoon twice a day, magnesium, and vitamin C for at least a week, then starts the Iodoral at 12.5 mg daily. (Personal communication) This is important to avoid the annoying symptoms of bromide excretion called "Bromism," which may be severe enough to cause the patient to stop taking Iodoral. (1-15)

Dermo Bromism Treatment with NaCl (Salt)

Bromine is an oily liquid and insoluble in water. Excretion is primarily through the oil glands in the skin. Since bromine is irritating, this may cause hair loss and acne. Table salt is the usual and customary treatment for bromine toxicity, also called "Bromism." Salt consists of sodium (Na+) and chloride (Cl-) ions. The chlorine atom is a halogen same as bromine, with the same number of electrons in the outer shell. The bromide ion exchanges for the chloride ion, forming sodium bromide, now soluble in water and excreted by the kidney into the urine. In 1925, Dr. Burgess discussed the treatment of dermobromism with salt, writing:

> The injection of sodium chloride intravenously, apparently results in a displacement of the stored-up bromides and their consequent elimination by the kidneys, and from the results reported, although there are only a small number of cases, its use in cases of bromoderma would appear to be a useful advance in the therapy of this condition. (5)

Here is a typical nutritional supplement protocol:

- Unrefined Celtic Sea Salt (Celtic) – Half teaspoon of salt in water twice a day
- Selenium: 200 – 400 mcg per day
- Magnesium: 400 – 1200 mg per day
- Vitamin C: 3,000 – 10,000 mg per day
- Vitamins B2: 100 mg riboflavin per day
- Vitamin B3: 500 mg inositol hexanicotinate once or twice a day

Note: the use of inositol is discussed in the previous Chapter 28 on Myo-Inositol for Hashimoto's.

Below are the symptoms which can be avoided with the Bromine Detox Protocol with Celtic Sea Salt:

Symptoms of Bromism and During Bromide Detoxification

Bromine is an oily liquid that is secreted by the oil glands at the base of the hair follicles. This irritates the oil glands which may then clog causing acne and hair loss. Bromoderma may manifest as an acneiform rash on the face and hands and hair loss. In 2016, Dr. Fumiko Oda described the usual presentation of bromoderma:

> Bromoderma occurs frequently on the face and limbs, which are rich with hair follicles and sebaceous glands, but it is not observed

on the palmoplantar regions. Therefore, it is possible that bromide ions are eliminated through hair follicles and sebaceous glands and that they cause neutrophil accumulation. (16)

In 2020, Dr Ahmad Nofal describes the usual presentation of bromoderma:

Clinically, patients with bromoderma usually present with acneiform pustular eruption, and vegetating nodules and plaques with or without exudation. However, panniculitis-like lesions, necrotic ulcers, hemorrhagic blisters, tuberous lesions, and pyoderma gangrenosum-like lesions have also been described. Face and upper body are the most commonly involved sites; however, involvement of the limbs, mucous membranes, and a generalized distribution have been also described in some patients as was the case in our patient. The skin lesions may be also associated with systemic symptoms of bromide toxicity (bromism) such as muscle weakness, fatigue, convulsions, ataxia, hallucinations, and personality changes. (17)

Note: although the most common symptoms of encountered in patients with dermobromism from starting high dose iodine are acne and hair loss, as mentioned above, many other mysterious atypical symptoms may be encountered, such as itchy skin rashes and a long list of bizarre symptoms. The physician must maintain a high index of suspicion, and advise a "holiday" from the iodine supplement, which in itself, is diagnostic of dermobromism when the symptoms promptly resolve.

Bromine in the Environment and Food

The environment has considerable bromine, which ends up in our food. When consumed, bromine accumulates in our tissues. You can find bromine in flame-retardants (used in electronics, furniture, mattresses, automobiles), brominated vegetable oils in food and soft drinks, bromine-containing over-the-counter medications, etc. In September 1970, BVO,

Brominated Vegetable Oil, was banned in the United Kingdom. BVO has also been banned in Japan, Europe, and India. Here in the U.S., we still have BVO in various soft drinks, Mountain Dew, Squirt, Fanta Orange, Sunkist Pineapple, Gatorade Thirst Quencher Orange, Powerade Strawberry Lemonade or Fresca Original Citrus, etc. These all contain bromine. (18-37)

Bromine Containing Medications

Bromine was the first medication useful in epilepsy, and over the years, many bromine-containing sedatives and anti-convulsant drugs have been marketed for human and veterinary use. These include potassium bromide, cold complex syrups, dextromethorphan, Robitussin HBr, Cordial De Monell for Baby Colic, Bromo-Seltzer, Dr. Miles' Nervine, pyridostigmine bromide, and many others. (38-43)

When Starting Iodoral, Bromine is Released

The adverse effects of taking iodine tablets are not due to the iodine, instead, they are caused by the release of bromine from the body, producing symptoms of bromism. Bromine is problematic since it is a toxic red liquid substance. We have been ingesting various forms of bromine our entire lives without realizing it. This excess bromine accumulates in the nooks and crannies of the body and is released when we start iodine supplements. This is more pronounced for the iodine-deficient patient, with a low spot urinary iodine test.

One way to avoid these symptoms is to start the Iodoral with a low dose, such as half a tablet (6.25 mg) every other day, to allow the body time to release the bromine. An added measure is unrefined sea salt, half a teaspoon in water once or twice a day, providing chloride ions for the renal excretion of bromine. Otherwise, the bromine is excreted by the skin and accumulates in the oil glands at the base of the hair follicles. This leads to the dermobromism symptoms of acne and hair loss. We have seen this in a few patients not taking sea salt who report dermobromism symptoms after starting

Iodoral. Once starting the sea salt, symptoms promptly resolve.

Conclusion

Bromine, a toxic halide, competes with iodine in the body and may cause symptoms of dermobromism. Common, everyday table salt containing sodium chloride is prevention and treatment. Ignoring bromine and bromine detoxification is another error of modern endocrinology. (42-43)

♦ References for Chapter 29

1) Brownstein, David. "Clinical Experience with Inorganic, Non-Radioactive Iodine/Iodide." The Original Internist 12.3 (2005): 105-108.

2) Buist, Stephanie, "The Guide to Supplementing with Iodine, What You Need to Know to Get Started," Dec. 2011.

3) Abraham, Guy E. "The Safe and Effective Implementation of Orthoiodosupplementation in Medical Practice." The Original Internist 11.1 (2004): 17-36.

4) Thornton, Christina S., and Jolene T. Haws. "Bromism in the Modern Day: Case Report and Canadian Review of Bromide Intoxication." Journal of General Internal Medicine 35.8 (2020): 2459-2461.

5) Burgess, J. F. "Some Recent Researches on Iodide and Bromide Eruptions." Canadian Medical Association Journal 15.2 (1925): 178.

6) Lugassy, Daniel M., and Lewis S. Nelson. "Case Files of the Medical Toxicology Fellowship at the New York City Poison Control: Bromism: Forgotten, But Not Gone." Journal of Medical Toxicology 5.3 (2009): 151-157.

7) Bechet, Paul E. "The Intravenous Administration of Sodium Chloride in Bromoderma" Journal of the American Medical Association 87.5 (1926): 320-321.

8) Nichol, R. W. "Bromism: The Sodium Chloride Treatment." British Medical Journal 1.3405 (1926): 636.

9) Fantinati, Marco, et al. "Bromide Toxicosis (Bromism) Secondary to a Decreased Chloride Intake After Dietary Transition in a Dog with Idiopathic Epilepsy: A Case Report." BMC Veterinary Research 17.1 (2021): 1-7.

10) Rossmeisl, John H., and Karen D. Inzana. "Clinical Signs, Risk Factors, and Outcomes Associated with Bromide Toxicosis (Bromism) in Dogs with Idiopathic Epilepsy." Journal of the American Veterinary Medical Association 234.11 (2009): 1425-1431.

11) Fukunaga, Koya, et al. "Effects of Three Infusion Fluids with Different Sodium Chloride Contents on Steady-State Serum Concentrations of Bromide in Dogs." Journal of Veterinary Pharmacology and Therapeutics 41.5 (2018): 684-690.

12) Trepanier, L. A., and J. G. Babish. "Effect of Dietary Chloride Content on the Elimination of Bromide by Dogs." Research In Veterinary Science 58.3 (1995): 252-255.

13) James, Laura P., et al. "Bromism: Intoxication from a Rare Anticonvulsant Therapy." Pediatric emergency care 13.4 (1997): 268-270.

14) Taylor, Brent R., et al. "Bromide Toxicity from Consumption of Dead Sea Salt." The American Journal of Medicine 123.3 (2010): e11-e12.

15) Sclare, A. Balfour. "Bromism." Scottish Medical Journal 7.3 (1962): 141-143.

16) Oda, Fumiko, et al. "Bromoderma Mimicking Pyoderma Gangrenosum Caused by Commercial Sedatives." The Journal of dermatology 43.5 (2016): 564-566.

17) Nofal, Ahmad, et al. "Disseminated Vegetating Infantile Bromoderma: A Dramatic Response to Systemic Steroids." Dermatologic Therapy 33.6 (2020): e14298

18) Rahimulddin, Sawsan Abdulaziz. "Perspective Review: Bromide, Ways of Exposure and Environmental Effects." Journal of King Abdulaziz University 30.2 (2018): 35-45.

19) Jin, Rong, et al. "Chlorinated and Brominated Polycyclic Aromatic Hydrocarbons: Sources, Formation Mechanisms, And Occurrence in the Environment." Progress in Energy and Combustion Science 76 (2020): 100803.

20) Feiteiro, Joana, et al. "Health Toxicity Effects of Brominated Flame Retardants: From Environmental to Human Exposure." Environmental Pollution 285 (2021): 117475.

21) Zuiderveen, Emma AR, et al. "Novel Brominated Flame Retardants-A Review of Their Occurrence in Indoor Air, Dust, Consumer Goods, and Food." Chemosphere 255 (2020): 126816.

22) Shi, Zhixiong, et al. "Legacy and Emerging Brominated Flame Retardants in China: A Review on Food and Human Milk Contamination, Human Dietary Exposure and Risk Assessment." Chemosphere 198 (2018): 522-536.

23) Pratt, Iona, et al. "Brominated and Fluorinated Organic Pollutants in the Breast Milk of First-Time Irish Mothers: Is There a Relationship to Levels in Food?" Food Additives & Contaminants: Part A 30.10 (2013): 1788-1798.

24) Fernandes, A. R., et al. "Polybrominated Diphenyl Ethers (Pbdes) and Brominated Dioxins (PBDD/Fs) In Irish Food of Animal Origin." Food Additives and Contaminants: Part B 2.1 (2009): 86-94.

25) Xiong, Ping, et al. "A Review of Environmental Occurrence, Fate, and Toxicity of Novel Brominated Flame Retardants." Environmental Science & Technology 53.23 (2019): 13551-13569.

26) Fernandes, A. R., et al. "Bromine Content and Brominated Flame Retardants in Food and Animal Feed from The U.K." Chemosphere 150 (2016): 472-478.

27) Shrader, S., et al. "Determination of Total and Inorganic Bromide in Foods Fumigated with Methyl Bromide." Industrial & Engineering Chemistry Analytical Edition 14.1 (1942): 1-4.

28) Getzendaner, Milton E., et al. "Bromide Residues from Methyl Bromide Fumigation of Food Commodities." Journal of Agricultural and Food Chemistry 16.2 (1968): 265-271.

29) Kaushik, R. D. "Methyl Bromide: Risk Assessment, Environmental, and Health Hazard." Hazardous Gases. Academic Press, 2021. 239-250.

30) De Wit, Cynthia A. "An Overview of Brominated Flame Retardants in the Environment." Chemosphere 46.5 (2002): 583-624.

31) Horowitz, B. Zane. "Bromism from Excessive Cola Consumption." Journal of Toxicology: Clinical Toxicology 35.3 (1997): 315-320.

32) Bendig, Paul, et al. "Brominated Vegetable Oil in Soft Drinks–An Underrated Source of Human Organobromine Intake." Food Chemistry 133.3 (2012): 678-682.

33) Munro, I. C., et al. "Toxic Effects of Brominated Vegetable Oils in Rats." Toxicology and Applied Pharmacology 22.3 (1972): 432-439.

34) Carroll, James E., et al. "Brominated Vegetable Oil Myopathy: Inhibition at Multiple Sites." Muscle & Nerve: Official Journal of the American Association of Electrodiagnostic Medicine 7.8 (1984): 642-646.

35) Crampton, R. F., et al. "The Bromine Content of Human Tissue." British Journal of Nutrition 25.2 (1971): 317-322.

36) Raymond, Lawrence W., and Marsha D. Ford. "Severe Illness in Furniture Makers Using a New Glue: 1-Bromopropane Toxicity Confounded by Arsenic." Journal Of Occupational and Environmental Medicine (2007): 1009-1019.

37) Jih, Debra M., et al. "Bromoderma After Excessive Ingestion of Ruby Red." New England Journal of Medicine 348.19 (2003): 1932-1934.

38) Pearce, J. M. S. "Bromide, the First Effective Antiepileptic Agent." Journal of Neurology, Neurosurgery & Psychiatry 72.3 (2002): 412-412.

39) Hung, Yao-Min. "Bromide Intoxication by the Combination of Bromide-Containing Over-The-Counter Drug and Dextromethorphan Hydrobromide." Human & Experimental Toxicology 22.8 (2003): 459-461.

40) Torosian, George, et al. "Hazards of Bromides in Proprietary Medication." American Journal of Health-System Pharmacy 30.8 (1973): 716-718.

41) Frances, C., et al. "Bromism from Daily Over Intake of Bromide Salt: Case Report." Journal of Toxicology: Clinical Toxicology 41.2 (2003): 181-183.

42) Shaw, N., et al. "High Dietary Chloride Content Associated with Loss of Therapeutic Serum Bromide Concentrations in an Epileptic Dog." Journal of the American Veterinary Medical Association 208.2 (1996): 234-236.

43) Togawa, Go, et al. "Effects of Chloride in the Diet on Serum Bromide Concentrations in Dogs." International Journal of Applied Research in Veterinary Medicine 16.3 (2018): 197-202.

Chapter 30

Maternal Iodine Supplements and Smarter Children

A Young Mom with Hashimoto's Thyroiditis and Low Iodine Levels

CHRISTINA IS A 32-YEAR-OLD MOM with Hashimoto's Thyroiditis. Unfortunately, the autoimmune thyroid disease has damaged her thyroid gland leaving her with a low thyroid condition. Her lab panel revealed elevated TPO antibodies and low Free T3 and Free T4 levels. When first seen a year ago, Christina complained of chronic fatigue, weight gain, a "puffy" appearance of the eyes and face, dry skin, and hair loss. Thankfully, these symptoms resolved over time on a treatment program with NDT, natural desiccated thyroid, 2 grains per day, selenium supplement, 200 mcg per day, and iodine supplement, potassium iodide 450 mcg/day. (1-4)

Christina's spot urine iodine test revealed a low iodine level of 49 mcg/L, indicating moderate iodine deficiency based on WHO Guidelines. (5)

2013 WHO World Health Organization Iodine Urinary Excretion Guidelines

50-99 mcg/L indicates mild deficiency,

20-49 mcg/L indicates moderate deficiency,

and less than 20 mcg/L indicates severe deficiency.

After twelve months of our treatment program, which includes iodine supplementation and prenatal vitamins containing methyl folate, Christina calls the office to share the good news. She is expecting a baby!

Raising I.Q. with Iodized Salt.

Based on the work of David Marine and David Cowie in 1924, iodized salt fortification was introduced into the United States as a public health measure. In 1942, eighteen years later, military recruits entering the army from iodine-deficient areas showed a dramatic 15-point increase in I.Q. This was entirely due to the introduction of iodized salt back in 1924. Our iodine-fortified soldiers had increased intelligence with the ability to improvise in the field. Later, over time, other countries instituted similar iodine fortification programs, seeking the same benefits for public health. (6-15)

In 2013, Dr. James Feyrer studied the benefits of salt iodization in the United States, writing:

> Iodine deficiency is the leading cause of preventable mental retardation in the world today. The condition, which was common in the developed world until the introduction of iodized salt in the 1920s, is connected to low iodine levels in the soil and water... We use military data collected during WWI and WWII to compare outcomes of cohorts born before and after iodization in localities that were naturally poor and rich in iodine... Interpreting our measure in terms of I.Q., our finding is that in iodine-deficient regions, iodization raised I.Q. scores by roughly one standard deviation or 15 points. Given that one-quarter of the population lived in such regions, this implies a nationwide increase in average I.Q. of 3.5 points. (7)

Low Maternal Iodine is Still a Problem

Maternal iodine deficiency is the single most common cause of preventable mental retardation in children and is a global health problem addressed by the World Health Organization. (5-7) (19-23)

Despite iodized salt in the U.S., one-third of young women have low iodine levels placing the baby at risk for neuro-developmental delay. Low maternal iodine level is a preventable cause of mental retardation. As noted above, low maternal iodine levels have a deleterious effect on the baby's brain development and I.Q. scores. In many countries, screening programs have been instituted to detect congenital hypothyroidism caused by iodine deficiency so the babies can be treated immediately. (16-21)

How Much Iodine for Women of Childbearing Age?

Our office program for the expectant mom with Hashimoto's thyroiditis is 450 mcg of potassium iodide daily. The spot urinary iodine excretion is monitored serially. We also monitor thyroid labs, TSH, Free T3, Free T4, and antibody levels at more frequent intervals, every 6 weeks or so. As the pregnancy progresses, we typically observe declining TPO antibody levels related to "immune tolerance" of pregnancy, as reported in 2013 by Dr. Balucan and in 2021 by Dr. Chuyu Li. (22-23)

Excess Maternal Iodine May Raise TSH in Newborn

Although iodine deficiency is the topic of this Chapter, we will now discuss the other side of the coin, "Maternal Iodine Excess" causing "Transient Congenital Hypothyroidism in the Newborn" reported in the pediatric literature. For this reason, we recommend maternal iodine intake of 450 mcg/day. This is well below the 1,100 mcg per day upper limit set by the Food and Nutrition Board (FNB) of the Institute of Medicine. (3)(24)

Asian Cultures Have High Dietary Iodine Intake

The above discussion was concerned with iodine deficiency. Now we turn to the opposite side of the coin, iodine excess during pregnancy. In Asian cultures such as Japan and Korea, mothers consume kombu soups containing seaweed with high iodine content, 2,000-3,000 mcg per day, or even higher. This may translate into elevated TSH levels in the newborn which alarms the neonatologist, who now suspects congenital hypothyroidism detected during congenital hypothyroidism screening. (25-26)

Iodine Is a Supplement Available at the Health Food Store

If you are considering supplementing with high-dose iodine, I recommend seeking out and working closely with a knowledgeable physician who can monitor iodine levels and do thyroid function testing.

53 Countries Have Mandatory Flour Fortification with Folate

Folate fortification of flour for the prevention of neural tube defects, anencephaly, microcephaly, and spina bifida is mandated in 53 countries. Fortification of flour with folic acid was mandated in the U.S. in 1998, the most successful public health measure in history, with a reduction of neural tube defects by 36%. In 2009, Dr. Oakley declared this success story a "modern miracle of epidemiology." (28-37)

Study Blood Folate Levels

In 1998, after folate fortification in the U.S., folate deficiency, defined as folate blood levels less than three ng/ml, decreased from 21% to less than 1% of the population. In Australia, mandatory fortification of bread with folate and iodine was introduced in 2009, resulting in a 50-80 percent reduction in neural tube defects in at-risk indigenous women and teenagers. (28-37)

Reducing Microcephaly in Brazil with Folate Fortification

Studies in Brazil show folate deficiency is severe, affecting 94% of people living under the poverty line. Folate fortification of flour in three South American countries, Brazil, Argentina, and Chile, resulted in a significant reduction in

52 different fetal anomalies, including microcephaly and anencephaly. Currently, all South American countries except Venezuela have mandatory folate fortification legislation. In populations using folate fortification, there have been decreases in neural tube defects from 30-50%. I would add here that methyl folate is the most biologically active form of the vitamin, and is preferred over folate, the precursor used in fortification programs. (28-37)

Conclusion

Iodine and folate supplementation in women of childbearing age represents two of the greatest public health achievements of all time, improving fetal I.Q. and reducing fetal neural tube defects (NTD).

◆ **References for Chapter 30**

1) Leung, Angela M., et al. "Sufficient Iodine Intake During Pregnancy: Just Do It." Thyroid 23.1 (2013): 7.

2) De Groot, Leslie, et al. "Management of Thyroid Dysfunction During Pregnancy and Postpartum: An Endocrine Society Clinical Practice Guideline." The Journal of Clinical Endocrinology & Metabolism 97.8 (2012): 2543-2565.

3) Connelly, Kara J., et al. "Congenital Hypothyroidism Caused by Excess Prenatal Maternal Iodine Ingestion." The Journal of Pediatrics 161.4 (2012): 760-762.

4) Brown, Benjamin, and Ciara Wright. "Safety and Efficacy of Supplements in Pregnancy." Nutrition Reviews 78.10 (2020): 813-826.

5) World Health Organization. Urinary Iodine Concentrations for Determining Iodine Status in Populations. No. WHO/NMH/NHD/EPG/13.1. World Health Organization, 2013.

6) Raffensperger, Lisa. "How Adding Iodine to Salt Boosted Americans' I.Q., "Discover Magazine, July 23, 2013.

7) Feyrer, James, et al. "The Cognitive Effects of Micronutrient Deficiency: Evidence from Salt Iodization in the United States." Journal of the European Economic Association 15.2 (2017): 355-387.

8) Tafesse, Wiktoria. "The Effect of Universal Salt Iodization on Cognitive Test Scores in Rural India." World Development 152 (2022): 105796.

9) Protzko, John. "Raising I.Q. Among School-Aged Children: Five Meta-Analyses and a Review of Randomized Controlled Trials." Developmental Review 46 (2017): 81-101.

10) Leung, Angela M., and Gregory A. Brent. "Children of Mothers with Iodine Deficiency During Pregnancy Are More Likely to Have Lower Verbal I.Q. and Reading Scores at 8–9 Years of Age." Evidence-Based Nursing 17.3 (2014): 86-86.

11) Giacalone, Massimiliano, et al. "Does the Iodized Salt Therapy of Pregnant Mothers Increase the Children's I.Q.? Empirical Evidence of a Statistical Study Based on Permutation Tests." Quality & Quantity 52.3 (2018): 1423-1435.

12) Politi, Dimitra. "The Effects of the Generalized Use of Iodized Salt on Occupational Patterns in Switzerland." Unpublished Manuscript (2015).

13) Zhang, Kaiwen, et al. "Trends in Iodine Status Among U.S. Children and Adults: A Cross-Sectional Analysis of National Health and Nutrition Examination Survey Data from 2001–2004 to 2017–2020." Thyroid 32.8 (2022): 962-971

14) Leung, Angela M., et al. "History of U.S. Iodine Fortification and Supplementation." Nutrients 4.11 (2012): 1740-1746.

15) Sistrunk, J. Woody, and Frits van der Haar. "A History of Iodine Deficiency Disorder Eradication Efforts." Iodine Deficiency Disorders a

16) Haddow, James E., et al. "Maternal Thyroid Deficiency During Pregnancy and Subsequent Neuropsychological Development of the Child." New England Journal of Medicine 341.8 (1999): 549-555.

17) Mayunga, K. Clara, et al. "Pregnant Dutch Women Have Inadequate Iodine Status and Selenium Intake." Nutrients 14.19 (2022): 3936.

18) Patriota, Erika SO, et al. "Prevalence of Insufficient Iodine Intake in Pregnancy Worldwide: A Systematic Review and Meta-Analysis." European Journal of Clinical Nutrition 76.5 (2022): 703-715.

19) Hollowell, Joseph G., et al. "Iodine Nutrition in The United States. Trends and Public Health Implications: Iodine Excretion Data from National Health and Nutrition Examination Surveys I and III (1971–1974 and 1988–1994)." The Journal of Clinical Endocrinology & Metabolism 83.10 (1998): 3401-3408.

20) Caldwell, Kathleen L., et al. "Iodine Status of the U.S. Population, National Health and Nutrition Examination Survey, 2005–2006 and 2007–2008." Thyroid 21.4 (2011): 419-427.

21) Hatch-McChesney, Adrienne, and Harris R. Lieberman. "Iodine and Iodine Deficiency: A Comprehensive Review of a Re-Emerging Issue." Nutrients 14.17 (2022): 3474.

22) Balucan, Francis S., et al. "Thyroid Autoantibodies in Pregnancy: Their Role, Regulation, And Clinical Relevance." Journal Of Thyroid Research 2013 (2013).

23) Li, Chuyu, et al. "Variations in the Antithyroid Antibody Titre During Pregnancy and After Delivery." Risk Management and Healthcare Policy (2021): 847-859.

24) Meyers, Linda D., et al., eds. Dietary Reference Intakes: The Essential Guide to Nutrient Requirements. National Academies Press, 2006.

25) Nishiyama, Soroku, et al. "Transient Hypothyroidism or Persistent Hyperthyrotropinemia in Neonates Born to Mothers with Excessive Iodine Intake." Thyroid 14.12 (2004): 1077-1083.

26) Emder, Phillip John, and Michelle Marion Jack. "Iodine-induced Neonatal Hypothyroidism Secondary to Maternal Seaweed Consumption: A Common Practice in Some Asian Cultures to Promote Breast Milk Supply." Journal of Paediatrics and Child Health 47.10 (2011): 750-752.

27) Chen, Wen, et al. "Neonatal Thyroid Function Born to Mothers Living with Long-Term Excessive Iodine Intake from Drinking Water." Clinical endocrinology (2014).

28) Crider, Krista S., Lynn B. Bailey, and Robert J. Berry. "Folic Acid Food Fortification—Its History, Effect, Concerns, and Future Directions." Nutrients 3.3 (2011): 370-384.

29) Cordero, A., et al. "CDC Grand Rounds: Additional Opportunities to Prevent Neural Tube Defects with Folic Acid Fortification." Morbidity and Mortality Weekly Report 59.31 (2010): 980-984.

30) López-Camelo, Jorge S., et al. "Folic Acid Flour Fortification: Impact on the Frequencies of 52 Congenital Anomaly Types in Three South American Countries." American Journal of Medical Genetics Part A 152.10 (2010): 2444-2458.

31) Oakley Jr, G. P. "The Scientific Basis for Eliminating Folic Acid-Preventable Spina Bifida: A Modern Miracle from Epidemiology." Annals of Epidemiology 19.4 (2009): 226.

32) Bekaert, Samir, et al. "Folate Biofortification in Food Plants." Trends in Plant Science 13.1 (2008): 28-35.

33) Crider, Krista S., et al. "Folic Acid Food Fortification—Its History, Effect, Concerns, and Future Directions." Nutrients 3.3 (2011): 370-384.

34) Crider, Krista S., et al. "Folic Acid and the Prevention of Birth Defects: 30 Years of Opportunity and Controversies." Annual Review of Nutrition 42 (2022): 423-452.

35) Rodrigues, Humberto Gabriel, et al. "Folic Acid Intake by Pregnant Women from Vale Do Jequitinhonha, Brazil, and the Contribution of Fortified Foods." Archivos Latinoamericanos De Nutricion 65.1 (2015): 27-35.

36) López-Camelo, Jorge S., et al. "Folic Acid Flour Fortification: Impact on the Frequencies of 52 Congenital Anomaly Types in Three South American Countries." American Journal of Medical Genetics Part A 152.10 (2010): 2444-2458.

37) Rosenthal, Jorge, et al. "Neural Tube Defects in Latin America and the Impact of Fortification: A Literature Review." Public Health Nutrition 17.3 (2014): 537-550.

Chapter 31

Breast Cancer Prevention with Iodine Supplementation

A GOOD FRIEND OF OURS just went through an ordeal with breast cancer. The incidence of breast cancer has increased to 1 in 8 women, with 4,000 new cases weekly. As of 2022, 43,250 women died annually from breast cancer in the U.S. Mortality for male breast cancer is considerably less. Approximately 500 males succumb to breast cancer annually. (1-2)

Does Screening Mammography Reduce Breast Cancer Mortality?

What about screening mammography? This is the practice of doing an annual mammogram on the entire population of healthy women in the United States. Can screening mammography prevent breast cancer? In 2009, Dr. Laura Esserman reviewed 20 years of U.S. national data on breast cancer mortality before the 1983 introduction of mammography compared to the years after. It is disappointing that the expected survival benefits of screening mammography have not materialized. Screening mammography does not reduce annual mortality from breast cancer, and instead, causes overdiagnosis and over-treatment with unnecessary (and lucrative) procedures. What is the reason for this? This is explained in 2011 in my book, Bioidentical Hormones 101. Dr. Jeffrey Dach writes:

> The reason why mammography has had little impact on breast cancer mortality is that mammography is an X-Ray imaging technique that finds small calcifications indicating DCIS, an indolent, non-aggressive lesion with a good prognosis. The data suggests that finding and aggressively treating DCIS does not reduce mortality rates from advanced breast cancer. Note: DCIS is Ductal Carcinoma in-Situ. (3-6)

You might ask, could it be possible that mainstream medicine has overlooked a breast cancer preventive that is safe, cheap, and widely available? The answer is yes, and it is the essential mineral iodine, added to table salt in 1924 as part of a national program to prevent thyroid enlargement (goiter) caused by iodine deficiency. (7)

Our Diet is Iodine Deficient

Iodized salt is the primary source of dietary iodine for Americans. Yet, many of us have been advised by our doctors to avoid salt because salt causes high blood pressure. If this advice is followed, one would have very little dietary iodine. Here in the U.S., we still have iodine deficiency in the population. Currently, 15% of the U.S. adult female population is classified by the World Health Organization (WHO) as iodine deficient. Although all processed foods contain a large quantity of salt, none of this added salt is iodized. For people using sea salt, make sure to purchase iodized sea salt, now available alongside the non-iodized version on the grocery shelf. (8-9)

The RDA for Iodine is Too Low for Optimal Health.

According to Guy Abraham, MD, our dietary intake of iodine is too low. This was set at 150 mcg per day as the government recommended RDA. In 2002, Dr. Guy Abraham recommended a higher daily iodine intake of 12.5 mg per day, inspired by the Japanese diet which contains seaweed, rich in iodine. Higher dietary iodine explains why the Japanese have the lowest breast, prostate, and thyroid cancer rates compared to ours here in the US with an RDA of only 150 mcg/day for iodine. Note: RDA is Recommended Dietary Allowance. (10-17)

In 2008, Dr. Lyn Patrick writes:

Japanese populations have historically consumed significant amounts of dietary iodine from seaweed intake, possibly consuming a minimum of 7,000 mcg of iodine daily from kombu alone. Estimates of the average daily Japanese iodine consumption vary from 5,280 mcg to 13,800 mcg; by comparison the average U.S. daily consumption is 167 mcg. (17)

How Safe is Iodine Supplementation?

Iodine is the only trace element that can be ingested safely in amounts up to 100,000 times the RDA. Potassium iodide has been prescribed safely to large numbers of pulmonary COPD patients in amounts of up to 2,400 milligrams per day for several years. This is called SSKI (Super Saturated Potassium Iodide), a well-known treatment for chronic obstructive pulmonary disease (COPD) which helps mobilize lung secretions. The commonly used anti-arrhythmia cardiology drug, amiodarone, contains 37.2% iodine by weight (37.2 mg iodine per 100 mg amiodarone tablet). The government protocol for a nuclear reactor leak provides two 65 mg iodine tablets (130 mg) to everyone in the surrounding area. Asian diets are high in iodine from the consumption of seaweed. Iodine supplements are widely available as Iodoral and Lugol's solution over the counter without a prescription. All the above considerations indicate iodine is generally regarded as safe. (17-21)

FDA Recommends 130 mg of iodine

The FDA has officially stated that iodine supplementation is safe and recommends 130 mg of potassium iodide for adults in case of radiation emergency to protect the population from thyroid cancer. (17)

Iodine Allergy?

"Iodine Allergy" is a misnomer since this name applies to allergy to iodinated radiographic contrast agents and not to elemental iodine, which has a different chemical structure. Elemental iodine is an essential mineral and is required for health. Deficiency of iodine in the developing embryo causes cretinism, and deficiency in the newborn child causes goiter. As such, any developing embryo allergic to iodine would not survive more than a few weeks, and therefore there can be no allergy to elemental iodine, just as there cannot be an allergy to oxygen or water, also essential nutrients. (22-23)

Iodine, a well-known topical antiseptic and antimicrobial agent, has anti-cancer effects and is the key player in our body's surveillance system for removing abnormal pre-cancer cells. As we will see below, considerable medical research supports this statement.

Iodine Deficiency Causes Fibrocystic Breast Disease, Breast Cancer, and Thyroid Cancer – Dr. Eskin

Dr. B.A. Eskin published 80 papers over 30 years researching iodine and breast cancer, finding iodine deficiency causes breast cancer and thyroid cancer in humans and animals. Iodine deficiency is also known to cause a precancerous condition called fibrocystic breast disease. In 1993, Dr. Ghent showed iodine supplementation effectively resolved fibrocystic breast disease, considered a precancerous condition. (24-35)

Despite its obvious potential, not much has been done with iodine treatment in the United States over the past 40 years. Iodine is a natural substance and not eligible for patent protection, making it unprofitable to market. As such, the drug industry is unlikely to fund studies for "FDA approval." However, FDA approval is not required since iodine is already an additive to table salt at the supermarket, and iodine supplements are available over the counter without a physician's prescription.

Ultrasound for Thyroid Cysts and Nodules

As an interventional radiologist working in the hospital for 25 years, a large part of my job was evaluating thyroid abnormalities, nodules, and cysts with ultrasound, radionuclide scans, and needle biopsy procedures. Although it was obvious these common thyroid abnormalities were due to iodine deficiency, I often wondered why none of the patients ever received iodine supplementation. The obvious answer is they should have been. The protective role of iodine is ignored by mainstream medicine.

Iodine Deficiency – Fibrocystic Breast Disease

Part of my day as a radiologist was spent reading mammogram and ultrasound breast imaging studies. When I say reading, I mean interpreting the images and trying to find cancer hiding in the dense tissue called fibrocystic breast disease. Many of these women would have needle aspiration procedures for the many breast cysts and needle biopsies of the solid nodules commonly seen in fibrocystic breast disease. Many women returned multiple times for these procedures because the medical system had no useful treatment to offer them. We now know an excellent medical treatment for fibrocystic breast disease exists. Iodine supplementation not only resolves breast cysts and fibrocystic breast disease but also resolves ovarian and thyroid cysts. Iodine supplementation has always been available, but this is ignored by mainstream medicine, and hospital-based physicians are unaware of it. (24-35) (41-69)

Goiter is Caused by Iodine Deficiency

Iodine deficiency is the direct cause of thyroid enlargement called goiter, thyroid nodules, and cysts. In severe cases, thyroid enlargement can be massive. Iodine deficiency is the direct cause of thyroid nodules as discussed in Chapter 33, The Thyroid Nodule Epidemic.

Lugol's Solution

There are many iodine supplements widely available without the need for a prescription. The oldest and best known is Lugol's Solution, available over the counter and contains five percent molecular iodine and ten percent potassium iodide. In 2017, Dr. Jan Calissendorff writes:

> Lugol's solution (L.S.) was developed in 1829 by the French physician Jean Guillaume August Lugol, initially as a cure for tuberculosis. It is a solution of elemental iodine (5%) and potassium iodide (K.I., 10%) together with distilled water. (36)

Iodoral from Optimox

Another commonly used tablet form of iodine is Iodoral from Optimox, a company founded by Guy Abraham, MD, a former professor of obstetrics and gynecology at UCLA who started "The Iodine Project" in 1997. Two family practice physicians Jorge Flechas, MD and David Brownstein, MD were engaged in the project and conducted clinical studies. Their hypothesis was the body needs 12.5 mg of iodine a day. Each 12.5 mg tablet of Iodoral contains 7.5 mg of potassium iodide (K.I.) and 5 mg of elemental iodine. This formula is remarkably similar to Lugol's Solution. (12).

More than 4,000 patients in this project consumed iodine supplements from 12 to 50 mg per day, and in those with diabetes, up to 100 mg a day. From observing this population taking iodine supplements, Drs. Flechas and Brownstein reported the resolution of fibrocystic disease; diabetic patients require less insulin; hypothyroid patients require less thyroid medication; symptoms of fibromyalgia and migraine headaches resolve as well. (37-38)

Dr. Albert Szent Györgi

The Nobel laureate Dr. Albert Szent Györgi (1893–1986), the physician who discovered vitamin C, used iodine freely in his medical practice. The standard dose of potassium iodide given in those days was one gram, which contains 770 mg of iodide (the other 230 mg is potassium). Dr. Albert Szent Györgi writes:

> When I was a medical student, iodine in the form of K.I. (potassium Iodide) was the

universal medicine. Nobody knew what it did, but it did something and did something good. We students used to sum up the situation in this little rhyme: If ye don't know where, what, and why, Prescribe ye then K and I. (12) (40)

Routine Iodine Laboratory Testing and Supplementation - The Spot Urine for Iodine

Iodoral is an essential part of our breast cancer prevention program and is widely available at health food stores and online without a prescription. Per office policy, we have chosen the random spot urine for iodine as our routine iodine test. This is more convenient than the 24-hour urine collection, as only one sample is required, at the same session as the blood draw. This is included on all routine lab panels because of its ease and convenience. Excluding patients with auto-immune thyroid disease, all other female patients are routinely advised to take an Iodoral tablet (12.5 mg) daily as a breast cancer preventive agent. Hashimoto's patients are the exception, given a low-dose iodine supplement, 225 mcg of potassium iodide daily, as described in Chapters 20-23.

For many specialized tests, we do not use the lab range. Spot urinary iodine testing is one of these tests in which the laboratory range is useful for detecting iodine deficiency in the population but not in following the patient on iodine supplements. The test result will always be above the lab range for those on iodine supplements. Above the lab reference range is a desired outcome for the spot urinary iodine test, and indicates the patient is taking iodine supplements with good results. The follow-up spot urine for iodine is useful to confirm the patient is indeed taking the iodine supplement.

Conclusion

Another error in modern endocrinology and women's health is ignoring iodine as our most important agent for preventing and treating fibrocystic breast disease and breast cancer. (41-69)

♦ References for Chapter 31

1) Giaquinto, Angela N., et al. "Breast Cancer Statistics, 2022." CA: A Cancer Journal for Clinicians 72.6 (2022): 524-541.

2) Wang, Fei, et al. "Overall Mortality After Diagnosis of Breast Cancer in Men Vs Women." JAMA Oncology 5.11 (2019): 1589-1596.

3) Esserman, Laura, et al. "Rethinking Screening for Breast Cancer and Prostate Cancer." JAMA 302.15 (2009): 1685-1692.

4) Welch, H. Gilbert. "Overdiagnosis and Mammography Screening." BMJ: British Medical Journal (Online) 339 (2009).

5) Welch, H. Gilbert, and William C. Black. "Using Autopsy Series to Estimate the Disease "Reservoir" for Ductal Carcinoma in Situ of the Breast: How Much More Breast Cancer Can We Find?" Annals of Internal Medicine 127.11 (1997): 1023-1028.

6) Dach, Jeffrey. Bioidentical Hormones 101. iUniverse, 2011.

7) Pearce, Elizabeth N., and Michael B. Zimmermann. "The Prevention of Iodine Deficiency: A History." Thyroid 33.2 (2023): 143-149.

8) Pennington, J. A., and S. A. Schoen. "Total Diet Study: Estimated Dietary Intakes of Nutritional Elements, 1982-1991." International Journal for Vitamin and Nutrition Research. 66.4 (1996): 350-362.

9) Blankenship, Jessica L., et al. "Effect of Iodized Salt on Organoleptic Properties of Processed Foods: A Systematic Review." Journal Of Food Science and Technology 55 (2018): 3341-3352.

10) Abraham, Guy E., et al. "Optimum Levels of Iodine for Greatest Mental and Physical Health." The Original Internist 9.3 (2002): 5-20.

11) Abraham, Guy E., Jorge D. Flechas, and J. C. Hakala. "Optimum Levels of Iodine for Greatest Mental and Physical Health." The Original Internist 9.3 (2002): 5-20.

12) Abraham, Guy E. "Iodine: The Universal Nutrient." Townsend Letter for Doctors and Patients 269 (2005): 85.

13) Ahad, Farhana, and Shaiq A. Ganie. "Iodine, Iodine Metabolism, and Iodine Deficiency Disorders Revisited." Indian Journal of Endocrinology and Metabolism 14.1 (2010): 13.

14) Stadel, Bruce V. "Dietary Iodine and Risk of Breast, Endometrial, and Ovarian Cancer." The Lancet 307.7965 (1976): 890-891.

15) Brown, Emma M., et al. "Seaweed and Human Health." Nutrition Reviews 72.3 (2014): 205-216.

16) Aceves, Carmen, et al. "Is Iodine a Gatekeeper of the Integrity of the Mammary Gland?" Journal of Mammary Gland Biology and Neoplasia 10.2 (2005): 189-196.

17) Patrick, Lyn. "Iodine: Deficiency and Therapeutic Considerations." Alternative Medicine Review 13.2 (2008).

18) Guidance on Potassium Iodide as a Thyroid Blocking Agent in Radiation Emergencies, U.S. Department of Health and Human Services, Food and Drug Administration, Center for Drug Evaluation and Research (CDER), December 2001

19) Bernecker, C. "Intermittent Therapy with Potassium Iodide in Chronic Obstructive Disease of the Airways. A Review of 10 Years Experience." Acta Allergologica 24.3 (1969): 216-225.

20) Chiovato, Luca, et al. "Studies on the in Vitro Cytotoxic Effect of Amiodarone." Endocrinology 134.5 (1994): 2277-2282.

21) Aakre, Inger, et al. "Commercially Available Kelp and Seaweed Products–Valuable Iodine Source or Risk of Excess Intake?" Food & Nutrition Research 65 (2021).

22) Stewart, Michael W. "Doctor I Have an Iodine Allergy." Ophthalmology and Therapy 11.3 (2022): 931-938.

23) Meunier, B., et al. "Iodinated Contrast Media and Iodine Allergy: Myth or Reality?" Revue Medicale De Liege 68.9 (2013): 465-469.

24) Eskin, Bernard A., et al. "Mammary Gland Dysplasia in Iodine Deficiency: Studies in Rats." JAMA 200.8 (1967): 691-695.

25) Eskin, Bernard A, and Bruce V Stadel. "Dietary Iodine and Cancer Risk." The Lancet 308.7989 (1976): 807-808.

26) Eskin, Bernard A. "Iodine and Mammary Cancer." Inorganic and Nutritional Aspects of Cancer. Springer, Boston, MA, 1978. 293-304.

27) Eskin, Bernard A. "Section of Biological and Medical Sciences: Iodine Metabolism and Breast Cancer." Transactions of the New York Academy of Sciences 32.8 Series II (1970): 911-947.

28) Eskin, Bernard A. "Iodine and Breast Cancer, a 1982 Update." Biological Trace Element Research 5.4 (1983): 399-412.

29) Eskin, Bernard A., et al. "Rat Mammary Gland Atypia Produced by Iodine Blockade with Perchlorate." Cancer Research 35.9 (1975): 2332-2339.

30) Ohshima, Masato, and Jerrold M. Ward. "Dietary Iodine Deficiency as a Tumor Promoter and Carcinogen in Male F344/Ncr Rats." Cancer Research 46.2 (1986): 877-883.

31) Hartmann, Lynn C., et al. "Benign Breast Disease and the Risk of Breast Cancer." New England Journal of Medicine 353.3 (2005): 229-237.

32) Ghent, W. R., et al. "Iodine Replacement in Fibrocystic Disease of the Breast." Canadian Journal of Surgery. 36.5 (1993): 453-460.

33) Gaby, Alan R. "Iodine Treatment of Fibrocystic Breast Disease." Townsend Letter for Doctors and Patients 256 (2004): 24-25.

34) Krouse, T. B., B. A., Eskin, and J. Mobini. "Age-Related Changes Resembling Fibrocystic Disease in Iodine-Blocked Rat Breasts." Archives of Pathology & Laboratory Medicine 103.12 (1979): 631-634.

35) Karpas, Charles M., et al. "Relationship of Fibrocystic Disease to Carcinoma of the Breast." Annals of Surgery 162.1 (1965): 1.

36) Calissendorff, Jan, and Henrik Falhammar. "Lugol's Solution and Other Iodide Preparations: Perspectives and Research Directions in Graves' Disease." Endocrine 58 (2017): 467-473

37) Brownstein, David. "Iodine: Why You Need It, Why You Can't Live Without It." Medical Alternatives Press, 2008.

38) Brownstein, David. "Clinical Experience with Inorganic, Non-Radioactive Iodine/Iodide." The Original Internist 12.3 (2005): 105-108.

39) Flechas, Jorge D. "Orthoiodosupplementation in a Primary Care Practice." The Original Internist 12.2 (2005): 89-96.

40) Miller, D. W. "Extrathyroidal Benefits of Iodine." Journal of American Physicians and Surgeons 11.4 (2006): 106.

41) Derry, D. "Breast Cancer and Iodine: How to Prevent and How to Survive Breast Cancer." Victoria, BC: Trafford Publishing (2002).

42) Miller, D. W. "Iodine in Health and Civil Defense." Proceeding of the Twenty-fourth Annual Meeting of Doctors for Disaster Preparedness. 2006.

43) Aceves, Carmen, et al. "Molecular Iodine Has Extrathyroidal Effects as an Antioxidant, Differentiator, and Immunomodulator." International Journal of Molecular Sciences 22.3 (2021): 1228.

44) Manjer, Jonas, et al. "Serum Iodine and Breast Cancer Risk: A Prospective Nested Case–Control Study Stratified for Selenium Levels." Cancer Epidemiology, Biomarkers & Prevention 29.7 (2020): 1335-1340.

45) Dijck-Brouwer, DA Janneke, et al. "Thyroidal and Extrathyroidal Requirements for Iodine and Selenium: A Combined Evolutionary and (Patho) Physiological Approach." Nutrients 14.19 (2022): 3886.

46) Cann, Stephen A., et al. "Hypothesis: Iodine, Selenium and the Development of Breast Cancer." Cancer Causes & Control 11.2 (2000): 121-127.

47) Smyth, Peter. "The Thyroid, Iodine, and Breast Cancer." Breast Cancer Research 5.5 (2003): 1-4.

48) Venturi, Sebastiano, et al. "Role of Iodine in Evolution and Carcinogenesis of Thyroid, Breast, and Stomach." Advances in Clinical Pathology 4 (2000): 11-18.

49) Venturi, Sebastiano. "Is There a Role for Iodine in Breast Diseases?" The Breast 10.5 (2001): 379-382.

50) Stoddard II, Frederick R., et al. "Iodine Alters Gene Expression in the MCF7 Breast Cancer Cell Line: Evidence for an Anti-Estrogen Effect of Iodine." International Journal of Medical Sciences 5.4 (2008): 189.

51) Kato, N., et al. "Suppressive Effect of Iodine Preparations on Proliferation of DMBA-induced Breast Cancer in Rat." Journal-Japan Society for Cancer Therapy 29 (1994): 582-582.

52) Funahashi, Hiroomi, et al. "Seaweed Prevents Breast Cancer?" Japanese Journal of Cancer Research 92.5 (2001): 483-487.

54) Tokudome, Shinkan, et al. "Seaweed and Cancer Prevention." Cancer Science 92.9 (2001).

55) Rappaport, Jay. "Changes in Dietary Iodine Explains the Increasing Incidence of Breast Cancer with Distant Involvement in Young Women." Journal of Cancer 8.2 (2017): 174.

56) Aceves, Carmen, et al. "Is Iodine a Gatekeeper of the Integrity of the Mammary Gland?" Journal of Mammary Gland Biology and Neoplasia 10.2 (2005): 189-196.

57) Torremante, Pompilio Elio, and Harald Rosner. "Anti-Proliferative Effects of Molecular Iodine in Cancers." Curr Chem Biol 5.3 (2011): 168-76.

58) Iwamoto, Keisuke S. "The Mechanistic Role of Iodine in Breast Carcinogenesis." California Univ Los Angeles, 2005. U.S. Army Medical Research and Materiel Command, Fort Detrick, Maryland, 21702-5012 Award Number: W81XWH-04-1-0684

59) Zuckier, Lionel S., et al. "The Endogenous Mammary Gland Na+/I– Symporter May Mediate Effective Radioiodide Therapy in Breast Cancer." Journal of Nuclear Medicine 42.6 (2001): 987-987.

60) Slebodzinski, A. B. "Ovarian Iodide Uptake and Triiodothyronine Generation in Follicular Fluid: The Enigma of the Thyroid Ovary Interaction." Domestic Animal Endocrinology 29.1 (2005): 97-103.

61) Monteleone, Patrizia, et al. "Thyroid Peroxidase Identified in Human Granulosa Cells: Another Piece to the Thyroid-Ovary Puzzle?" Gynecological Endocrinology 33.7 (2017): 574-576.

62) Mutinati, M., et al. "Localization of Thyrotropin Receptor and Thyroglobulin in the Bovine Corpus Luteum." Animal Reproduction Science 118.1 (2010): 1-6.

63) Ravera, Silvia, et al. "The Sodium/Iodide Symporter (NIS): Molecular Physiology and Preclinical and Clinical Applications." Annual Review of Physiology 79 (2017): 261.

64) Kogai, Takahiko, et al. "Retinoic Acid Induces Sodium/Iodide Symporter Gene Expression and Radioiodide Uptake in the MCF-7 Breast Cancer Cell Line." Proceedings of the National Academy of Sciences 97.15 (2000): 8519-8524.

65) Tazebay, Uygar H., et al. "The Mammary Gland Iodide Transporter Is Expressed During Lactation and in Breast Cancer." Nature Medicine 6.8 (2000): 871-878.

66) Zuckier, Lionel S., et al. "The Endogenous Mammary Gland Na+/I– Symporter May Mediate Effective Radioiodide Therapy in Breast Cancer." Journal of Nuclear Medicine 42.6 (2001): 987-987.

67) Yao, Chen, et al. "Effect of Sodium/Iodide Symporter (NIS)-Mediated Radioiodine Therapy on Estrogen Receptor-Negative Breast Cancer." Oncology Reports 34.1 (2015): 59-66.

68) Elliyanti, Aisyah, et al. "Analysis Natrium Iodide Symporter Expression in Breast Cancer Subtypes for Radioiodine Therapy Response." Nuclear Medicine and Molecular Imaging 54.1 (2020): 35-42.

69) Elliyanti, Aisyah, et al. "An Iodine Treatments Effect on Cell Proliferation Rates of Breast Cancer Cell Lines; In Vitro Study." Open Access Macedonian Journal of Medical Sciences 8. B (2020): 1064-1070.

Chapter 32

Iodine Treats Breast Cancer, Overwhelming Evidence

FOR ANYONE INTERESTED IN IODINE supplementation for health, I recommend Dr. David Brownstein's book, "Iodine, Why You Need It, Why You Can't Live Without It". (1)

On page 63, Dr. Brownstein reports three cases of spontaneous regression of breast cancer in women taking an iodine supplement called Iodoral. Each 12.5 mg Iodoral tablet contains 5 mg of molecular iodine (I2) and 7.5 mg of potassium iodide (K.I.).

Joan, an English Teacher

The first patient, Joan, a 63-year-old English teacher, was diagnosed with breast cancer in 1989, declined conventional treatment, and took 50 mg of Iodoral per day. Six weeks later, a PET scan showed "all of the existing tumors were disintegrating."

Delores

The second patient, 73-year-old Delores, was diagnosed with breast cancer in 2003. She declined conventional treatment with radiation and chemotherapy. Instead, Delores took 50 mg of Iodoral daily. A follow-up ultrasound of the breast 18 months later showed, "It appears that these malignancies have diminished in size since the last examination. Interval improvement is definitely seen." Two years later, a follow-up mammogram and ultrasound failed to show any abnormality and were read by the radiologist as normal.

Joyce

The third patient, 52-year-old Joyce, was diagnosed with breast cancer two years prior and was started on Iodoral, 50 mg per day. Three years later, her follow-up mammograms and ultrasound exams showed decreasing size of the tumor with no progression. (1)

Although these cases are "anecdotal" evidence and do not rise to the level of a clinical trial, I found them remarkable. The medical literature has much more evidence, as we will see below.

Iodine Deficiency Causes Breast Cancer – The Overwhelming Evidence

Studies of Iodine Deficiency in Animals and Humans

Iodine deficiency is associated with a higher rate of goiter and breast cancer. Similarly, higher dietary iodine intake is associated with less goiter and breast cancer. For example, Japan has the highest dietary intake of iodine based on seaweed in the diet, 1,000 to 3,000 mcg per day, and the lowest rates for goiter and breast cancer. However, when Japanese women immigrate to America and change their dietary intake of iodine to the lower 150 mcg/day, breast cancer rates increase. Animal studies show that iodine-deficient diets induce breast cancer and goiter in animals. (1-8)

Fishing Industry in Iceland

Iceland is another country with high iodine intake and low goiter and breast cancer rates. Before 1914, the First World War, high dietary iodine content originated from the fishing industry in Iceland. In those days, the fish meal was fed to dairy cows providing milk with high iodine content. After the war, the fish meal was eliminated from the dairy cows, and breast cancer rates soared ten-fold. (9)

Iodine Research from Mexico, India, and Japan.

India - Shrivastava Group

In 2006, the Shrivastava group in India reported molecular iodine causes regression of breast cancer xenografts in mice, induces apoptosis, programmed cell death in human breast cancer cell cultures, and is beneficial for fibrocystic disease, writing:

> The iodine-induced apoptotic mechanism was studied in MCF-7 [breast cancer] cells. DNA fragmentation analysis confirmed internucleosomal DNA degradation. Terminal deoxynucleotidyl transferase-mediated dUTP nick-end labeling established that iodine-induced apoptosis in a time- and dose-dependent manner in MCF-7 [breast cancer] cells...We propose a detailed mechanism of the **molecular iodine (I2)-induced apoptosis in human breast cancer cells that may explain iodine-induced breast cancer regression in experimental rat models as well as beneficial effects observed in human fibrocystic breast subjects. Iodine showed cytotoxic effects in cultured human breast cancer cells.** (10)

Note: Terminal deoxynucleotidyl transferase-mediated dUTP nick-end labeling is called the TUNEL assay, an established technique for detecting DNA fragments indicating apoptosis, programmed cell death and a marker of cancer treatment efficacy.

Mexico - Carmen Aceves Velasco Group

In 2009, the Carmen Aceves Velasco Group from Mexico reported iodine as safe, with no harmful effects on thyroid function. Their study showed iodine has an anti-proliferative effect on human breast cancer cell cultures. They reported the mechanism by which iodine works as an anti-cancer agent. Iodine binds to membrane lipids called lactones, forming iodo-lactones which regulate apoptosis, also called programmed cell death. In other words,

iodine makes cancer cells undergo apoptosis. Dr. Aceves concluded that continuous molecular iodine treatment has a "potent antineoplastic effect" on the progression of mammary cancer, writing:

> This report confirms our previous observations that I2 [molecular iodine] treatment reduces mammary cancer incidence, decreases the proliferative rate (PCNA), and induces apoptosis (TUNEL and caspases) in cancerous mammary cells in vitro or in vivo without any secondary adverse effect on the thyroid or general health... Our previous observation that tumor growth resumes if I2 treatment is suspended...In conclusion, these data support our notion that I2 supplement could be an adjuvant in the therapy of mammary cancer, where the high concentration of A.A. [Arachadonic Acid] characteristic of tumoral cells serves as substrate to form 6-IL [6-Iodolactone], which in turn triggers the activation of apoptotic and anti-invasive pathways by modulating PPAR receptors. (11-15)

Note: 6 iodo-lactone is also involved in thyroid auto-regulation, as discussed in Chapter 14 on the Production of Thyroid Hormone.

Japan – Dr. Funahashi

In 2001, Dr. Funahashi from Japan induced breast cancer by treating mice with a carcinogenic chemical called DMBA, causing large visible breast cancer masses in the mice. However, when the mice were pretreated with iodine-containing seaweed (Wakame-mekabu) and then treated with DMBA, these mice were protected and had no visible tumor masses. Dr. Funahashi found a common seaweed food containing high iodine content is more beneficial than chemotherapy for breast cancer, writing:

> Administration of Lugol's iodine or iodine-rich Wakame seaweed to rats treated with the carcinogen dimethyl benzanthracene [DMBA] suppressed the development of mammary tumors. The same group

demonstrated that seaweed induced apoptosis in human breast cancer cells with greater potency than that of fluorouracil, a chemotherapeutic agent used to treat breast cancer. (16)

Note: DMBA is polycyclic aromatic hydrocarbon 7,12-dimethylbenz[a]anthracene, a chemical carcinogen and an established research model for inducing breast cancer in animals. Another established animal model of breast cancer is the MPA mouse breast cancer model. MPA is medroxyprogesterone, also called Provera, still widely used by gynecologists who freely prescribe this carcinogenic drug to women with dysfunctional uterine bleeding. (17-22)

Iodine Mechanism of Action-Altering Gene Expression

In 2008, Drs. Frederick R. Stoddard and Bernard A. Eskin studied the effect of Lugol's Solution on gene expression in MCF-7 breast cancer cell line in-vitro, using micro-array analysis, showing that iodine altered gene expression in breast cancer cells, modulated the estrogen pathway, and regulated cell cycle progression, growth, and differentiation. The first author, Dr. Frederick R. Stoddard, writes:

> The protective effects of iodine on breast cancer have been postulated from epidemiologic evidence and described in animal models...laboratory evidence suggests that iodine may inhibit cancer promotion through modulation of the estrogen pathway. To elucidate the role of iodine in breast cancer, the effect of Lugol's iodine solution (5% I2, 10% K.I.) on gene expression was analyzed in the estrogen-responsive MCF-7 breast cancer cell line. Microarray analysis identified 29 genes that were up-regulated and 14 genes that were down-regulated in response to iodine/iodide treatment. The altered genes included several involved in hormone [estrogen] metabolism as well as genes involved in the regulation of cell cycle progression, growth, and differentiation... this work suggests that

iodine/iodide may be useful as adjuvant therapy in the pharmacologic manipulation of the estrogen pathway in women with breast cancer. (23)

Note: Lugol's iodine solution is 5% molecular Iodine (I2) and 10% potassium iodide (K.I.).

6-Iodolactone Mediated Apoptosis

In 2008 Dr. Arroyo-Helguera studied the effect of molecular iodine on breast cancer cells in vitro finding 6-iodolactone (6-IL) mediates apoptotic effects (programmed cell death). The conversion of iodine to 6-IL is mediated by A.A. (Arachidonic Acid), found in high concentrations in breast cancer cells. Another finding is molecular iodine exerts apoptotic effects in breast cancer cells at lower concentrations than in normal breast tissue cells. Dr. Arroyo-Helguera writes:

> Previous reports have documented the **anti-proliferative properties of I2 [molecular iodine]** and the arachidonic acid (A.A.) derivative 6-iodolactone (6-IL) in both thyroid and mammary glands. In this study, we characterized the cellular pathways activated by these molecules and their effects on cell cycle arrest and apoptosis in normal (MCF-12F) and cancerous (MCF-7) breast cells...Low-to-moderate concentrations of I2 (10–20 µM) cause G1 and G2/M phase arrest in MCF-12F and caspase-dependent apoptosis in MCF-7 cells. In normal cells, only high doses of I2 (40 µM) induced apoptosis, and this effect was mediated by poly (ADP-ribose) polymerase-1 (PARP1) and the apoptosis-induced factor, suggesting an oxidative influence of iodine at high concentrations. Our data indicate that both I2 and 6-IL trigger the same intracellular pathways and suggest that **the antineoplastic effect of I2 in mammary cancer involves the intracellular formation of 6-IL.** Mammary cancer cells are known to contain high concentrations of A.A., which might explain why I2 exerts apoptotic effects at lower concentrations only in tumoral cells. (14)

Dr. Aceves Group in Mexico on Iodolactones

In 2014, Dr. Carmen Aceves Group in Mexico did further work on 6-iodolactone (6-IL), an iodinated derivative of arachidonic acid as a key mediator of thyroid autoregulation and anti-cancer properties of iodine via potent activation of nuclear receptor PPAR gamma, an anti-inflammatory effect by inhibiting inflammatory cytokines. Similar anti-cancer effects are seen in extrathyroidal tissues such as breast, prostate, colon, and nervous system. Dr. Carmen Aceves writes:

> An iodinated derivative of arachidonic acid, 5-hydroxy-6-iodo-8,11,14-eicosatrienoic acid lactone (6-IL) has been implicated as a possible intermediate in the autoregulation of the thyroid gland by iodine. In addition to anti-proliferative and apoptotic effects observed in thyrocytes, this iodolipid could also exert similar actions in cells derived from extrathyroidal tissues like mammary gland, prostate, colon, or the nervous system. In mammary cancer (solid tumors or tumor cell lines), 6-IL has been detected after molecular iodine (I2) supplement and is a potent activator of peroxisome proliferator-activated receptor type gamma (PPAR gamma). These observations led us to propose an I2 supplement as a novel coadjutant therapy which, by inducing differentiation mechanisms, decreases tumor progression and prevents chemoresistance. Some kinds of tumoral cells, in contrast to normal cells, contain high concentrations of arachidonic acid, making the I2 supplement a potential "magic bullet" that enables local, specific production of 6-IL, which then exerts antineoplastic actions with minimal deleterious effects on normal tissues. (24-26)

Note: PPAR is a Peroxisome Proliferator-Activated Receptor, a family of steroid receptors located in the nucleus involved in regulating energy production, lipid metabolism, and inflammation. PPAR alpha represses NFkB (Nuclear Factor Kappa B) and is strongly anti-inflammatory. PPAR gamma activation is anti-inflammatory, inhibiting inflammatory cytokines tumor necrosis factor-alpha (TNF-α), and interleukin 6 (IL-6).

Extrathyroidal Tissues with NIS Sodium Iodide Symporter

The birth of nuclear medicine was made possible by Dr. Saul Hertz, who used radioactive iodine (I-131) to treat the first patient with hyperthyroidism in 1941 at Massachusetts General Hospital. Since then, nuclear medicine imaging has added many other isotopes such as I-123, technetium 99M, and Fluorine-18, to name a few. (27-29)

Radionuclide imaging of the thyroid gland is made possible by the sodium iodide symporter (NIS), the active transport protein embedded in the basolateral membrane of the thyrocyte. The NIS takes up and concentrates iodine in the thyrocytes 20-40 times that of plasma and 100 times greater in Graves' disease. Routine radionuclide scans show radioiodine uptake in non-thyroidal tissues such as the salivary glands, breast tissue, and gastric mucosa. About 80 percent of breast cancers express NIS, the sodium iodide symporter. In 2003, Dr. Geeta Upadhyay studied human breast tumors, finding high expression of the NIS, sodium iodide symporter, thus explaining the ability of breast cancer cells to take up and concentrate iodine. Dr. Geeta Upadhyay suggests the same radioactive iodine (I-131) used in thyroid ablation for thyroid cancer, can be also be used to treat breast cancer, writing:

> We report high NIS expression at both transcriptional and translational levels and its ability to transport iodine in human breast tumors. The in vivo iodine transport ability was confirmed by scintigraphy... The unequivocal demonstration of NIS expression, its functionality, and retention of iodine by organification further provides supportive evidence for the use of radioiodine as an additional treatment modality of human breast carcinoma. (30)

Various other extrathyroidal tissues contain the NIS and take up iodine. These are lacrimal sac and nasolacrimal duct, salivary glands, choroid plexus, stomach, intestine, lactating breast, kidney, placenta, ovary, and prostate. In 2017, Dr. Silvia Ravera writes:

> NIS function is traditionally associated with the thyroid. However, active I– [iodide] transport has also been also demonstrated in other organs, including the lacrimal sac and nasolacrimal duct, salivary glands, choroid plexus, stomach, intestine, and lactating breast. Reverse transcription polymerase chain reaction (RT-PCR) and immunodetection have further uncovered NIS expression in the kidney, placenta, and ovary. (31-36)

Potent Inhibitory Effect on Breast Cancer

A 2017 study by Dr. Zack Xu further elucidated the mechanism of action of molecular iodine on MCF7 breast cancer cell lines, as well as triple negative cell lines, using gene expression analysis, finding potent inhibitory effects on cancer cell growth and dramatic increase in cancer cell death, writing:

> Data from this study indicated that molecular iodine had potent inhibitory effects on cell growth and showed a dramatic increase in cell death in both breast cancer cell lines. Gene expression analysis using quantitative RT-PCR further confirmed that cell cycle genes controlling G1-S phase transition were largely up-regulated. Changes were not seen in Cyclin B expression levels, which further suggest that cells were arrested before entry into cell division. BCL-2, PPAR-α, and PPAR-γ were also up-regulated along with down-regulation of Caspase 3, suggesting molecular iodine-induced cell death through activation of a caspase-independent apoptosis pathway. Interestingly, mesenchymal-epithelial transition (MET) occurrence was noticed upon molecular iodine treatment as indicated by a sharp increase of GATA3 and E-Cadherin and significant down-regulation of Vimentin in invasive MDA-MB231 [breast cancer] cells. Our current study enables us to understand

a molecular mechanism controlling tumor cell growth and demonstrates potent cellular effects of molecular iodine on breast cancer cell lines. These results also demonstrate the promising effects of molecular iodine for the regulation of breast cancer EMT [epithelial to mesenchymal transition] differentiation, which is required for tumor initiation and metastasis. (37)

A 2020 in-vitro study by Dr. Aisyah Elliyanti investigated the effect of iodine (I2), Lugol (I3K), and the combination of both types of iodine on cell proliferation rate of three different types of breast cancer cell lines (luminal A, HER2+, and triple-negative), finding a considerable reduction in proliferation rate, writing:

> In MCF7 cells, I2 [molecular iodine] reduced cell proliferation by 54–94%, and I3K [Lugol's] reduced the proliferation by 74–94%. The effectiveness of I3K treatments in slowing cell proliferation rate was dose-dependent. In SKBR3 cells, I2 reduced proliferation cells up to 85% and I3K 4%-94% depending on the dose. Clonogenic assay results showed discontinuation of the cell proliferation by all doses of I2 and I3K (10 μM and 20 μM)... CONCLUSION: Breast cancer cell lines, representing subtypes of luminal A, HER2+, and triple-negative, show an excellent response to iodine treatments and I3K response shows in a dose-dependent manner. (38)

Note: MCF7 and SKBR3 are breast cancer cell types used in research.

Lung Cancer and Iodine

A 2003 study by Dr. Ling Zhang showed that molecular iodine caused lung cancer cells to undergo programmed cell death, also called apoptosis. These lung cancer cells had been genetically modified to increase iodine uptake. Similarly, a 1993 case report by Dr. Aleck Hercbergs describes spontaneous remission of lung cancer in a patient incidentally treated with amiodarone which contains iodine (about 9 mg per tablet/day). (39-40)

Iodine Combined with Chemotherapy

In 2013 Dr. Alfaro studied breast cancer in mice showing the synergy of molecular iodine combined with conventional chemotherapy (doxorubicin). Dr. Alfaro writes:

> The DOX-I2 (Doxorubicin / Iodine) combination exerts antineoplastic, chemosensitivity, and cardioprotective effects and could be a promising strategy against breast cancer progression. (41)

In 2018, Dr. Zambrano-Estrada studied the Molecular Iodine/Doxorubicin combination in dogs with canine mammary carcinoma finding excellent synergy. Dr Zambrano-Estrada writes:

> The mDOX+I2 (Doxorubicin/Iodine) scheme improves the therapeutic outcome, diminishes the invasive capacity, attenuates the adverse events, and increases disease-free survival. These data led us to propose mDOX+I2 as an effective treatment for canine mammary cancer. (42)

In 2021, Dr. Olga Cuenca-Micó studied the immune component of breast cancer tumor samples in patients treated with combined molecular iodine (5 mg a day oral) and chemotherapy. The study showed molecular iodine activates the immune response with stimulation of the Th1 pathways, i.e., cell-mediated immunity. Dr. Olga Cuenca-Micó writes:

> Molecular iodine (I2) induces apoptotic, antiangiogenic, and anti-proliferative effects in breast cancer cells…. We studied the effect of oral (5 mg/day) I2 supplementation alone (I2) or together with conventional chemotherapy (Cht+I2) on the immune component of breast cancer tumors from a previously published pilot study conducted in Mexico. RNA-seq, I2, and Cht+I2 samples showed significant increases in the expression of Th1 and Th17 pathways. Tumor immune composition determined by deconvolution analysis revealed significant increases in M0 macrophages and B lymphocytes in both I2 groups… In conclusion, our data showed that I2

supplements induce the activation of the immune response and that when combined with Cht, the Th1 pathways are stimulated. (44)

Breast Cancer Xenografts in Mice, Iodine Actives Immune Response

In 2019, Dr. Irasema Mendieta studied triple-negative breast cancer xenografts, finding molecular iodine activates the anti-tumor immune response. Two human breast cancer cell lines with low and high metastatic potential were studied in vitro and in vivo mouse xenografts, finding that iodine decreases the proliferation rate and invasive potential of the cancer cells. Dr. Irasema Mendieta writes:

> The immune system is a crucial component in cancer progression or regression…In vitro analysis showed that the 200 µM I2 supplement decreases the proliferation rate in both cell lines and diminishes the epithelial-mesenchymal transition (EMT) profile and the invasive capacity in MDA-MB231 [breast cancer]. In immunosuppressed mice, the I2 supplement impairs implantation (incidence), tumoral growth, and proliferation of both types of cells. Xenografts of the animals treated with I2 decrease the expression of invasion markers like CD44, vimentin, urokinase plasminogen activator and its receptor, and vascular endothelial growth factor; and increase peroxisome proliferator-activated receptor gamma. Moreover, in mice with xenografts, the I2 supplement increases the circulating level of leukocytes and the number of intratumoral infiltrating lymphocytes, some of them activated as CD8+, suggesting the activation of anti-tumor immune responses….I2 decreases the invasive potential of a triple-negative breast cancer cell line, and under in vivo conditions the oral supplement of this halogen [iodine] activates the anti-tumor immune response, preventing progression of xenografts from laminal and basal mammary cancer cells. These effects allow us to propose iodine supplementation as a possible adjuvant in breast cancer therapy. (45)

Adjuvant Treatment with Iodine in Breast Cancer

In 2019, Dr. Moreno-Vega completed a randomized human study on 60 breast cancer patients treated with adjuvant use of iodine combined with chemotherapy for breast cancer. Thirty women were in the early stage, and thirty women advanced stage breast cancer. Dr. Moreno-Vega writes:

> Five-year disease-free survival rate was significantly higher in patients treated with the I2 [molecular iodine] supplement before and after surgery compared to those receiving the supplement only after surgery (82% versus 46%). I2-treated tumors exhibit less invasive potential and significant increases in apoptosis, estrogen receptor expression, and immune cell infiltration. Transcriptomic analysis indicated activation of the anti-tumoral immune response. The results led us to register a phase III clinical trial to analyze chemotherapy + I2 treatment for advanced breast cancer. (46)

Iodine Combined with Zoledronic Acid for Breast Cancer Bone Metastasis

Breast cancer has a predilection for metastatic spread to the bone, frequently to the ribs in the chest wall. This is routinely treated by mainstream oncology with an IV bisphosphonate drug called Zoledronate. A 2016 study by Dr. Tripathi used a mouse xenograft model to show molecular iodine (Iodoral) has good synergy when combined with Zoledronate. Dr. Tripathi writes:

> We analyzed the effect of the combination of I2 (molecular iodine) with Zol (Zoledronate) as a potent adjuvant therapeutic agent for triple-negative breast cancer cells (MDA-MBA-231) and in the mice model of breast cancer... We report that Zol potentiates the efficacy of I2 by inducing non-mitochondrial intrinsic apoptosis by increasing intracellular calcium and E.R. stress. We show that MDA-MB-231 cells [breast cancer] register minimal hypodiploidy in response to

individual treatment with either I2 or Zol but synergistically enhances apoptosis when given in combination. A similar potentiating effect, as reflected by enhanced apoptotic index on I2-mediated cell death, was also reported in these cells by the addition of chloroquine and by the addition of doxorubicin in other animal tumor models and cancer cells. (43)

Safety of Iodine for Breast Cancer Treatment

In 2007, Dr. Anguiano studied the chronic administration of iodine, finding iodine will diminish mammary fibrosis (fibrocystic disease), reduce chemically induced breast cancer in mice, and has in-vitro anti-cancer effects on breast cancer cell cultures. Dr. Anguiano reports moderately high I2 supplement dosage causes characteristic "Wolff-Chaikoff effect", namely, reduction in sodium/iodide symporter expression, reduction in pendrin, and reduction in thyroperoxidase (TPO) activity. These effects compensate for the high iodine intake and prevent the thyroid gland from converting the excess iodine into dangerously high thyroid hormone levels. Dr. Anguiano found no harmful effects of iodine on thyroid physiology, writing:

> Several studies have demonstrated that moderately high concentrations of molecular iodine (I2) diminish the symptoms of mammary fibrosis in women, reduce the occurrence of mammary cancer induced chemically in rats (50–70%), and have a clear anti-proliferative and apoptotic effect in the human tumoral mammary cell line MCF-7...Nevertheless, the importance of these effects has been underestimated, in part because of the notion that exposure to excess iodine represents a potential risk to thyroid physiology. In the present work, we demonstrate that uptake and metabolism of iodine differ in an organ-specific manner and also depend on the chemical form of the iodine ingested (potassium iodide vs. I2). Further, we show that a moderately high I2 supplement causes some of the characteristics of the "acute Wolff-Chaikoff effect"; namely, it lowers expression of

the sodium/iodide symporter, pendrin, thyroperoxidase (TPO), and deiodinase type 1 in thyroid gland without diminishing circulating levels of thyroid hormone... Finally, we confirm that I2 metabolism is independent of TPO, and we demonstrate that, at the doses used here, which are potentially useful to treat mammary tumors, **chronic I2 supplement is not accompanied by any harmful secondary effects on the thyroid or general physiology.** Thus, we suggest that I2 could be considered for use in clinical trials of breast cancer therapies...I2 increases expression of NIS, PEN, and lactoperoxidase (LPO) in tumoral mammary tissue without any alteration in thyroid physiology. These data indicate that the uptake and metabolism of iodine are organ-specific and differ depending on the chemical form in which it is ingested, and they provide additional evidence that a chronic, moderately high I2 supplement causes no harmful secondary effects on health (e.g., body weight, thyroid economy, or reproductive cycle). **Thus, we propose that I2 supplementation should be considered for use in clinical trials of breast cancer therapies.** (12)

Type of Iodine Supplement for Cancer Prevention and Treatment

One might ask which type of iodine to use, potassium iodide or molecular iodine? For anti-cancer effects, molecular iodine (I2) is recommended, found in Lugol's and Iodoral, rather than potassium iodide (K.I.). Molecular Iodone (I2) is used for breast cancer, while potassium iodide (KI) is used for Grave's disease, and iodine deficiency.

How to Enhance Anti-Cancer Effects of Iodine-Autophagy Inhibitors

In 2011, Dr. Preeti Singh studied the effect of autophagy inhibition with chloroquine on estrogen receptor-negative breast cancer In vitro and in vivo, finding enhanced efficacy, writing:

These data indicate that inhibition of autophagy renders E.R. (-ve) breast tumor cells more sensitive to I(2) induced apoptosis. Thus, I(2), together with autophagy inhibitor, could have a potential monostatic role in E.R. (-ve) aggressive breast tumors that may be evaluated in future studies. (47)

A widely available over-the-counter antihistamine, loratadine, is a "cationic amphiphilic antihistamine" that accumulates in lysosomes and serves as an autophagy inhibitor. Studies show loratadine has anti-cancer effects for breast cancer. Rather than use chloroquine, one might speculate on the synergy of autophagy inhibitor loratadine combined with iodine in breast cancer. Another class of drugs, PPI antiacids such as omeprazole, may serve as autophagy inhibitors for breast cancer treatment. (48-52)

Cracking Cancer Toolkit Molecular Iodine Treatment for Breast Cancer

My previous 2020 book, Cracking Cancer Toolkit discusses the use of iodine for breast cancer treatment. Here is a quote from my book:

Over the years, a number of studies have accumulated evidence that molecular iodine is effective treatment for breast cancer. The mechanism of action (MOA) involves activation of peroxisome proliferator-activated receptors (PPAR) and production of iodolactones, which mediate apoptotic effects. ...A drop of the 2% iodine Lugol's solution contains 1 mg of molecular iodine (I2) and 2 mg of potassium iodide (I-). An iodine supplement called Iodoral® is available for people who prefer Lugol's iodine in tablet form. The tablet avoids annoying yellow stains on clothing from accidental spills of the liquid product.... The anti-cancer effects of iodine are thought to be related to the type of iodine used, with molecular iodine (I2) and not iodide (I-) considered the effective anti-cancer agent, via increasing expression of PPAR-gamma (peroxisome proliferator-activated receptor gamma), which in turn induces cancer cell apoptosis…Activation of the PPAR nuclear receptor family requires a vitamin A cofactor such as ATRA. In 2020, Dr. Irasema Mendeita found that molecular iodine (which activates PPARgamma) augmented the anti-cancer activity of ATRA in a neuroblastoma model. Similarly, fenofibrate activates PPAR by forming a heterodimer with the retinoid X receptor (RXR)…Iodine treatment has a dual anti-cancer effect. It has a direct anti-cancer effect by inducing apoptosis of the cancer cells, and secondarily, iodine "activates the anti-tumor immune response." In 2019, Dr. Aura Morena-Vega et al. studied the use of molecular iodine in thirty breast cancer patients, either alone or as adjuvant with chemotherapy, in two groups— early and advanced. In the early group, thirty women were treated with either 5 mg per day of molecular iodine (I2) or placebo for 7 to 35 days before surgery. For the advanced group, all patients received chemotherapy (5-fluorouracil/epirubicin/cyclophosphamide or Taxotere/epirubicin (FEC/TE) and were randomized to receive either molecular iodine 5mg/day or placebo before and 170 days after surgery. Five-year disease-free survival was significantly higher for patients treated with molecular iodine (I2) before and after surgery compared to placebo—82 percent vs. 46 percent. Examination of histology of tissue samples showed Iodine-treated patients had "activation of the anti-tumoral immune response."…Dr. Moreno-Vega et al. write: I2 supplementation showed a significant attenuation of the [chemotherapy] side effects and an absence of tumor chemoresistance … I2-treated tumors exhibit less invasive potential, and significant increases in apoptosis, estrogen receptor expression, and immune cell infiltration….Transcriptomic analysis indicated activation of the anti-tumoral immune response…In 2019, further studies by Dr. Irasema Mendieta et al. using human breast cancer cell lines in vitro and in vivo animal xenografts confirm Dr. Morena's conclusions, finding that supplementation with I2 reduced the ability to implant tumor cells into immunosuppressed mice and reduced the proliferation rate and invasive capacity of the cancer cells. Various cancer markers, such as CD44 and vascular endothelial growth factor (VEGF), were reduced by iodine, and PPAR-gamma was increased. In the mouse xenograft model, evidence of immune enhancement was seen with increased levels of circulating immune cells (leukocytes) and increased intra-tumor infiltration of CD8+ lymphocytes (anti-tumor lymphocytes). Dr. Mendieta proposes iodine supplementation as a possible adjuvant in breast cancer therapy, writing: I2 [iodine] decreases the invasive potential of a triple-negative basal cancer cell line, and under in vivo conditions the oral supplement of this halogen [iodine] activates the anti-tumor immune response, preventing progression of xenografts from laminal and basal mammary cancer cells. These effects allow us to propose iodine supplementation as a possible adjuvant in breast cancer therapy. (53)

Note: this the above quote is taken from my previous book, Cracking Cancer Toolkit by Jeffrey Dach, MD.

How to Obtain Iodine Tablets

Iodine supplements in the form of Lugol's Solution and Iodoral tablets are widely available without a prescription. However, it is advisable to work with a knowledgeable physician who can monitor the patient and perform serial laboratory studies.

Iodine Adverse Effects

Extremely large quantities of iodine are routinely prescribed by physicians in the form of SSKI for COPD (chronic obstructive lung disease) and amiodarone for cardiac arrhythmias. These are well tolerated for the most part, with a few adverse events reported, such as metallic taste, headache, G.I. upset, and skin rash thought to be related to dermo-bromism. Iodine is contra-indicated in a few relatively rare thyroid conditions, such as toxic multi-nodular goiter and autonomous thyroid nodule, in which case the administration of iodine supplements, such as iodized salt, may induce hyperthyroidism which can be fatal in some cases. These are all good reasons to be under the care of a competent healthcare professional who can monitor the patient during such treatment. High-dose iodine supplementation during pregnancy is important for fetal development, yet may influence fetal thyroid function on prenatal testing, so caution is advised. In addition to iodine supplementation, a typical breast cancer prevention program includes DIM (di-indole-methane) and calcium-D-glucarate while avoiding xeno-estrogens in food and plastics. Testing for selenium and vitamin D3 is also useful.

Conclusion

Ignoring the role of iodine in breast cancer prevention and treatment is another error in modern endocrinology. Abundant medical research suggests the use of molecular iodine for the prevention and adjuvant treatment of breast cancer. Iodine may also benefit lung cancer, melanoma, and prostate cancer. Iodine may be an adjunct in breast cancer treatment combined with conventional chemotherapy or I.V. Zoledronate. Further research on iodine for breast cancer should receive priority for NIH funding. (54-75)

Financial Disclosure: The author has no financial interest in books or iodine supplements mentioned above, except for the author's book, Cracking Cancer Toolkit.

♦ References for Chapter 32

1) Brownstein, David. Iodine: Why You Need It, Why You Can't Live Without It. Medical Alternatives Press, 2008.

2) Nagataki, Shigenobu. "The Average of Dietary Iodine Intake Due to the Ingestion of Seaweeds is 1.2 mg/day in Japan." Thyroid 18.6 (2008): 667-668.

3) Zava, Theodore T., and David T. Zava. "Assessment of Japanese Iodine Intake Based on Seaweed Consumption in Japan: A Literature-Based Analysis." Thyroid Research 4.1 (2011): 14.

4) Smyth, Peter. "The Thyroid, Iodine, and Breast Cancer." Breast Cancer Research 5.5 (2003): 1-4.

5) Rappaport, Jay. "Changes in Dietary Iodine Explains the Increasing Incidence of Breast Cancer with Distant Involvement in Young Women." Journal of Cancer 8.2 (2017): 174

6) Cann, Stephen A., et al. "Hypothesis: Iodine, Selenium and the Development of Breast Cancer." Cancer Causes and Control 11.2 (2000): 121-127.

7) Smyth, Peter PA. "Iodine, Seaweed, and the Thyroid." European Thyroid Journal 10.2 (2021): 101-108.

8) Venturi, Sebastiano, et al. "Role of Iodine in Evolution and Carcinogenesis of Thyroid, Breast, and Stomach." Advances in Clinical Pathology 4 (2000): 11-18.

9) Derry, David Michael. Breast Cancer and Iodine. Bloomington, IN: Trafford, 2001.

10) Shrivastava, Ashutosh, et al. "Molecular Iodine Induces Caspase-Independent Apoptosis in Human Breast Carcinoma Cells Involving the Mitochondria-Mediated Pathway." Journal of Biological Chemistry 281.28 (2006): 19762-19771.

11) Aceves, Carmen, et al. "Antineoplastic Effect of Iodine in Mammary Cancer: Participation of 6-Iodolactone (6-IL) and Peroxisome Proliferator-Activated Receptors (PPAR)." Molecular Cancer 8.1 (2009): 1-9.

12) Anguiano, B., et al. "Uptake and Gene Expression with Anti-Tumoral Doses of Iodine in Thyroid and Mammary Gland: Evidence That Chronic Administration Has No Harmful Effects." Thyroid: Official Journal of the American Thyroid Association 17.9 (2007): 851.

13) Arroyo-Helguera, O., et al. "Uptake and Anti-Proliferative Effect of Molecular Iodine in the MCF-7 Breast Cancer Cell Line." Endocrine-Related Cancer 13.4 (2006): 1147-1158.

14) Arroyo-Helguera, O., et al. "Signaling Pathways Involved in the Anti-Proliferative Effect of Molecular Iodine in Normal and Tumoral Breast Cells: Evidence That 6-Iodolactone Mediates Apoptotic Effects." Endocrine-Related Cancer 15.4 (2008): 1003-1011.

15) Rillema, James A., and Melissa A. Hill. "Pendrin Transporter Carries Out Iodide Uptake Into MCF-7 Human Mammary Cancer Cells." Experimental Biology and Medicine 228.9 (2003): 1078-1082.

16) Funahashi, Hiroomi, et al. "Seaweed Prevents Breast Cancer?" Japanese Journal of Cancer Research 92.5 (2001): 483-487.

17) Lanari, Claudia Lee Malvina, et al. "The MPA Mouse Breast Cancer Model: Evidence for a Role of Progesterone Receptors in Breast Cancer." (2009).

18) Molinolo, A. A., et al. "Mouse Mammary Tumors Induced by Medroxyprogesterone Acetate: Immunohistochemistry and Hormonal Receptors." Journal of the National Cancer Institute 79.6 (1987): 1341-1350.

19) Pazos, Patricia, et al. "Mammary Carcinogenesis Induced by N-Methyl-N-Nitrosourea (MNU) and Medroxyprogesterone Acetate (MPA) in BALB/C Mice." Breast Cancer Research and Treatment 20 (1991): 133-138.

20) Lanari, Claudia, et al. "Induction of Mammary Adenocarcinomas by Medroxyprogesterone Acetate in Balbc Female Mice." Cancer letters 33.2 (1986): 215-223.

21) Bender, Rukiye Ada. "Medroxyprogesterone Acetate for Abnormal Uterine Bleeding Due to Ovulatory Dysfunction: The Effect of 2 Different-Duration Regimens." Medical Science Monitor: International Medical Journal of Experimental and Clinical Research 28 (2022): e936727-1.

22) Munro, Malcolm G., et al. "Oral Medroxyprogesterone Acetate and Combination Oral Contraceptives for Acute Uterine Bleeding: A Randomized Controlled Trial." Obstetrics & Gynecology 108.4 (2006): 924-929.

23) Stoddard II, Frederick R., et al. "Iodine Alters Gene Expression in the MCF7 Breast Cancer Cell Line: Evidence for an Anti-Estrogen Effect of Iodine." International Journal of Medical Sciences 5.4 (2008): 189.

24) Nava-Villalba, Mario, and Carmen Aceves. "6-Iodolactone, a Key Mediator of Anti-Tumoral Properties of Iodine." Prostaglandins & Other Lipid Mediators 112 (2014): 27-33.

25) Álvarez-León, Winniberg, et al. "Molecular Iodine/Cyclophosphamide Synergism on Chemoresistant Neuroblastoma Models." International Journal of Molecular Sciences 22.16 (2021): 8936.

26) Mendieta, Irasema, et al. "Molecular Iodine Synergized and Sensitized Neuroblastoma Cells to the Antineoplastic Effect of ATRA." Endocrine-Related Cancer 27.12 (2020): 699-710.

27) Fahey, Frederic H., and Frederick D. Grant. "Celebrating Eighty Years of Radionuclide Therapy and the Work of Saul Hertz." Journal of Applied Clinical Medical Physics 22.1 (2021): 4-10.

28) Hertz, Barbara. "Dr. Saul Hertz Discovers the Medical Uses of Radioiodine (RAI)." J Radiol Oncol 2 (2018): 3-54.

29) Hertz, Saul, and Arthur Roberts. "Radioactive Iodine in the Study of Thyroid Physiology: VII. The Use of Radioactive Iodine Therapy in Hyperthyroidism." Journal of the American Medical Association 131.2 (1946): 81-86.

30) Upadhyay, Geeta, et al. "Functional Expression of Sodium Iodide Symporter (NIS) in Human Breast Cancer Tissue." Breast Cancer Research and Treatment 77 (2003): 157-165.

31) Ravera, Silvia, et al. "The Sodium/Iodide Symporter (NIS): Molecular Physiology and Preclinical and Clinical Applications." Annual Review of Physiology 79 (2017): 261-289.

32) Chung, June-Key. "Sodium Iodide Symporter: Its Role in Nuclear Medicine." Journal Of Nuclear Medicine 43.9 (2002): 1188-1200.

33) Wapnir, Irene L., et al. "The Na+/I− Symporter Mediates Iodide Uptake in Breast Cancer Metastases and Can Be Selectively Down-Regulated in the Thyroid." Clinical Cancer Research 10.13 (2004): 4294-4302.

34) Micali, Salvatore, et al. "Sodium Iodide Symporter (NIS) in Extrathyroidal Malignancies: Focus on Breast and Urological Cancer." BMC Cancer 14.1 (2014): 1-12.

35) Lacroix, Ludovic, et al. "Na (+)/I (-) Symporter and Pendred Syndrome Gene and Protein Expressions in Human Extra-Thyroidal Tissues." European Journal of Endocrinology 144.3 (2001): 297-302.

36) Aranda, Nuri, et al. "Uptake and Anti-Tumoral Effects of Iodine and 6-Iodolactone in Differentiated and Undifferentiated Human Prostate Cancer Cell Lines." The Prostate 73.1 (2013): 31-41.

37) Xu, Zack, et al. "Elucidating the Mechanism of Action of Molecular Iodine on Breast Cancer Cells." Cancer Research 77.13_Supplement (2017): 2243-2243.

38) Elliyanti, Aisyah, et al. "An Iodine Treatments Effect on Cell Proliferation Rates of Breast Cancer Cell Lines; In Vitro Study." Open Access Macedonian Journal of Medical Sciences 8.B (2020): 1064-1070.

39) Zhang, Ling, et al. "Nonradioactive Iodide Effectively Induces Apoptosis in Genetically Modified Lung Cancer Cells." Cancer Research 63.16 (2003): 5065-5072.

40) Hercbergs, Aleck, and John T. Leith. "Spontaneous Remission of Metastatic Lung Cancer Following Myxedema Coma—An Apoptosis-Related Phenomenon?" JNCI: Journal of the National Cancer Institute 85.16 (1993): 1342-1343.

41) Alfaro, Yunuen, et al. "Iodine and Doxorubicin, a Good Combination for Mammary Cancer Treatment: Antineoplastic Adjuvant, Chemoresistance Inhibition, and Cardioprotection." Molecular cancer 12.1 (2013): 1-11.

42) Zambrano-Estrada, Xóchitl, et al. "Molecular Iodine/Doxorubicin Neoadjuvant Treatment Impair Invasive Capacity and Attenuate Side Effect in Canine Mammary Cancer." BMC Veterinary Research 14.1 (2018): 1-14.

43) Tripathi, Ranu, et al. "Zoledronate and Molecular Iodine Cause Synergistic Cell Death in Triple-Negative Breast Cancer Through Endoplasmic Reticulum Stress." Nutrition and Cancer 68.4 (2016): 679-688.

44) Cuenca-Micó, Olga, et al. "Effects of Molecular Iodine/Chemotherapy in the Immune Component of Breast Cancer Tumoral Microenvironment." Biomolecules 11.10 (2021): 1501.

45) Mendieta, Irasema, et al. "Molecular Iodine Exerts Antineoplastic Effects by Diminishing Proliferation and Invasive Potential and Activating the Immune Response in Mammary Cancer Xenografts." BMC Cancer 19.1 (2019): 261.

46) Moreno-Vega, Aura, et al. "Adjuvant Effect of Molecular Iodine in Conventional Chemotherapy for Breast Cancer. Randomized Pilot Study." Nutrients 11.7 (2019): 1623.

47) Singh, Preeti, et al. "Inhibition of Autophagy Stimulate Molecular Iodine-Induced Apoptosis in Hormone-Independent Breast Tumors." Biochemical and Biophysical Research Communications 415.1 (2011): 181-186.

48) Olsson, Hakan Lars, et al. "Effects of Antihistamine Use on Survival in Breast Cancer." (2018): e12527-e12527.

49) Ellegaard, Anne-Marie, et al. "Repurposing Cationic Amphiphilic Antihistamines for Cancer Treatment." EBioMedicine 9 (2016): 130-139.

50) Olsson, Håkan Lars, et al "Abstract P5-06-07: Desloratadine and Loratadine Increase Breast Cancer Survival." (2020): P5-06.

51) Lu, Zhen-Ning, et al. "Repositioning of Proton Pump Inhibitors in Cancer Therapy." Cancer Chemotherapy and Pharmacology 80 (2017): 925-937.

52) Ihraiz, Worood G., et al. "Proton Pump Inhibitors Enhance Chemosensitivity, Promote Apoptosis, and Suppress Migration of Breast Cancer Cells." Acta Pharmaceutica 70.2 (2020): 179-190.

53) Dach, Jeffrey. Cracking Cancer Toolkit: Using Repurposed Drugs for Cancer Treatment. Medical Muse Press. 2020.

54) Cann, Stephen A., et al. "Hypothesis: Iodine, Selenium and the Development of Breast Cancer." Cancer Causes and Control 11.2 (2000): 121-127.

55) Tazebay, Uygar H., et al. "The Mammary Gland Iodide Transporter Is Expressed During Lactation and in Breast Cancer." Nature Medicine 6.8 (2000): 871-878.

56) Venturi, Sebastiano, et al. "Role of Iodine in Evolution and Carcinogenesis of Thyroid, Breast, And Stomach." Advances in Clinical Pathology 4 (2000): 11-18.

57) Venturi, Sebastiano. "Is There a Role for Iodine in Breast Diseases?" The Breast 10.5 (2001): 379-382.

58) Kessler, Jack H. "The Effect of Supraphysiologic Levels of Iodine on Patients with Cyclic Mastalgia." The Breast Journal 10.4 (2004): 328-336.

59) Ghent, W. R., et al. "Iodine Replacement in Fibrocystic Disease of the Breast." Canadian Journal of Surgery. 36.5 (1993): 453-460.

60) Dwyer, Roisin M., et al. "In Vivo Radioiodide Imaging and Treatment of Breast Cancer Xenografts After MUC1-Driven Expression of the Sodium Iodide Symporter." Clinical Cancer Research 11.4 (2005): 1483-1489.

61) Carroll, Candace E., et al. "Curcumin Delays the Development Of MPA-Accelerated DMBA-Induced Mammary Tumors." Menopause (New York, NY) 17.1 (2010): 178.

62) Aldaz, C. Marcelo, et al. "Medroxyprogesterone Acetate Accelerates the Development and Increases the Incidence of Mouse Mammary Tumors Induced by Dimethylbenzanthracene." Carcinogenesis 17.9 (1996): 2069-2072.

63) Lanari, Claudia, et al. "The MPA Mouse Breast Cancer Model: Evidence for a Role of Progesterone Receptors in Breast Cancer." Endocrine-Related Cancer 16.2 (2009): 333-350.

64) Aceves, Carmen, et al. "Is Iodine a Gatekeeper of the Integrity of the Mammary Gland?" Journal of Mammary Gland Biology and Neoplasia 10.2 (2005): 189-196.

65) Anguiano, Brenda, and Carmen Aceves. "Iodine In Mammary and Prostate Pathologies." Current Chemical Biology 5.3 (2011): 177-182.

66) Elliyanti, Aisyah, et al. "An Iodine Treatments Effect on Cell Proliferation Rates of Breast Cancer Cell Lines; In Vitro Study." Open Access Macedonian Journal of Medical Sciences 8.B (2020): 1064-1070.

67) Vega-Riveroll, L. et al. "The Antineoplastic Effect of Molecular Iodine on Human Mammary Cancer Involves the Activation of Apoptotic Pathways and the Inhibition of Angiogenesis." Cancer Research 69.2_Supplement (2009): 3082.

68) Rösner, Harald, et al. "Anti-Proliferative/Cytotoxic Effects of Molecular Iodine, Povidone-Iodine and Lugol's Solution in Different Human Carcinoma Cell Lines." Oncology Letters 12.3 (2016): 2159-2162.

69) Patrick, Lyn. "Iodine: Deficiency and Therapeutic Considerations." Alternative Medicine Review 13.2 (2008).

70) Aceves, Carmen, et al. "Molecular Iodine Has Extrathyroidal Effects as an Antioxidant, Differentiator, and Immunomodulator." International Journal of Molecular Sciences 22.3 (2021): 1228.

71) Torremante, Pompilio Elio, and Harald Rosner. "Anti-Proliferative Effects of Molecular Iodine in Cancers." Curr Chem Biol 5.3 (2011): 168-76.

72) Malya, Fatma Umit, et al. "The Correlation Between Breast Cancer and Urinary Iodine Excretion Levels." Journal of International Medical Research 46.2 (2018): 687-692.

73) Bontempo, Alexander, et al. "Molecular Iodine Impairs Chemoresistance Mechanisms, Enhances Doxorubicin Retention and Induces Downregulation of the CD44+/CD24+ And E-Cadherin+/Vimentin+ Subpopulations In MCF-7 Cells Resistant to Low Doses of Doxorubicin." Oncology Reports 38.5 (2017): 2867-2876.

74) Bigoni-Ordóñez, Gabriele Davide, et al. "Molecular Iodine Inhibits the Expression of Stemness Markers on Cancer Stem-Like Cells of Established Cell Lines Derived from Cervical Cancer." BMC Cancer 18.1 (2018): 1-12.

75) Cuenca, Olga, et al. "Molecular Iodine Activates Cytotoxic Immune Response in Breast Cancer Tumor Microenvironment." The Journal of Immunology 204.1_Supplement (2020): 241-8.

Chapter 33

The Thyroid Nodule Epidemic

A 36-Year-Old Female with Hypothyroidism After Thyroidectomy for Papillary Thyroid Cancer

LISA IS A 36-YEAR-OLD MODEL and actress who underwent total thyroidectomy for small papillary thyroid cancer. After the surgery, Lisa's endocrinologist prescribed a small dose of levothyroxine which did not help Lisa's low thyroid symptoms with continuing fatigue, muscle pain, hair loss, and dry skin.

Finding Thyroid Nodules on Screening Ultrasound

How did Lisa end up with a thyroidectomy? Her family doctor palpated her thyroid gland and was not sure if he felt a nodule, so he ordered a thyroid ultrasound which showed a small nodule, 9 mm in size. The doctor then recommended an ultrasound-guided needle biopsy "just to be sure." The biopsy report came back as "papillary carcinoma of the thyroid." As you can imagine, Lisa was distraught to learn she had thyroid cancer. "Not to worry," said her doctor, "You have an excellent prognosis and a high likelihood for cure after surgery followed by radioactive iodine treatment."

Lisa Undergoes Surgery and Radiation – Complete Thyroidectomy

Grateful to her doctors, Lisa underwent thyroid surgery and radiation. Since the neck surgeon removed the entire thyroid gland, Lisa now takes thyroid medication every day. She also returns for screening tests every year to check for recurrent cancer.

Adverse Effects of Treatment

Unfortunately, Lisa was not spared the adverse effects of her treatment. The surgery had disturbed her recurrent laryngeal nerve, leaving her with chronic hoarseness, cough, and voice change. The surgery also removed the parathyroid glands leaving her at risk for osteoporosis. The radioactive iodine treatment caused salivary gland damage, leaving her with a chronic dry mouth and bad taste. The radioactive iodine also carried an increased generalized cancer risk over her lifetime and, of course, a detrimental effect on the ovaries and fertility, which may influence her decision to have a family.

Switching from Levothyroxine to Natural Thyroid

I explained to Lisa that her symptoms of hypothyroidism were caused by inadequate dosage of thyroid medication. Her levothyroxine (generic Synthroid) dosage was insufficient. We switched Lisa to NDT, natural desiccated thyroid. In addition, Lisa was given iodine supplements. Three weeks later, Lisa called to report a dramatic improvement, relief from chronic fatigue, and better energy.

A Cancer with No Biological Significance

Twenty years ago, while working as an interventional and diagnostic radiologist in the hospital, I performed many ultrasound needle biopsies of thyroid nodules on patients sent to me by primary care doctors and endocrinologists. Thyroid nodules are quite common and can be easily found using ultrasound imaging in 60 percent of the population. Most nodules are benign; however, occasionally, the biopsy shows a small papillary carcinoma, a relatively benign tumor with an excellent prognosis of no clinical significance. Despite the benign nature of these tumors, conventional medicine treats them aggressively with thyroidectomy and radioactive iodine (I-131). (1-3)

A Frustrated Radiologist Says: Turn Off the Ultrasound Machines

In June 2008, an exasperated radiologist, John J. Cronan, MD, published his opinion in the journal, Radiology, writing: "We should turn off the ultrasound machines." Dr. Cronin questioned this entire medical enterprise of detecting thyroid nodules and small cancers with ultrasound-guided biopsy, writing:

> From the patient perspective, we have hung the psychological stigma of cancer on these patients and the dependency on daily thyroid supplementation... We accept all these consequences to control a cancer with a 99% 10-year survival. (2)

A Normal Finding in Finland

Dr. H. Rubén Harach says occult papillary carcinoma of the thyroid is a "normal finding" in Finland and does not cause biologically significant disease. Dr. Louise Davies agrees with Dr. Harach and says in JAMA, "Papillary cancers smaller than 1 cm could be classified as a normal finding". (5-7)

Our Quixotic Approach to Thyroid Nodules

In 2006 at the Hayes Martin lecture, Dr. Keith Heller, a neck surgeon with a 28-year career during which he performed 1,000 thyroidectomies for thyroid cancer, addressed his colleagues, saying he did not believe the epidemic of thyroid cancer is real. Here is an excerpt from his 2006 talk:

> I do not believe that this epidemic of (thyroid cancer) is real. It is due to... the increasing use of ultrasound-guided needle biopsy of thyroid nodules. We

may be diagnosing and treating cancers that have no clinical significance... We have embarked on a quixotic quest to rid our patients of microscopic and probably clinically unimportant thyroid cancer... We are performing far too many unnecessary thyroidectomies. (4)

Japan to the Rescue – Watchful Waiting

In 2003, Dr. Yasuhiro Ito of Kobe, Japan, agreed with Dr. Heller, proposing a thyroid-sparing approach for papillary thyroid cancer, and has several studies to back up his statements. Patients may choose observation rather than surgery if their tumors are not progressing. Dr. Ito published this article in thyroid, writing:

> Our preliminary data suggest that papillary microcarcinomas do not frequently become clinically apparent and that patients can choose observation while their tumors are not progressing, although they are pathologically multifocal and involve lymph nodes in high incidence. (8)

Dr. Ito observed 162 patients with papillary thyroid microcarcinoma less than 10 mm size (< 10 mm) over 8 years. 70% of tumors either remained stable or decreased in size. Only 10% enlarged by more than 10 mm. Only 1.2% of patients developed neck node metastasis over the eight years of observation. Because of this study, Dr. Ito says the patient can opt for watchful waiting with serial ultrasound follow-up studies. Dr. Ito says that if follow-up ultrasound shows enlarging tumor, or enlarging metastatic neck nodes, then more aggressive surgical treatment is indicated with an excellent prognosis. (8)

In another study of 52 cases, Dr. Ito found when papillary thyroid cancer is found incidentally after thyroid surgery while examining the histology slides; then no further surgery is needed. (9-10)

It is the Pathologist's Fault – Just Stop Calling It Cancer

Perhaps this whole problem is caused by incorrect terminology used by the pathologist who reviews the biopsy slide and uses the word "cancer," which strikes fear and creates undue stress. Once a pathology report with the word "cancer" is placed on the desk, rationality gets thrown out the window, and the patient demands aggressive treatment, usually out of proportion to the actual pathology.

In the 2003 issue of the International Journal of Surgical Pathology, Dr. Rosai presented the Porto Proposal, in which he proposed a change in terminology. Instead of "cancer," he suggested the wording "papillary microtumor". Others, Dr. Hazard et al., proposed a "nonencapsulated thyroid tumor" because "the surgeon may become unduly alarmed when the pathologist reports the presence of carcinoma." Dr. Harach et al. proposed the term occult papillary tumor "in order to avoid unnecessary operations and serious psychologic effects on patients." (11-12)

Is Treatment of Papillary Micro-Carcinoma Overly Aggressive?

Over the years, surgical treatment for breast cancer evolved from the overly aggressive and debilitating radical mastectomy procedure to the current-day simple lumpectomy for many small breast cancers. Perhaps treatment for thyroid cancer is going in this same direction and is playing "catch-up" with the more limited breast cancer treatments.

No Improvement in Long Term Outcome over 40 Years

In 2008, Dr. Ian Hay from the Mayo Clinic, Rochester, Minnesota, published in Endocrine Abstracts his study of 900 patients followed with papillary thyroid microcarcinoma over 54 years. Dr. Ian Hay writes:

> Neither total thyroidectomy nor postoperative Radioactive Iodine Ablation improved long-term outcomes during 40 years, in terms of either tumor recurrence or cause-specific mortality. (13)

Dr. Ian Hay advocates the removal of the tumor with unilateral lobectomy, saying that it was unnecessary to perform total thyroidectomy, nor radioactive iodine treatment, since neither improves prognosis compared to unilateral thyroid lobectomy alone. (13)

The Role of Iodine Supplementation

You might ask the obvious question, "Thyroid nodules are found in 67% of the population. What is causing this?" As discussed in previous chapters of this book, iodine deficiency in the population causes thyroid enlargement (goiter), thyroid nodules, and thyroid cancer. Thyroid cancer appears to be linked to iodine deficiency in both animal models and humans. Studies have shown that iodine deficiency is associated with increased anaplastic thyroid cancer, the aggressive type unresponsive to treatment, with a high mortality rate. Population studies in which iodine supplements are given showed reduced mortality from thyroid cancer. Incidentally, this reduced mortality was also associated with an increase in well-differentiated papillary cancers, suggesting the papillary type is associated with a better outcome. Make sure to take iodine supplements to reduce the risk of dangerous types of thyroid cancer. (14-19)

JAMA - Thyroid Cancer Epidemic is Due to Over-Diagnosis

In 2014, Drs. Welch and Davies wrote in JAMA Otolaryngology the incidence of thyroid cancer has tripled. They state this is not an epidemic of disease but rather an epidemic of overdiagnosis. Drs. Welch and Davies write:

> Since 1975, the incidence of thyroid cancer has now nearly tripled, from 5 to 15 per 100,000 population, mostly from papillary thyroid cancer. The ongoing epidemic of thyroid cancer in the United States is not an

epidemic of disease but rather an epidemic of diagnosis. The problem is particularly acute for women. (1)

In 2015: Dr. Cosimo Durante reported on the natural history of benign thyroid nodules, writing:

Among patients with asymptomatic, sonographically, or cytologically benign thyroid nodules, the majority of nodules **exhibited no significant size increase during five years of follow-up**, and thyroid cancer was rare. These findings support consideration of revision of current guideline recommendations for follow-up of asymptomatic thyroid nodules. (20) Emphasis Mine.

Large or Increasing Size of Thyroid Nodule

For patients with nodules that are large or increasing in size on serial sonograms, aspiration needle biopsy is recommended, and if the biopsy is positive for cancer diagnosis, then the patient is referred for thyroid surgery, usually partial or total thyroidectomy. If needle biopsy is negative or inconclusive, then the nodule is followed with serial ultrasound while the patient is treated medically with TSH suppression using thyroid medication, either NDT or levothyroxine. Iodine supplements are also used as needed. The etiology of thyroid nodules is thought to be the mutagenic effect of excess hydrogen peroxide generation arising from long-term iodine deficiency. TSH suppression inhibits hydrogen peroxide generation, thus removing mutagenic stimulus. In addition, myo-inositol may be useful for reducing the size of thyroid nodules. See Chapter 28 on Myo-Inositol for further discussion. (27-35)

In 2020, Dr. Giorgio Grani studied contemporary thyroid nodule evaluation and management, writing:

More recently, however, a prospective study found that nodules displaying significant growth during follow-up (diameter increases exceeding 2 mm per year) [on ultrasound follow-up] are significantly more likely to be malignant than slower-growing nodules and, therefore, warrant repeat biopsy. (33)

Post-Op Thyroidectomy Follow Up

Mainstream endocrinologists typically treat postoperative thyroid cancer patients with TSH suppression using adequate doses of thyroid medication, usually levothyroxine. In my office, we prefer to use NDT. In addition, all post-op thyroid cancer patients are followed with the serum thyroglobulin test, as discussed by Dr. Keith Heller. This test is excellent for the detection of recurrent thyroid cancer. We do not routinely do postoperative neck ultrasound studies as we have found high false positive rates; the detection of benign cervical lymph nodes makes this test relatively useless. In 2019, Dr. Lauren Orr agreed with this conclusion in post-thyroidectomy patients, yearly neck ultrasounds can be avoided, and only blood tests for thyroglobulin are needed. (4) (36)

Anaplastic Thyroid Cancer

Quite the opposite of the benign indolent nature of papillary thyroid cancer, anaplastic thyroid cancer is rare and one of the most aggressive cancers known, with a median survival of 3.16 months. Approximately 350 to 700 people die from anaplastic thyroid cancer annually in the US. Anaplastic thyroid cancer is so aggressive that surgery and radioactive iodine treatment is considered futile, having no effect on the dismal prognosis. (37-42)

In 2020, Dr. Simone De Leo reviewed the management of anaplastic thyroid cancer and writes:

Anaplastic thyroid cancer (ATC) is the rarest type of thyroid cancer but also the deadliest. Its incidence has been constant during the last four decades and it accounts for around 1–2% of all thyroid cancer diagnoses...Anaplastic thyroid cancer (ATC) is undoubtedly the thyroid cancer histotype with the poorest prognosis. ATC is generally managed with a combination of surgery, chemotherapy, and radiotherapy; however, its prognosis is still dire...the improvement in the survival of these patients seems still to be a very difficult task, since to date even the molecules [drugs] with the best results reported a not significantly durable disease control, apart from some anecdotal cases. (42)

A 15-Year Update by Dr. Davies

In 2021, Dr. Louise Davies provides an update on thyroid cancer overdiagnosis since awareness was first raised 15 years earlier. Dr. Davies notes a 240 percent increase in detection and diagnosis of thyroid cancer between 1973 and 2002. This is an incidence rate of 7.7 people per 100,000. However, mortality due to thyroid cancer is and had not changed, 0.5 per 100,000 population. Although mortality from thyroid cancer is 0.0005 percent, autopsy studies show an 11.2 percent incidence of thyroid cancer found in people dying from other causes, indicating a large reservoir of clinically insignificant disease. Of the 11.2 percent of autopsies revealing thyroid cancer, 11.1995 percent are clinically insignificant. Dr. Davies writes:

> Nearly 15 years has passed since the Davies and Welch publication first raised broad awareness about overdiagnosis of thyroid cancer in the USA. Overdiagnosis is the detection of subclinical disease that would have been unlikely to go on to become clinically apparent had it not been found through testing. Between 1973 and 2002, annual incidence of detected thyroid cancer cases increased 240% to 7·7 per 100 000 people. Mortality due to thyroid cancer during that time period was low and had not changed significantly, at 0·5 per 100 000 population. The majority of the incident cases were due to papillary histology, and this was also the type of thyroid cancer that had been responsible for virtually the entire increase in incidence. Davies and Welch suggested the detection of subclinical disease was likely the reason for the increase, because papillary thyroid cancer is commonly found at autopsy in people who

have died of other causes, never knowing they had a thyroid cancer. A meta-analysis of autopsy studies has since shown that the prevalence of thyroid cancer in people who have died of other causes is 11·2%. (43-45)

In 2016, Dr. Luis Furuya-Kanamori conducted a meta-analysis of autopsy studies over 6 decades showing the prevalence of incidental differentiated thyroid cancer (iDTC) is common at autopsy, and most likely reflects increasing diagnostic detection of papillary thyroid cancer using thyroid ultrasound, unlikely to reflect a true population increase in tumorgenesis, meaning this is an epidemic of diagnosis, not an epidemic of disease. Dr. Luis Furuya-Kanamori writes:

> The current study confirms that iDTC [incidental differentiated thyroid cancer] is common, but the **observed increasing incidence is not mirrored by prevalence within autopsy studies** and, therefore, is unlikely to reflect a true population-level increase in tumorigenesis. This strongly suggests that the **current increasing incidence of iDTC most likely reflects diagnostic detection increasing over time**. (45)

Conclusion: Our Clinical Experience with Thyroid Nodules

Over the years, many patients have arrived in our office after having declined needle aspiration for small thyroid nodules, wishing to avoid unnecessary thyroid surgery. In such cases, we follow the thyroid nodule with serial ultrasound exams and medical treatments such as TSH suppression with NDT, natural desiccated thyroid, iodine, myo-inositol, and selenium supplements. In all cases in which we have followed such nodules, they have decreased or remained stable in size over time, rendering surgery unnecessary. Many endocrinologists will routinely perform a thyroid sonogram to screen for small nodules in their office. Based on the advice of John Cronan MD and Gilbert Welch MD, we intentionally do not do this. We do not perform routine screening thyroid ultrasound on the general population. However, for patients already presenting with a documented nodule, these are followed serially for any change in size, and any increase in size is referred for a repeat needle biopsy. Over the last 20 years of clinical practice using ultrasound for follow-up of thyroid nodules under medical management, none have required surgical intervention. Let me repeat that: None have required surgical intervention. (2) (46-79)

♦ **References for Chapter 33**

1) Davies, Louise, and H. Gilbert Welch. "Current Thyroid Cancer Trends in the United States." JAMA Otolaryngology–Head & Neck Surgery 140.4 (2014): 317-322.

2) Cronan, John J. "Thyroid Nodules: Is It Time to Turn Off the US Machines?" Radiology 247.3 (2008): 602-604.

3) Ross, Douglas S. "Nonpalpable Thyroid Nodules—Managing an Epidemic." The Journal of Clinical Endocrinology & Metabolism 87.5 (2002): 1938-1940.

4) Heller, Keith S. "Do All Cancers Need to Be Treated? The Role of Thyroglobulin in the Management of Thyroid Cancer: the 2006 Hayes Martin Lecture." Archives of Otolaryngology–Head & Neck Surgery 133.7 (2007): 639-643.

5) Davies, Louise, and H. Gilbert Welch. "Increasing Incidence of Thyroid Cancer in the United States, 1973-2002." JAMA 295.18 (2006): 2164-2167.

6) Harach, H. Rubén, et al. "Occult Papillary Carcinoma of the Thyroid. A "Normal" Finding in Finland. A Systematic Autopsy Study." Cancer 56.3 (1985): 531-538.

7) Harach, H. R., et al. "Occult Papillary Microcarcinoma of The Thyroid--A Potential Pitfall of Fine Needle Aspiration Cytology?" Journal of Clinical Pathology 44.3 (1991): 205-207.

8) Ito, Yasuhiro, et al. "An Observation Trial Without Surgical Treatment in Patients with Papillary Microcarcinoma of The Thyroid." Thyroid 13.4 (2003): 381-387.

9) Ito, Yasuhiro, et al. "Papillary Microcarcinoma of the Thyroid: How Should It Be Treated?" World Journal of Surgery 28.11 (2004): 1115-1121.

10) Ito, Yasuhiro, et al. "Long-Term Follow-Up for Patients with Papillary Thyroid Carcinoma Treated as Benign Nodules." Anticancer Research 27.2 (2007): 1039-1043.

11) Rosai, Juan, et al. "Renaming Papillary Microcarcinoma of The Thyroid Gland: The Porto Proposal." International Journal of Surgical Pathology 11.4 (2003): 249-251.

12) Hazard, JB, et al. "Nonencapsulated Sclerosing Tumors of the Thyroid." The Journal of Clinical Endocrinology and Metabolism 9.11 (1949): 1216.

13) Hay, Ian, et al. "Neither Total Thyroidectomy nor Radioiodine Remnant Ablation Improved Long-Term Outcome in 900 Patients with Papillary Thyroid Microcarcinoma Treated During 1945 Through 2004." Endocrine Abstracts. Vol. 16. Bioscientifica, 2008.

14) Huszno, B., et al. "Influence of Iodine Deficiency and Iodine Prophylaxis on Thyroid Cancer Histotypes and Incidence in Endemic Goiter Area." Journal of Endocrinological Investigation 26.2 Suppl (2003): 71-76.

15) Bacher-Stier, C., et al. "Incidence and Clinical Characteristics of Thyroid Carcinoma After Iodine Prophylaxis in An Endemic Goiter Country." Thyroid 7.5 (1997): 733-741.

16) Patrick, Lyn. "Iodine: Deficiency and Therapeutic Considerations." Alternative Medicine Review 13.2 (2008).

17) Belfiore, Antonino, et al. "The Frequency of Cold Thyroid Nodules and Thyroid Malignancies in Patients from an Iodine-Deficient Area." Cancer 60.12 (1987): 3096-3102.

18) Knobel, Meyer, and Geraldo Medeiros-Neto. "Relevance of Iodine Intake as a Reputed Predisposing Factor for Thyroid Cancer." Arquivos Brasileiros de Endocrinologia & Metabologia 51 (2007): 701-712.

19) Kasagi, Kanji. "Epidemiology of Thyroid Tumors: Effect of Environmental Iodine Intake." Nihon into. Japanese Journal of Clinical Medicine 65.11 (2007): 1953-1958.

20) Durante, Cosimo, et al. "The Natural History of Benign Thyroid Nodules." JAMA 313.9 (2015): 926-935.

21) Cheema, Yusra, et al. "What Is the Biology and Optimal Treatment for Papillary Microcarcinoma of the Thyroid?" Journal of Surgical Research 134.2 (2006): 160-162.

22) Ito, Yasuhiro, and Akira Miyauchi. "Appropriate Treatment for Asymptomatic Papillary Microcarcinoma of the Thyroid." Expert Opinion on Pharmacotherapy 8.18 (2007): 3205-3215.

23) Ito, Yasuhiro, and Akira Miyauchi. "A Therapeutic Strategy for Incidentally Detected Papillary Microcarcinoma of the Thyroid." Nature Clinical Practice Endocrinology & Metabolism 3.3 (2007): 240-248.

24) Davies, Louise, et al. "Patient Experience of Thyroid Cancer Active Surveillance in Japan." JAMA Otolaryngology–Head & Neck Surgery 145.4 (2019): 363-370.

25) Ito, Yasuhiro, et al. "Preoperative Ultrasonographic Examination for Lymph Node Metastasis: Usefulness When Designing Lymph Node Dissection for Papillary Microcarcinoma of the Thyroid." World Journal of Surgery 28.5 (2004): 498-501.

26) Ito, Yasuhiro, et al. "Papillary Microcarcinoma of the Thyroid: How Should It Be Treated?" World Journal of Surgery 28.11 (2004): 1115-1121.

27) Woyke, S., et al. "Occult Papillary Microcarcinoma of the Thyroid: A Potential Pitfall of Fine Needle Aspiration Cytology? Is It Possible to Avoid It?" Journal of Clinical Pathology 48.2 (1995): 185.

28) Papini, E., et al. "Long-Term Changes in Nodular Goiter: A 5-Year Prospective Randomized Trial of Levothyroxine Suppressive Therapy for Benign Cold Thyroid Nodules." The Journal of Clinical Endocrinology & Metabolism 83.3 (1998): 780-783.

29) Clark, Orlo H. "TSH Suppression in The Management of Thyroid Nodules and Thyroid Cancer." World Journal of Surgery 5.1 (1981): 39-46.

30) Nordio, M., and S. Basciani. "Evaluation of Thyroid Nodule Characteristics in Subclinical Hypothyroid Patients Under a Myo-Inositol Plus Selenium Treatment." Eur Rev Med Pharmacol Sci 22.7 (2018): 2153-9.

31) Gharib, Hossein, and Ernest L. Mazzaferri. "Thyroxine Suppressive Therapy in Patients with Nodular Thyroid Disease." Annals of Internal Medicine 128.5 (1998): 386-394.

32) Pemayun, Tjokorda Gde Dalem. "Current Diagnosis and Management of Thyroid Nodules." Acta Medica Indonesiana 48.3 (2017): 247-257.

33) Grani, Giorgio, et al. "Contemporary Thyroid Nodule Evaluation and Management." The Journal of Clinical Endocrinology & Metabolism 105.9 (2020): 2869-2883.

34) Rassael, H., L. D. R. Thompson, and C. S. Heffess. "A Rationale for Conservative Management of Microscopic Papillary Carcinoma of The Thyroid Gland: A Clinicopathologic Correlation of 90 Cases." European Archives of Oto-Rhino-Laryngology 255.9 (1998): 462-467.

35) Burman, Kenneth D. "Micropapillary Thyroid Cancer: Should We Aspirate All Nodules Regardless of Size?" The Journal of Clinical Endocrinology & Metabolism 91.6 (2006): 2043-2046.

36) Orr, Lauren E., et al. "Do Patients with Low-and Intermediate-Risk Thyroid Cancer Need Continuing Postoperative Neck Surveillance Ultrasounds?" Clinical Thyroidology 31.8 (2019): 343-345.

37) Tuttle, R. Michael, Eric J. Sherman, and Douglas S. Ross. "Anaplastic Thyroid Cancer." Cooper DS, Ross DS. [Internet] Waltham MA: UpToDate (2016).

38) Quiros, Roderick M., et al. "Evidence That One Subset of Anaplastic Thyroid Carcinomas Are Derived from Papillary Carcinomas Due to BRAF And P53 Mutations." Cancer: Interdisciplinary International Journal of the American Cancer Society 103.11 (2005): 2261-2268.

39) Voutilainen, Petri E., et al. "Anaplastic Thyroid Carcinoma Survival." World Journal of Surgery 23.9 (1999): 975-979.

40) McIver, Bryan, et al. "Anaplastic Thyroid Carcinoma: A 50-Year Experience at a Single Institution." Surgery 130.6 (2001): 1028-1034.

41) Lin, Bo, et al. "The Incidence and Survival Analysis for Anaplastic Thyroid Cancer: A SEER Database Analysis." American Journal of Translational Research 11.9 (2019): 5888.

42) De Leo, Simone, et al. "Recent Advances in the Management of Anaplastic Thyroid Cancer." Thyroid Research 13.1 (2020): 1-14.

43) Davies, Louise, and Jenny K. Hoang. "Thyroid Cancer in the USA: Current Trends and Outstanding Questions." The Lancet Diabetes & Endocrinology 9.1 (2021): 11-12.

44) Davies, Louise, and H. Gilbert Welch. "Increasing Incidence of Thyroid Cancer in The United States, 1973-2002." JAMA 295.18 (2006): 2164-2167.

45) Furuya-Kanamori, Luis, et al. "Prevalence of Differentiated Thyroid Cancer in Autopsy Studies Over Six Decades: A Meta-Analysis." Journal of Clinical Oncology: Official Journal of the American Society of Clinical Oncology 34.30 (2016): 3672-3679.

46) Welker, Mary Jo, and Diane Orlov. "Thyroid Nodules." American Family Physician 67.3 (2003): 559-566.

47) How, Jacques, and Roger Tabah. "Explaining the Increasing Incidence of Differentiated Thyroid Cancer." CMAJ 177.11 (2007): 1383-1384.

48) Mazzaferri, Ernest L. "Managing Small Thyroid Cancers." JAMA 295.18 (2006): 2179-2182.

49) Lin, Harrison W., and Neil Bhattacharyya. "Survival Impact of Treatment Options for Papillary Microcarcinoma of the Thyroid." The Laryngoscope 119.10 (2009): 1983-1987.

50) Mazzaferri, Ernest L. "What Is the Optimal Initial Treatment of Low-Risk Papillary Thyroid Cancer (And Why Is It Controversial)?" Oncology 23.7 (2009): 579.

51) Tan, Gerry H., and Hossein Gharib. "Thyroid Incidentalomas: Management Approaches to Nonpalpable Nodules Discovered Incidentally on Thyroid Imaging." Annals of Internal Medicine 126.3 (1997): 226-231.

52) Kakudo, K1, et al. "Papillary Carcinoma of the Thyroid in Japan: Subclassification of Common Type and Identification of Low-Risk Group." Journal of clinical pathology 57.10 (2004): 1041-1046.

53) Sakorafas, G. H., et al. "Microscopic Papillary Thyroid Cancer as an Incidental Finding in Patients Treated Surgically for Presumably Benign Thyroid Disease." Journal of Postgraduate Medicine 53.1 (2007): 23.

54) Ito, Yasuhiro, and Akira Miyauchi. "Active Surveillance of Low-Risk Papillary Thyroid Microcarcinomas in Japan and Other Countries: A Review." Expert Review of Endocrinology & Metabolism 15.1 (2020): 5-12.

55) Drake, Tyler. "Should Small Low-Risk Papillary Thyroid Cancer Be Called Cancer at All?" Clinical Thyroidology 33.1 (2021): 25-28.

56) Vaccarella, Salvatore, et al. "Worldwide Thyroid-Cancer Epidemic? The Increasing Impact of Overdiagnosis." New England Journal of Medicine 375.7 (2016): 614-617.

57) Pearce, Elizabeth N. "Thyroid Cancer Overdiagnosis is a Result of Screening Programs in South Korea." Clinical Thyroidology 29.1 (2017): 8-10.

58) Durante, Cosimo, and Giorgio Grani. "Clinically Silent Thyroid Cancers: Drop Those Needles and Scalpels!" The Journal of Clinical Endocrinology & Metabolism 105.3 (2020): e889-e890.

59) Krajewska, Jolanta, et al. "Early Diagnosis of Low-Risk Papillary Thyroid Cancer Results Rather in Overtreatment Than a Better Survival." Frontiers in Endocrinology 11 (2020): 571421.

60) Pereira, Malesa, et al. "Thyroid Cancer Incidence Trends in The United States: Association with Changes in Professional Guideline Recommendations." Thyroid 30.8 (2020): 1132-1140.

61) Papaleontiou, Maria, and Megan R. Haymart. "Too Much of a Good Thing? A Cautionary Tale of Thyroid Cancer Overdiagnosis and Overtreatment." Thyroid 30.5 (2020): 651.

62) Genere, Natalia, et al. "Incidence of Clinically Relevant Thyroid Cancers Remains Stable for Almost a Century: A Population-Based Study." Mayo Clinic Proceedings. Vol. 96. No. 11. Elsevier, 2021.

63) El Sheikh, Reem, and Spyridoula Maraka. "The Incidence of Clinically Relevant Thyroid Cancers Remains Stable." Clinical Thyroidology 34.1 (2022): 26-28.

64) Solis-Pazmino, Paola, et al. "Thyroid Cancer Overdiagnosis and Overtreatment: A Cross-Sectional Study at a Thyroid Cancer Referral Center in Ecuador." BMC Cancer 21.1 (2021): 1-10.

65) Barrett, Kaitlyn V., et al. "Predictors and Consequences of Inappropriate Thyroid Ultrasound in Hypothyroidism." Cureus 13.8 (2021).

66) Fish, Stephanie A. "Too Many Thyroid Ultrasound Exams Lead to an Increase in the Diagnosis of Low-Risk Thyroid Cancer." Clinical Thyroidology 30.11 (2018): 519-522.

67) Grani, Giorgio. "Inappropriate Use of Thyroid Ultrasound Is Common in Clinical Practice." Clinical Thyroidology 34.1 (2022): 23-25.

68) Haymart, Megan R., et al. "Thyroid Ultrasound and the Increase in Diagnosis of Low-Risk Thyroid Cancer." The Journal of Clinical Endocrinology & Metabolism 104.3 (2019): 785-792.

69) Haymart, Megan R., et al. "The Relationship Between Imaging and Thyroid Cancer Diagnosis and Survival." The Oncologist 25.9 (2020): 765-771.

70) Peiling Yang, Samantha, et al. "Frequent Screening with Serial Neck Ultrasound Is More Likely to Identify False-Positive Abnormalities Than a Clinically Significant Disease in the Surveillance of Intermediate-Risk Papillary Thyroid Cancer Patients Without Suspicious Findings on Follow-Up Ultrasound Evaluation." The Journal of Clinical Endocrinology & Metabolism 100.4 (2015): 1561-1567.

71) Hegedüs, Laszlo. "Down-Sizing the Overzealous Search for Low-Risk Thyroid Malignancy." Endocrine 52.3 (2016): 408-410.

72) Shakhtarin, V. V., et al. "Iodine Deficiency, Radiation Dose, and the Risk of Thyroid Cancer Among Children and Adolescents in the Bryansk Region of Russia Following the Chernobyl Power Station Accident." International Journal of Epidemiology 32.4 (2003): 584-591.

73) Patrick, Lyn. "Iodine: Deficiency and Therapeutic Considerations." Alternative Medicine Review 13.2 (2008).

74) Schaller Jr, Robert T., and John K. Stevenson. "Development of Carcinoma of the Thyroid in Iodine-Deficient Mice." Cancer 19.8 (1966): 1063-1080.

75) Park, Sohee, et al. "Association Between Screening and the Thyroid Cancer "Epidemic" in South Korea: Evidence from a Nationwide Study." BMJ 355 (2016).

76) Haugen, Bryan R., et al. "2015 American Thyroid Association Management Guidelines for Adult Patients with Thyroid Nodules and Differentiated Thyroid Cancer: The American Thyroid Association Guidelines Task Force on Thyroid Nodules and Differentiated Thyroid Cancer." Thyroid 26.1 (2016): 1-133.

77) Ito, Yasuhiro, and Akira Miyauchi. "Active Surveillance of Low-Risk Papillary Thyroid Microcarcinomas." Gland Surgery 9.5 (2020): 1663.

78) Shin, Ji Hoon, et al. "Radiofrequency Ablation of Thyroid Nodules: Basic Principles and Clinical Application." International Journal of Endocrinology 2012 (2012): 934-940.

79) Cho, Se Jin, et al. "Long-Term Follow-Up Results of Ultrasound-Guided Radiofrequency Ablation for Low-Risk Papillary Thyroid Microcarcinoma: More Than 5-Year Follow-Up for 84 Tumors." Thyroid 30.12 (2020): 1745-1751.

Chapter 34

Adrenal Insufficiency, HPA Dysfunction, and Fatigue

IGNORED BY MAINSTREAM MEDICINE, ADRENAL fatigue is a common problem I see every day at the office. The paramount symptom is fatigue unrelieved by sleep. Other symptoms include craving for salty foods, hypoglycemic episodes, decreased libido, stress intolerance, lightheaded upon standing (postural hypotension), depression, memory loss and cognitive decline, allergies, sinus problems, and prolonged recovery from flu-like illnesses. The basic underlying cause is low cortisol output by the adrenal glands.

A Self-Help Book for Chronic Burn-Out called Adrenal Fatigue

The definitive book on adrenal fatigue is by James L Wilson, Ph.D., a self-help guide for all of us chronically stressed-out members of the "rat race" suffering from this new 21st-century epidemic. In his book, Wilson outlines how to diagnose and treat adrenal fatigue, a syndrome not recognized by mainstream medicine, and it should be. Dr. Wilson's book describes findings of adrenal fatigue on physical examination, such as the unstable pupil, blood pressure reduction upon standing, and Sergent's white line test, first described in 1917 by Emil Sergent, a French endocrinologist. (1-3)

Cortisol Testing

Chapter eleven of Wilson's book covers the different cortisol testing methods available for cortisol in saliva, blood, and urine, as well as the ACTH stimulation test. Wilson favors the 4-sample salivary cortisol test as the easiest and most convenient method, with the advantage that salivary testing can be done at home without a doctor's prescription. Home salivary testing kits are widely available online without a prescription. Another chapter in the book covers treatment and recovery from adrenal fatigue with diet and lifestyle modifications, avoiding food allergies, and the use of hormone replacement and dietary supplements. Dr. Wilson also discusses using Cortef (cortisol) versus adrenal cortical extracts. (4-8)

Results from Years of Chronic Stress

Adrenal fatigue is the net result of years of continuous high cortisol output by the adrenals caused by chronic stress from job, family, illness, injury, and poor diet and lifestyle associated with high-tech modern living. After years of chronic stress, the two small triangular supra-renal glands poop out, and we become another casualty of adrenal fatigue, the 21st-century epidemic. Since mainstream doctors cannot help, either ignoring the syndrome or prescribing anti-depressants for it, this self-help book is a lifesaver. In 2001, Dr. James L Wilson defined adrenal fatigue, writing:

> Adrenal Fatigue is a collection of signs and symptoms that results from low function of the adrenal glands. The paramount symptom is fatigue, which is not relieved by sleep. The syndrome may be caused by intense or prolonged stress or after acute or chronic infections, especially respiratory infections such as influenza, bronchitis, or pneumonia…. People suffering from Adrenal Fatigue often have to use coffee, colas, and other stimulants to get going in the morning and to prop themselves up during the day. (1)

Symptoms and Conditions Associated with Adrenal Fatigue:

Anxiety, Asthenia – lack of, or loss of strength, generalized weakness, Asthma, Autoimmune problems, Bronchitis – recurrent, chronic, Chemical Sensitivity, Chronic fatigue syndrome (CFS), Chronic infections, Chronically run down – with early morning fatigue and low blood pressure, Chronic mental and/or physical exhaustion, Cravings for carbohydrates, sweets or salt, Depression, Fatigue – severe, disabling early morning fatigue, Feeling tired despite sufficient hours of sleep, Fibromyalgia, Hair loss, Hypoglycemia, Immune System dysfunction – frequent illnesses, insomnia – or non-restful sleep, Low Blood Pressure, Nervous breakdown (nervous exhaustion), Pneumonia, Respiratory infections – recurrent, chronic or slow recovery from, Rheumatoid arthritis, Reliance on stimulants like caffeine, Slow recovery following acute infectious diseases, especially influenza, pneumonia, or other respiratory infections, Weight gain. (1)

The Important Role of Cortisol

Cortisol is the stress hormone and is produced in response to stress. Cortisol is important for blood sugar regulation by mobilizing glycogen stores in the liver to maintain blood glucose levels. Symptoms of hypoglycemia are common in low cortisol adrenal fatigue. Postural hypotension, low blood pressure or inability to maintain blood pressure upon standing is a common symptom. Another finding of the physical exam is the unstable pupil response to light. The pupil at first contracts and then opens and closes after a few seconds. Physical findings may also include skin hyperpigmentation, orthostatic hypotension, hyperkalemia (high serum potassium), and hyponatremia (low serum sodium). (9)

The Adrenal Glands Make the Cortisol

The two small triangular adrenal glands are located just above the kidneys and secrete the hormone cortisol in response to physical, emotional, or traumatic stress. The cortex of the adrenal glands makes the hormone cortisol in response to ACTH secretion by the pituitary. The cortex also makes the mineralocorticoid aldosterone, which maintains blood pressure, sodium, and potassium levels. The adrenal medulla secretes catecholamines, epinephrine, and norepinephrine following activation of the sympathetic nervous system in a "fight or flight" response to a perceived threat.

Cortisol, the Stress Hormone

Like all the other steroidal hormones, cortisol is made from cholesterol. Cholesterol, in turn, is made from Vitamin B5 and Acetyl CoA. The manufacture of steroidal hormones can be best understood by referring to a steroidal pathway chart.

4 Sample Salivary Cortisol Test

Although cortisol can be measured in a blood sample, the best way to measure cortisol levels is with four saliva samples taken throughout the day. Hundreds of medical research studies validate the usefulness of salivary cortisol measurements. A 2008 study by Dr. Urs Nater showed that a low value for early morning salivary cortisol is associated with chronic fatigue syndrome in women but not men. (10-21)

Diagnosis with Salivary Cortisol Test

Four salivary cortisol samples are taken at 8 AM, Noon, 4 PM, and Midnight. The four results are plotted on a chart with the normal channel drawn as dotted lines. If the four samples fall within the normal channel, this is considered a normal cortisol response. If all four salivary cortisol samples fall below the normal channel, this is a "flat line pattern" indicating adrenal fatigue, a pattern identified in childhood trauma and breast cancer survivors. If the morning samples are low and the evening samples are high, this indicates a reversed pattern usually associated with insomnia, and the treatment is phosphatidylserine. (22-28)

Nutritional Supplement Recovery Program for Stress and Adrenal Fatigue

The keystone of the treatment program for stress and adrenal fatigue is a nutritional supplement program to relieve stress and restore adrenal function. This includes vitamin C, B5, magnesium, and adaptogenic herbs. Phosphatidylserine is useful to correct the reversed pattern of high cortisol at night, which may cause insomnia. These are all widely available online or at the local health food store. Many of these products contain various combinations of supplements, and might include such items as Rhodiola Rosea, Magnolia, Ashwagandha, and phosphatidyl serine. Lithium orotate, 5-HTP, L-theanine, Phellodendron Chinensis, and Holy Basil are also commonly used. Typical recovery time is about 6 -12 weeks. De-stressing with good-quality sleep, exercise, diet, and lifestyle modification is important and should not be ignored. I frequently suggest to the patient, read one of the hundreds of books on how to de-stress a lifestyle with meditation, yoga, music, relaxing sessions, therapeutic massage, hot baths, walks in the park, etc. In some cases, the patient may be stuck in a stressful job or family environment, which seems impossible to change, forcing the patient to resort to psychoactive drugs or anti-depressants. This is the unfortunate byproduct of modern civilization. Psychoactive drugs temporarily act as a crutch to allow the continuation of a stressful environment, job, or family member. However, digging the patient into a deeper hole is not worth it in the long run, and inevitably, drastic changes to eliminate stressful people, jobs or environments may be the best path forward. (2) (29-36)

Cortef for Severe Cases of Adrenal Fatigue

In very severe cases of adrenal failure, Cortef tablets are available and dramatically improve the clinical condition. See the book, Safe Uses of Cortisol by William McK Jefferies, MD. Cortef is the name for bio-identical cortisol, widely available by prescription at the local drug store. According to Dr. McK Jefferies, cortef dosage below 30 mg. a day is a physiologic replacement and not associated with adverse side effects commonly found with high-dose synthetic prednisone. Higher doses of cortef or synthetic forms of cortisol such as prednisone are not recommended as they can be associated with adverse side effects such as cataract formation, thinning of the skin with easy bruising, osteoporosis, glaucoma, HPA suppression, etc. (36-41)

Other Useful Treatments Routinely Used

Dr. Wilson's book advises other modifications of diet to avoid excess caffeine, refined carbohydrates, alcohol, and sugar. Get plenty of sleep. Take steps to reduce stress with gentle exercise, meditation, and yoga. Bio-identical hormones may be useful, as determined by the lab profile. (2)

Jacob Teitelbaum MD

Another excellent book is From Fatigued to Fantastic by Jacob Teitelbaum, MD, which covers adrenal fatigue and other related conditions causing chronic fatigue. (21)

Cortisol's Relation to Thyroid Function – Avoiding A Common Pitfall

Low cortisol adrenal fatigue will place the body into a protective state in which the metabolic rate is reduced to cope with the low cortisol production. The body accomplishes this reduction in metabolic rate by reducing thyroid function, usually by shunting thyroid hormone production into the reverse T3 pathway. This mechanism converts T4 to its inactive form, reverse T3, creating a functional low thyroid state. Thyroid labs will typically show low thyroid hormone levels and elevated reverse T3, and giving thyroid hormone in this scenario is a common pitfall to be avoided. Giving thyroid hormone to a patient with Addison's Disease or low cortisol adrenal fatigue will only make the patient feel worse or trigger an Addisonian crisis in the worst-case scenario. (42-49)

In patients with adrenal fatigue or Addison's Disease, the low adrenal function must first be addressed before giving thyroid hormone medication. This can be done with a 4-sample salivary cortisol test and a nutritional supplement program over six weeks, as described above. If the patient is already taking thyroid hormone medication that does not seem to be working or is not tolerated, then one must consider the possibility of Addison's Disease, low cortisol output, or adrenal fatigue. Once this is addressed, the patient will then be able to tolerate thyroid medication. (42-49)

The HPA in Adrenal Fatigue and Fibromyalgia

In 2007, Dr. Kent Holtorf found adrenal fatigue is commonly associated with fibromyalgia with underlying dysfunction of the HPA, the hypothalamic-pituitary axis. Dr. Kent Holtorf also found hypothalamic-pituitary dysfunction results in low pituitary hormone output, including low TSH, low ACTH, low growth hormone, etc. Some cases may not be detected with conventional testing. Associated symptoms include insomnia, immune dysfunction with chronic infections, autonomic nervous system dysfunction, and gastrointestinal distress. Dr. Holtorf's multifaceted treatment approach includes low-dose cortisol (5-15 mg per day) as initially advocated by William McK Jefferies, MD, and Jacob Teitelbaum, MD. The low dose of cortisol is only one part of a multifaceted treatment approach which includes nutritional supplementation, diet, and lifestyle modification. (2)(20-21)(36)

In 2007, Dr. Kent Holtorf, MD, writes:

> There is controversy regarding the incidence and significance of hypothalamic-pituitary-adrenal (HPA) axis dysfunction in chronic fatigue syndrome (CFS) and fibromyalgia (FM). Studies...have demonstrated that HPA axis dysfunction of central origin is present in a majority of these patients... Because treatment with low physiologic doses of cortisol (<15 mg) has been shown to be safe and effective and routine dynamic ACTH testing does not have adequate

diagnostic sensitivity, it is reasonable to give a therapeutic trial of physiologic doses of cortisol to the majority of patients with CFS and FM, especially to those who have symptoms that are consistent with adrenal dysfunction, have low blood pressure or have baseline cortisol levels in the low or low-normal range. (20)

Food Sensitivities, Leaky Gut and HPA Dysfunction

We have found that many patients with chronic fatigue/ fibromyalgia syndrome have, in addition to all the above, problems with gluten sensitivity, leaky gut, and other food sensitivities. There may be malabsorption of vitamins, minerals, and amino acids. A leaky gut with leakage of LPS (lipo-saccharides from enteric bacteria) into the bloodstream may contribute to the syndrome or may play a causative role in HPA dysfunction. For example, low testosterone from HPA dysfunction may be found in marathon runners and athletes whose high-intensity exercise causes reduced splanchnic blood flow and hyperthermia, which then leads to endotoxemia and gastrointestinal symptoms. (50-56)

Adrenal Fatigue Does Not Exist!

For those who claim that adrenal fatigue does not exist, I would simply point to the life work of Dr. Hans Selye, a Hungarian-Canadian endocrinologist working in 1936 with a stress model in mice, who first described the three stages of adaptation to stress, the initial brief alarm reaction, followed by a prolonged period of resistance and then a terminal stage of exhaustion and death. Over his 80-year career devoted to the endocrinology of stress, Dr. Hans Selye wrote over 1,500 scientific articles and 32 books and trained 40 Ph.D. students, one of whom won a Nobel Prize. Dr. Hans Selye's studies on animal models of stress defined the field for over 80 years. (57-62)

In 2014, Dr. Mark Jackson writes:

> Selye's notion of biological stress and its

impact on health was adopted and adapted by researchers in a variety of adjacent fields, including military medicine, veterinary medicine, clinical allergy, sociobiology, population studies, cybernetics, and psychiatry. (57)

Conclusion

Adrenal insufficiency may be unmasked by the use of thyroid hormone, and in severe cases, levothyroxine may trigger an Addisonian crisis. For the unsuspecting physician, this is a pitfall to avoid. HPA dysfunction may be associated with adrenal, thyroid, and gonadal hormonal abnormalities, chronic fatigue, sleep disturbance, and fibromyalgia. Four-sample salivary cortisol is a useful test for HPA dysfunction. The most commonly used test for adrenal insufficiency is the ACTH stimulation test. In anabolic steroid abusers, a useful test for HPA dysfunction is the clomiphene stimulation test. (44-49) (63-105)

♦ **References for Chapter 34**

1) Wilson, James L., and Jonathan V. Wright. Adrenal fatigue: The 21st-century Stress Syndrome. Vol. 4. Petaluma: Smart Publications, 2001.

2) Cook, Sarah Bedell. "Current Controversy: Does Adrenal Fatigue Exist?" Natural Medicine Journal 9.10 (2017).

3) Sergent, Emile. "The White Adrenal Line: Its Production and Diagnostic Significance." Endocrinology 1.1 (1917): 18-23.

4) Sad, Eduardo F., et al. "Salivary Cortisol in Critical Care Patients." Chest 132.4 (2007): 555A.

5) Vining, Ross F., et al. "Salivary Cortisol: A Better Measure of Adrenal Cortical Function than Serum Cortisol." Annals of Clinical Biochemistry 20.6 (1983): 329-335.

6) Laudat, M. H., et al. "Salivary Cortisol Measurement: A Practical Approach to Assess Pituitary-Adrenal Function." The Journal of Clinical Endocrinology & Metabolism 66.2 (1988): 343-348.

7) Nicolson, Nancy A., and Rob van Diest. "Salivary Cortisol Patterns in Vital Exhaustion." Journal of Psychosomatic Research 49.5 (2000): 335-342.

8) Roberts, Amanda DL, et al. "Salivary Cortisol Response to Awakening in Chronic Fatigue Syndrome." The British Journal of Psychiatry 184.2 (2004): 136-141.

9) Papierska, Lucyna, and Micha B Rabijewski. "Delay in Diagnosis of Adrenal Insufficiency Is a Frequent Cause of Adrenal Crisis." (2013). International Journal of Endocrinology (2013): 482370-482370.

10) Nater, Urs M., et al. "Attenuated Morning Salivary Cortisol Concentrations in a Population-Based Study of Persons with Chronic Fatigue Syndrome and Well Controls." The Journal of Clinical Endocrinology & Metabolism 93.3 (2008): 703-709.

11) Portella, Maria J., et al. "Enhanced Early Morning Salivary Cortisol in Neuroticism." American Journal of Psychiatry 162.4 (2005): 807-809.

12) Nijhof, Sanne L., et al. "The Role of Hypocortisolism in Chronic Fatigue Syndrome." Psychoneuroendocrinology 42 (2014): 199-206.

13) Nater, Urs M., et al. "Alterations in Diurnal Salivary Cortisol Rhythm in a Population-Based Sample of Cases with Chronic Fatigue Syndrome." Psychosomatic Medicine 70.3 (2008): 298-305.

14) Gaab, Jens, et al. "Low-Dose Dexamethasone Suppression Test in Chronic Fatigue Syndrome and Health." Psychosomatic Medicine 64.2 (2002): 311-318.

15) Di Giorgio, Annabella, et al. "24-hour Pituitary and Adrenal Hormone Profiles in Chronic Fatigue Syndrome." Psychosomatic Medicine 67.3 (2005): 433-440.

16) McBurnett, Keith, et al. "Low Salivary Cortisol and Persistent Aggression in Boys Referred for Disruptive Behavior." Archives of general psychiatry 57.1 (2000): 38-43.

17) Kos-Kudla, B. "Iatrogenic Adrenal Cortex Failure in Patients with Steroid-Dependent Asthma in Relation to Different Methods of Glucocorticoid Treatment." Endocrine regulations 32 (1998): 99-106.

18) Klein, Laura Cousino, et al. "Sex Differences in Salivary Cortisol Levels Following Naltrexone Administration 1." Journal of Applied Biobehavioral Research 5.2 (2000): 144-153.

19) Roberts, Amanda DL, et al. "Salivary Cortisol Response to Awakening in Chronic Fatigue Syndrome." The British Journal of Psychiatry 184.2 (2004): 136-141.

20) Holtorf, Kent. "Diagnosis and Treatment of Hypothalamic-Pituitary-Adrenal (HPA) Axis Dysfunction in Patients with Chronic Fatigue Syndrome (CFS) and Fibromyalgia (FM)." Journal of Chronic Fatigue Syndrome 14.3 (2007): 59-88.

21) Teitelbaum, Jacob. From Fatigued to Fantastic! A Proven Program to Regain Vibrant Health, Based on a New Scientific Study Showing Effective Treatment for Chronic Fatigue and Fibromyalgia. Penguin, 2001.

22) Bush, Bradley, and T. Hudson. "The Role of Cortisol in Sleep." Natural Medicine Journal 2.6 (2010): 2010-06.

23) Tori Hudson, N. D., and N. D. Bradley Bush. "The Role of Cortisol in Sleep." Nat Medi J 2 (2010): 6.

24) Monteleone, Palmiero, et al. "Blunting by Chronic Phosphatidylserine Administration of the Stress-Induced Activation of the Hypothalamic-Pituitary-Adrenal Axis in Healthy Men." European Journal of Clinical Pharmacology 42 (1992): 385-388.

25) Starks, Michael A., et al. "The Effects of Phosphatidylserine on Endocrine Response to Moderate Intensity Exercise." Journal of the International Society of Sports Nutrition 5.1 (2008): 11.

26) Hellhammer, Juliane, et al. "A Soy-Based Phosphatidylserine/Phosphatidic Acid Complex (PAS) Normalizes the Stress Reactivity of Hypothalamus-Pituitary-Adrenal-Axis in Chronically Stressed Male Subjects: A Randomized, Placebo-Controlled Study." Lipids in Health and Disease 13 (2014): 1-11.

27) Suzuki, Akiko, et al. "Long-Term Effects of Childhood Trauma on Cortisol Stress Reactivity in Adulthood and Relationship to the Occurrence of Depression." Psychoneuroendocrinology 50 (2014): 289-299.

28) Kamen, Charles, et al. "Effects of Childhood Trauma Exposure and Cortisol Levels on Cognitive Functioning Among Breast Cancer Survivors." Child Abuse & Neglect 72 (2017): 163-171.

29) Simpson, Kathryn. Overcoming Adrenal Fatigue: How to Restore Hormonal Balance and Feel Renewed, Energized, and Stress-Free. New Harbinger Publications, 2011.

30) Meletis, Chris D., and Wayne A. Centrone. "Adrenal Fatigue: Enhancing Quality of Life for Patients with a Functional Disorder." Alternative & Complementary Therapies 8.5 (2002): 267-272.

31) Head, Kathleen A., and Kelly, Gregory S. "Nutrients and Botanicals for Treatment of Stress: Adrenal Fatigue, Neurotransmitter Imbalance, Anxiety, and Restless Sleep." Altern Med Rev 14.2 (2009): 114-40.

32) Wilson, James L. "Clinical Perspective on Stress, Cortisol, and Adrenal Fatigue." Advances in Integrative Medicine 1.2 (2014): 93-96.

33) Anderson, D. "Assessment and Nutraceutical Management of Stress-Induced Adrenal Dysfunction." Integrative Medicine 7.5 (2008): 18-25.

34) Kariatsumari, Bob. "Understanding Adrenal Fatigue: Nutritional and Lifestyle Strategies to Effectively Restore Proper Adrenal Function." Nutritional Perspectives: Journal of the Council on Nutrition 42.1 (2019).

35) Teitelbaum, Jacob, and Sarah Goudie. "An Open-Label, Pilot Trial of HRG80™ Red Ginseng in Chronic Fatigue Syndrome, Fibromyalgia, And Post-Viral Fatigue." Pharmaceuticals 15.1 (2022): 43.

36) Jefferies, William McK. Safe Uses of Cortisol. Charles C Thomas Publisher, 2004.

37) Yasir, Muhammad, et al. "Corticosteroid Adverse Effects." StatPearls Publishing, 2022.

38) Manson, Stephanie C., et al. "The Cumulative Burden of Oral Corticosteroid Side Effects and the Economic Implications of Steroid Use." Respiratory Medicine 103.7 (2009): 975-994.

39) Satyanarayanasetty, Divya, et al. "Multiple Adverse Effects of Systemic Corticosteroids: A Case Report." Journal of Clinical and Diagnostic Research: JCDR 9.5 (2015): FD01.

40) Dahl, Ronald. "Systemic Side Effects of Inhaled Corticosteroids in Patients with Asthma." Respiratory Medicine 100.8 (2006): 1307-1317.

41) Cave, Alison, et al. "Inhaled and Nasal Corticosteroids: Factors Affecting the Risks of Systemic Adverse Effects." Pharmacology & therapeutics 83.3 (1999): 153-179.

42) Shaikh, M. G., et al. "Thyroxine Unmasks Addison's Disease." Acta Pediatrica 93.12 (2004): 1663-1665.

43) Sabih, Durr E., and Mohammad Inayatullah. "Managing Thyroid Dysfunction in Selected Special Situations." Thyroid Research 6 (2013): 1-7.

44) Davis, Julian, and Michael Sheppard. "Acute Adrenal Crisis Precipitated by Thyroxine." British Medical Journal (Clinical Research Ed.) 292.6535 (1986): 1595.

45) Graves 3rd, L., et al."Addisonian Crisis Precipitated by Thyroxine Therapy: A Complication of Type 2 Autoimmune Polyglandular Syndrome." Southern Medical Journal 96.8 (2003): 824-827.

46) Patel, Dhruvkumar M., et al. "Adrenocortical Crisis Triggered by Levothyroxine in an Unrecognized Autoimmune Polyglandular Syndrome Type-2: A Case Report with Review of the Literature." Current Drug Safety 16.1 (2021): 101-106.

47) Rajput, Rajesh, et al. "Reversible Thyrotropin Elevation in Case of Primary Addison's Disease." Thyroid Research and Practice 18.1 (2021): 31-33.

48) Gharib, Hossein, et al. "Reversible Hypothyroidism in Addison's Disease." The Lancet 300.7780 (1972): 734-736.

49) Murray, Jonathan Stephen, et al. "Deterioration of Symptoms After Start of Thyroid Hormone Replacement." BMJ 323.7308 (2001): 332-333.

50) Dach, Jeffrey. "Gut–Brain: Major Depressive Disorder, Hypothalamic Dysfunction, and High Calcium Score Associated with Leaky Gut." Alternative Therapies in Health and Medicine 21 (2015): 10-15.

51) Deuschle, Michael, et al. "Hypothalamic-Pituitary-Adrenocortical Dysfunction in Elderly, Male Marathon Runners: Feedback Sensitivity, Stress Response, And Effects on Verbal Memory." Neuroendocrinology 105.2 (2017): 150-156.

52) Bell, Lee M., and Lee Ingle. "Psycho-Physiological Markers of Overreaching and Overtraining in Endurance Sports: A Review of the Evidence." Medicina Sportiva 17.2 (2013).

53) Stuempfle, Kristin J., et al. "Nausea is Associated with Endotoxemia During a 161-Km Ultramarathon." Journal of Sports Sciences 34.17 (2016): 1662-1668.

54) Pires, Washington, et al. "Association Between Exercise-Induced Hyperthermia and Intestinal Permeability: A Systematic Review." Sports Medicine 47 (2017): 1389-1403.

55) Lambert, G. Patrick. "Intestinal Barrier Dysfunction, Endotoxemia, And Gastrointestinal Symptoms: The Canary in The Coal Mine During Exercise-Heat Stress?" Thermoregulation and Human Performance 53 (2008): 61-73.

56) Pugh, Jamie N., et al. "Four Weeks of Probiotic Supplementation Reduces GI Symptoms During a Marathon Race." European Journal of Applied Physiology 119 (2019): 1491-1501.

57) Jackson, Mark, et al. "Evaluating the Role of Hans Selye in The Modern History of Stress." Stress, Shock, and Adaptation in the Twentieth Century (2014).

58) Szabo, Sandor, et al. "Stress" Is 80 Years Old: From Hans Selye's Original Paper in 1936 to Recent Advances in GI Ulceration." Current Pharmaceutical Design 23.27 (2017): 4029-4041.

59) Szabo, Sandor, et al. "The Legacy of Hans Selye and the Origins of Stress Research: A Retrospective 75 Years After His Landmark, Brief "Letter" to the Editor of Nature." Stress 15.5 (2012): 472-478.

60) Selye, Hans. "A Syndrome Produced by Diverse Nocuous Agents." Nature 138.3479 (1936): 32-32.

61) Selye, Hans. "Stress and the General Adaptation Syndrome." British Medical Journal 1.4667 (1950): 1383.

62) Selye, Hans. "The Evolution of the Stress Concept: The Originator of the Concept Traces Its Development from the Discovery In 1936 of the Alarm Reaction to Modern Therapeutic Applications of Syntoxic and Catatoxic Hormones." American Scientist 61.6 (1973): 692-699.

63) Kasperlik-Załuska, A. A., et al. "Secondary Adrenal Insufficiency Associated with Autoimmune Disorders: A Report of Twenty-Five Cases." Clinical Endocrinology 49.6 (1998): 779-783.

64) Kasperlik-Zaluska, A. A., et al. "Association of Addison's Disease with Autoimmune Disorders–A Long-Term Observation of 180 Patients." Postgraduate Medical Journal 67.793 (1991): 984-987.

65) Pazderska, Agnieszka, and Simon HS Pearce. "Adrenal Insufficiency–Recognition and Management." Clinical Medicine 17.3 (2017): 258.

66) Osman, I. A., and Peter Leslie. "Addison's Disease. Adrenal Insufficiency Should Be Excluded Before Thyroxine Replacement Is Started." BMJ: British Medical Journal 313.7054 (1996): 427.

67) Banitt, P. F., and A. K. Munson. "Addisonian Crisis After Thyroid Replacement." Hospital Practice (Office ed.) 21.5 (1986): 132-134.

68) Stryker, Timothy D., and Mark E. Molitch. "Reversible Hyperthyrotropinemia, Hyperthyroxinemia, and Hyperprolactinemia Due to Adrenal Insufficiency." The American Journal of Medicine 79.2 (1985): 271-276.

69) Medras, M., et al. "Clomiphene Stimulation Test in Men Abusing Anabolic-Androgenic Steroids for Long Time." J Steroids Hormon Sci 4 (2014).

70) Bickelman, Carol, Laura Ferries, and R. Philip Eaton. "Impotence Related to Anabolic Steroid Use in a Body Builder. Response to Clomiphene Citrate." Western Journal of Medicine 162.2 (1995): 158.

71) Ospina, Naykky Singh, et al. "ACTH Stimulation Tests for the Diagnosis of Adrenal Insufficiency: Systematic Review and Meta-Analysis." The Journal of Clinical Endocrinology & Metabolism 101.2 (2016): 427-434.

72) Javorsky, Bradley R., et al. "New Cutoffs for the Biochemical Diagnosis of Adrenal Insufficiency After ACTH Stimulation Using Specific Cortisol Assays." Journal of the Endocrine Society 5.4 (2021): bvab022.

73) Nanzer, Alexandra M., et al. "Diagnosing Adrenal Insufficiency Using ACTH Stimulation Test." European Respiratory Journal 56.2 (2020).

74) Guilliams, Thomas G. "Adrenal Stress: Measuring and Treating." The Standards 30 (2000): 1-7.

75) Haussmann, Mark F., et al. "A Laboratory Exercise to Illustrate Increased Salivary Cortisol in Response to Three Stressful Conditions Using Competitive ELISA." Advances in Physiology Education 31.1 (2007): 110-115.6)

76) Randall, Michael. "The Physiology of Stress: Cortisol and the Hypothalamic-Pituitary-Adrenal Axis." Dartmouth Undergraduate Journal of Science 13.1 (2010): 22-24.

77) Edwards, Lena D., et al. "Hypocortisolism: An Evidence-Based Review." Integrative Medicine 10.4 (2011): 30.

78) Tsigos, Constantine, and George P. Chrousos. "Hypothalamic–Pituitary–Adrenal Axis, Neuroendocrine Factors and Stress." Journal of Psychosomatic Research 53.4 (2002): 865-871.

79) Raison, Charles L., and Andrew H. Miller. "When Not Enough Is Too Much: The Role of Insufficient Glucocorticoid Signaling in the Pathophysiology of Stress-Related Disorders." American Journal of Psychiatry 160.9 (2003): 1554-1565.

80) Papadopoulos, Andrew S., and Anthony J. Cleare. "Hypothalamic–Pituitary–Adrenal Axis Dysfunction in Chronic Fatigue Syndrome." Nature Reviews Endocrinology 8.1 (2012): 22-32.

81) Schuder, Suzie E. "Stress-Induced Hypocortisolemia Diagnosed as Psychiatric Disorders Responsive to Hydrocortisone Replacement." Annals of the New York Academy of Sciences 1057.1 (2005): 466-478.

82) Cleare, Anthony J. "The Neuroendocrinology of Chronic Fatigue Syndrome." Endocrine Reviews 24.2 (2003): 236-252.

83) Kaufman, Eliaz, and Ira B. Lamster. "The Diagnostic Applications of Saliva—A Review." Critical Reviews in Oral Biology & Medicine 13.2 (2002): 197-212.

84) De Bellis, Annamaria, et al. "Hypothalamic-Pituitary Autoimmunity and Related Impairment of Hormone Secretions in Chronic Fatigue Syndrome." The Journal of Clinical Endocrinology & Metabolism 106.12 (2021): e5147-e5155.

85) Lewis, Alexander, et al. "Diagnosis and Management of Adrenal Insufficiency." Clinical Medicine 23.2 (2023): 115-118.

86) Libianto, Renata, et al. "Adrenal Disease: An Update." Australian Journal of General Practice 50.1/2 (2021): 9-14.

87) Irwig, Michael S., et al. "Off-Label Use and Misuse of Testosterone, Growth Hormone, Thyroid Hormone, and Adrenal Supplements: Risks and Costs of a Growing Problem." Endocrine Practice 26.3 (2020): 340-353.

88) McDermott, Michael T. "Adrenal Fatigue." Management of Patients with Pseudo-Endocrine Disorders: A Case-Based Pocket Guide (2019): 127-137.

89) Mullur, Rashmi S. "Making a Difference in Adrenal Fatigue." Endocrine Practice 24.12 (2018): 1103-1105.

90) Ross, I. L., J. Jones, and M. Blockman. "We Are Tired of Adrenal Fatigue'." SAMJ: South African Medical Journal 108.9 (2018): 724-725.

91) Cadegiani, Flavio A., and Claudio E. Kater. "Adrenal Fatigue Does Not Exist: A Systematic Review." BMC Endocrine Disorders 16.1 (2016): 1-16.

92) Papadopoulos, Andrew S., and Anthony J. Cleare. "Hypothalamic–Pituitary–Adrenal Axis Dysfunction in Chronic Fatigue Syndrome." Nature Reviews Endocrinology 8.1 (2012): 22-32.

93) Demitrack, Mark A., et al. "Evidence for Impaired Activation of the Hypothalamic-Pituitary-Adrenal Axis in Patients with Chronic Fatigue Syndrome." The Journal of Clinical Endocrinology & Metabolism 73.6 (1991): 1224-1234.

94) Van Den Eedea, Filip, et al. "Hypothalamic-Pituitary-Adrenal Axis Function in Chronic Fatigue Syndrome." Neuropsychobiology 55 (2007): 112-120.

95) Tanriverdi, Fatih, et al. "The Hypothalamic–Pituitary–Adrenal Axis in Chronic Fatigue Syndrome and Fibromyalgia Syndrome." Stress 10.1 (2007): 13-25.

96) Demitrack, Mark A., and Leslie J. Crofford. "Evidence for and Pathophysiologic Implications of Hypothalamic-Pituitary-Adrenal Axis Dysregulation in Fibromyalgia and Chronic Fatigue Syndrome." Annals of the New York Academy of Sciences 840.1 (1998): 684-697.

97) Cleare, A. J., et al. "Hypothalamo-Pituitary-Adrenal Axis Dysfunction in Chronic Fatigue Syndrome, and the Effects of Low-Dose Hydrocortisone Therapy." The Journal of Clinical Endocrinology & Metabolism 86.8 (2001): 3545-3554.

98) Cleare, Anthony J. "The HPA Axis and the Genesis of Chronic Fatigue Syndrome." Trends in Endocrinology & Metabolism 15.2 (2004): 55-59.

99) Tomas, Cara, Julia Newton, and Stuart Watson. "A Review of Hypothalamic-Pituitary-Adrenal Axis Function in Chronic Fatigue Syndrome." International Scholarly Research Notices 2013 (2013).

100) Giebels, V., et al. "Severe Fatigue in Patients with Adrenal Insufficiency: Physical, Psychosocial and Endocrine Determinants." Journal of Endocrinological Investigation 37 (2014): 293-301.

101) King, Mitchell S. "Adrenal Insufficiency: An Uncommon Cause of Fatigue." The Journal of the American Board of Family Practice 12.5 (1999): 386-390.

102) Sharpley, Christopher F., et al. "The Association Between Cortisol: C-Reactive Protein Ratio and Depressive Fatigue Is a Function of CRP Rather Than Cortisol." Neuropsychiatric Disease and Treatment 15 (2019): 2467-2475.

103) Hinchado, María Dolores, et al. "Synbiotic Supplementation Improves Quality of Life and Inmunoneuroendocrine Response in Patients with Fibromyalgia: Influence of Codiagnosis with Chronic Fatigue Syndrome." Nutrients 15.7 (2023): 1591.

104) Takeshita, Kaori, et al. "Clinical Investigation of a Unique Type of Hypothalamic Adrenal Insufficiency." Medicine 101.41 (2022): e30597.

105) Tattersall, R. B. "Hypoadrenia or "a Bit of Addison's Disease." Medical History 43.4 (1999): 450-467.

Index

M

SSRI anti-depressant 39, 49

statin 48, 83, 84, 85, 94

Stress 73, 80, 89, 91, 122, 124, 125, 148, 190, 223, 229, 288, 299, 300, 301, 303, 304, 305, 306, 307

stress test 82, 235

subacute thyroiditis 31, 132, 202

subclinical hypothyroidism 96, 104, 108, 245, 254, 256

suppress 31, 48, 49, 54, 55, 56, 109, 110, 139, 152, 159, 169, 210, 219, 220

supra-physiologic dosing 41

supraphysiologic dosing 41, 70, 71

symptoms of hypothyroidism 14, 29, 36, 37, 70, 116, 119, 181, 290

synthetic 13, 18, 19, 22, 29, 58, 63, 71, 72, 73, 79, 167, 301

Synthetic Combination 63, 71

Synthroid 11, 14, 18, 19, 20, 21, 24, 29, 33, 35, 36, 42, 43, 48, 49, 50, 51, 63, 64, 65, 77, 79, 94, 95, 214, 216, 219, 290

T

T3 predominant synthesis 154

T4-monotherapy 11, 18, 63, 68

T4 Monotherapy 42, 74

T4-only 18, 24, 25, 29, 31, 33, 34, 35, 42, 43, 48, 50, 51, 53, 68, 69, 72, 79, 240

T4-Only 35

T4 only-monotherapy 11

Teprotumumab 134, 147, 191

Thanh D. Hoang 29

thiamine 83

Thierry Hertoghe 56

thioamides 129, 157, 168, 169

thiocyanate 10, 114, 115

thioredoxin reductase 9, 10, 35, 114, 115, 211, 215

thymoquinone 83

Thyrocyte 102, 121, 124, 145

thyroglobulin antibodies 9, 15, 43, 106, 139, 159, 175, 220, 228, 244, 253, 254

thyroglobulin antibody 104, 106, 160, 199, 215, 239

thyroglobulin hydrolysis 128

Thyroid 4, 5, 6, 7, 8, 10, 11, 12, 13, 14, 15, 16, 17, 18, 20, 21, 22, 23, 24, 25, 26, 27, 28, 29, 32, 33, 34, 35, 36, 37, 38, 41, 43, 44, 45, 46, 47, 48, 49, 50, 51, 52, 53, 54, 55, 56, 59, 60, 61, 62, 63, 64, 65, 66, 67, 68, 70, 71, 73, 74, 75, 76, 77, 78, 79, 80, 81, 82, 85, 86, 87, 89, 91, 92, 93, 94, 95, 97, 98, 99, 100, 101, 102, 103, 105, 108, 110, 111, 112, 114, 119, 120, 121, 122, 123, 124, 125, 126, 128, 130, 132, 133, 134, 136, 137, 145, 146, 147, 148, 149, 150, 153, 156, 158, 159, 160, 161, 162, 163, 164, 167, 170, 171, 172, 173, 174, 175, 176,

182, 183, 185, 186, 187, 188, 189, 190, 191, 192, 193, 195, 196, 197, 198, 199, 200, 201, 203, 204, 205, 206, 207, 208, 209, 210, 211, 213, 214, 215, 216, 217, 218, 220, 221, 222, 223, 225, 226, 227, 228, 229, 230, 231, 232, 233, 234, 235, 236, 237, 238, 239, 240, 241, 242, 243, 244, 247, 248, 249, 250, 251, 252, 253, 255, 256, 258, 259, 262, 269, 270, 272, 273, 274, 275, 276, 278, 286, 287, 288, 290, 291, 292, 293, 294, 295, 296, 297, 298, 301, 304, 305, 306

thyroid ablation 68, 70, 82, 133, 144, 154, 201, 280

thyroid acropachy 133

thyroidectomy 3, 23, 24, 25, 29, 30, 37, 38, 49, 50, 54, 55, 65, 104, 126, 129, 133, 134, 138, 142, 144, 153, 155, 168, 169, 170, 196, 198, 203, 206, 225, 255, 290, 291, 292, 293

Thyroid Hormone Receptor Mutation 56

thyroiditis 8, 9, 10, 13, 23, 24, 31, 36, 37, 56, 57, 60, 90, 91, 103, 104, 105, 107, 109, 110, 111, 112, 113, 114, 115, 116, 119, 128, 129, 131, 132, 135, 137, 138, 139, 140, 142, 143, 157, 158, 159, 167, 175, 176, 177, 179, 180, 181, 182, 197, 198, 200, 201, 202, 203, 210, 211, 212, 214, 215, 216, 218, 219, 220, 221, 225, 228, 231, 232, 235, 238, 239, 240, 244, 245, 246, 247, 248, 253, 254, 255, 256, 258, 268

thyroid-releasing hormone 39

Thyroid Stimulatory Immune Globulin 132

Thyroperoxidase antibody 82, 83, 90, 109, 110, 116, 132, 137, 138, 139, 157, 159, 160, 178, 195, 197, 200, 203, 210, 211, 216, 219, 221, 226, 229, 232, 238, 239, 240, 244, 245, 255, 280

thyrotoxicosis 12, 27, 35, 38, 39, 42, 46, 53, 54, 57, 59, 62, 76, 86, 94, 102, 105, 109, 116, 118, 124, 126, 127, 128, 129, 130, 131, 132, 135, 136, 137, 138, 139, 140, 144, 145, 146, 149, 150, 151, 157, 158, 159, 161, 162, 163, 164, 165, 166, 167, 168, 169, 170, 171, 172, 177, 180, 194, 195, 196, 197, 198, 199, 200, 201, 202, 203, 204, 205, 207, 208, 209, 216, 227, 232, 233, 244, 245, 249, 250

thyrotropin 25, 27, 31, 51, 57, 59, 60, 62, 66, 79, 80, 90, 92, 97, 100, 108, 110, 112, 123, 129, 147, 148, 161, 162, 183, 204, 207, 220, 227, 229, 236, 237, 248, 249, 252, 276, 305

thyroxine 14, 18, 25, 29, 31, 33, 38, 55, 56, 58, 64, 71, 79, 103, 110, 128, 130, 153, 156, 166, 168, 198, 199, 215, 227, 238, 256

Thyroxine Suppression Test 192

Tissue Transglutaminase 187, 241

tissue transglutaminase antibody 175

Townsend Letter 16, 17, 22, 41, 46, 56, 60, 71, 73, 170, 274, 275

Toxic Nodular Goiter 53, 129, 131, 132

toxic nodule 130

TPO antibodies 49, 104, 106, 160, 174, 183, 214, 218, 220, 227, 267

TPO antibody 106, 179, 214, 220, 239, 268

TPO enzyme 35, 38, 103, 105, 107, 110, 138, 158, 165, 211, 215